Idiopathic generalized epilepsies:
clinical, experimental and genetic aspects

Idiopathic generalized epilepsies: clinical, experimental and genetic aspects

Edited by

Alain Malafosse
Pierre Genton
Edouard Hirsch
Christian Marescaux
Dominique Broglin
Raymond Bernasconi

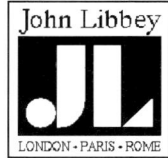

British Library Cataloguing in Publication Data

Idiopathic generalized epilepsies: clinical, experimental and genetic aspects

1. Epilepsy
I. Malafosse, Alain.

616.853
ISBN: 0 86196 436 5
ISSN: 0950 4591

Published by

John Libbey & Company Ltd, 13 Smiths Yard, Summerley Street, London SW18 4HR, England.

Telephone: 0181-947 2777 – Fax: 0181-947 2664

John Libbey Eurotext Ltd, 6 rue Blanche, 92120 Montrouge, France

John Libbey – CIC s.r.l., via Lazzaro Spallanzi 11, 00161 Rome, Italy

©1994 John Libbey & Company Ltd. All rights reserved.
Unauthorised duplication contravenes applicable laws.
Printed in Great Britain by Biddles Ltd, Guildford, UK.

Contents

Part I Current approaches

Chapter 1 – Historical aspects: the concept of idiopathy
Peter Wolf   3

Chapter 2 – Clinical and electroencephalographic characteristics of idiopathic generalized epilepsies
Joseph Roger, Michelle Bureau, Luis Oller Ferrer-Vidal, Luis Oller Daurella, Amalia Saltarelli and Pierre Genton   7

Chapter 3 – Epidemiology of idiopathic generalized epilepsies
Isabelle Desguerre, Catherine Chiron, Jérôme Loiseau, Jean-François Dartigues, Olivier Dulac and Pierre Loiseau   19

Chapter 4 – Molecular and statistical methods for mapping human epilepsy genes
Alain Malafosse, Jean-Louis Mandel, David Greenberg and Michel Baldy-Moulinier   27

Part II Familial neonatal and infantile convulsions

Chapter 5 – Benign familial neonatal convulsions
Perrine Plouin   39

Chapter 6 – Benign infantile familial convulsions
Federico Vigevano, Rosella Sebastianelli, Lucia Fusco, Matteo Di Capua, Stefano Ricci, Pierpaolo Lucchini, Benedetto Dordi, Antonio Chindemi, Olivier Dulac, Corinne Beck and Alain Malafosse   45

Chapter 7 – Developmental aspects of experimental generalized seizures induced by pentylenetetrazol, bicuculline and flurothyl
S.L. Moshé, L. Velíšek and G.L. Holmes   51

Part III Absence seizures and absence epilepsy

Chapter 8 – Gene mapping for benign familial neonatal convulsions and related syndromes
V. Elving Anderson, Mark Leppert, Dick Lindhou, Alain Malafosse and Ortrud Steinlein   65

Chapter 9 – The clinical spectrum of typical absence seizures and absence epilepsies
C.P. Panayiotopoulos   75

Chapter 10 – What are the relevant criteria for a better classification of epileptic syndromes with typical absences?
E. Hirsch, A. Blanc-Platier and C. Marescaux   87

Chapter 11 – Late-onset absence status epilepticus is most often situation-related
Pierre Thomas and Frederick Andermann   95

Chapter 12 – Physiopathogenesis of feline generalized penicillin epilepsy: the role of thalamocortical mechanisms
M. Avoli and P. Gloor   111

Chapter 13 – Thalamocortical rhythm generation *in vitro*: physiological mechanisms, pharmacological control and relevance to generalized absence epilepsy
Douglas A. Coulter and Yun-fu Zhang   123

Chapter 14 – Pathophysiological mechanisms of experimental generalized absence seizures in rats
O. Carter Snead III   133

Chapter 15 – Pathophysiological mechanisms underlying genetic absence epilepsy in rats
M. Vergnes and C. Marescaux   151

Chapter 16 – Brain metabolism and blood flow in models of generalized idiopathic epilepsies in rodents
A. Nehlig, M. Vergnes, E. Hirsch and C. Marescaux   169

Chapter 17 – Characteristics of $GABA_B$-receptor binding sites in genetic absence epilepsy rats from Strasbourg (GAERS) and in non-epileptic control rats
Pascal Mathivet, Raymond Bernasconi, Jean de Barry, Stuart Mickel, Wolfgang Froestl and Helmut Bittiger   177

Chapter 18 – The role of $GABA_B$-receptor activation in the lethargic (*lh/lh*) mouse model of primary generalized absence seizures
David A. Hosford, Fu-hsiung Lin, Zhen Cao, Diana L. Kraemer, Alex Huin, Eric Akawie, Yin Yin and John T. Wilson   187

Chapter 19 – Potential role of intrinsic and $GABA_B$ IPSP-mediated oscillations of thalamic neurons in absence epilepsy
Vincenzo Crunelli, Jonathan P. Turner, Stephen R. Williams, Alice Guyon and Nathalie Leresche   201

Chapter 20 – Genetic and phenotypic heterogeneity of inherited spike-and-wave epilepsies
Jeffrey L. Noebels   215

Part IV Juvenile myoclonic epilepsy and related syndromes

Chapter 21 – Impulsive petit mal
D. Janz and W. Christian   229

Chapter 22 – Juvenile myoclonic epilepsy and related syndromes: clinical and neurophysiological aspects
Pierre Genton, Xavier Salas Puig, A. Tunon, C. H. Lahoz, Maria Del Socorro and Gonzalez Sanchez   253

Chapter 23 – Idiopathic generalized epilepsies with myoclonus in infancy and childhood
Renzo Guerrini, Charlotte Dravet, Giuseppe Gobbi, Stefano Ricci and Olivier Dulac   267

Chapter 24 – Juvenile myoclonic epilepsy: is there heterogeneity?
A.V. Delgado-Escueta, A. Liu, J. Serratosa, K. Weissbecker, M.T. Medina, M. Gee, L.J. Theiman and R.S. Sparkes   281

Chapter 25 – Phenotypic variability of idiopathic generalized epilepsies and refinement of the map position of EJM1 in JME families
D. Janz, G. Beck-Managetta, T. Hildman, T. Sander and H. Neitzel   287

Part V Photosensitivity

Chapter 26 – Photosensitivity – a human 'model' of epilepsy
D.G.A. Kasteleijn-Nolst Trenité, W. van Emde Boas and C.D. Binnie   297

Chapter 27 – Pathophysiological mechanisms of photosensitivity in IGEs
Takeo Takahashi   305

Part VI Pathophysiology of convulsive seizures

Chapter 29 – The epileptic and nonepileptic generalized myoclonus of the *Papio papio* baboon
C. Menini, C. Silva-Barrat and R. Naquet — 331

Chapter 30 – Forebrain convulsive mechanisms examined in the primate model of generalized epilepsy: emphasis on the claustrum
Juhn A. Wada — 349

Chapter 31 – Genetic epilepsy in chicken: new approaches and concepts
N. Guy, M.A. Teillet, G. Le Gal La Salle, N. Fadlallah, N.M. Le Douarin, R. Naquet and C. Batini — 375

Chapter 32 – The GEPR model of the epilepsies
Phillip C. Jobe, Pravin K. Mishra, Leah E. Adams-Curtis, Kwang Ho Ko and John W. Dailey — 385

Chapter 33 – Anatomy of generalized convulsive seizures
Ronald A. Browning — 399

Chapter 34 – Propagation of generalized seizures from brain-stem to forebrain networks
E. Hirsch, M.Vergnes, S. Simler, B. Maton, A. Nehlig and C. Marescaux — 415

Part VII Fundamental and therapeutic aspects

Chapter 35 – Influence of drugs on the outcome of idiopathic generalized epilepsies
Pierre Loiseau — 425

Chapter 36 – Seizures induce molecular and morphological changes in rat brain
Alfonso Represa, Jérôme Niquet, Hélène Pollard, Joëlle Moreau, Michel Khrestchatisky and Yehezkel Ben-Ari — 433

Chapter 37 – Possible mechanisms of action of first choice drugs for the treatment of idiopathic generalized epilepsies
P.E. Keane & D. Broglin — 447

Chapter 38 – New anti-epileptic drugs and idiopathic generalized epilepsies
Mogens Dam — 455

Chapter 39 – Therapeutic prospects for novel excitatory amino acid antagonists in idiopathic generalized epilepsy
Astrid G. Chapman — 463

Chapter 40 – Antiepileptic drugs modulate the seizure threshold for excitatory amino acids in mice
Lechoslaw Turski & David N. Stephens — 473

Chapter 41 – Nitric oxide (NO) and epilepsy
Gérard Rondoin, Marguerite Vergnes and Mireille Lerner-Natoli — 485

Chapter 42 – Relevance of the nigral control of seizures in the treatment of generalized epilepsies
Antoine Depaulis — 497

Chapter 43 – Gene therapy: perspectives in epilepsy
Gildas Le Gal La Salle and Jacques Mallet — 511

List of Contributors

DEDICATION
The editors wish to dedicate this volume to Joseph Roger, Elving Anderson and Robert Naquet.

Preface

In the past few years, epileptologists witnessed a rapid growth of knowledge in the field of clinical, genetic and basic sciences, which challenged many entrenched opinions. A new International Classification of Epilepsies and Epileptic Syndromes was adopted by clinicians in 1989, while chromosomal localizations were being proposed for some epileptic entities and both new and older models of inherited epilepsy were intensively studied in various animal species. Being themselves active in one or another of these various approaches of epileptology, the editors of this volume met informally during the Rio International Epilepsy Congress, in the fall of 1991, and began to plan an International Workshop that would gather scientists from different branches of epileptology. Idiopathic generalized epilepsies clearly constitute a topic on which clinicians, geneticians and basic or experimental scientists would want to exchange observations, data and ideas for future research.

The meeting took place in Alsace, not far from Strasbourg, on 22–25 April, 1993. The working conditions were ideal and the atmosphere friendly. In spite of the many tourist temptations surrounding the Bischenberg, a beautifully located hillside resort overlooking the Alsace, participants from nearly 20 countries managed to stay there and work during three full days.

The success of the meeting was due to the constant, longstanding help the organizers received from their mentors, namely Joseph Roger, Elving Anderson and Robert Naquet, who supported it not only in word, but also by their relentless work. We acknowledge here the important part they have been playing for many years in our interest in epilepsy, and in the scientific organization of this meeting. All participants were active, whether they were speakers or otherwise involved: we thank all of them for the consistently high quality of their participation. The location of the meeting was chosen as a tribute to Professor Francis Rohmer and Professor Maurice Collard, from the Strasbourg University Hospital. The meeting was held under the auspices of the International League Against Epilepsy, of the Ligue Française Contre l'Epilepsie, the Association Française Contre les Myopathies and the Fondation Française pour la Recherche sur l'Epilepsie.

Many pharmaceutical firms helped us organize this meeting: we are greatly indebted to them, as they made our project become a reality. We wish to express our thanks to all for their generous sponsoring.

The meeting would have been impossible without the dedicated participation and enthusiasm of our respective colleagues and staff; our special thanks go to Violette Ottenad from Strasbourg, Charlotte Billerey and Nicole Lieutier from Marseille and Martine Bonnefoy from Montpellier, who, at the meeting secretariat, resolved with energy and friendliness the multiple problems arising from our own shortcomings; they were also a great help when it came to handling the manuscripts for this volume. So many others helped that we cannot list them here, but we remember their goodwill and dedication.

The meeting reaches its logical conclusion in this volume, carefully reviewed and edited by John Libbey and his staff. This publication has been made possible by a grant from Sanofi Pharma International, which we gratefully acknowledge.

The Editors

The meeting that inspired this volume would not have been possible without the support from the following companies and institutions:

   Laboratoires Sanofi-Winthrop, France
   Laboratoires Schering-Plough
   Laboratoires Merrell–Dow, France
   Laboratoires Ciba–Geigy France
   Association Française contre les Myopathies
   Fondation pour la Recherche sur l'Epilepsie
   Laboratoires Wellcome
   Laboratoires Biocodex
   Laboratoires UCB, Belgium
   Laboratoires Therval Médical
   Laboratoires Sandoz, Switzerland
   Laboratoires Ciba–Geigy, Switzerland
   Laboratoires Hoffmann–Laroche, Switzerland
   Laboratoires Cilag
   Laboratoires Duphar
   Laboratoires Roche France

The publication of the proceedings of the meeting in book form was made possible by a grant from Sanofi International.

Colour Plates

The illustrations on the following pages are reproduced in full colour and relate to the chapters in this volume to which they are referred. To preserve the integrity of individual chapters, a black and white reproduction of these figures also appears in the text pages.

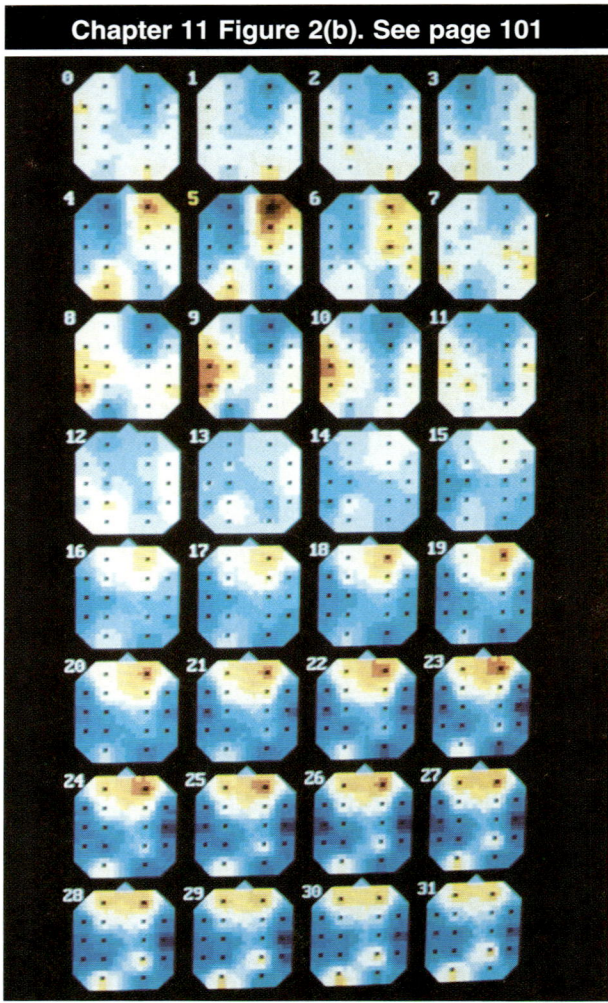

Fig. 2(b). Brain mapping of EEG activity during absence seizure in same patients. Twenty polyspike-waves have been averaged on the peak of their spiky component. Amplitude mapping was performed every 8 ms. Map no. 5 shows the distribution of potentials at the moment of maximum spike amplitude, clearly showing a dipolar distribution with maximal negativity focused over the right frontal area. The slow-wave component spreads over both anterior areas after onset over the right frontal lobe. Dark red: maximum negativity; dark blue: maximum positivity.

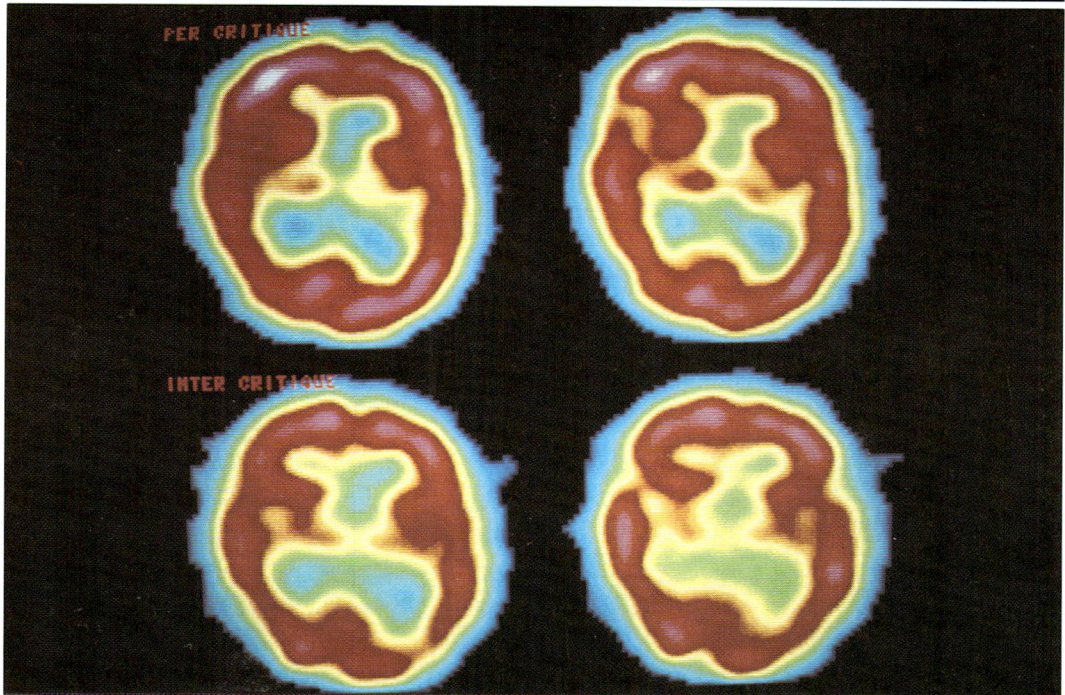

Fig. 3 (c). 99 Tc HMPAO SPECT, first performed during status, at the beginning of a seizure (top), then post-ictally (bottom). During absence status, there is a significantly increased perfusion over the right frontal area (top left of the figure).

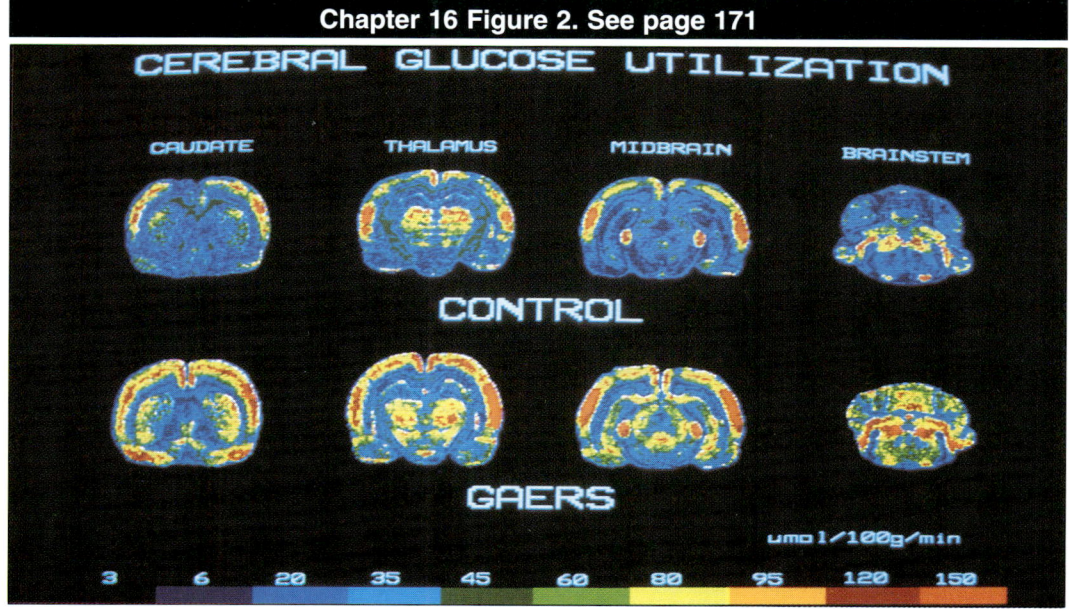

Fig. 2. Colour-coded autoradiographs of GAERS and control rat brain sections taken at the level of the caud-ate nucleus, thalamus, midbrain and brain-stem. By reference to the colour scale located at the right, the diffuse metabolic increase in epileptic rats compared to controls is striking in all cerebral regions.

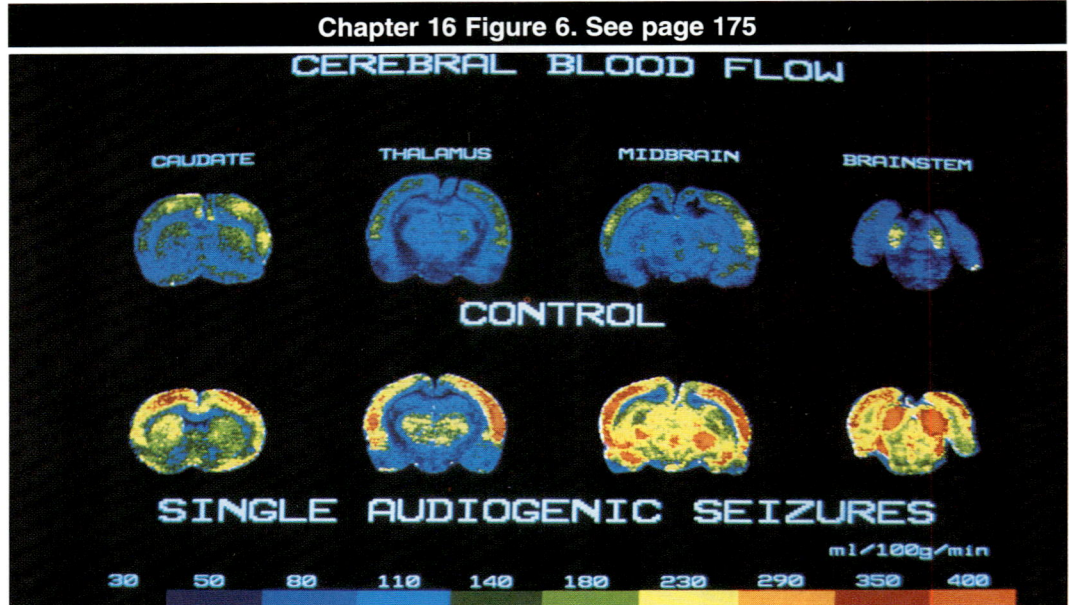

Fig. 6. Colour-coded autoradiographs of audiogenic and control rat brain sections taken at the level of the caudate nucleus, thalamus, midbrain and brain-stem. By reference to the colour scale located at the bottom, the generalized metabolic increase in audiogenic rats compared to controls is striking in all cerebral areas and of markedly higher amplitude in posterior than in anterior regions.

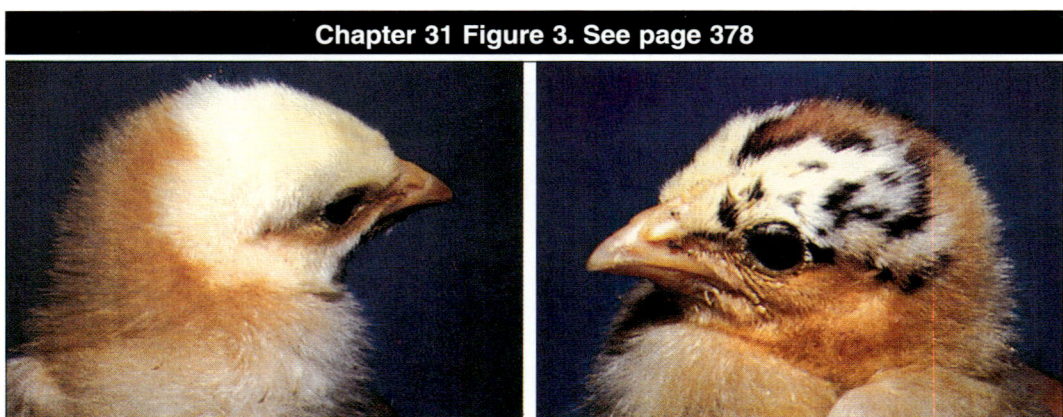

Fig. 3. Ten days old epileptic chimeras, constructed by transplanting prosencephalic, mesencephalic and metencephalic vesicles from FEpi to normal chick embryos at 2 days of incubation. The white pigmentation (left view) or variegated pigmentation (right view) at the level of the graft is due to melanoblasts of neural crest origin transplanted along with the neural anlage. Both of these pigmentations are found in the FEpi

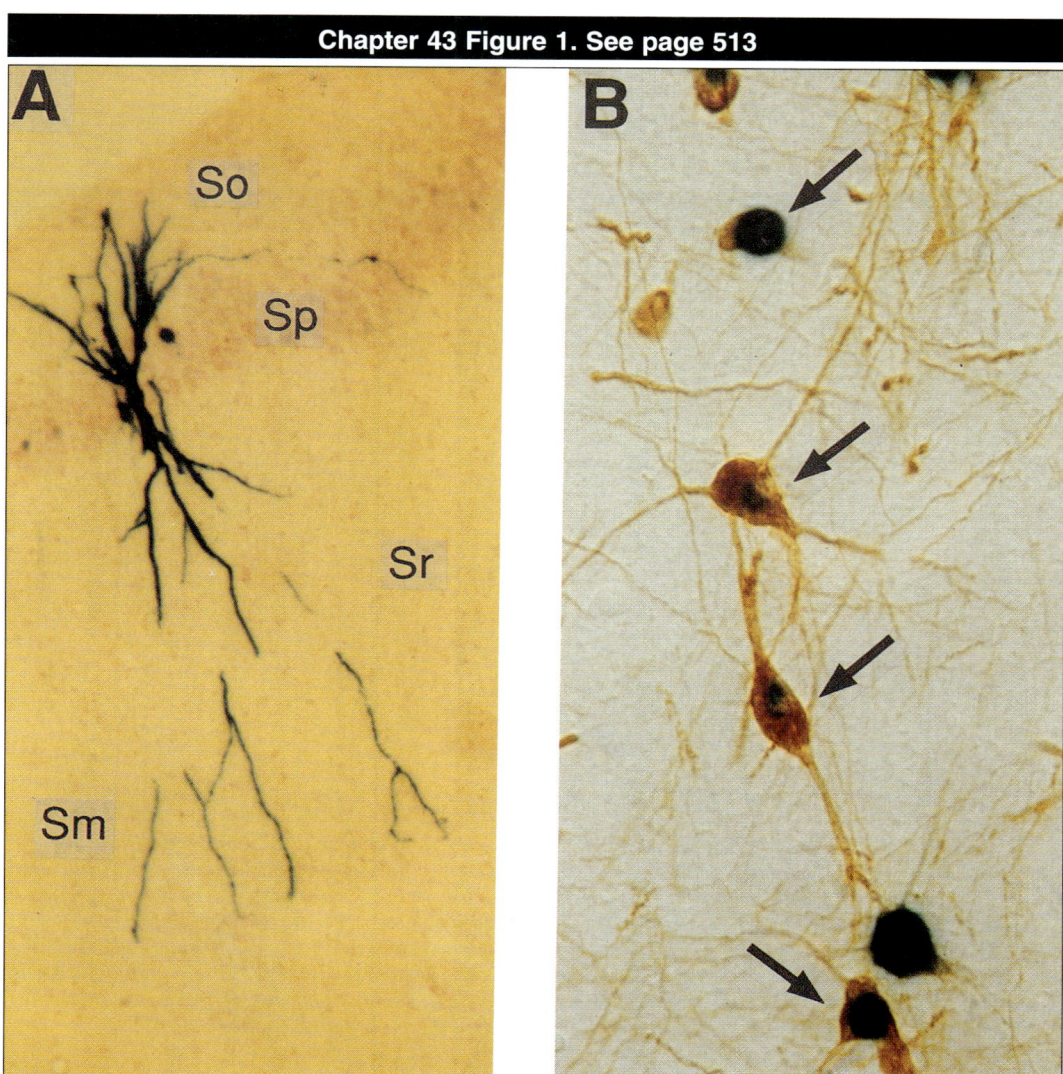

Fig. 1. Example of neurons infected by direct in vivo inoculation with an adenovirus carrying a reporter gene encoding β-galactosidase. Dense blue staining was detectable in a pyramidal cell of the CA1 stratum pyramidale of the dorsal hippocampus (a) and in nigral cells, most of which were also labelled with tyrosine hydroxylase monoclonal antibodies. Abbreviations: sm, stratum moleculare, so, stratum oriens; sp, stratum pyramidale, sr, stratum radiatum.

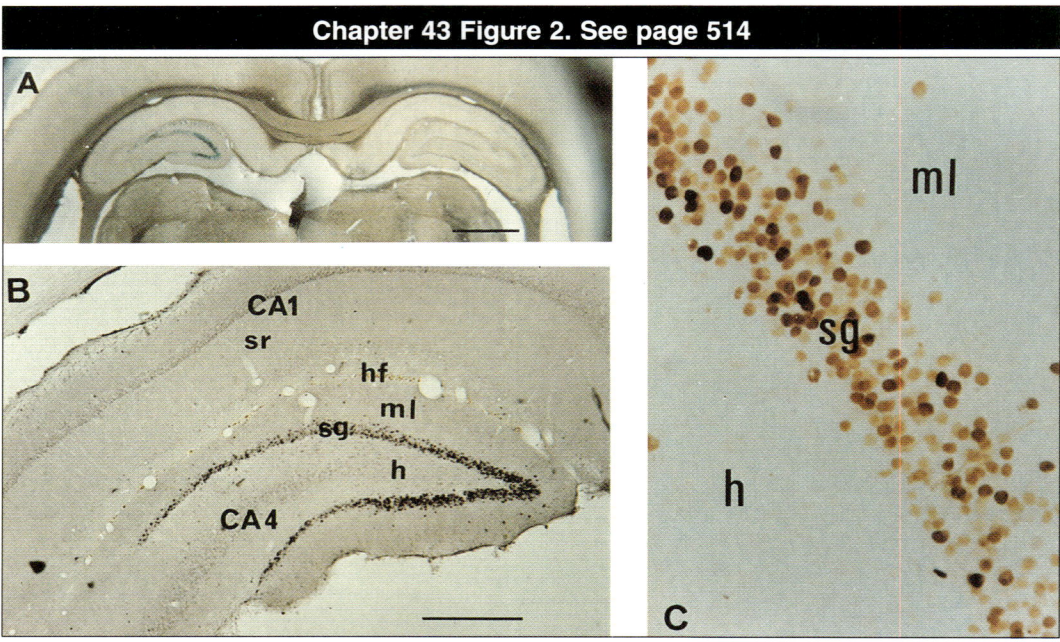

Fig. 2. Distribution of β-galactosidase-positive cells in the dorsal hippocampus 1 month after stereotaxic inoculation with recombinant adenovirus. (A) Photomicrograph stained for β-galactosidase expression with X-gal histochemistry. The cells that are stained blue were observed in the dentate gyrus of the injected left hippocampus. Scale bar, 1 mm. (B) Dentate localization of the infected cells was confirmed immunohistochemically using an antibody against β-galactosidase. Scale bar, 300 μm. (C) High magnification view showing the large number of densely packed immunoreactive (anti-β-gal antibodies) cells in the granular cell layer of the dentate gyrus. Abbreviations: h, hilus; hf, hippocampal fissure; ml, molecular layer; sg, stratum granulosum; sr, stratum radiatum. (From Le Gal La Salle et al., 1993)

Introduction

The concept of idiopathic generalized epilepsy (IGE): an introduction to the clinical, experimental and genetic study of IGEs

The 1989 International Classification of Epilepsies, Epileptic Syndromes and Related Disorders defines 'idiopathic' epilepsies as those in which *'there is no underlying cause other than a possible inherited predisposition. [. . . .] [They] are defined by age-related onset, clinical and electroencephalographic characteristics, and usually a genetic background.'* This recent statement already appears to be obsolete: it has been shown that several syndromes of idiopathic generalized epilepsies (IGEs) are indeed associated with a definite genetically transmitted trait: this is either a putative chromosomal localization, still to be confirmed (as in juvenile myoclonic epilepsy), or a definite, proven localization confirmed by several teams (as in benign familial neonatal convulsions (BFNNC); such *syndromes* may thus be considered as discrete *diseases*, that can be defined by a genetic marker – and possibly, in the near future, by a characteristic biochemical trait that is the consequence of the genetic anomaly underlying these conditions.

The body of knowledge is moving fast, very fast, and the challenges to clinicians, experimentalists and geneticians are many.

Idiopathic generalized epilepsies: the clinical spectrum

As all clinicians with some amount of experience in clinical epileptology know, IGEs are frequent. Many patients who are neurologically normal experience generalized seizures and exhibit a generalized EEG pattern. However, it may be difficult, in many cases, to make a precise diagnostic classification into one of the syndromic categories. The 1989 International Classification states that the various types of IGEs vary mainly in their age of onset: as many as seven distinct entities have been validated by this classification effort, which, besides, leaves the door open to other types that have yet to be defined. Thus two main questions remain open for the clinicians:

– is there only one 'disease', with various clinical presentations that depend mostly on the age of clinical appearance of the epileptic and EEG symptoms (possibly due to environmental factors), or are there different diseases, each based on a distinct, specific, probably inherited defect ?
– to what extent are the criteria proposed for the diagnosis of IGE and of the various syndromes of IGE valid? To what extent is it possible to differentiate between the various syndromes listed as IGEs ?

The first question can already be answered: evidence is mounting that indicates the existence of several, distinct, unrelated conditions. This evidence stems from experimental data that have shown the existence of several, different animal models and/or mechanisms of generalized 'non-lesional' epilepsy, and from the emerging genetic data that have separated benign familial neonatal convulsions from the rest of the group of IGEs, and have stressed the heterogeneity of the category of IGEs. The syndromic approach of the IGEs is thus validated, and the existence of a 'continuum' of IGEs invalidated. However, the precise limits between syndromes (especially among myoclonic IGEs and among epilepsies with onset in adolescence) are open to discussion.

The second question will probably not receive a definite answer in the near future: all the clinical

Table 1. Genetic models of spontaneous and chronic absence epilepsies

Species	Genetic transmission	Seizures EEG	Network	Other neurological deficits
GAERS rats	Multigenic, dominant	Bilateral SWD Behavioural arrest	Thalamocortical loop	No
WAG:Rij rats	Multigenic, dominant	Bilateral SWD Behavioural arrest	Thalamocortical loop	No
Tottering mice	Single gene, recessive	Bilateral SWD Behavioural arrest	Thalamocortical loop	Yes
Stargazer mice	Single gene, recessive	Bilateral SWD Behavioural arrest	Thalamocortical loop	Yes
Lethargic mice	Single gene, recessive	Bilateral SWD Behavioural arrest	Thalamocortical loop	Yes

and neurophysiological markers that have been proposed for the differentiation between IGE syndromes can be criticized. There is a vacuum here; clinicians, who at times may feel that they have reached the limits of clinical differentiation, need objective, biological diagnostic tools. It is their hope that the geneticians will provide one in the near future.

Idiopathic generalized epilepsies: animal models and neurophysiological mechanisms

The pathophysiological mechanisms underlying IGEs are still one of the basic puzzles of epileptology. Many data concerning focal epilepsies are obtained thanks to presurgical and surgical procedures in humans, but obvious ethical considerations rule out the use of any of the modern neuroscientist's tools in children or adolescents with IGE. The study of IGEs is dependent on animal models, and the validity of the results are correlated with the adequacy of these models.

There are many models of acute generalized seizures induced in normal animals by chemical or electrical stimulation. Such models may provide a great deal of information regarding the neural networks and the cellular and molecular mechanisms involved in the genesis of generalized seizures. However, the capacity of a normal brain to produce seizures following stimulation is not relevant to the fundamental basis of IGEs, characterized by chronically recurrent spontaneous seizures, that are a response to a multifacted process in which genetically determined susceptibility plays a crucial part. Only the genetic animal models of IGE provide the means for examining the mechanisms of seizure predisposition in a spontaneously epileptic brain. Many animal species, including chicken, mice, rats, and primates, develop inherited generalized epilepsies (Tables 1 and 2). These models are important for two reasons:

- first, they present an abnormal epileptic nervous system that does not need artifical perturbation, and thus the information obtained care more relevant to the human IGEs;
- second, genetic mutations can be studied on an otherwise unaffected background with controlled breeding of many individuals in a large number of generations.

Thus important information can be obtained from acute and chronic models in relation to networks underlying genetic seizures and to the genetic transmission of generalized epilepsies.

The question of the cortical vs subcortical origin of the discharges underlying seizures in IGEs has been addressed by the study of these various models during the past few decades. Evidence reported in this volume supports the concept that generalized clonic or myoclonic seizures are driven by abnormal activity within the forebrain, whereas tonic seizures are generated within brain-stem circuits. During tonic–clonic seizures, both brain-stem and forebrain mechanisms are involved; connections between forebrain and brain-stem networks occur through specific structures, such as the claustrum in primates and the amygdala in rodents. According to the data presented in several chapters of this volume, generalized non-convulsive seizures depend on different mechanisms and

Table 2. Genetic models of reflex chronic generalized convulsive epilepsies

Species	Provocative factors	Seizures	Cortical EEG	Networks
Epileptic fowl	Light, sound, stress	Tonic–clonic	Flattening	Brain-stem + forebrain
Baboon *Papio papio*	Light	Myoclonic (tonic–clonic)	Spikes and spike-wave discharges	Forebrain ± brain-stem
GEPR rats	Sound and other epileptogenic stimuli	Tonic (tonic–clonic after repetition)	Flattening (flattening, then spike-wave discharges after repetition)	Brain-stem (+forebrain after repetition)
Wistar audiogenic susceptible rats	Sound only	Tonic (tonic–clonic after repetition)	Flattening (flattening, then spike-wave discharges after repetition)	Brain-stem (+forebrain after repetition)

circuits: absences are provoked by an abnormal oscillatory pattern within a thalamo-cortical loop that includes the reticular nucleus of the thalamus, the specific thalamic nuclei and the neocortex. Whether the generation of absences is the result of an excessive cortical excitability, as was proposed in the feline penicillin model, or of an excessive thalamic synchronization possibly under the control of $GABA_B$ mechanisms, remains debatable.

In this volume, the genetic background of IGEs has been studied mainly in the absence models in rodents. In rats, bilateral and synchronous spike-and-wave discharges are inherited in a dominant way and are apparently controlled by several distinct genes. It seems likely that there are genes that control predisposition, expression, modulation and temporal sequence of seizures. In mice, absences are transmitted in a recessive way, and may result from several different mutations affecting distinct chromosomes. The concept of genetic heterogeneity is thus strikingly demonstrated by these animal models: similar seizure phenotypes can result from different genetic defects. Current research on genetic models of IGEs focuses on three main questions:

(1) what are the monogenic or polygenic mutations that cause generalized epilepsies?

(2) What are the nature and properties of the abnormal epilepsy proteins? Are they expressed in neuronal or glial cells? Are they involved in connectivity within specific circuits?

(3) Why are these inborn errors expressed only at a certain age, after completion of some maturational steps in the central nervous system?

Defining the functional consequences of the mutations in an *in vitro* expression system will be a logical first step towards the understanding of how the mutant genes result in epilepsy. This in turn may provide, in the future, some clues towards new therapeutic approaches.

Idiopathic generalized epilepsies: a challenge for geneticists

Clinical evidence for the genetic aetiology of IGEs includes (1) the increased familial incidence of IGEs, with frequent homophenic transmission; (2) the results of twin studies; and (3) the absence of apparent exogenous causes. Since several lines of evidence suggest an important genetic contribution to the aetiology of human IGEs, gene mapping is potentially an important experimental approach for understanding the molecular basis of these disorders. Gene mapping studies, however, work best when the phenotype can be determined accurately and when the disease gene is highly penetrant. Consequently, genetic linkage analysis of epileptic syndromes with a Mendelian mode of inheritance is now the most promising approach for the identification of the pathogenetic mechanisms that underly epilepsies; this approach is the first step towards the cloning of the responsible gene and the identification of the pathogenic protein product.

The localization of the genes responsible for benign familial neonatal convulsions has demonstrated the power of this new approach. In this rare epileptic entity, the mode of inheritance is dominant, the penetrance is high and the clinical phenotype is quite easy to assess: this made things comparatively easy. In the very close future, the identification of the genes of benign familial neonatal convulsions will be one of the major steps of contemporary epileptology.

However, the identification of the genes responsible for other types of IGE is a more complex challenge, because of the clinical heterogeneity of these other epileptic syndromes, even within pedigrees, and because of the uncertainty surrounding the genetic parameters of comparatively common types of IGE, such as childhood absence epilepsy and juvenile myoclonic epilepsy. New genetic strategies exist so-called non-parametric methods of linkage analysis that will allow the study of such complex inherited disorders. The success of the genetic approach is now largely dependent on the accuracy of the clinical analysis of IGE patients and of their families.

Idiopathic generalized epilepsies: the present and the future of treatment

The 'anti-seizure' efficacy of the currently used 'antiepileptic' drugs (AEDs) is unquestionable for many patients, especially for those who have an idiopathic generalized epilepsy: here, seizures are relatively easy to control using classical antiepileptic drugs, especially in comparison with other, non-idiopathic or focal types of epilepsies. However, the benefit/risk ratio of the antiepileptic drugs is not always optimal, and their therapeutic effect consists in the prevention of the recurrence of seizures, and is, as such, strictly symptomatic, not ætiological. At this time, we do not know whether the antiepileptic drugs have in fact a true *curative* effect, *a fortiori* a preventative *antiepileptogenic* effect, against the underlying epileptogenic process. Finally, the mechanism of action of the classical antiepileptic drugs remains poorly understood; it is well-known that almost all have been discovered serendipitously or, at best, after a systematic and rather empirical screening of the anticonvulsant properties of thousands of compounds.

It is no longer unrealistic to anticipate the availability of new drugs that are designed and not discovered by chance. In the relatively near future, it should be possible to elaborate such new compounds thanks to the parallel and reciprocal advances in molecular biology and molecular pharmacology. Such advances result in a better understanding of the mechanisms of epileptic discharges and epileptogenesis on one hand, of the mechanisms of action of the drugs on the other hand, and finally of the precise nature of the relationships between the former and the latter. Compared to classical compounds, such new compounds could be classical 'antiseizure' drugs, characterized by greater efficacy and/or better benefit/risk ratio. New drugs could also usher in a new era of the treatment of epilepsies, with true antiepileptic and even antiepileptogenic properties. Such drugs might have simultaneously an antiseizure effect and constitute a classical, chronic treatment or could be prescribed over a relatively short time.

The correction of the neurobiological basis of the propensity to have seizures – i.e. in the specific case of idiopathic, genetically determined epilepsies the prevention of the occurrence of the epilepsy itself – is still out of reach. However, the perspectives opened by gene therapy may make this utopia come true in the next decades.

Such advances in theoretically very different therapeutic approaches will be based both on progress in basic research and on a better, more pragmatic knowledge of the epilepsies by the clinicians who treat patients with epilepsy.

How this volume is organized

In this volume, the clinical, experimental and genetic approaches have been used together, or in succession, to try and sum up the state of current knowledge.

The first part reviews the current concepts and working tools used by the various approaches. P. Wolf goes back into history and tells us how the concept of idiopathy came to light. J. Roger and co-workers outline the basic concepts that are at the base of the current clinical classification of epilepsies and explain how this classification can be used in clinical practice. The Paris and

Bordeaux teams have undertaken large, syndrome-based epidemiological studies; their experience on the epidemiology of IGEs is the subject of another chapter. The various models of generalized epilepsy studied in different laboratories around the world have been briefly reviewed in this Introduction (Tables 1 & 2). The methods used by geneticians to study the epilepsies are described by Malafosse, Mandel & Greenberg.

In the following parts of the book, the clinical situations encountered in patients with IGE are assessed against their experimental and genetic background.

Part II is devoted to the uncommon, yet characteristic syndrome of benign familial neonatal convulsions and related conditions: the electro-clinical features have been summarized by Plouin and Vigevano *et al.*, the specific features of the neonatal and developing brain by Moshe *et al.*, and the already well-established genetic mechanisms by Anderson *et al.*

Part III tackles a vast, controversial subject: human absence epilepsies are not too well understood, and the clinical controversies are the subject of three chapters by C. P. Panayiotopoulos, E. Hirsch *et al.*, and P. Thomas & F. Andermann. The electrophysiological and biochemical mechanisms underlying absence (or 'generalized spike-and-wave' (SW) epilepsy) in animal models are the subjects of eight further papers, while the genetics of genetic SW epilepsy in the mouse are reviewed by J. Noebels.

Part IV covers another group of IGEs, i.e. those that are characterized, clinically, by myoclonic seizures. Myoclonic epilepsies can be found at all ages, some belong to the groups of the IGEs; there are no animal models for these epilepsies, but they are at the centre of many controversies among geneticians. The most frequent type is juvenile myoclonic epilepsy (JME): the original, complete description of this syndrome was published in Germany in 1957 by D. Janz & W. Christian. With the agreement and the support of D. Janz, we chose to translate this milestone of modern epileptology into English and to include a practically unabridged version in this volume. An update on juvenile myoclonic epilepsy by Genton *et al.* shows how little has changed from the clinical point of view and stresses how the clinical and EEG presentation can be misleading. Guerrini *et al.* discuss the nosography of myoclonic epilepsies found in young children. The present state of the ongoing genetic studies performed in juvenile myoclonic epilepsy by the American and European groups are summarized in the papers by Delgado-Escueta *et al.* and by Janz *et al.*.

Photosensitivity, the subject of Part V, is a clinical and neurophysiological trait that can be found in several syndromes of IGE, but that is considered by many as a genetic trait that can be transmitted independently. The clinical significance and symptomatology of photosensitivity has been reviewed, in the light of their vast personal experience, by D. Kasteleijn & C. Binnie and their co-workers, and by T. Takahashi.

Generalized convulsive seizures, typically of the tonic–clonic type, but also of the myoclonic type, can be found in many types of epilepsies and are not specific to IGEs. Part VI reviews the basic mechanisms, both electrophysiological, biochemical and genetic, that underly these seizure types and some more specific types of epilepsies found in animal models.

The last part of the book (Part VII) encompasses both classical data and advances that can reasonably be foreseen for the next decade. Both the clinical and the fundamental approaches have been used. The clinical efficacy of the drugs of first choice used in IGEs (P. Loiseau), their presumed mechanism of action (P. Keane & D. Broglin) and the therapeutic impact of the newer antiepileptic drugs (M. Dam) are reviewed. Some of the leading hypotheses on the mechanisms underlying the self-recurrence of spontaneous epileptic discharges and their propagation are described by A. Represa *et al.*, and by Depaulis *et al.* Other chapters deal with hypotheses of neurotransmitter implication, especially excitatory amino-acids (receptors, antagonizing agents) (A. Chapman, and L. Turski & D. Stephens), and second messengers, such as nitric oxide (G. Rondoin *et al.*). The future perspectives offered by gene therapy of epilepsies are discussed by G. Le Gal La Salle & J. Mallet.

Conclusions

Idiopathic generalized epilepsies are better understood now than they were only a few years ago. In this particular field of epileptology, the data provided by clinical experience and by ongoing genetic and experimental research need to be integrated. Such is the ambition of this volume. It is clear that the huge and fast progress that looms ahead will quickly challenge many of the opinions expressed here: it was our aim to stimulate the collaboration between the various branches of modern epileptology, and to allow most of us to change their opinion in the light of the data provided by others.

The Editors:
Alain Malafosse
Pierre Genton
Edouard Hirsch
Christian Marescaux
Dominique Broglin
Raymond Bernasconi

Part I
Current approaches

Chapter 1

Historical aspects: the concept of idiopathy

Peter Wolf

Klinik für Anfallskranke Mara, Epilepsiezentrum, Bethel Maraweg 21, 33617 Bielefeld, Germany

Of the terms which have been used for the major classes of epilepsy in recent times, idiopathic is the one with the longest history. 'Idios' (Greek) signifies 'self' or 'proper', and the term refers to the brain where according to Hippocrates epileptic seizures originated. Galen in the second century introduced 'idiopathic' as a term for those cases where the epilepsy was considered to be caused by a disorder of the brain itself, as opposed to 'sympathetic' epilepsy where the brain was only secondarily involved whereas the seat of the disorder was elsewhere.

With small modifications, this distinction prevailed throughout the Middle Ages and the Renaissance.

When autopsies began to be used, intracranial pathological findings were taken as a confirmation of idiopathy. At the same time, however, it became apparent that there were presumed idiopathic cases where no brain pathology whatsoever could be discovered, and this called for terminological changes. Tissot (1728–1797) (Fig. 1), who discussed this problem at length, concluded that, in these cases, the only cause was the 'epileptic disposition of the brain, which is without any doubt a fault in its organization, but a fault which escapes our senses.' (Tissot, 1770). For these cases, he used the term 'essential epilepsy' in distinction from idiopathic cases with definite brain pathology. Our present knowledge about both genetic predispositions, the functional disorders as they are expressed in the interictal EEG, and micro-dysgenesias all confirm Tissot's astonishing foresight. The terminology, however, has changed, and idiopathic today is used exactly for the conditions which Tissot called 'essential'.

This was above all the consequence of the redefinition of terms by Delasiauve in his 1854 monograph. He saw no reason to differentiate appreciable cerebral lesions from other causes of symptomatic epilepsy, so consequently included such cases in the symptomatic epilepsies, and used idiopathic and essential epilepsy as synonyms.

It seems that, in about the same period, 'genuine epilepsy' came into use as an additional synonym (meaning 'true' or 'proper' in contrast to 'epileptiform fits') which would eventually replace 'essential' in common use. This, however, relates to a nosological rather than an aetiological problem, namely to the question what is epilepsy, and what is only epileptiform.

In all discussions in the mid-19th century, it was highly important what seizures could be accepted as epileptic or not, and the terms idiopathic, essential or genuine epilepsy were usually reserved for

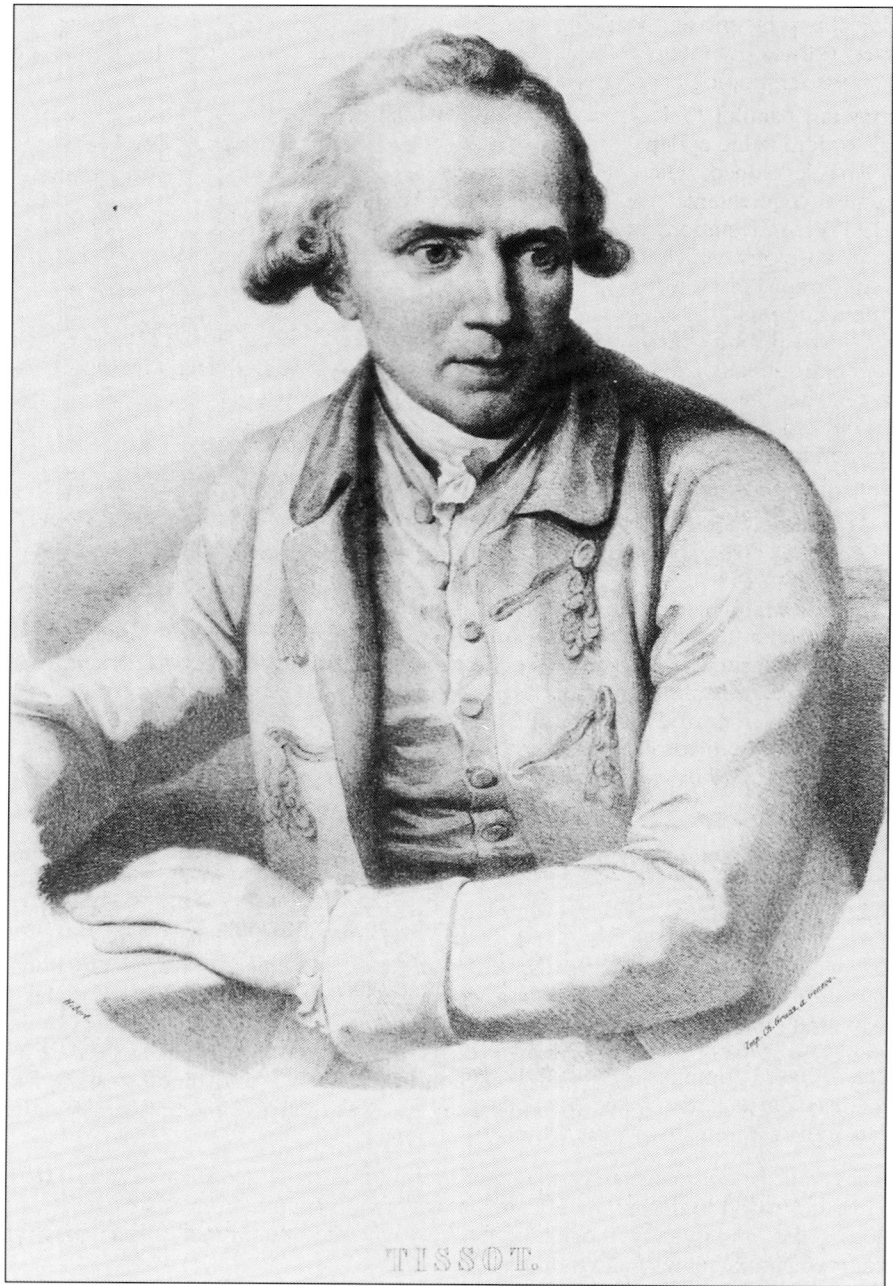

Fig. 1. Samuel-Auguste-André-David Tissot (1728–1797). Lithograph after a portrait by Angelica Kauffmann (1782)

grand mal seizures. Jackson (*Selected Writings* I, p 5f, 8) was little interested in this discussion. He found that these terms and concepts had become an obstacle to research progress, and suggested that it was more useful to study convulsions in their 'simplest varieties', and then proceed further.

In following this principle and studying 'epileptiform fits' rather than 'genuine epilepsy' or 'epilepsy proper' (all his own words), he became the father of modern epileptology, but gained little influence on the terminological discussion.

As a contrasting parallel to Jackson's proposal, a mainstream of writings on genuine epilepsy, 'functional' or idiopathic epilepsy (Gowers, 1881) or 'idiopathic' as opposed to 'organic' epilepsy (Turner, 1907) developed, where auras and, under the influence of French and German psychiatrists, psychical 'equivalents' came to be accepted as possible, common, or even characteristic (Stauder, 1938) manifestations of 'genuine' epilepsy. This had probably to do with the high level of interest in nosology which was prevalent around the turn of the century and resulted in the classical monographs of Gowers (1881), Binswanger (1899) and Turner (1907). Thus, for the last of these authors, idiopathic epilepsy was 'a chronic progressive disease of the brain', and had as an 'essential', 'predisposing' cause an 'inherited neuropathic disposition'. However, 'determining causes of epileptic attacks' could contribute to what later would be called a multifactorial pathogenesis. He noted that the seizures of organic and idiopathic epilepsy could be indistinguishable in appearance but did not yet conclude that this similarity could be due to the secondary rather than the primary pathogenetic factors in the idiopathic cases.

In the middle of our century, the beginnings of a new clinical syndromatology of epilepsy (the 'petit mal triad' (Lennox, 1945); epilepsy with grand mal on awakening (Janz 1953); the 'impulsive petit mal' of Janz & Christian (1957), together with the new and often surprising information provided by electroencephalography called for another reform of epilepsy classification and terminology.

As many of the traditional terms had become equivocal and subject to confusion due to the new developments, the first Commission on Classification and Terminology of the ILAE (Merlis, 1970) opted for a radical change and suggested calling those generalized epilepsies which were not the consequence of recognizable diseases or brain damage, 'primary generalized epilepsies' and the others, 'secondary generalized epilepsies'. This distinction remained restricted to generalized epilepsies, as epilepsies with focal seizures which are primary in this sense had not yet been clearly perceived. It turned out, however, that this terminology gave rise to new misunderstandings as it was frequently confounded with the concept of primarily or secondarily generalized tonic–clonic seizures.

A later League commission reintroduced therefore the terms symptomatic and idiopathic, the latter defined as epilepsies *sui generis*, of their own pathology, 'not preceded or occasioned by another disorder' (Commission, 1985). This now also included a group of idiopathic epilepsies with focal seizures, the first of which had been described in 1958 by Nayrac and Beaussart.

A possible misunderstanding remained, as idiopathic was now sometimes used for all cases where no definite symptomatic origin could be demonstrated, a use of idiopathy which essentially is a return to medieval concepts. The last revision of the *International Classification of Epilepsies and Epileptic Syndromes* (Commission, 1989) therefore clarified that the term was only to be applied if a symptomatic origin is neither detected nor suspected. For epilepsies with a suspected symptomatic cause which, however, remains obscure, the term 'cryptogenic' should be used, meaning 'of hidden origin'.

A genetic predisposition is consistent with this definition of idiopathy because the development of an epilepsy *sui generis* very well can originate in a genetic defect. This, however, applies only to genetic disorders where epileptic seizures are the only primary clinical symptoms.

The term 'genuine' epilepsy has been dropped altogether along with its counterpart 'epileptiform', as now all seizure types are accepted as epileptic which are characterized by the occasional, sudden, excessive and rapid discharges of grey matter postulated by Jackson.

References

Binswanger, O. (1899): *Die Epilepsie*. Wien: Hölder.

Commission on Classification and Terminology of the ILAE (1985): Proposal for classification of epilepsies and epileptic syndromes. *Epilepsia* **26,** 268–278.

Commission on Classification and Terminology of the ILAE (1989): Proposal for revised classification of epilepsies and epileptic syndromes. *Epilepsia* **30,** 389–399.

Delasiauve (1854): *Traité de l'épilepsie.* Paris: Masson.

Gowers, W.R. (1881): *Epilepsy and other chronic convulsive diseases.* London: Wood.

Jackson, J.H. (1931): *Selected writings.* London: Hodder and Stoughton.

Janz, D. (1953): Aufwach-Epilepsien. *Arch. Psychiat. Nervenkrh.* **191,** 73–98.

Janz, D. & Christian, W. (1957): Impulsiv-petit mal. *J. Neurol.* **176,** 346–386.

Lennox, W.G. (1945): The petit mal epilepsies. *J.A.M.A.* **129,** 1069–1073.

Merlis, J.K. (1970): Proposal for an International Classification of the Epilepsies. *Epilepsia* **11,** 114–119.

Nayrac, P. & Beaussart. M. (1958): Les pointe-ondes prérolandiques: expression EEG très particulière. *Rev. Neurol.* **99,** 201–206.

Stauder, J.H. (1938): *Konstitution und Wesensänderung der Epileptiker.* Leipzig: Thieme.

Tissot, S.A. (1770): *Traité de l'épilepsie.* Lausanne: Chapuis.

Turner, W.A. (1907): *Epilepsy – a study of the idiopathic disease.* London: Macmillan.

Chapter 2

Clinical and electroencephalographic characteristics of idiopathic generalized epilepsies

Joseph Roger[*], Michelle Bureau[*], Luis Oller Ferrer-Vidal[†], Luis Oller Daurella[†], Amalia Saltarelli[*] and Pierre Genton[*]

[*]Centre Saint Paul, 13258 Marseille 09, France; [†]Escuelas Pias 89, 08017 Barcelona, Spain

Introduction

Although the existence of cases in which epilepsy was not associated with organic brain damage was recognized a long time ago, idiopathic generalized epilepsies (IGEs) are a comparatively recently individualized category of epileptic syndromes: in the wake of an international workshop organized in Marseille in 1983 (Roger *et al.*, 1985, 1992), the Commission on Classification and Terminology submitted a tentative classification of epilepsies and epileptic syndromes in 1985 (Commission, 1985), that was completed in 1989 (Commission, 1989) (Table 1). Among these, several syndromes of IGE were recognized, each with a distinct age-dependency and/or clinical expression (Table 2).

As no clear aetiology is present in patients with IGE, other than a genetic predisposition, these epilepsies are likely to be due to genetically transmitted defects that express themselves in an age-related manner and result in various phenotypes. Several distinct genetic defects are involved, resulting in several distinct epileptic conditions. The differences (or possibly lack of difference) between the syndromes individualized by the currently accepted International Classification will be discussed at length in other chapters of this volume.

The purpose of this chapter is to delineate, for basic scientists and geneticists involved in the search for the genetic defects responsible for the various forms of IGE, the clinical and electroencephalographic (EEG) criteria that led physicians to diagnose these conditions. A good knowledge of these criteria will make the selection of patients and families for genetic studies easier and more reliable. Most points raised here are subjected to detailed discussion in other chapters of this book: the reader is kindly referred to the respective chapters.

It must be kept in mind that IGEs are a heterogeneous group of epileptic conditions, and that the criteria defined and used by clinicians rely on uncertain premisses. Both clinicians and basic scientists should benefit from the present progress in this field.

IDIOPATHIC GENERALIZED EPILEPSIES

Table 1. International classification of epilepsies, epileptic syndromes and related disorders (synopsis) (adapted from Commission, 1989)

Localization-related (focal, local, partial) epilepsies and syndromes

  Idiopathic (with age-related onset):
    Benign childhood epilepsy with centro-temporal spikes
    Childhood epilepsy with occipital paroxysms
    Primary reading epilepsy
  Symptomatic
    Chronic progressive epilepsia partialis continua of childhood
    Seizures characterized by specific modes of precipitation
    Other syndromes based on localization or aetiology
  Cryptogenic

Generalized epilepsies and syndromes

  Idiopathic (with age-related onset – listed in order of age):
    Benign neonatal familial convulsions
    Benign neonatal convulsions
    Benign myoclonic epilepsy in infancy
    Childhood absence epilepsy
    Juvenile absence epilepsy
    Juvenile myoclonic epilepsy
    Epilepsy with grand mal seizures on awakening
    Other generalized idiopathic epilepsies not defined above
    Epilepsies with seizures characterized by specific modes of precipitation (photogenic epilepsy)
  Cryptogenic and/or symptomatic (in order of age)
    West syndrome (infantile spasms)
    Lennox–Gastaut syndrome
    Epilepsy with myoclonic–astatic seizures
    Epilepsy with myoclonic absences
  Symptomatic
    Non-specific aetiology
      Early myoclonic encephalopathy
      Early infantile epileptic encephalopathy with suppression-bursts
      Other symptomatic generalized epilepsies not defined above
    Specific syndromes.

Epilepsies and syndromes undetermined whether focal or generalized

  With both generalized and focal seizures
    Neonatal seizures
    Severe myoclonic epilepsy in infancy
    Epilepsy with continuous spike-waves during slow sleep
    Acquired epileptic aphasia
    Other undetermined epilepsies not defined above
  Without unequivocal generalized or focal features.

Special syndromes

  Situation-related seizures
    Febrile convulsions
    Seizures occurring only in the context of acute metabolic or toxic events
  Isolated seizures or isolated status epilepticus.

Table 2. Definitions of the epileptic syndromes of IGE (adapted from Commission, 1989)

Benign neonatal familial convulsions	Benign neonatal familial convulsions are rare, dominantly inherited disorders manifesting mostly on the second and third days of life, with clonic or apnoeic seizures and no specific EEG criteria. History and investigations reveal no aetiological factors. About 14 per cent of these patients later develop epilepsy.
Benign neonatal convulsions	Benign neonatal convulsions are very frequently repeated clonic or apnoeic seizures occurring at about the fifth day of life, without known aetiology or concomitant metabolic disturbance. Interictal EEG often shows alternating sharp θ(theta) waves. There is no recurrence of seizures and the psychomotor development is not affected.
Benign myoclonic epilepsy in infancy	This syndrome is characterized by brief bursts of generalized myoclonus associated with generalized spike-waves, that occur during the first or second year of life in otherwise normal children who often have a family history of convulsions or epilepsy. Generalized tonic–clonic seizures may occur during adolescence.
Childhood absence epilepsy (pyknolepsy)	Pyknolepsy occurs in children of school age (peak manifestation age 6–7 years) in otherwise normal children, more frequently in girls than in boys. It is characterized by very frequent (several to many per day) absences. The EEG reveals bilateral, synchronous symmetrical spike-waves, usually at 3 Hz, on a normal background activity. During adolescence, generalized tonic–clonic seizures often develop. Otherwise, absences may remit, or, more rarely, persist as the only seizure type.
Juvenile absence epilepsy	The absences of juvenile absence epilepsy are the same as in pyknolepsy, but they occur around puberty and the seizure frequency is lower than in pyknolepsy, with absences occurring mostly sporadically. Association with generalized tonic–clonic seizures and myoclonic seizures is frequent. Sex distribution is equal. The spike-waves are often > 3 Hz.
Juvenile myoclonic epilepsy (impulsive petit mal)	Juvenile myoclonic epilepsy appears around puberty and is characterized by seizures with bilateral, single or repetitive, arrhythmic, irregular myoclonic jerks, predominantly in the arms, without disturbance of consciousness. The sex distribution is equal. Often, there are generalized tonic–clonic seizures and, less often, infrequent absences. The seizures usually occur shortly after awakening and may be precipitated by sleep deprivation. Interictal and ictal EEGs show generalized, often irregular spike-waves and polyspike-waves, usually > 3 Hz. The patients may be photosensitive.
Epilepsy with generalized tonic–clonic seizures on awakening	Epilepsy with generalized tonic–clonic seizures on awakening is a syndrome with onset mostly in the second decade of life. The generalized tonic–clonic seizures occur exclusively or predominantly (> 90 per cent of the time) shortly after awakening or around a second peak in the evening period of relaxation. Absence or myoclonic seizures may occur. Seizures may be precipitated by sleep deprivation. The EEG shows one of the patterns of idiopathic generalized epilepsy. The patients may be photosensitive.
Other generalized epilepsies not defined above	
Epilepsies with seizures precipitated by specific modes of activation	Most of the photosensitive epilepsies (photogenic epilepsies) belong to the group of idiopathic generalized epilepsies

Clinical criteria of IGEs

In the 1989 International Classification, the criteria of IGEs were defined in the following words:

> 'Idiopathic generalized epilepsies are forms of generalized epilepsies in which all seizures are initially generalized, with an EEG expression that is a generalized, bilateral, synchronous, symmetrical discharge (such as is described in the seizure classification of the corresponding type). The patient usually has a normal interictal state, without neurological or neuroradiologic signs. In general, interictal EEGs show normal background activity and generalized discharges, such as spikes, polyspike, spike-wave, and polyspike-waves ≥ 3 Hz. The discharges are increased by slow sleep. The various syndromes of idiopathic generalized epilepsies differ mainly in age of onset'. (Commission, 1989)

These criteria can be summarized: (1) only three types of seizures are found in IGEs: absences, massive myoclonias (myoclonic jerks) and generalized tonic–clonic seizures (GTCS) (Commission, 1981); (2) no aetiology can be found besides a genetic predisposition towards these disorders.

The International Classification lists a number of syndromes (Table 2) that have been recognized and accepted worldwide: this does not mean that other epileptic entities should not be added to the list.

The age of onset of these epilepsies may pose a problem:

– benign neonatal convulsions, in their familiar or sporadic form, do not strictly fulfil the criteria of IGEs: the convulsions are not necessarily generalized and the patients fail to exhibit the typical trait of generalized spike-wave discharges. It can be argued that the immaturity of the neonatal brain prevents these conditions from expressing themselves in a fully generalized manner.

– myoclonic forms of IGEs may appear in children after the age of benign myoclonic epilepsy of infancy and before the age of juvenile myoclonic epilepsy, making it thus impossible to classify them properly according to the present guidelines.

– in elderly patients, the onset of myoclonias (Gram *et al.*, 1988, Case 2) or of absences, often in the form of absence status, may lead the clinician to diagnose IGE: many clinical data militate against the onset of IGE in the elderly. According to Gastaut (1981), less than 1 per cent of all epilepsies with onset in the elderly should be considered to be IGEs, and these are mostly represented by absence status in post-menopausal women.

The existence of a known or probable anatomical lesion of the brain may also pose a problem when the diagnosis of IGE is suspected. It should be stressed that IGEs are comparatively frequent forms of epilepsy, and that they may, by sheer coincidence, coexist with some form of brain pathology. This type of situation is probably not uncommon, and most series reporting large numbers of patients with IGEs have mentioned a proportion of cases where mental retardation and/or severe personality disorders were present. We shall cite two instances of such coincidences:

– one is a patient with Down's syndrome who had a typical form of benign myoclonic epilepsy in infancy (Dravet *et al.*, 1992);

– the other is a patient with both tuberous sclerosis (TS) and childhood absence epilepsy (CAE); he had probably inherited the genetic trait of CAE from his father, who had typical absences, and had a sporadic form of tuberous sclerosis (Roger *et al.*, 1984). This was the only case of IGE in a series of 126 patients with tuberous sclerosis.

We must thus admit that IGE can coexist with a brain lesion – which is probably a chance simultaneous occurrence – and with significant mental or psychiatric disturbances: in the latter cases, the relationship between epilepsy and the associated disorders may be significant.

The Classification does not explicitly cite another category of epilepsies that does fulfil the criteria of IGEs. A large number of patients experience only infrequent generalized tonic–clonic seizures, sometimes after some febrile convulsions during early childhood; the age of onset is very variable from case to case, it ranges between early childhood and adulthood. There is no clear relationship between the timing of the seizures and the sleep–wake cycle. Interictal changes are represented, on the EEG, by generalized spike-wave discharges. Diagnosis may be difficult with some forms of frontal lobe epilepsy, and if the EEG criteria are not present, the accurate diagnosis would rather be a focal type of epilepsy, especially when the generalized tonic–clonic seizures occur during sleep. Most authors have included these in the category of epilepsy with generalized tonic–clonic seizures on awakening, but others prefer to individualize these patients as having a nonsyndromic grand mal epilepsy or, according to a recent collaborative study, 'benign adult-onset grand mal' (Oller-Daurella & Sorel, 1989). However, this terminology sounds somewhat restrictive, as these patients may experience their first generalized tonic–clonic seizures during childhood.

Electroencephalographic criteria of IGEs

According to the International Classification of Epilepsies and Epileptic Syndromes (Commission, 1989), the EEG criteria of IGE are as follows:
- normal background activity,
- normal organization of sleep with bilateral and symmetrical sleep patterns,
- presence of interictal abnormalities such as generalized spikes, polyspikes, spike-wave (SW) and polyspike-wave (PSW) discharges at 3 Hz or more,
- increase of interictal abnormalities during slow wave sleep,
- ictal discharges are generalized at their onset, bilateral, synchronous and symmetrical.

These diagnostic criteria are strict; in some clinical situations, these criteria will not strictly apply:
- the background activity will be markedly slowed in the wake of a generalized tonic–clonic seizure; such slowing may be found hours and in some cases days after the seizure;
- some drugs, particularly benzodiazepines, may interfere with the physiological sleep patterns and decrease both the number of sleep transients (such as spindles and K complexes) and slow delta waves during sleep stages 3 and 4; they may also cause a decrease in the number of eye movements during rapid-eye movement (REM) sleep;
- the ictal and interictal abnormalities are usually of higher voltage over the frontal and vertex areas; sometimes they can be slightly asymmetrical; however, whenever the discharges are irregular in their morphology or their frequency, or are slower than 2.5 Hz, or constantly asymmetrical, the diagnosis of IGE must be reappraised.

A point not mentioned in the International Classification is the presence of photosensitivity: this may be found in about 20 per cent of all IGE cases, and even in up to 40 per cent of IGEs diagnosed in children.

Most EEG criteria must be seen as age-related and they can be addressed according to the different syndromes of IGE occurring in infancy, childhood, adolescence or adulthood. We will only insist on the EEG features of three distinct syndromes, with ages of onset typically in infancy, childhood and adolescence, respectively.

Benign myoclonic epilepsy of infancy (BMEI)

The background is normal for age. Some slow waves may be found over the central areas. Most of the time, there are no interictal abnormalities during waking. Intermittent light stimulation (ILS) does not provoke subclinical spike-wave discharges – i. e. spike-wave discharges are constantly associated with myoclonic jerks on EEG recordings performed in the waking state. Sleep recordings show a normal, age-related organization of sleep, normal sleep transients, and generalized spike-waves with or without associated myoclonias can be found during drowsiness and in the early stages of slow sleep, while they tend to decrease during slow wave sleep.

The ictal EEG consists of brief bursts of generalized spike-waves associated with more or less massive myoclonic jerks (Fig. 1). Jerks may be followed by a brief atonia. Sometimes, the discharge is not generalized at its onset and may begin over the frontal areas.

Childhood absence epilepsy (CAE)

The background activity is normal, but some children can exhibit a rather particular posterior delta rhythm, usually in the form of long bursts of high-amplitude, sinusoidal around 3 Hz, that may be symmetrical or (more often) asymmetrical over the occipital or parieto-occipital areas (Fig. 2). This

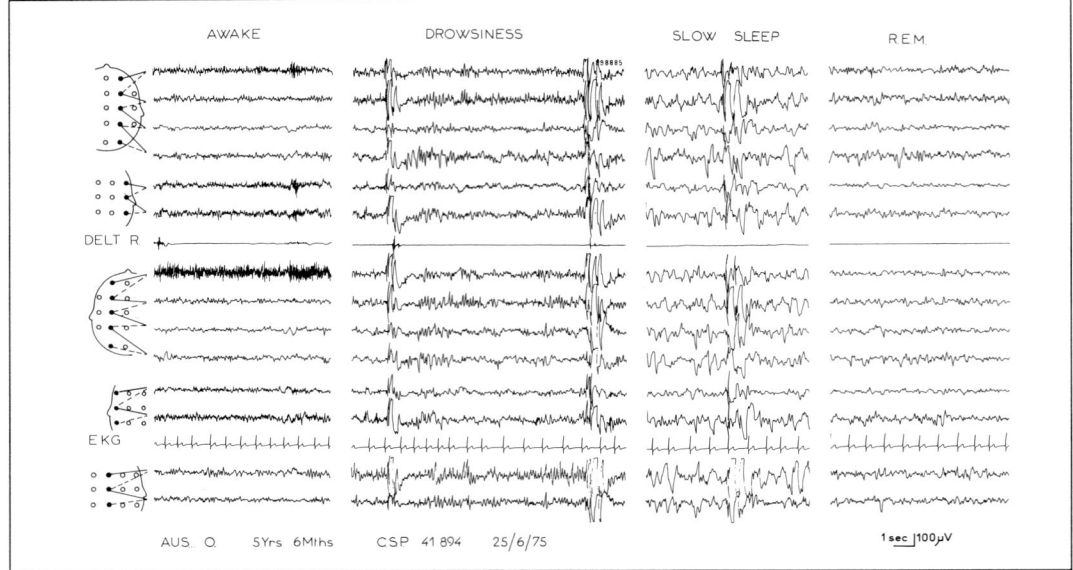

Fig. 1. Benign myoclonic epilepsy of infancy. Boy aged 5 years 6 months. Left: awake; normal background activity without paroxysmal anomalies. Middle left: drowsiness; presence of generalized spike-wave and polyspike-wave discharges associated with myoclonias recorded on the right deltoid muscle. Middle right: slow wave sleep; subclinical generalized spike-wave. Right: REM sleep; no paroxysmal anomaly.

slow rhythm is blocked by eye opening and is enhanced by hyperventilation. This particular trait persists even if absence seizures disappear following efficient therapy; they can be considered a genetic marker of childhood absence epilepsy.

The interictal abnormalities consist in generalized spike-wave discharges, but in some cases one can find spikes of spike-waves that are asymmetrical and predominate over the frontal areas. During sleep, generalized polyspike-waves can appear, but one never finds runs of rapid rhythms, such as in the Lennox–Gastaut syndrome.

The ictal EEG shows a rhythmic discharge of spike-waves at 3 Hz or more, associated with the clinical absence (Fig. 2). As a rule, the onset is sudden and the end is abrupt. In longer absences, the frequency of spike-waves can decrease below 3 Hz towards the end of the discharge.

When absences persist into adulthood, the interictal abnormalities can change and become more irregular (Fig. 3).

A very important diagnostic criterion is the effect of hyperventilation: this procedure is the easiest way to provoke an absence and the diagnosis of absence epilepsy should be questioned if an untreated patient does not have an absence during a well-performed hyperventilation.

However, the unity of the syndrome now recognized as childhood absence epilepsy is questionable: the relative importance played by myoclonic components of seizures and by photosensitivity, as well as by the genetic background, may lead to the individualization of discrete syndromes; at present, there is no consensus on these points, and the respective changes of the EEG criteria concerning such possible distinct entities will be discussed elsewhere in this volume.

Juvenile myoclonic epilepsy (JME)

There are few interictal abnormalities. They consist of fast, 4–6 Hz generalized spike-waves or polyspike-waves that are often irregular; they may appear only at sleep onset, or, more charac-

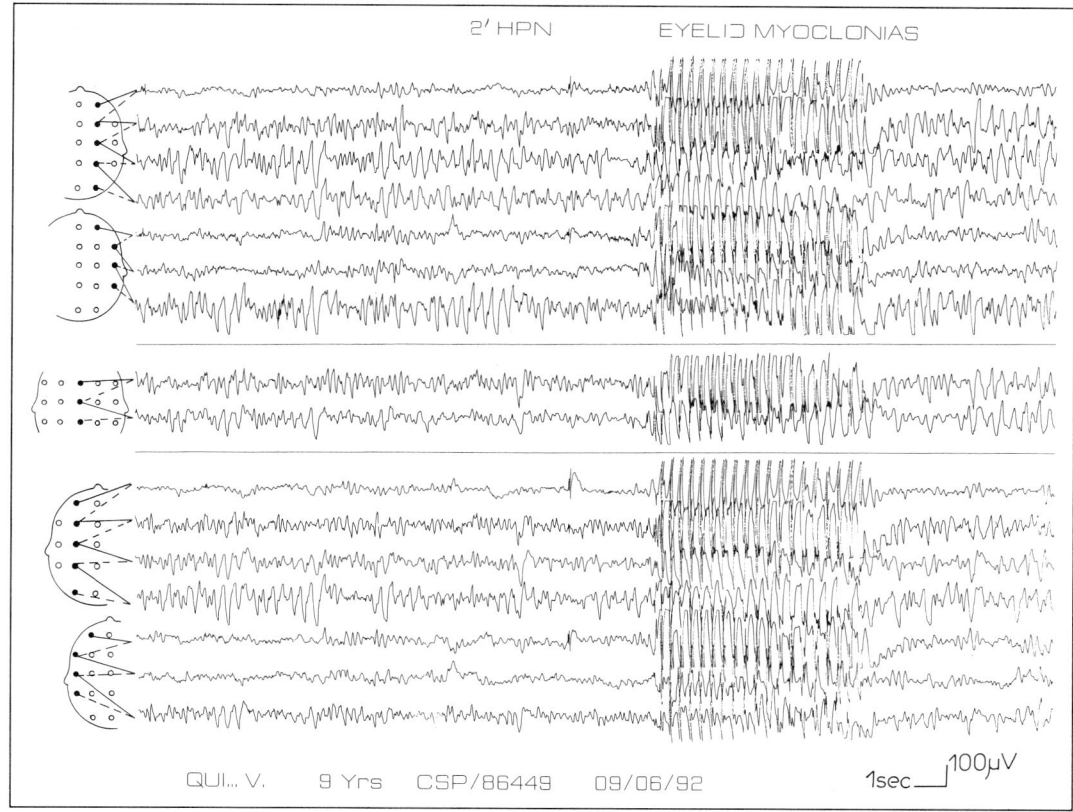

Fig. 2. Childhood absence epilepsy. Girl aged 9 years. After 2 min of hyperventilation, appearance of a slow rhythm over the posterior leads followed by a discharge of 3 Hz spike-waves associated with a clinical absence with slight eyelid myoclonias.

teristically, during intermediate awakenings or after the final, morning awakening. Photosensitivity is frequently found, and intermittent light stimulation may provoke discharges of spike-waves and polyspike-waves that may be associated with myoclonic jerks. Both interictal and ictal changes are enhanced by sleep deprivation. Sleep recordings, performed if possible after sleep deprivation, are very useful in the diagnosis of this condition. Particular attention should be paid to the EEG tracings recorded after awakening from the night-time sleep or from a daytime sleep episode: such recordings may show increased discharges of spike-waves and polyspike-waves associated with myoclonic jerks (Fig. 4).

However, the EEG changes found in patients with juvenile myoclonic epilepsy may be very misleading. In some cases, it may be difficult to find interictal abnormalities and the tracings are repeatedly normal; in such patients, a sleep EEG should be performed. In other cases, focal or atypical changes will be found during short, routine EEG recordings. These particular aspects will be discussed in another chapter of this volume.

The classification of idiopathic generalized epilepsies in clinical practice

The criteria defined by the 1985 and 1989 Classifications have been used in daily practice by many epileptologists. They allowed us to classify our patients over the years and to estimate the pre-

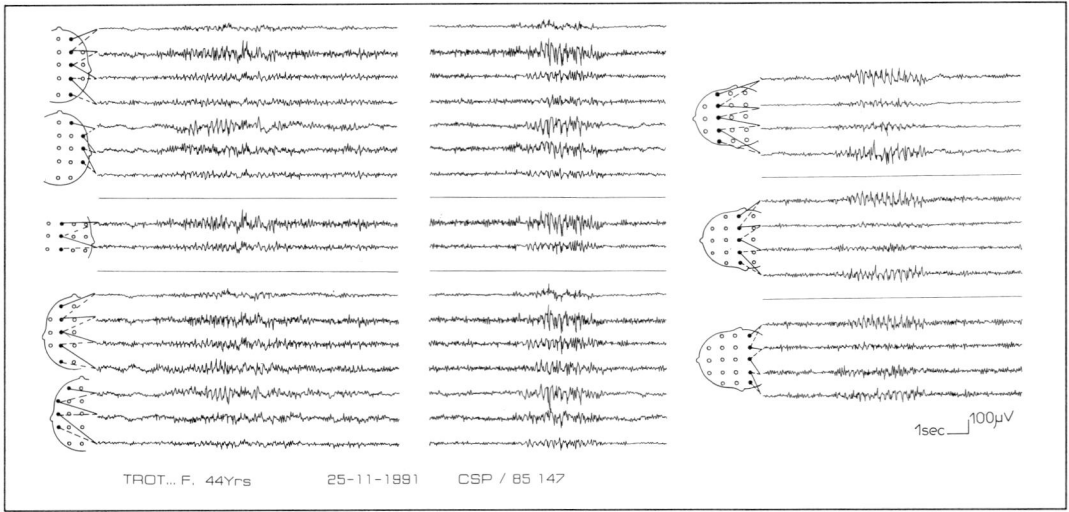

Fig. 3. Childhood absence epilepsy, with onset of absences at age 8. Persisting absences in a 44-year-old woman. Note the irregular pattern of the interictal changes.

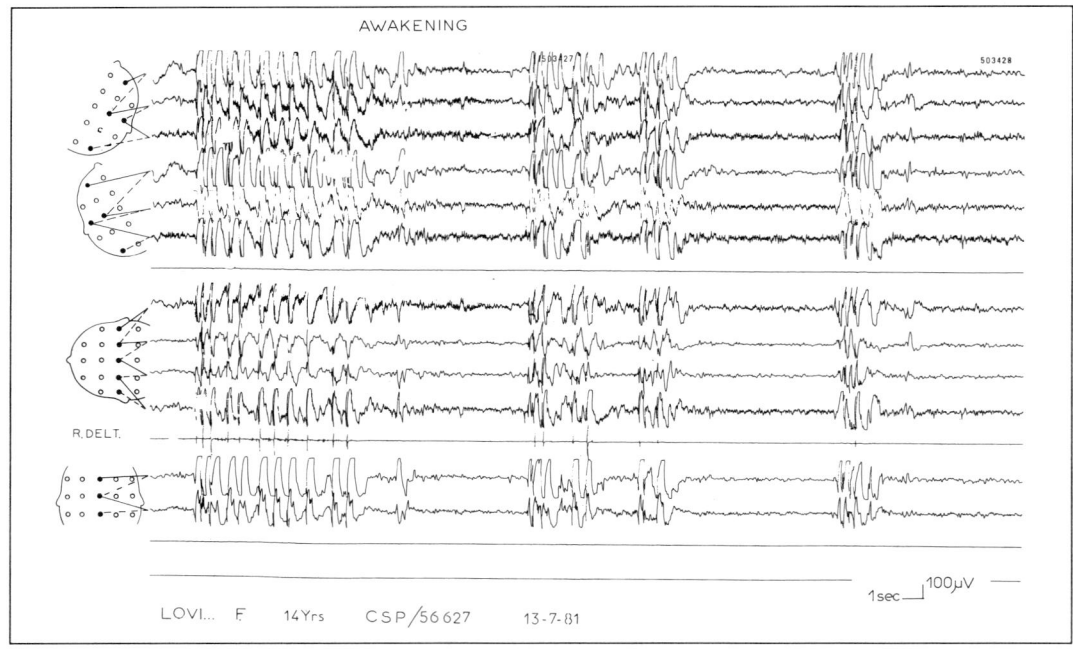

Fig. 4. Juvenile myoclonic epilepsy. Boy aged 14 years. EEG performed after awakening showing a discharge of more or less irregular spike-wave associated with myoclonic jerks recorded on the right deltoid muscle.

valence of IGEs in our centres, and we shall report here our experience in two different patient populations:
– a specialized epilepsy centre (Marseille),

– a private epilepsy outpatient clinic (Barcelona).

At the Centre Saint Paul, we prospectively classified 1486 consecutive, newly referred patients, first seen between 1986 and 1992, using the 1985 Classification project criteria (Commission, 1985) and updating the classification in 1989 in the light of the definitive version of the International Classification (Commission, 1989). All patients had had unprovoked recurring seizures. A vast majority of cases were classified into one of the recognized categories and syndromes: only 170 cases (11.4 per cent) were not classified, mostly due to lack of precise data; 268 patients (18 per cent) were considered to have IGE. The data were reviewed in 1993: 15 cases of suspected IGE were considered insufficiently documented

We thus consider that 253 patients had a firm diagnosis of IGE, i.e. 17 per cent of the total sample or 19.6 cent of the cases that were classified.

It appears that childhood absence epilepsy and juvenile myoclonic epilepsy are the most frequently encountered types of IGE, representing 28.9 per cent and 23.3 per cent of IGEs respectively. Other syndromes were less frequently encountered (Table 3).

Table 3. *Generalized idiopathic epilepsies: classification of 253 consecutive cases newly referred to the Centre Saint Paul, Marseille (1986–1992)*

	n	%	Sex ratio M/F	Age of onset (years) mean	range
Benign neonatal convulsions	0	0			
Benign familial neonatal convulsions	1	0.4	0/ 1	0	
Benign myoclonic epilepsy	4	1.6	2/ 2	1.2	0.8–1.4
Childhood absence epilepsy	73	28.9	34/39	6.0	0.8–13
Juvenile absence epilepsy	28	11.1	14/14	13.5	10–23
Juvenile myoclonic epilepsy	59	23.3	27/32	14.5	3–33
Awakening grand mal	30	11.9	12/18	15.3	9.5–23
Isolated GTC seizures	39	15.4	15/14	19.6	1–46
Photogenic epilepsy	8	3.2	2/ 6	10.0	4–20
Not further classified/overlap	11	4.3	5/ 6	11.6	4–21

Three categories of patients merit a special mention:

– a group of patients had clinical and electrophysiological photosensitivity, in association with a generalized pattern of EEG abnormalities; they were classified into a separate category of photosensitive IGEs because they did not fulfil the clinical and EEG definitions of one of the other syndromes; there was a female predominance in this group (6/8 patients, i.e. 75 per cent). The limits between this category and the syndromes of IGE where photosensitivity is a common finding (especially benign myoclonic epilepsy of infancy and juvenile myoclonic epilepsy, but also some forms of childhood absence epilepsy) are unclear.

– a comparatively large group of patients had a mild form of IGE characterized by infrequent generalized tonic–clonic seizures and generalized interictal EEG changes. This group represents a sizeable proportion of IGE patients (15.4 per cent in our experience). We consider these cases to represent a different, probably mild form of IGE, a 'non-syndromic grand mal'.

– a last group of 11 patients (4.3 per cent of the IGEs) was not further classified: although these patients undoubtedly belonged to the category of IGEs, a precise syndromic classification could not be reached either because of insufficient clinical and EEG data, especially concerning the possible existence of absence seizures during childhood or adolescence, or the precise age of onset of seizures, or because the age

Table 4. Classification of seizure types in 1033 cases of IGE observed in Barcelona

Seizure types	n	%
One seizure type	517	50.0
Absence (A)	190	18.4
Generalized tonic–clonic (GTCS)	265	25.7
Myoclonic (M)	62	6.0
Several seizure types	516	50.0
A + GTCS	329	31.8
A + M	21	2.0
A + GTCS + M	61	5.9
GTCS + M	105	10.2
Total	1033	100.0

of onset was very atypical for the most likely syndrome of IGE. However, these patients represented only a small minority within the group of IGEs.

A longstanding private epileptologic outpatient practice allowed two of us to establish a computerized database on the clinical data observed in 5000 consecutive epilepsy patients seen over the past 20 years (Oller-Daurella & Oller, 1994). Due to the fact that this database was started well before the present classifications were used, the seizure types and the interictal EEG changes were the most reliable classification criteria, although ictal data were available in some patients; routinely performed hyperventilation was particularly useful in provoking typical absences.

Among 5000 patients with epilepsy, 1102 were diagnosed as having IGE; however, 69 cases had other types of seizures besides those found in IGE, and these cases will not be considered further. We thus established a reliable diagnosis of IGE in 1033 patients (20.6 per cent of the whole sample).

The different seizure types and the various associations of seizure types have been reported in Table 4. The data show that half of the sample had experienced only one seizure type; generalized tonic–clonic seizures were the most frequent, and myoclonic seizures the rarest seizure type.

Table 5. Syndromic classification of IGEs among 1033 cases of IGE observed in Barcelona

Syndrome of IGE	n	%classified	% total IGEs
Benign myoclonic epilepsy (onset before age 3 in all)	20	2.7	1.9
Childhood absence epilepsy			
Onset between ages 3 and 11	219		
Onset before age 4	9		
Total	228	30.6	22.1
Juvenile absence epilepsy			
Onset between ages 12–18	30		
With onset ≥ age 19	2		
Total	32	4.3	3.1
Juvenile myoclonic epilepsy			
Onset between ages 8–18	101	13.6	9.8
Epilepsy with GTCS only	138	18.5	13.4
Epilepsy with GTCS preceding the onset of absences	225	30.2	21.8
Total	744	100.0	72.0

The syndromic classification of these cases is reported in Table 5. This classification only concerns 744 patients, i.e. 72 per cent of the sample, as the criteria for the syndromes outlined in the International Classification could not lead to a precise categorization in the remaining 28 per cent. Typical syndromes of benign myoclonic epilepsy of infancy and of juvenile myoclonic epilepsy were ascertained in relatively few patients. The largest group of patients were those with absence seizures: when the absences preceded the onset of other seizure types, they were considered to have childhood or juvenile absence epilepsy, according to the age of onset of absences.

There is however a large group of patients who had absences only after having experienced generalized tonic–clonic seizures; these were put into a separate category which represents 30.2 per cent of the classified cases or 21.8 per cent of the total sample. In these patients, the age of onset was before age 3 in 19 cases, between ages 3 and 11 in 116, between ages 12 and 18 in 78 and after age 18 in 12.

In this study, we also individualized a group of patients who experienced only generalized tonic–clonic seizures. These represented 18.5 per cent of the classified cases or 13.4 per cent of the total sample. The age of onset of generalized tonic–clonic seizures was spread over several age classes: 15 had begun before age 3, 45 between ages 3 and 11, 51 between ages 12 and 18 and 27 after age 18.

Taken together, these data, collected either in a specialized epilepsy centre or in a private outpatient clinic show that most patients can be classified according to the ILAE criteria into one of the recognized syndromes. However, a significant amount of cases does not fulfil these strict criteria, either because pertinent clinical and/or EEG data are missing or because the proposed categories do not correspond to the clinical reality observed. It appears that some of the borders between syndromes are arbitrary: the three syndromes of juvenile IGEs, i.e. juvenile absence epilepsy, juvenile myoclonic epilepsy and epilepsy with awakening generalized tonic–clonic seizures, are difficult to distinguish in some patients; childhood and juvenile absence epilepsies are usually distinguished mostly according to their respective ages of onset, but other criteria may be necessary in order to further separate or 'split' these entities. Lastly, the large number of patients experiencing only generalized tonic–clonic seizures, usually as a benign epilepsy with infrequent seizures, seems to justify a separate category; however, this group does not exhibit a particular age- dependency.

Conclusions

In order to distinguish IGEs from other types of epilepsies, strict clinical and EEG criteria have been proposed by the International Classification of Epilepsies and Epileptic Syndromes. However, clinical experience shows that these criteria are not fulfilled by all patients all of the time: it must be kept in mind that the epileptic conditions considered as representative of 'idiopathic generalized epilepsy' are in fact a heterogeneous group, and that their clinical and EEG correlates may vary slightly, due to many factors, such as age, interfering drugs, time of day, state of vigilance . . .

If one considers screening patients for genetic studies, the criteria reported above should nevertheless be adhered to. Both the clinical and the EEG criteria of these conditions are relative, and not absolute: once very reliable genetic or biochemical markers have been individualized thanks to studies performed using the imperfect criteria that we now have, we may have to change our minds slightly and admit a greater variability of clinical and EEG phenotypes.

These criteria have been very helpful in the clinical management of patients and have allowed us to classify a large group of patients we consider to have one or the other form of idiopathic generalized epilepsy. It must be stressed that a proportion of patients with IGE does not fit into the categories of the ILAE classification: this is especially the case of patients with infrequent generalized tonic–clonic seizures, who do not necessarily fulfil the criteria of 'epilepsy with awakening grand mal'.

For the time being, genetic studies have to rely on what we have: both the clinical criteria – i.e.

seizure type, age of onset, personal and family background, evolution over time, sensitivity to drug therapy . . . – and the EEG criteria should be upheld as long as no other diagnostic tool is at hand. Strict observation of these criteria will probably avoid a lot of waste in the search for the genetic and biochemical mechanisms of idiopathic generalized epilepsies. The precise clinical and EEG phenotype of a single patient is often difficult to ascertain; the significance of subclinical EEG abnormalities in relatives is often debatable. From a strictly clinical and neurophysiological point of view, genetic studies comparing well-ascertained IGE patients with well-ascertained normal controls seem easier to carry out than those performed among siblings and/or multi-generational family members, in whom the phenotype is much more difficult to assess.

References

Commission on Classification and Terminology of the International League Against Epilepsy (1981): Proposal for revised clinical and electroencephalographic classification of epileptic seizures. *Epilepsia* **22,** 489–501.

Commission on Classification and Terminology of the International League Against Epilepsy (1985): Proposal for classification of epilepsy and epileptic syndromes. *Epilepsia* **26,** 268–278.

Commission on Classification and Terminology of the International League Against Epilepsy (1989): Proposal for revised classification of epilepsies and epileptic syndromes. *Epilepsia* **30,** 389–399.

Dravet, C., Bureau, M. & Roger, J. (1992): Benign myoclonic epilepsy in infants. In: *Epileptic syndromes in infancy, childhood and adolescence*, 2nd edn, eds. J. Roger, M. Bureau, C. Dravet, F.E. Dreifuss, P. Wolf & A. Perret, pp. 67–74. London: John Libbey.

Gastaut, H. (1981): Individualisation des epilepsies dites 'bénignes' ou 'fonctionnelles' aux différents âges de la vie. Appréciation des variations corréspondantes de la prédisposition épileptique à ces âges. *Rev. EEG Neurophysiol.* **11,** 346–366.

Gram, L., Alving, J., Sagild, J.C. & Dam, M. (1988): Juvenile myoclonic epilepsy in unexpected age groups. *Epilepsy Res.* **2,** 137–140.

Hirsch, E., Velez, A., Sellal, F. *et al.* (1993): Electroclinical signs of benign neonatal familial convulsions. *Ann. Neurol.* **34,** 835–841.

Oller-Daurella, L. & Sorel, L. (1989): L'épilepsie Grand Mal bénigne de l'adulte. *Acta Neurol. Belg.* **89,** 38–45.

Oller-Daurella, L.F-V. & Oller, L. (1994): *5000 epilepticos. Clinica y evolucion*. Barcelona: Ciba-Geigy, 1994. 317 pages.

Roger, J., Dravet, C., Boniver, C., Magaudda, A., Bureau, M., Fernandez-Alvarez, E., Sanmarti, F.X., Fabregust, I., Cenraud, B. & Larrieu, J.L. (1984): L'épilepsie dans la sclerose tubéreuse de Bourneville. *Boll. Lega. It. Epi.* **45/46,** 33–38.

Roger, J., Dravet, C., Bureau, M., Dreifuss, F.E. & Wolf, P. (1985): *Epileptic syndromes in infancy, childhood and adolescence.*. London: John Libbey.

Roger, J., Dravet, C., Bureau, M., Dreifuss, F.E., Perret, A. & Wolf, P. (1992): *Epileptic syndromes in infancy, childhood and adolescence*, 2nd edn. London: John Libbey.

Chapter 3

Epidemiology of idiopathic generalized epilepsies

Isabelle Desguerre*, Catherine Chiron*, Jérôme Loiseau†, Jean-François Dartigues‡, Olivier Dulac* and Pierre Loiseau†

*Department of Neuropediatrics and INSERM U29, Hôpital Saint Vincent de Paul, Paris, †Department of Neurology and ‡Department of Epidemiology, Bordeaux University Hospital, Bordeaux, France.

The criteria of idiopathic generalized epilepsies and their application to epidemiological studies

Idiopathic generalized epilepsies (IGEs) are newly described disorders: they were defined in 1985 and 1989 by the Commission on Classification and Terminology of the International League against Epilepsy (Commission, 1985, 1989), and the definitions of the various types of IGE imply both clinical and EEG criteria. Epidemiological data are scarce, and often unreliable, as most studies were either based solely on seizure types or were performed before the description of the syndromes now considered to represent IGEs.

Prior to 1985, idiopathic generalized epilepsy cases were classified as 'primary generalized epilepsy'. Looser diagnostic criteria were used: generalized convulsive or non-convulsive seizures and the absence of evidence of brain lesion were considered sufficient, whatever the EEG. For instance, Wagner (1983) wrote that epilepsy with clinical primary generalized seizures had the highest incidence of normal EEG findings. In a series of 90 adult patients diagnosed as having primary generalized epilepsy, interictal bilateral spike-wave complexes were present in only 36 patients (Oller-Daurella, 1988). In another series, they were found in only 48 of 80 patients (Sorel, 1988). However, Sorel based diagnosis on more than one criteria: grand mal seizures plus bilateral spike-waves or, when absent, myoclonic seizures or other idiopathic generalized epilepsies in the family. Other studies were far less restrictive and most epidemiological studies are flawed for this reason. Surely patients were included who would now be diagnosed as having undetermined epilepsy or other types of epilepsy.

Conversely, narrow diagnostic criteria may lead to an underestimation of IGEs. In a retrospective study of 1054 patients, aged 16 to 66 years, epilepsy with clinically primary generalized seizures represented 32 per cent of all epileptic syndromes (Wagner, 1983). But only half of these patients fulfilled the positive criteria for IGE, i.e. absence or myoclonic seizures, with or without grand mal seizures, or epilepsy with awakening grand mal.

The EEG criterion may, in incidence surveys, lead to an underestimation of IGEs. EEG recordings cannot be performed in some countries. Even when an EEG has been performed, it may remain inconclusive. Absence and myoclonic seizures are probably very seldom misdiagnosed, because of numerous interictal and/or ictal epileptiform EEG abnormalities. Interictal spike-wave discharges are less frequent in patients with only generalized tonic–clonic seizures. They may be lacking on one or even on several routine recordings. For instance, in an incidence survey undertaken in the French Southwest (Loiseau *et al.*, 1990), 66 patients immediately fulfilled the diagnosis criteria for IGE. Within one year, 13 patients who had been previously classified under the heading of undetermined epilepsy or isolated seizures were reclassified as IGEs, because bilateral spike-and-wave discharges were found on later EEGs. The characteristic EEG abnormalities were found only within the second or third year of follow-up in four further patients.

Although the outcome is not a primary element of the definition of IGEs, it is supposed to be favourable for epilepsy and for mental status, especially when compared to the outcome of symptomatic and cryptogenic epilepsies. The rate of seizure remission has been extensively studied and a score predictive for a remission from seizures has even been proposed (Camfield *et al.*, 1993). However, few long-term data are currently available concerning the mental and social or schooling outcome (Sillanpää, 1992). IGEs constitute a heterogeneous group and the various syndromes included among IGEs are suspected to have different levels of 'benignity'.

Other methodological problems

Definition of IGEs is a crucial point but other facts make the evaluation of their incidence and prevalence difficult.

(1) Some time may elapse between onset of absence or myoclonic seizures and the first medical contact with the patient. This time-lag was estimated to be one year or longer in 37 per cent of patients with absence seizures (Olsson, 1988).

(2) IGEs encompass several distinct syndromes, but quite a few patients shift from one phenotype to another. Children with absence seizures may develop juvenile myoclonic epilepsy; generalized tonic–clonic seizures may become the prominent feature in patients who initially had absence epilepsy.

(3) Recently described and comparatively uncommon syndromes such as benign neonatal convulsions (BNC) and benign myoclonic epilepsy of infancy (BMEI) should be considered among the IGEs. Benign myoclonic epilepsy of infancy is characterized by the association of myoclonic seizures and bilateral spike-and-wave discharges; benign neonatal convulsions have a demonstrated genetic origin in their familial form. It may be argued that seizures and EEG abnormalities remain focal in benign neonatal convulsions because of the incomplete functional development of the newborn brain.

(4) IGEs are age-dependent syndromes, with various durations of active epilepsy. For instance, Hedström & Olsson (1991) collected all new cases of absence epilepsy during the period 1978 to 1982 and reviewed the patients until December 1985. They described several subgroups with regard to the clinical profile. A subgroup of 56 patients was characterized by response to therapy within six months and little risk of relapse after the withdrawal of medication. Such patients clearly fit the diagnosis of childhood absence epilepsy. In a subgroup of 10 children already treated for absence seizures who later experienced generalized tonic–clonic seizures, the remission rate was only 50 per cent. In the past, this group would have been called mixed petit mal. We know this is often a long-lasting condition. A subgroup of 12 patients had experienced both absence and generalized tonic–clonic seizures before the start of therapy. As the median age of onset was 12 years, these patients obviously belong to the category of juvenile absence epilepsy. The remission rate under therapy was very high (91 per cent), but the risk of relapse was also very high when medication was withdrawn. Lastly, a less homogeneous group of 12 patients, with various ages at onset of generalized tonic–clonic seizures followed by absence seizures, was reported by these authors. A remission rate of 73 per cent was noted.

This study illustrates an important point: incidence and prevalence rates for active epilepsy must be specifically related to age. The numerator is the number of affected persons in a given population. The denominator is the number of subjects at risk. Most IGEs begin in childhood or adolescence. Rates are clearly different when the denominator is the number of children, or young adults, or the whole population.

Literature data on the epidemiology of IGEs

With these restrictions in mind, one can find some interesting data in the literature. We chose to select modern, well-documented studies. Two of them address the prevalence of IGEs and the others the incidence or prevalence of various idiopathic generalized syndromes.

In a survey of 5- to 14-year-old children in schools of Northern Italy, the prevalence rate of epilepsy was 4.53/1000. Primary generalized epilepsy was diagnosed in 30.8 per cent of the cases (Cavazzuti, 1980.) In a survey of males aged 17–18 years who were called for selection for military service in Northern Italy, IGEs represented 28.3 per cent of the cases (Cornaggia et al., 1990). In an Italian population of children 6–14 years old, the prevalence of absence seizures with or without generalized tonic–clonic seizures was 0.4/1000 (Pazzaglia & Franck, 1976). In Sweden, among children under 16 years of age, the annual incidence rate of 'petit mal' was 8/100 000 (Blom et al., 1978).

The National Child Development Study conducted in the United Kingdom included all children who were born during one week in 1958 and experienced two or more nonfebrile seizures before the age of 11 years. The prevalence rate of epilepsy was in keeping with data from the literature: 4.1/1000. The prevalence rate for absence seizures, with or without associated grand mal seizures, was 0.6/1000 (Ross et al., 1980).

In Germany, among children aged up to 8 years, the prevalence rate for absence seizures was 0.7/1000 (Doose & Sitepu, 1983).

In an epidemiological survey in Northern Italy, including patients of all ages, the prevalence rate of epilepsy was higher than in the above studies: 6.2/1000, and the annual incidence rate was 33/100 000. Prevalence and incidence rates for absence seizures were 0.7/1000 and 4.6/100 000, respectively (Granieri et al., 1983).

In a retrospective study in the Faroes Islands, the annual incidence rate was found to be 42/100 000 and the point-prevalence rate was 7.63/1000 for epileptic patients of all ages. The prevalence and incidence rates were 2.9/1000 and 14.8/100 000, respectively, for primary generalized epilepsies; for grand mal, 2.5/1000 and 13/100 000; for absence seizures, 0.2/1000 and 0.7/1000, and for juvenile myoclonic epilepsy, 0.2/1000 and 1.1/100 000, respectively (Joensen, 1986).

In a district of Sweden all new cases of absence seizures in persons under 16 years of age were collected. The incidence rate for absence seizures with or without myoclonic or tonic–clonic seizures was 6.3/100 000 (Olsson, 1988).

In an American survey of persons under 20 years of age, all sources of medical care yielded a prevalence rate for epilepsy of 4.7/1000. The prevalence rates for generalized tonic–clonic seizures, absence and myoclonic seizures were 1.14, 0.10, and 0.4/1000, respectively (Cowan et al., 1989).

In a population-based study carried out in Sweden, the age-specific prevalence rates per 1000 persons were estimated for absence seizures as follows: 0.14 in the group 17–19 years; 0.13 in the group 20–29; 0.04 in the group 30–39, and none in older persons (Forsgren, 1992).

These figures illustrate the age-dependency of IGEs and their favourable outcome. They also show some of the limits of epidemiological surveys: in clinical practice, it is possible to see patients with an onset of absence seizures after the age of 30, or persistent absence seizures after the age of 40.

To our knowledge, only one population-based case control study of risk factors for absence seizures has been published (Rocca et al., 1987). None of the previously suggested factors, such as perinatal events, reached statistical significance.

The two syndrome-oriented French surveys

An epidemiological survey of epileptic seizures was initiated in 1984 in the French Southwest (Loiseau *et al.*, 1990). During a 12-month period, all neurologists and electroencephalographers of an administrative district with slightly more than one million residents collected all persons aged over two months who experienced a first epileptic seizure. The cohort was followed and the diagnosis updated five years after the first seizure. Eighty-three cases of IGE were diagnosed, 73 of whom had an onset under 25 years of age. The total annual incidence rate was estimated at 9.2/100 000 in persons under 60 years and 18.4/100 000 under 25 years of age. The annual incidence rate of childhood absence epilepsy was 5.9/100 000 in the population under 15 years. Annual incidence rates for juvenile myoclonic epilepsy, grand mal on awakening and photosensitive epilepsies in the population under 25 years of age were 2.8, 1.8, and 1.5/100 000, respectively.

Another epidemiological survey performed in France was specifically dedicated to epilepsy with onset under 10 years of age (Chiron, 1986; Luna *et al.*, 1987). It had three main objectives: (1) to evaluate the respective incidence of epileptic syndromes in childhood with particular emphasis for the neonatal and infantile periods, (2) to test the reliability of the classification given at first visit by reviewing the cases several years later, and (3) to follow the cohort over a long period in order to assess the outcome of epilepsy and the performance at school.

The study was performed in the North of France, in a well-defined area, the 'departement de l'Oise', in which the population characteristics and health care can be considered as representative for the whole of France. Inclusion criteria were as follows: (1) at least two seizures with at least one nonfebrile, (2) onset of seizures before 10 years of age, (3) onset of seizures during the period 1980–1984, and (4) living in the 'departement de l'Oise' at seizure onset. A systematic procedure was used to avoid loss of cases; the cases of all the physicians likely to see epileptic patients (in hospital or private practice, paediatricians, neurologists, electroencephalographers, general physicians) were reviewed in the 'departement de l'Oise' as well as in bordering areas. Data were retrospectively recorded and doubtful cases were discussed with the local physicians. Each case was then classified according to the International Classification of the ILAE (1989) by two neuropaediatricians different from the local physicians. The incidence of each epileptic syndrome was finally determined. Six years later (1991), the cohort was reexamined by another investigator in order to complete epilepsy data, to validate the previous syndromic classification, to study seizure outcome, and to evaluate social and school performance.

Two hundred and twenty cases were initially collected. The global incidence was 40/100 000, and not surprisingly, it was age-related; the highest rate was observed during the first two years of life, reaching 100/100 000, consistent with the curve of incidence of seizures published by Hauser & Kurland (1975). Such a dramatic incidence of epilepsy in infants highly justifies the inclusion of the early period of life in epidemiological samples. Idiopathic generalized epilepsies (IGE) represented 25 per cent of the global population, in the same range as the 28 and 30 per cent previously reported (Cavazzuti, 1980; Cornaggia *et al.*, 1990; Viani *et al.*, 1988).

Among IGEs, childhood absence epilepsy (CAE) was the most frequently recognized syndrome (44 per cent), reaching 11 per cent of the whole population, then benign neonatal convulsions (24 per cent) and 'other IGE with generalized tonic–clonic seizures (GTCS)' (28 per cent), or respectively 6 per cent and 7 per cent of the whole population; benign myoclonic epilepsy in infancy and juvenile myoclonic or juvenile absence epilepsy were the least frequent (2 per cent each). Incidence varied according to age (Fig. 1). Comparison with published studies is difficult because the age of the population is different. However the incidence of childhood absence epilepsy at 9 years (6/100 000) is similar to Loiseau's rate under 15 years. Our group 'other IGE with GTCS' which exhibits a peak of incidence to 4.5/100 000 at 3 years is different from the classical grand mal on awakening or from other epilepsies of teenagers with GTC seizures. It is heterogeneous and not precisely defined; further studies focusing on this specific group are needed.

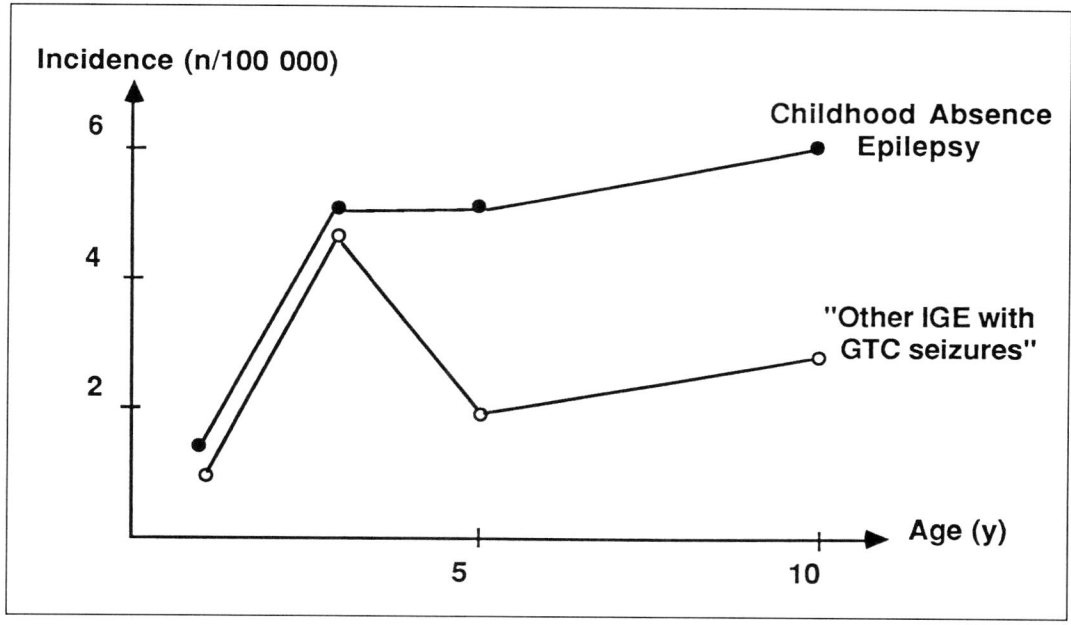

Fig. 1. Age-related incidence of idiopathic generalized epilepsies.

Six years later, the cohort was reexamined by two other investigators. One hundred and thirty three cases (60 per cent) could be studied; 6 per cent had died from encephalopathy; the other 31 per cent refused to contribute or were lost to follow-up. Despite the reduction of the size of the cohort, the proportion of idiopathic epilepsies was similar at onset and at follow-up. Reliability of the International Classification is good since for 88 per cent of the cases the initial diagnosis was confirmed at the end of follow-up. A few patients (4 per cent) had been initially misdiagnosed: four proved not to have been epileptic and four not to have IGE (initially classified childhood absence epilepsy or benign neonatal convulsions). Only two patients (1 per cent) switched from one syndrome to another. Nine patients (4 per cent) who were unclassifiable initially became classifiable thanks to an interview with the parents or to further EEG recordings. The major changes involved IGEs whose global rate rose to 27 per cent of the whole remaining sample. The proportion of childhood absence epilepsy and benign neonatal convulsions decreased (36 per cent and 14 per cent of IGE respectively) but that of 'other IGE with GTC seizures' increased (34 per cent). These findings confirm the reliability of the syndromic classification. They also point out the need to rely on strict diagnostic criteria and the diagnostic contribution of the EEG. The incidence of benign neonatal convulsions was probably overestimated before the 1990s, when the syndrome had just been described. The high incidence of the peculiar group 'other IGE with GTC seizures' is interestingly confirmed.

The cohort was also followed according to epilepsy outcome and schooling. Three-quarters (72 per cent) of the cases had become seizure free for periods ranging from 4.5 to 11 years. This is the same proportion as in Cavazutti's study (1980). IGE had a high rate of persisting seizures (13 per cent), not only higher than idiopathic partial epilepsy but also higher than cryptogenic partial epilepsy and unclassificable cases. Most of the IGE cases with persisting seizures had 'other IGE with GTC seizures' (8 per cent) whereas only one patient with childhood absence epilepsy and one with benign myoclonic epilepsy of infancy had persisting seizures. All the patients with benign neonatal convulsions were seizure free.

The same discrepancy was found as regards schooling. Schooling was classified into three categories, 'normal', 'adapted', or 'impossible', the latter associated with severe learning impairment. Surprisingly, 11 per cent of the IGE cases were in the category of 'impossible schooling'. They all exhibited 'other IGE with GTC seizures'. On the contrary, all cases of benign neonatal convulsions and all but one case of benign myoclonic epilepsy of infancy and childhood absence epilepsy had 'normal' schooling. The persistence of seizures was not found to be a statistically significant parameter to explain the differences between IGE subgroups with regard to school performance. But behavioural disorders and difficulties generated by low socio-economic conditions appeared to be more frequent in patients suffering from 'other IGE with GTC seizures' than in other groups of IGE. Further statistical studies are needed to evaluate whether these factors play a role in the impaired schooling of these patients.

Conclusions

An overall estimate of epidemiological indices may be as follows: in the population under 25 years of age, the prevalence of idiopathic generalized epilepsies is approximately 2/1000, and its annual incidence rate 15/100 000; the prevalence of absence epilepsies, essentially childhood absence epilepsy, is approximately 0.6/1000 and its incidence 7/100 000; the prevalence of juvenile myoclonic epilepsy is not clearly documented and its annual incidence rate is approximately 3/100 000. When focusing on the group under 10 years, the incidence of childhood absence epilepsy remains the same but two other syndromes have to be considered: benign neonatal convulsions, with an incidence of about 3 per cent during the first month of life and the insufficiently defined category of 'other IGE with GTC seizures', with a peak of incidence of about 5 per cent by 3 years. Among the usually benign IGEs, the latter group carries a remarkable 10 per cent level of persisting seizures and severe schooling impairment.

References

Blom, J., Heijbel, J. & Bergfors, P.G. (1978): Incidence of epilepsy in children: a follow-up study three years after the first seizure. *Epilepsia* 19, 343–350.

Camfield, C., Camfield, P., Gordon, K., Smith, B. & Dooley, J. (1993): Outcome of childhood epilepsy: a population-based study with a simple predictive scoring system for those treated with medication. *J. Pediatr.* 122, 861–868.

Cavazzuti, G.B. (1980): Epidemiology of different types of epilepsy in school age children in Modena, Italy. *Epilepsia* 21, 57–62.

Chiron, C., Luna, D., Dulac, O. & Jallon, P. (1986): Problémes méthodologiques d'une enquête épidémiologique rétrospective des épilepsies de l'enfant à l'échelle d'un département français. *Boll. Lega. It. Epil.* 54/55, 269–275.

Commion on Classification and Terminology of the International League Against Epilepsy (1985): Proposal for classification of epilepsies and epileptic syndromes. *Epilepsia* 26, 268–278.

Commission on Classification and Terminology of the International League Against Epilepsy (1989): Proposal for revised classification of epilepsies and epileptic syndromes. *Epilepsia* 30, 389–399.

Cornaggia, C.M., Canevini, M.P., Christe, W., Giuccioli, D., Facheris, M.A., Sabbadini, M. & Canger, R. (1990): Epidemiologic survey of epilepsy among army draftees in Lombardy, Italy. *Epilepsia* 31, 27–32.

Cowan, L.D., Bodensteiner, J.B., Leviton, A. & Doherty, L. (1989): Prevalence of the epilepsies in children and adolescents. *Epilepsia* 30, 94–106.

Doose, H. & Sitepu, B. (1983): Childhood epilepsy in a German city. *Neuropediatrics* 14, 220–224.

Forsgren, L. (1992): Prevalence of epilepsy in adults in Northern Sweden. *Epilepsia* 33, 450–458.

Granieri, E., Rosati, G., Tola, R., Pavoni, M., Paolino, E., Pinna, L. & Monetti, V.C. (1983): A descriptive study of epilepsy in the district of Copparo, Italy; 1964–1978. *Epilepsia* 24, 502–514.

Hauser, A. & Kurland, L. (1975): The epidemiology of epilepsy in Rochester, Minnesota, 1935 through 1969. *Epilepsia* 16, 1–66.

Hedström, A. & Olsson, I. (1991): Epidemiology of absence epilepsy: EEG findings and their predictive value. *Pediatr. Neurol.* **7,** 100–104.

Joensen, P. (1986): Prevalence, incidence, and classification of epilepsy in the Faroes. *Acta Neurol. Scand.* **74,** 150–155.

Loiseau, J., Loiseau, P., Guyot, M., Duche, B., Dartigues, J.F. & Aublet, B. (1990): Survey of seizure disorders in the French Southwest. 1. Incidence of epileptic syndromes. *Epilepsia* **31,** 391–396.

Luna, D., Chiron, C., Pajot, N., Dulac, O. & Jallon, P. (1987): Epidémiologie des épilepsies de l'enfant dans le département de l'Oise (France). In: *Epidemiologie des épilepsies*, pp. 41–53. Paris: John Libbey Eurotext.

Oller-Daurella, L. (1988): El sindrome gran mal del adulto. *Rev. Esp. Epilepsia* **3,** 88–93.

Olsson, I. (1988): Epidemiology of absence epilepsy. I. Concept and incidence. *Acta Paediatr. Scand.* **77,** 860–866.

Pazzaglia, P. & Frank, L. (1976): Record in grade school of pupils with epilepsy. An epidemiological study. *Epilepsia* **17,** 361–366.

Rocca, W.A., Sharbrough, F.W., Hauser, W.A., Annegers, J.F. & Schoenberg, B.S. (1987): Risk factors for absence seizures: a population-based case-control study in Rochester, Minnesota. *Neurology* **37,** 1309–1314.

Ross, E.M., Peckham, C.S., West, P.B. & Butler, N.R. (1980): Epilepsy in childhood: findings from the National Child Development Study. *Br. Med. J.* **i,** 207–210.

Sillanpää M. (1992): Epilepsy in children: prevalence, disability and handicap. *Epilepsia* **33,** 444–449.

Sorel, L. (1988): Las epilepsias generalizadas primarias de instauration tardia. *Rev. Esp. Epilepsia* **3,** 86–87.

Viani, F., Beghi, E., Atza, M.G. & Gulotta, M.P. (1988): Classification of epileptic syndromes: advantages and limitations for evaluation of childhood epileptic syndromes in clinical practice. *Epilepsia* **29,** 440–445.

Wagner, A.L. (1983): A clinical and epidemiological study of adult patients with epilepsy. *Acta Neurol. Scand. Suppl.* **94,** 63–72.

Chapter 4

Molecular and statistical methods for mapping human epilepsy genes

Alain Malafosse[*], Jean-Louis Mandel[†], David Greenberg[‡] and Michel Baldy-Moulinier[*]

[*]*Laboratoire de Médecine Expérimentale, INSERM U249, CNRS UPR 9008, Institut de Biologie, 34060 Montpellier, France;* [†]*INSERM U184, Faculté de Médecine, Institut de Chimie Biologique, 67085 Strasbourg, France;* [‡]*Department of Psychiatry, Mount Sinai School of Medicine, New York, NY 10029, USA*

Introduction

The application of polymorphic DNA markers to the study of inherited human disease has brought spectacular advances for medicine since the approach was proposed in 1980 by Botstein *et al.* These genetic markers, which have replaced earlier protein markers for localizing suspected disease genes to specific chromosomal regions, are small differences in DNA between individuals and are spread throughout the human genome.

Historically, the first DNA polymorphisms which have been described were the presence or absence of restriction endonuclease recognition sites (restriction fragment length polmorphisms, RFLPs) (Kan & Dozy, 1978). More recently variation in the number of tandem nucleotide sequences at a particular region of a chromosome have been detected. Two kinds of such a repeat length polymorphism have been observed here, their mean difference being the length of the repeat unit (Nakamura *et al.*, 1987; Tautz *et al.*, 1986). Variable number of tandem repeats (VNTRs) have units from 11 to 60 base pairs, whereas so-called short tandem repeats (STRs) are most frequently di-, tri- or tetranucleotide repeats. The discovery and development of such markers have accelerated so rapidly that more than 3000 markers distributed across the human genome are now available for mapping disease genes. This new approach, initially called reverse genetics and also known now as positional cloning, corresponds to the identification of mutant genes causing diseases by determining their precise location in the genome. Yet several recent sucesses in identifying mutant genes for both dominant diseases (e.g., neurofibomatosis and Huntington's disease) and recessive disease (e.g. cystic fibrosis) have shown the technical feasibility of such an approach. Hence, linkage analysis, the first step is positional cloning, has taken on new significance, as detection of linkage now offers the possibility of identifying the causative gene and thus the aetiological basis for a disease. This approach has the greatest potential impact on a disease for which the biochemical basis is unknown or poorly understood. This certainly applies to quite all the epilepsies, the aetiology of which remains elusive. In this chapter, we explore how these recent developments in molecular genetics are likely to impact on epilepsies. But before discussing techniques for approaching these questions, we believe that it may be worthwhile to briefly review what is currently known about human genetics.

IDIOPATHIC GENERALIZED EPILEPSIES

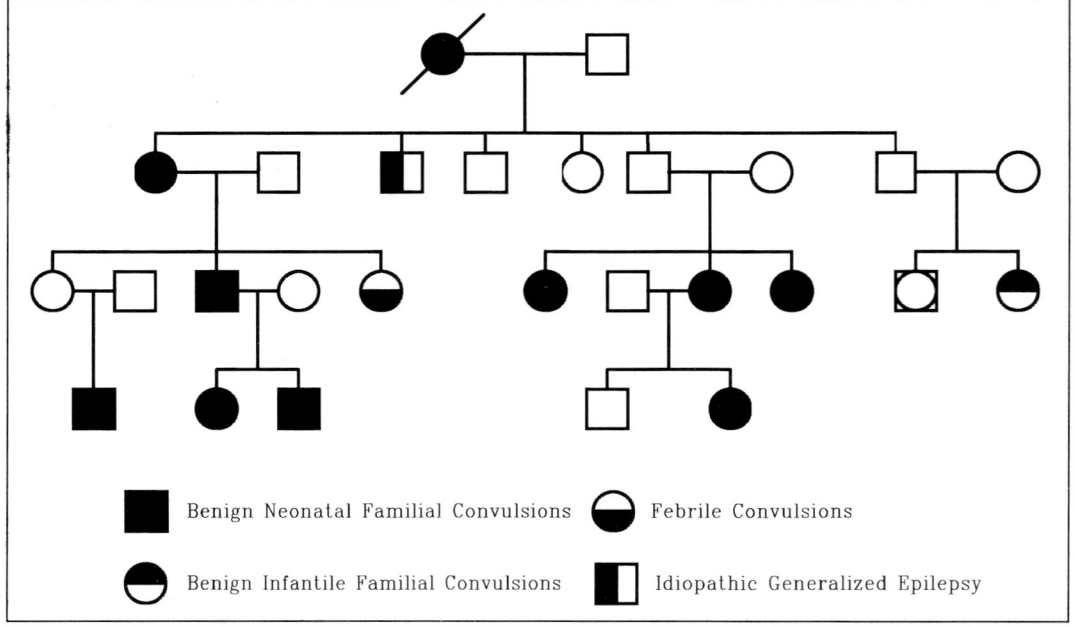

Fig. 1. A example of an autosomal dominant disease with reduced penetrance and variable expressivity: the benign familial neonatal convulsion (BFNC).

Formal genetics

Most, if not all, human diseases have some degree of heritability, ranging from minimal to large. A disease that is due entirely to the effect of a simple mutated gene is referred to as Mendelian. Mendelian diseases follow very specific patterns of inheritance in families. These patterns arise from the fact that genes are inherited in pairs, and one member of each pair is passed on from each parent. The human genome consists of 46 chromosomes 22 pairs of autosomal chromosomes and one pair of sex-determining chromosomes, labelled either X or Y. Females possess two X chromosomes and male possess X and Y chromosomes.

When possession of only a single copy of a mutant gene is sufficient for disease expression, the disease is referred to as dominant. If compatible with reproduction, dominant diseases are transmitted directly from parent to child, with half of the children, on average, carrying the same mutation. If the mutant gene is located on an autosome, males and females are affected with equal frequency. An example of such an autosomal dominant disease, the benign familial neonatal convulsion (BFNC), is shown in Fig. 1.

When two copies of a mutant gene are required for disease expression, it is referred to as recessive. In this case, disease transmission occurs in a horizontal, rather than vertical, fashion; that is, affected individuals appear together in sibships, whereas the parents and offspring of affected individuals are generally unaffected. Parents are usually unaffected carriers of the mutant gene, whereas the affected children are homozygotes. If the disease is rare, one can expect to find an increased frequency of parental consanguinity (i.e. parental relatedness), because the chances of both parents carrying the same rare mutant gene may be significantly increased when they are related. A pedigree of an autosomal recessive disease, Unverricht–Lundborg disease (ULD), with consanguinity is shown in Fig. 2.

The above are the seminal characteristics of a Mendelian disease. A number of features may lead

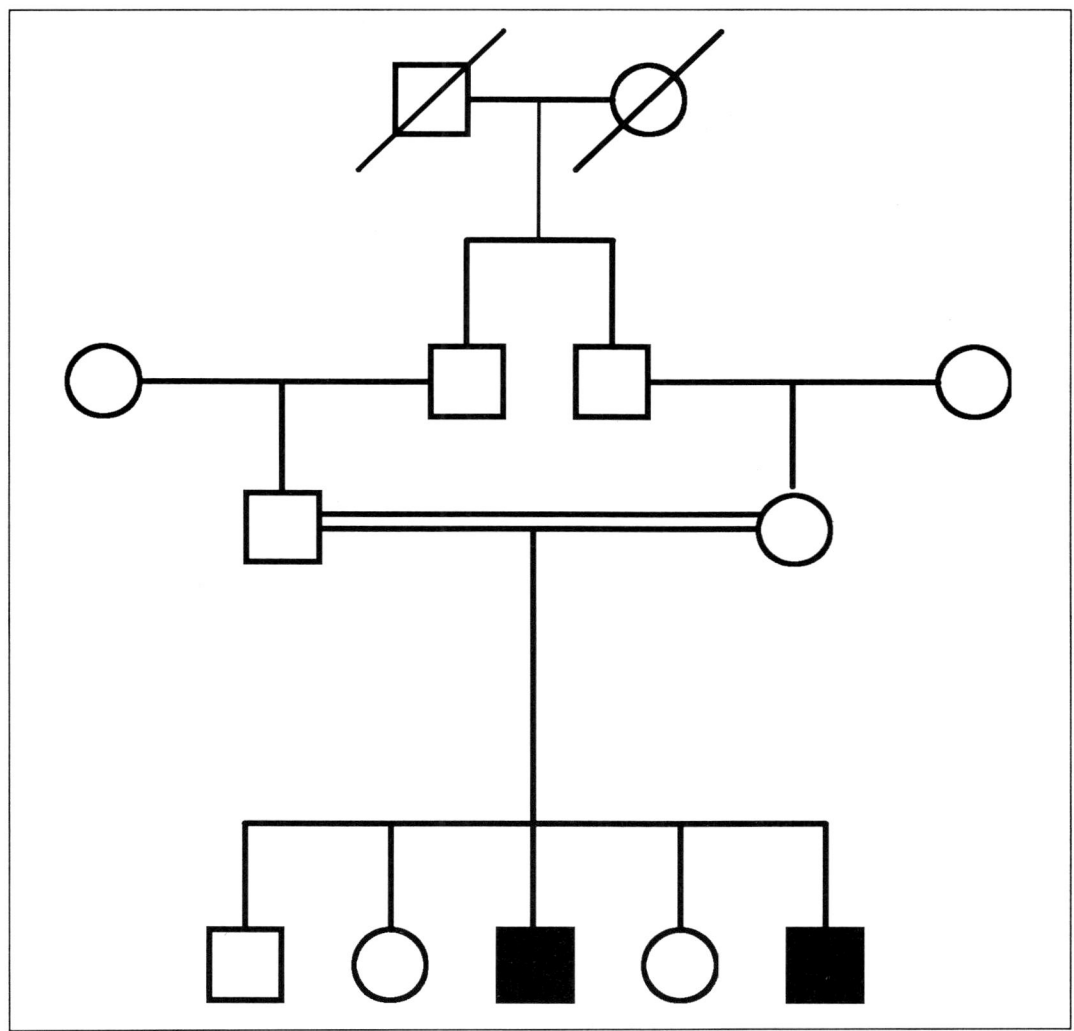

Fig. 2. A example of an autosomal recessive disease with consanguinity: the Unverricht Lundborg disease (ULD).

to deviation from precise conformance to the above rules. For example, not all individuals who possess a disease-predisposing phenotype may be affected. This phenomenon is referred to as reduced penetrance. Indeed, in some cases, the gene for a dominant disease may 'pass through' an individual, who remains unaffected, although he or she has an affected parent (and/or sibling) and an affected child. This may give the appearance of a 'skipped' generation. Akin to reduced penetrance is variable expressivity, in which the expression of disease among those carrying the genotype can vary greatly, ranging from extremely severe to extremely mild or even undetectable. Examples of reduced penetrance and variable expressivity are shown in Fig. 1. A further complication can arise when a similar disease phenotype can arise from non-genetic, or environmental, causes (referred to as phenocopies). This means that individuals without the disease-predisposing genotype may present with a disease quite similar to the genetic form. Although reduced penetrance and phenocopies eliminate the precise one-to-one correspondence between genotype and phenotype, neither phenomenon abrogates the Mendelian nature of a disease. The essential characteristic of a Mendelian disease is that the familial nature is attributable primarily to the effect of a single genetic locus. Other genetic loci may contribute to the expression of the disease, but they are neither necessary nor sufficient and play a 'modifying' role.

In some cases, what appears to be a single Mendelian disease may in fact be attributable to many different mutations. This phenomenon is referred to as genetic heterogeneity. For example, for benign familial neonatal convulsions, at least two different mutant alleles, one on chromosome 20 and the other on chromosome 8, run in different families (Lewis et al., 1993). This kind of genetic heterogeneity, occuring at different genetic loci, is called non-allelic or interlocus heterogeneity. Such heterogeneity can also be caused by mutations occuring at the same genetic locus, and is referred to as allelic or intralocus heterogeneity, an example being Unverricht–Lundborg disease, whose Baltic and Mediterranean forms may be due to an identical locus (Malafosse et al., 1991) but are caused by at least two different mutations (Lehesjoki et al., 1993; Beck et al., submitted).

In fact, many epilepsies of interest tend to be familial but do not conform to Mendelian patterns as observed in juvenile myoclonic epilepsy (Greenberg et al., 1988). Most epilepsies tend indeed to be far more common than typical Mendelian diseases, and the ratio of risk to first-degree relatives compared with population frequency are far below Mendelian rates. The answer to the critical question: What is the genetic basis for these disorders? is crucial for designing and interpreting linkage studies to map genes for such disorders. Classical families and twin studies have suggested that multiple loci contribute towards susceptibility to the main idiopathic generalized epilepsies (IGEs), with no one locus predominating. This type of interactive effect among loci contributing to risk for common, familial disorders appears to be a recurring theme among various diseases. However, that the general familial patterns of a disease may appear consistent with multiple, common interacting genes (so-called epistasis) does not automatically preclude the possible existence of a single locus with a very large, or even deterministic, effect. Classically, it is considered that if such loci do exist, they would be quite rare (as is typical for Mendelian genes) and account for only a small proportion of all cases. The demonstration that such genes exist may be obtained either on clinical or statistical grounds. The first, and perhaps most convincing, is the case in which a subset of disease can be determined on clinical characteristics, such as age at onset, in which early-onset disease appears to have an Mendelian bases. Benign familial neonatal convulsions (Rett, 1964) and, more recently, benign familial infantile convulsions (BFIC, Vigevano et al., 1992) are two such examples. The implication of the genes responsible for these disorders in the more common; IGEs is, however, not so straightforward as hoped (Schmitz et al., 1993). The second line of evidence that can be employed to detect a Mendelian subgroup is segregation analysis. Very few such analyses have been performed for epilepsies, and no evidence for the existence of a rare Mendelian subgroup of IGEs has yet been demonstrated (Greenberg et al., 1988). Another statistical possibility that exists to detect a major gene (i.e. responsible for a Mendelian disease) is linkage analysis. The demonstration, and the conformation, of a linkage between a disease and one or several genetic marker(s) allows us to detect a Mendelian subgroup of this disease, as shown for Alzheimer's disease.

Positional cloning

Our focus in the current situation is on identifying by linkage a region of the genome of aetiological significance for each disorder. However, that is not the ultimate goal. Eventually, we want to identify the actual gene involved and understand its normal and abnormal function. Linkage is simply the first step in the positional cloning strategy that has recently been so successful for many genetic diseases, particularly disroders of the nervous system (Martin, 1993). Thus, our objective is not to exclude 100 per cent of the genome, but to find a region containing a relevant gene.

Linkage analysis, lod-scores and significance tests

In family material, the traditional method for a linkage analysis has involved utilization of maximum likelihood with significance determined by the lod score, basically the logarithm of a likelihood ratio. Based on the prior likelihood of two loci chosen at random being on completely separate chromosomes, Morton (1955) initially choose a lod score of +3 as the desired significance level. However, among pairs of loci giving a lod score of +3, one in 20 (5 per cent) will be false positives. From any laboratory where extensive linkage analysis for DNA polymorphisms is being done, several examples of lod scores greater than 3 for loci that are not located on the same chromosome can be cited. The question of multiple tests becomes very significant during initial stages of a linkage study because each locus tested is essentially unlinked to all other markers. Thus, by chance alone, at least one of those is more likely to surpass a lod score of +3 than if only a single locus were being tested. A simple correction is to increase the lod score for significance by $\log_{10} n$, where n is the number of independent markers tested (Kidd & Ott, 1984). However, the confirmation of linkage, after a first suggestion has been obtained with an intermediate lod score, may be obtained by analysing other closely linked markers and/or new families.

Correcting lod scores for multiple tests, whether multiple markers or multiple diagnostic schemes, is not one of the primary concerns when interpreting data on a complex disorder. One must also recognize that the analysis is parametric and so based on requisite assumptions. The primary concern is that the statistical premiss for use of lod scores in this situation is wrong – the phenotype is not stable.

A linkage analysis compares two hypotheses: whether the phenotypes in the pedigree can be better explained (1) by assuming linkage when inferring patterns of segregation of alleles at the hypothesized trait locus and at the marker loci or (2) by assuming independent segregation. Note, one infers transmission patterns for both a hypothetical trait locus and the marker loci. One step can be taken to shore up this virtual house of cards: making the transmission patterns for the markers loci as unambiguous as possible by studying multiple highly informative markers; many such are available (see below). That step does not address the real issue, however, since the transmission pattern inferred for the trait locus can change dramatically with a single change of phenotype (Hodge and Greenberg, 1992). Consequently, not only do we not know what to use as a significance level, but it is also unclear whether statistical significance in the conventional sense is relevant.

Rather than rely on lod scores alone, of whatever significance level, one might consider the alternative of relying on the stability of the lod score to changes in diagnosis. One method for evaluating the stability of a lod score in a given family is a series of reanalyses of the data with, in twin, each of the relatives being reclassified (Hodge & Greenberg, 1992).

Concerning linkage analysis issues in complex diseases (i.e. with an unknown mode of inheritance), the evidence for single-locus inheritance apart from linkage is not compelling. Consequently, there is no defined prior probability that any of the epilepsies with complex inheritance are linked to any single locus marker. It has been argued that therefore no theoretical justification exists for pursuing genomic mapping studies in this type of disorder, and that the prior probability may be zero (Edwards, 1990; Green et al., 1982). The successes that have been achieved from linkage mapping studies of complex disorders, particularly the Alzheimer's linkages on chromosome 14, 21 and 19 (St. Georges-Hyslop et al., 1987, 1992; Pericak-Vance et al., 1991), offer a pragmatic argument against this line of reasoning. However, different kinds of error in modeling the genetic component of a disease when using the lod-score method in case of a complex disease must be keep in mind (Clerget-Darpoux & Bonaiti-Pellie, 1980; Clerget-Darpoux, 1982; Clerget-Darpoux et al., 1986). These authors have more specifically studied the effect of:

- using the wrong genetic parameters for the disease locus (allele frequencies, penetrance values);
- ignoring an interaction between the disease locus and the marker locus;

– ignoring an association between alleles for the disease and the marker locus.

These authors have showed that the recombination fraction Θ may be very biased when the genetic model is badly specified. Besides the great sensitivity of the recombination fraction estimation to the genetic modelling of the disease, erroneous modelling can also decrease the maximum lod score (or at least the expected one). This effect is particularly important when a gametic disequilibrium between alleles at the disease and marker loci is ignored. Two consequences can result from this observation. Using the wrong genetic model for the disease may lead to an erroneous rejection of linkage for a given recombination fraction Θ, but it does not artificially increase evidence for linkage. This last remark is particularly important with respect to the adequacy of performing a lod-score analysis between a disease with an unknown mode of inheritance and a genetic marker.

Nonparametric method

At a family level linkage can also be tested with nonparametric methods such as the affected sib pair (ASP) method (Penrose, 1935) and the affected pedigree method (APM) (Weeks & Lange, 1988). In addition, at a population level, marker information can be used by association studies.

The affected sib pair method has been widely used for testing linkage between HLA or other markers and many diseases. The distribution of the number of shared haplotypes in a sample of affected sib pairs is compared with the one expected under independent transmission of the disease and the marker. In the case of the HLA marker, which is highly polymorphic, each parent of a sib pair can be assumed to be HLA heterozygous (ab) and different from his or her spouse (cd). In the case for independent transmission of the marker and the disease, if one of the affected sibs is ac, the probability for the second sib of sharing two HLA haplotypes (i.e. to be ac) is 1/4, that of sharing one haplotype (ad or bc) is 1/2 and that of sharing no haplotype is 1/4. An HLA halpotype shared by two sibs corresponds necessarily to a unique haplotype found in one parent. Two sibs with the same HLA genotype can be considered as identical descent.

On the other hand, if we consider a less polymorphic marker with two alleles, A1 and A2, two sibs having A1A2 have not necessarily inherited the same alleles A1 and A2. For example, if both parents are A1A2, one of the sibs may have inherited the maternal A1 and the paternal A2, but the other sib the reverse. For a less polymorphic marker, the information used is not the identity by descent, but the identity by state. Weeks & Lange (1988) have proposed the use of a variable Z, measuring the degree of identity by state observed between all affected members of the same pedigree. Note that the probability of identity by state for one allele is a function of the identity by descent and of the probability of random identity. For a sample of pedigrees with affected individuals, the observed value of Z may be compared with its value expected with independent segregation.

In an association study between a genetic marker and a disease, the distribution in a sample of unrelated affected individuals is compared with its distribution in a sample of unrelated control individuals. If we consider, for example, a marker with two alleles A1 and A2, the contingency table (Table 1) shows the number (expressed by a, b, c and d) of alleles A1 and A2 in samples of both affected and controls individuals.

Table 1. Contengency table for testing allocation between the marker allele A1 and A2 and a given disease.

	A1	A2	
Affected	a	b	a+b
Control	c	d	c+d
	a+c	b+d	

To determine if A1 is associated with the disease, the frequency of A1 in affected individuals a/(a+b) is compared with the frequency of A1 in control individuals c/(c+b). The equality of these frequencies a/(a+b) = c(c+d) is tested using a homogeneity χ^2-test with one degree of freedom. If the equality is rejected, association between A1 and the disease is concluded and a relative risk may be calculated. This risk indicates how much more frequently the disease occurs in individuals carrying A1 versus those not carrying A1. An approximation of the relative risk (RR) is given by ad/bc.

Generally, the association test is done not only for one marker and one allele, but for multiple markers with several alleles. In this eventuality, several tests are performed simultaneously on the same sample, and this has to be taken into account when evaluating the significance of the observed differences. Indeed, testing Ho with type 1 error $\alpha = 5$ per cent means that, when Ho is correct, one result in 20 (five in 100) is expected to fall outside the confidence limits. Similarly when performing 20 independent comparisons on one sample, one can expect a difference in one of these comparisons to be significant. A replication study on a different sample is often necessary to attain a good significance level for any given association. Furthermore, one must be cautious in interpreting an association between a marker allele and a trait. Differences in the distribution of marker alleles may be due to a stratification in the population (noncomplete random mating) from which the samples were drawn. Comparison of frequencies in HLA antigens between dark-haired and blond-haired individuals in Caucasian populations will reveal differences which illustrate a stratification effect. One possible explanation for an association between a disease and a genetic marker is the existence of a disease susceptibility locus very close to the marker, with a gametic disequilibrium between the marker alleles and the alleles at the disease locus.

Another approach, derived from the previous one, has been recently described (Sobell *et al.*, 1992). Here, genes of neurobiological interest are first examined at the DNA level in a subset of patient to search for changes that result in the alteration of either the protein structure or the level of expression. These variants, given the acronym VAPSE for 'variant affecting protein structure or expression', have a reasonable likelihood of being functionally aberrant. Once a VAPSE is found, the prevalence of the sequence change in a large group of patients and control subjects can be determined. If the VAPSE is significantly more prevalent among the affected individuals than among the control subjects, an aetiological association with disease is suggested. Conversely, if no VAPSEs are identified in a sufficiently large sample, this would suggest that the gene is not commonly associated with the disease of interest.

These parametric and nonparametric approaches each have their advantages and inconveniences. As mentioned above, an erroneous specification of the genetic model in the lod-score method decreases the power for detecting linkage. Similarly, the information provided by nonaffected individuals is lost in nonparametric methods. In particular, let us consider two individuals from the same pedigree having the same allele. The probability for this allele to be identical by descent or randomly identical will be computed without considering if intermediate linked individuals in the pedigree have or do not have this allele. Comparisons of the loss of power in different approaches are only possible in specific situations.

DNA polymorphisms

The human gene map has developed extensively over the past 20 years. At the 11th International Workshop on Human Gene Mapping (Human Gene Mapping 11, 1991), held in London in August 1991, the number of mapped genes was 2325, a substantial increase over the 1631 reported at the 10th workshop (Human Gene Mapping 10, 1989). A major thrust forward for gene mapping came in 1980 with the realization that extensive variation could be detected in anonymous DNA segments (Botstein *et al.*, 1980). The potential for mapping by linkage analysis was thus greatly enhanced through the availability of large numbers of polymorphic markers.

The polymorphisms first used for linkage analysis were those found in red cell antigens, proteins (revealed by electrophoresis and isoelectric focusing), and cytogenetic heteromorphisms. It was not until the development of DNA polymorphisms, however, that linkage analysis became a powerful technique for gene mapping. Any detectable variation provides a potential marker for linkage analysis. Several different types of DNA polymorphisms have been developped, with emphasis on those with high heterozygosity: RFLPs, VNTRs, STRs.

Initially, nucleotide differences were detected as single-base-pair substitutions within the sequences, known as restriction sites, that are recognized for cleavage by certain bacterial enzymes. These variation in DNA sequences are revealed in agarose-gel systems; they behave as stable, i.e. from generation to generation, inherited traits (for details, see Treiman, 1993). Such genetic markers, so-called RFLPs became powerful tools because any arbitrary stretch of DNA could be expected to function as a potential marker.

A second class of anonymous DNA markers, i.e. segments that are not part of a known coding sequence – has been developed on the basis of variation in the number of tandem repeats of a short sequence of nucleotides present at some loci, rather than on single-base-pair substitutions. These markers are termed VNTRs. The majority of them contain repeating units 14–70 base pairs long and contain a core consensus sequence. VNTR markers are valuable for genetic linkage studies because they are not limited to two allelic forms as are site-substituted RFLP markers. It is possible to resolve a difference of a single repeat unit between two alleles if conditions for gel separation are optimized. A typical VNTR marker will contain 10-20 repeating units, and thus as many as 20 different alleles at that locus may be seen in a random population sample (see Treiman, 1993).

A special class of variable tandem repeat polymophisms has recently been described in which the tandem repeat is $(dC-dA)n.(dG-dT)n$. This class is of interest to gene mappers not only because of the relatively high number of allelic variants that may be found at a single site but also because of the estimated 50 000–100 000 blocks of such repeats that exist within the human genome. Thus, such markers, if they turn out to be evenly dispersed throughout the genome, would exist every 30–50 kilobases. Abundant, interspersed tracts of $(dC-dA)n.(dG-dT)n$ sequences had been known in mammals since 1981 (Miesfeld et al., 1981; Hammada et al., 1982), but it was not until the development of the polymerase chain reaction (PCR) using thermostable DNA polymerase (Saiki et al., 1988) that analysis of these sequences became practical (Treiman, 1993). Shortly after the discovery of polymorphic $(dC-dA)_n.(dG-dT)_n$ sequences, other types of short tandem repeats, such as $(dA)_n.(dT)_n$, $(dG-dA)_n.(dC-dT)_n$ and $(dAAAT)_n.(dTTTA)_n$ were also found to exhibit length polymorphisms (Economou et al., 1990; Tautz, 1989; Zuliani & Hobbs, 1990).

Once linkage analysis, based on a large number of polymorphic DNA markers has unambiguously assigned the disease locus to a specific region of the genome, the next step is the identification of closely linked flanking markers (less than 2cM) in the subset of pedigrees so-called 'family recombinant set'. This makes possible to use various gene cloning strategies to pinpoint the disease gene. These methods include chromosome jumping from the flanking markers, cloning of DNA fragments from a defined physical region with the use of pulse-field electrophoresis, a combination of somatic cell hybrid and molecular-cloning techniques designed to isolate DNA fragments from undemethylated CpG islands near the disease gene, chromosome microdissection and cloning, exon-trapping and saturation cloning of a large number of DNA markers from the disease gene region. New methods are regurlaly described and the strategy to use is different from one disease to another.

Conclusion

Genetic strategies are not the same for diseases with simple modes of inheritance and for those with complex modes of inheritance. In the first case, the information provided by the segregation of the disease within families is sufficient to establish the role of a disease gene. The marker information will enable us to locate the disease locus. It may then be possible to determine the defective DNA sequence, and even to determine its activity. For diseases with complex aetiology, the trait segregation is not sufficient for inferring the way the susceptibility to the disease is inherited. The additional information provided by genetic markers may be useful in making evident the role of one factor and in subdividing a heterogeneous group of patients into subgroups which are homogeneous for at least one factor. In this way it becomes more realistic to study the role of other potential factors.

References

Botstein, D., White, R., Skolnick, M. & Davis, R.W. (1980): Construction of a genetic linkage map using restriction fragment length polymorphisms. *Am. J. Hum. Genet.* **32**, 314–331.

Clerget-Darpoux, F. (1982): Bias of the estimated recombination fraction and lod score due to an association between a disease gene and a marker gene. *Ann. Hum. Genet.* **46**, 363–372.

Clerget-Darpoux, F. & Bonaiti-Pellie, C. (1980): Epistasis effect: an alternative to the hypothesis of linkage disequilibrium in HLA-associated diseases. *Ann. Hum. Genet.* **44**, 195–204.

Clerget-Darpoux, F., Bonaiti-Pellie, C. & Hochez, J. (1986): Effects of misspecifying genetic parameters in lod score analysis. *Biometrics* **42**, 393–399.

Economou, E.P., Bergen, A.W. & Warren A.C. et al. (1990): The polydeoxy adenylate tract of Alu repetitive elements is polymorphic in the human genome. *Proc. Natl. Acad. Sci. USA* **87**, 2951–2954.

Edwards, J.H. (1990): Genetic linkage and psychiatric disease. *Nature* **344**, 298–299.

Green, A., Morton, N.E. & Iselius, L. (1982) Genetic studies of insulin-dependent diabetes mellitus: segregation and linkage analyses. *Tissue Antigens* **19**, 213–221.

Greenberg, D.A., Delgado-Escueta, A.V., Maldonado, H.M. & Widelitz, H. (1988): Segregation analysis of juvenile myoclonic epilepsy. *Genet. Epidemiol.* **5**, 81–94.

Hamada, H., Petrino, M.G. & Kakunaga, T. (1982): A novel repeated element with Z-DNA-forming potential is widely found in evolutionarily diverse eukaryotic genomes. *Proc. Natl. Acad. Sci. USA* **79**, 6465–6469.

Hodge, S.E. & Greenberg, D.A. (1992): Sensitivity of lod scores to changes in diagnostic status. *Am. J. Hum. Genet.* **50**, 1053–1066.

Kan, Y.W. & Dozy, A.M. (1978): Polymorphism of DNA sequence adjacent to human β-globin structural gene: relationship to sickle mutation. *Proc. Natl. Acad. Sci. USA* **75**, 5631–5635.

Kidd, K.K. & Ott, J. (1984): Power and sample size in linkage studies. HGM7: Seventh International Workshop on Human Gene Mapping. *Cytogenenet Cell. Genet.* **37**, 510–511.

Lehesjoki, A.E., Koskiniemi, M., Norio, R. et al. (1993): Localization of the EPM1 gene for progressive myoclonus epilepsy on chromosome 21: linkage disequilibrium allows high resolution mapping. *Hum. Molec. Genet.* **2**, 1229–1234.

Lewis, T.B., Leach, R.J., Ward, K. et al. (1993): Genetic heterogeneity in benign familial neonatal convulsions: identification of a new locus on chromosome 8q. *Am. J. Hum. Genet.* **53**, 670–675.

Malafosse, A., Lehesjoki, A.E., Genton, P. et al. (1991): Identical genetic locus for Baltic and Mediterranean myoclonus. *Lancet* **339**, 1080–1081.

Martin, G. (1993): Molecular genetics in neuro9logy: a decade of progress. *Ann. Neurol.* **34**, 758–766.

Miesfeld, R., Krystal, M. & Arnheim, N. (1981): A member of a new repeated sequence family which is conserved throughout eucaryote evolution is found between the human delta and beta globin genes. *Nucleic Acids Res.* **9**, 5931–5947.

Morton, N.E. (1955): Sequential tests for the detection of linkage. *Am. J. Hum. Genet.* **7**, 277–318.

Nakamura, Y., Leppert, M., O'Connell, P. et al. (1987): Variable number of tandem repeat (VNTR) markers for human gene mapping. *Science* **235**, 1616–1622.

Penrose, L.S. (1935): The detection of autosomal linkage in data which consist of pairs of brothers and sisters of unspecified parentage. *Ann. Eugen.* **6**, 133–138.

Pericak-Vance, M.A., Bebout, J.L., Gaskell, P.C. et al. (1991): Linkage studies in familial Alzheimer disease: evidence for chromosome 19 linkage. *Am. J. Hum. Genet.* **48**, 1034–1050.

Rett, A. & Teubel, R. (1964): Neugeboreneakrämpfe In Rahmn einer epileptisch belasteten Familie. *Wien Klin. Wochenschr.* **76**, 609–612.

Saiki, R.K., Gelfand, D.H. & Stoffel, S. (1988): Primer-directed enzymatic amplification of DNA with a thermostable DNA polymerase. *Science* **239**, 487–491.

Schmitz, B., Sander, T., Hildmann, T., Neitzel, H., Beck-Mannagetta, G. & Janz, D. (1993): Exclusion of linkage between D20S19 and idiopathic generalized epilepsies in juvenile myoclonic epilepsy families. International Worshop on Idiopathic Generalized Epilepsies. Le Bischenberg, Alsace, France. 22–25 April, 1993.

Sobell, J.L., Heston, L. & Sommer, S.S. (1992): Delineation of genetic predisposition to multifactorial disease: a general approach on the threshold of feasability. *Genomics* **12**, 1–6.

St. Georges-Hyslop, P., Tanzi, R, Polinsky, R.J. *et al.* (1987): The genetic defect causing familial Alzheimer's disease maps on chromosome 21. *Science* **235**, 885–890.

St. Georges-Hyslop, P., Haines, J., Rogaev, E. *et al.* (1992): Genetic evidence for a novel familial Alzheimer's disease locus on chromosome 14. *Nature Genet.* **2**, 330–334.

Tautz, D., Trick, M. & Dover, G.A. (1986): Cryptic simplicity in DNA is a major source of genetic variation. *Nature* **322**, 652–656.

Tautz, D. (1989): Hypervariability of simple sequences as a general source for polymorphic DNA markers. *Nucleic Acids Res.* **17**, 6463–6471.

Treiman, L.J. (1993): Genetics of epilepsy: an overview. *Epilepsia* **34 (Suppl.3)**, S1–S11.

Vigevano, F., Fusco, L., DiCapua, M., Ricci, S., Sebastianelli, R. & Lucchini, P. (1992): Benign infantile familial convulsions. *Eur. J. Pediatr.* **117**, 1–5.

Weeks, D.E. & Lange, K. (1988): The affected-pedigree-member method of linkage analysis. *Am. J. Hum. Genet.* **42**, 315–326.

Zuliani, G. & Hobbs, H.H. (1990): A high frequency of length polymorphisms in repeated sequences adjacent to Alu sequences. *Am. J. Hum. Genet.* **46**, 963–969.

Part II
Familial neonatal and infantile convulsions

Chapter 5

Benign familial neonatal convulsions

Perrine Plouin

Hôpital Saint Vincent de Paul, 82 avenue Denfert-Rochereau, INSERM U29, 75014 Paris, France

Benign neonatal convulsions (BNC) are neonatal convulsions showing a favourable neurological outcome, i.e. normal psychomotor development without secondary epilepsy. This seemingly plain definition may raise practical difficulties in the individual patient. Whereas psychomotor development can be easily assessed in infancy and childhood, the absence of subsequent epilepsy makes benign neonatal convulsions a retrospective diagnosis and raises the following question: how long should an affected child be followed up to confirm safely that his neonatal convulsions had been benign (Matsumoto *et al.*, 1983)? In addition, it may be difficult to document or exclude a causative link between neonatal convulsions and the eventual occurrence of subsequent convulsions.

Benign familial neonatal convulsions (BFNC) were first described by Rett & Teubel (1964). Following a symposium held in Marseille in 1983 on epileptic syndromes in infancy, childhood and adolescence, the Commission on Classification and Terminology of the International League Against Epilepsy decided to include this subtype in the classification of epilepsies and epileptic syndromes (1989). Benign familial neonatal convulsions belong to the second chapter, and are classified among idiopathic generalized epilepsies (age related).

Three hundred and forty cases of benign familial neonatal convulsions have been reported in the literature since the first paper by Rett & Teubel (1964). These neonates belong to 40 families. The number of generations affected varies from 1 to 5 (Table 1). It is not possible to define the prevalence of these benign familial neonatal convulsions as they are not compared with other neonatal convulsions in any study.

In 80 per cent of cases, seizures start on the second and third days of life. But some infants begin to convulse later, during the first month of life or even up to the third month of life. Ronen *et al.* (1993) report in their wide family that two of the individuals in whom the first seizures occurred at one month of age were premature.

In documented cases, birth was always at full-term (except for three cases of Ronen *et al.* 1993), with normal birth weight and an APGAR score above 7 at the first minute of life. None of these neonates was in an intensive care unit. There was always a free interval between birth and occurrence of convulsions. The sex ratio shows an equal partition between boys and girls.

In most cases biological radiological work-up had been performed and failed to disclose any aetiology except for a single case with transitory hypomagnesaemia.

Table 1. Benign familial neonatal convulsions

Author	No. of cases per family	No. of generations per family
Rett & Teubel, 1964	8	3
Bjerre & Corelius, 1968	14	5
Steejohnsen, 1968	8	?
Rose & Lombroso, 1975	3	3
Goutières, 1977	8	3
	2	1
Carton, 1978	9	4
Quattelbaum, 1979	15*	4
Pettit & Fenichel, 1980	5	3
Tibbles, 1980	2	2
	6	2
	3	2
Pavone et al., 1982	7	2
Giacoia, 1982	7	4
Plouin, 1992	2	2
	2	1
Kaplan & Lacey, 1983	12	4
Palencia & Berjon, 1985	4	2
Shevell et al., 1986	5	3
	4	3
Nieto Barrera et al., 1986	14	3
Calero Garcia et al., 1988	17	4
Cunniff et al., 1988	8	2
Giroud et al., 1989	2	2
	2	2
	2	1
Malafosse, 1990	6*	3
	4*	3
	4*	2
Webb & Bobel, 1990	9	5
Camfield et al., 1991	5	2
Ryan et al., 1991	14*	3
	15	3
Schiffmann et al., 1991	4	1
Wakai et al., 1991	5	2
Aso & Watanabe, 1992	3	2
Malafosse et al., 1992	9*	4
	3*	2
	9*	4
Mami et al., 1993	4	2
Ronen et al., 1993	69*	5
Hirsch et al., 1993	6*	2

Total 1964–1993: 340 cases, 40 families. *Families with BFNC mapped in chromosome 20 (linkage analysis of Quattelbaum's family was done by Leppert et al. (1989)).

Seizures were of the clonic type, sometimes with apnoeic spells. Tonic seizures were reported in two cases. Clonic or tonic seizures were short (lasting from 1 to 3 min), and frequently repeated over 7 days, whereas isolated seizures could occur in some cases during the following weeks. We

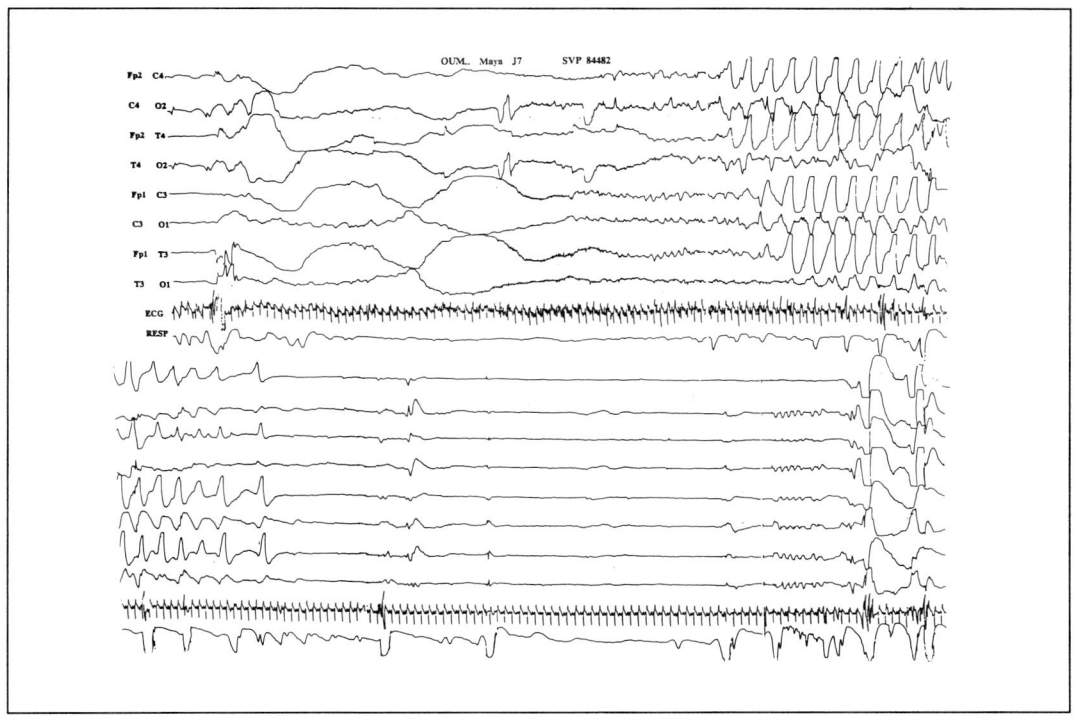

Fig. 1. BFNC: seizure recorded in a 7-day-old neonate; diffuse flatenning of the tracing, followed by theta rhythms and by high amplitude one Hz generalized delta waes during 30 s. Marked generalized depression of the tracing at the end of the seizure. Note the central apnoea at the beginning of the seizure.

had the opportunity to record seizures in one case (family 1 in the paper by Malafosse *et al.* (1992)): seizures were stereotyped, starting with a diffuse hypertonia with a short apnoea, followed by clonic movements of the limbs. In previous reports, seizures had already been described (Giacoia, 1982; Crispen & Kelly, 1985; Shevell *et al.*, 1986; Camfield *et al.*, 1991), but there was no evidence in these cases for a homogeneous presentation. More recently, Ronen *et al.* (1993) have listed all the clinical components of the 70 seizures they could analyse in their wide family. They concluded that most of the times seizures started with tonic, autonomic or oculo-facial features, being of a mixed type. Hirsch *et al.* (1993) recorded 14 seizures in three neonates with video-EEG monitoring. All seizures started with a tonic phase, with a right or left maximum, varying from one seizure to the next in a given baby, always accompanied by tachycardia and a short apnoea. The clonic phase (focal or generalized) was introduced by vocalization or chewing. No myoclonic seizure has been reported, nor a spasm.

When described, interictal EEG was normal, discontinuous including focal or multifocal abnormalities or with 'théta pointu alternant' pattern. Patterns suggesting poor prognosis such as paroxysmal or inactive EEG were never reported.

In previous reports some seizures were recorded but the EEG were not published or were incomplete. In the case we recorded, (Fig. 1) the ictal pattern is very similar to the one published by Ronen *et al.* (1993), and to the cases of Hirsch *et al.* (1993) who studied the ictal EEG very carefully and found that the length of the flattening could vary from 5 to 19 s and that the complete seizure lasted from 59 to 155 s. All these individuals had benign familial neonatal convulsions mapped in chromosome 20.

The electro-clinical presentation of these seizures suggests that they are of a generalized type. Aso & Watanabe, (1992) discussed this point because they recorded a unilateral seizure in a 3-month-old infant who had had benign familial neonatal convulsions. However, the recent publication of Hirsch *et al.* (1993), emphasizes that the initial flattening of the EEG is generalized from the start and that the successive symptoms occurring during a seizure (tonic, apnoea, clonic phases) are identical to those reported in generalized tonic–clonic seizures in children and adults. The same authors suggest that the asymmetrical character of some clinical and EEG signs during the tonic or the clonic phase could be related to the absence of maturation of the corpus callosum during the first weeks of life (Bardovick & Kjos, 1988).

Infants with such benign familial neonatal convulsions had a favourable psychomotor developmental outcome. In some cases (11 per cent), however, epileptic seizures subsequently occurred in infancy, in childhood, and in adulthood. When present, seizures were described as isolated, rare, and easily controlled by medication; some of these seizures were provoked. No case of severe epilepsy was reported. In addition 5 per cent of the children presented one or more simple febrile convulsions at the usual age. Consequently, overall rates of secondary epilepsy and febrile convulsions were 11 and 5 per cent respectively, the rate for febrile convulsions being comparable to that of general population.

Studies of pedigrees with several affected generations and a sufficient number of siblings show a 1/1 sex-ratio and a probability of around 1/2, confirming a dominant autosomal transmission. In 1989, Leppert *et al.* studied a family of four generations including 48 individuals, 19 of them having the characteristics of benign familial neonatal convulsions. They localized the gene to the long arm of chromosome 20, possibly to 20q13.2. A similar study concerning three families was published in 1990 by Malafosse *et al.* They used the same polymorphic DNA marker loci (RMR6 and CMM6) as Leppert *et al.* to determine the restriction fragment length polymorphism. Their results suggested the same localization to 20q13.2 of the gene linked to benign familial neonatal convulsions. They could not draw any conclusions from their own data only, but when adding their lod-scores to those reported by Leppert *et al.*, Malafosse *et al.* (1990) could establish a reliable linkage and suggest the single-gene origin of benign familial neonatal convulsions.

More recently Ryan *et al.* (1990) have studied two new families of benign familial neonatal convulsions; in the first one with only cases of benign familial neonatal convulsions they found that both markers (RMR6 and CMM6) were informative; in the second one with a different evolution of secondary epilepsy, only marker CMM6 was informative. They concluded that the syndrome of benign familial neonatal convulsions was genetically heterogeneous. Schiffmann *et al.* (1991) reported an autosomal recessive form of benign familial neonatal convulsions in a consanguineous sibship leading to the same conclusion. In another study, Sander *et al.* (1990) have demonstrated that there is an exclusion of linkage in susceptibility locus for benign familial neonatal convulsions with idiopathic generalized epilepsies in juvenile myoclonic epilepsy families. At the present time (Malafosse, personal communication), 25 families have been genetically studied: in 21 of them benign familial neonatal convulsions are linked to chromosome 20 whereas they are not in four. In one family there is a linkage to chromosome 8 (benign familial neonatal convulsions only). In the three remaining ones (one benign familial neonatal convulsions only, two benign familial neonatal convulsions associated with other seizures) no linkage has been found either to chromosome 20 or to chromosome 8. It appears then that Ryan's hypothesis is no more relevant and brings in the question of another locus. These data must be confirmed by testing additional families.

Benign familial neonatal convulsions are a familial disease with an autosomal mode of inheritance linked to genetic markers localized to the long arm of chromosome 20, at least in the majority of cases. Seizures start early (D2, D3) and may persist during 2 or 3 weeks. These seizures are of a generalized type and can be compared to generalized tonic–clonic seizures. Other types of seizures may appear later in life in 11 per cent of cases but no severe epilepsy has been reported. In other members of the families, other types of generalized or partial seizures may be present, again of a benign type.

Even if some questions remain open about this syndrome, it must be identified and recognized because it allows the forecast of a favourable neurological outcome from the neonatal period.

References

Aso, K. & Watanabe, K. (1992): Benign familial neonatal convulsions: generalized epilepsy? *Pediatr. Neurol.* **8**, 226–228.

Bardovick, A.J. & Kjos, B.O. (1988): Normal post natal development of the corpus callosum as demonstrated by MR imaging. *AJNR* **3**, 487–491.

Bjerre, I. & Cornelius, E. (1968): Benign neonatal familial convulsions. *Acta Paediatr. Scand.* **57**, 557–561.

Calero Garcia, J.L., Nieto Barrera, M., Moruno Tirado, A. & Gozalvez Bueno, I. (1988): Convulsiones neonatales familiares benignas. Aportacion de una nueva familia. *Rev. Esp. Epilepsia* **4**, 32–35.

Camfield, P.R., Dooley, J., Gordon, K. & Orlik, P. (1991): Benign familial neonatal convulsions are epileptic. *J. Child Neurol.* **6**, 340–342.

Carton, D. (1978): Benign neonatal familial convulsions. *Neuropädiatrie* **9**, 167–171.

Commission on Classification and Terminology of the International League Against Epilepsy (1989): Proposal for Revised Classification of Epilepsies and Epileptic Syndromes. *Epilepsia* **30**, 389–399.

Crispen, C. & Kelly, T. (1985): Benign familial neonatal convulsions. *Iowa Med.* **75**, 397–401.

Cunniff, C., Wieldlin, N. & Lyons Jones, K. (1988): Autosomal dominant benign neonatal seizures. *Am. J. Med Genet.* **30**, 963–966.

Giacoia, G.P. (1982): Benign familial neonatal convulsions. *Southern Med. J.* **75**, 629–630.

Giroud, M., Soichot, P., Nivelon-Chevalier, A., Gouyon, J.B., Nivelon, J.L. & Dumas, R. (1989): Les convulsions néo-natales familiales: leurs aspects électrocliniques et génétiques. *Neurophysiol. Clin.* **19**, 47–54.

Goutières, F. (1977): Convulsions néonatales familial bénignes. In: *Congrès de la société de neurologie infantile*, pp. 281–286. Marseille: Diffusion générale de librairie.

Hirsch, E., Velez, A., Sellal, F. *et al.* (1993): Electroclinical signs of benign neonatal familial convulsions. *Ann. Neurol.* **34**, 835–841.

Kaplan, R.E. & Lacey, D.J. (1983): Benign familial neonatal-infantile seizures. *Am. J. Med. Genet.* **16**, 595–599.

Leppert, M., Anderson, V.E., Quattlebaum, T. Stauffer, D., O'Connell, P., Nakamura, Y., Lalouel, J.M. & Whitr, R. (1989): Benign familial neonatal convulsions linked to genetic markers on chromosome 20. *Nature* **337**, 647–648.

Malafosse, A., Leboyer, M., Dulac, O., Plouin, P., Navelet, Y., Feinglold, J. & Mallet, J. (1990): Convulsions néonatales familiales bénignes: un modèle d'étude des bases moléculaires des facteurs génétiques des épilepsies. *Epilepsies* **2**, 64–71.

Malafosse, A., Leboyer, M., Dulac, O. *et al.* (1992): Confirmation of linkage of benign familial neonatal convulsions to D20S19 and D20S20. *Hum. Genet.* **89**, 54–58.

Mami, C., Tortorella, R., Manganaro, R. & Gemelli, M. (1993): Les convulsions néonatales familales bénignes. *Arch. Franc. Pediatr.* **50**, 31–33.

Matsumoto, A., Watanabe, K., Sigiura, M., Negoro, T., Takaesu, E. & Iwase, K. (1983): Longterm prognosis of convulsive disorders in the first year of life: mental and physical development and seizures persistance. *Epilepsia* **24**, 321–329.

Nieto Barrera, M., Borrego, S. & Aguilar Quero, F. (1986): Convulsiones neonatales familiares benignas y crisis asociadas. *Rev. Esp. Epilepsia.* **2**, 66–70.

Palencia, R. & Berjon, M.C. (1985): Convulsiones neonatales familiares benignas, crises febriles y epilepsia. Su coincidencia en una familia. *An. Esp. Pediatr.* **23**, 65–67.

Pavone, L., Mazzone, D., La Rosa, M., Livolti, S. & Mollica, F. (1982): Le convulsioni familiari benigne. Studio di una famiglia. *Ped. Oggi* **11**, 375–378.

Pettit, R.E. & Fenichel, G.M. (1980): Benign familial neonatal seizures. *Arch. Neurol.* **37**, 47–48.

Plouin, P. (1992): Benign idiopathic neonatal convulsions (familial and non-familial). In: *Epileptic syndromes in infancy, childhood and adolescence*, eds. J. Roger, M. Bureau, Ch. Dravet, F.E. Dreifuss, A. Perret & P. Wolf, pp. 3–11. London: John Libbey.

Quattelbaum, T.G. (1979): Benign familial convulsions in the neonatal period and early infancy. *J. Pediatr.* **95**, 257–259.

Rett, A. & Teubel, R. (1964): Neugeborenen Krampfe im Rahmen einer epileptisch belasten Familie. *Wien. Klin. Wochenschr.* **76,** 609–613.

Ronen, G.M., Rosales, T.O., Connolly, M.E., Anderson, V.E. & Leppert, M. (1993): Seizure characteristics in chromosome 20 benign familial neonatal convulsions. *Neurology* **43**, 1355–1360.

Rose, A.L. & Lombroso, C.T. (1975): Neonatal seizure states. A study of clinical pathology and EEG features in 137 full-term babies with a long-term follow-up. *Pediatrics* **47**, 405–425.

Ryan, S.G., Wiznitzer, M., Hollman, C., Torres, C., Szekeresova, M. & Schneider, S. (1991): Benign familial neonatal convulsions: evidence for clinical and genetic heterogeneity. *Ann. Neurol.* **29**, 469–473.

Sander, T., Johnson, K. & Janz, D. (1990): Exclusion of linkage between the susceptibility locus for benign familial neonatal convulsions with idiopathic generalized epilepsies in juvenile myoclonic epilepsy. *Epilepsia* **31,** 818.

Shevell, M.I., Sinclair, D.B. & Metrakos, K. (1986): Benign familial neonatal seizures: clinical and electroencephalographic characteristics. *Pediatr. Neurol.* **2,** 272–275.

Schiffmann, R., Shapira, Y. & Ryan, G. (1991): An autosomal recessive form of benign familial neonatal seizures. *Clin. Genet.* **40,** 467–470.

Steejohnsen (1968): Cited in Bjerre and Cornelius (1968).

Tibbles, J.A.R. (1980): Dominant benign neonatal seizures. *Dev. Med. Child Neurol.* **22,** 664–667.

Wakai, S., Tachi, N., Chiba, S., Ishikawa, Y., Okabe, M., Minami, R. & Kibayashi, M. (1991): Benign familial neonatal convulsions: clinical features of the propositus and comparison with the previously reported cases. *Acta Paediatr. Jpn* **33,** 77–82.

Webb, R. & Bobele, G. (1990): 'Benign' familial neonatal convulsions. *J. Child Neurol.* **5,** 295–298.

Chapter 6

Benign infantile familial convulsions

Federico Vigevano, Rosella Sebastianelli, Lucia Fusco, Matteo Di Capua, Stefano Ricci, Pierpaolo Lucchini, Benedetto Dordi, Antonio Chindemi, Olivier Dulac, Corinne Beck and Alain Malafosse

Benign Infantile Familial Convulsions Multicenter Group, Section of Neurophysiology, Bambino Gesù Children's Hospital, Piazza S. Onofrio 4, 00165 Rome, Italy

Introduction

If the idiopathic epilepsies reported in the current Classification of Epilepsies and Epileptic Syndromes of the International League Against Epilepsy (1989) are analysed according to increasing age, after neonatal convulsions we find, toward the end of the first year of life, benign myoclonic epilepsy. There would not seem to be any more idiopathic forms during the first year of life.

We have paid particular attention to studying the epilepsies of this age and believe that other idiopathic forms do exist. For example, there are some cases of West syndrome that fulfil the criteria for an idiopathic epilepsy (Vigevano *et al.*, 1993).

Recently we reported (Vigevano *et al.*, 1990, 1992) an undescribed form of epileptic disorder: familial, with seizures first appearing between 4 and 8 months and favourable outcome. At first we called it 'sixth-month benign familial convulsions', but later preferred the term 'benign infantile familial convulsions' (BIFC) because of its similarity to the neonatal familial form.

Material and methods

In the original paper, data was presented on five infants, three girls and two boys. Prenatal and perinatal history and psychomotor development were normal. All diagnostic tests, including cerebral computed tomography, were normal.

All patients had one or more paternal relatives with a history of benign seizures at the same age. In four families the affected member was the infant's father. Analogous seizures were identified in 13 relatives. In the probands, the age at onset ranged from 4 to 7 months; in the relatives it ranged from 4 to 8 months and peaked around the sixth month. None of them had seizure onset in the neonatal age or after the eighth month of life.

The attacks occurred mainly in a cluster, lasting for 2 to 4 days, with five to ten episodes a day, both while awake and asleep. The duration of each cluster was strictly correlated with the start of therapy. In two patients, the cluster was the only seizure manifestation, and occurred respectively at 6 and 4 months.

In the other three patients, the cluster was preceded by isolated seizures, lasting from 1 to several min. Initial seizures were usually longer, even as long as 10 to 15 min, and became shorter as the treatment took effect.

Clinically, the seizures were characterized by psychomotor arrest, slow deviation of the head and eyes to one side, diffuse hypertonia, cyanosis, and unilateral limb jerks, which became bilateral and were synchronous or asynchronous. Although the seizures were highly stereotyped, the direction of the head and eye deviation sometimes changed from seizure to seizure in the same patient. Oral automatisms were occasionally observed. The ictal EEG was characterized by a recruiting rhythm, beginning in the left or right central–occipital areas, spreading over the hemisphere and then involving the entire brain and increasing in amplitude. The alternating clinical pattern was confirmed by the demonstration of seizures originating sometimes in the right, sometimes in the left hemisphere. Interictal EEG in sleep and while awake was always normal.

The patients underwent treatment with phenobarbital or sodium valproate only when seizures occurred in a cluster. The seizures were under control within 24 to 48 h and the same drugs were then given orally.

Follow-up has now reached 4–5 years. None of the children had further seizures; their EEGs and psychomotor development are normal. All patients stopped therapy after 1 or 2 years.

Multicentre study

Following our report, others published reports or informed us about similar cases. At present with a multicentre study, we have data on 17 probands, 15 Italian and two French. Observation of a greater number of cases allows us to define the syndrome better. The results are summarized in Table 1.

Table 1. Results of the multicentre study on 17 families

Sex of Probands:	6 M 11 F
Relatives with:	
– BIFC	31 (21M, 10F)
– Other epilepsies	4
– Febrile convulsions	5
– Neonatal convulsions	0
Seizure characteristics:	
Onset	3 months 20 days – 7 months
Seizures in a cluster	16
Semeiology	Psychomotor arrest, cyanosis, head/eye deviation to one side (often variable), tonic contraction, bilateral clonic jerks
EEG characteristics:	
Interictal	Normal
Postictal	Lateralized occipito-parietal delta waves and spikes
Ictal (8 pts)	Fast activity originating in the occipito-parietal areas of the one hemisphere with subsequent involvement of the other hemisphere

The disorder seems to be most frequent among females, the ratio being 2:1 with respect to males. Among the 17 families, there were 31 relatives of first and second degree with benign infantile convulsions, with a clear prevalence of males (21 males to 10 females). This could be a consequence of the fact that in more than half the cases (9/17) it was the father who had the same

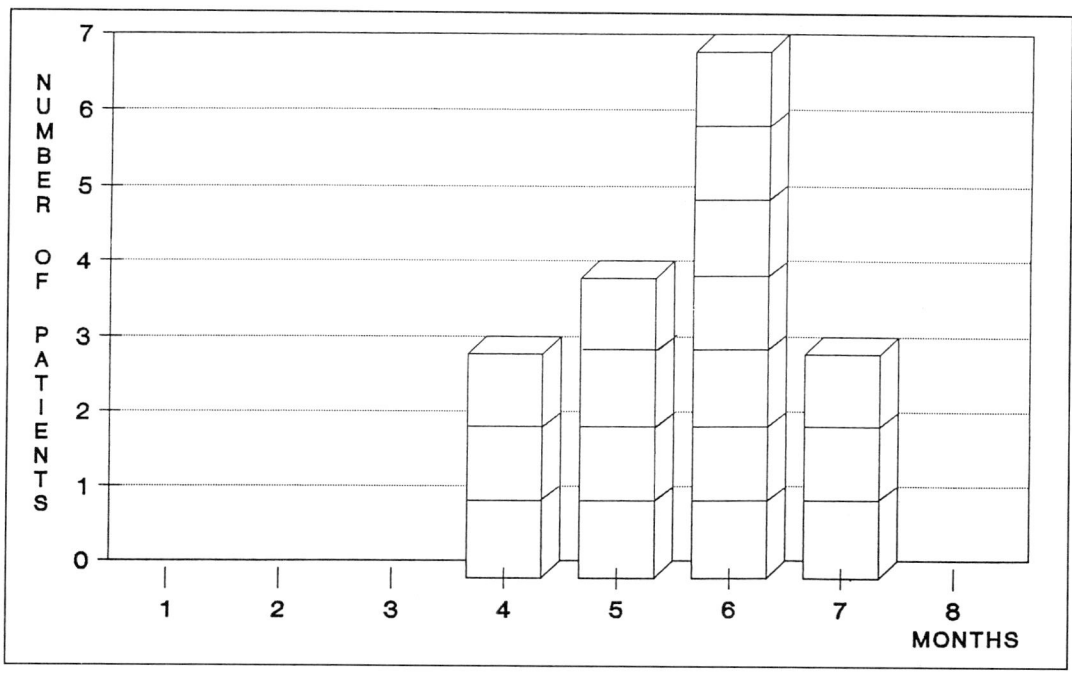

Fig. 1. Age at onset of seizures in 17 probands.

convulsions. There were also three siblings in this group. None of these relatives later developed other forms of epilepsy.

Among the 17 families, there were also four relatives with other forms of epilepsy: one case of hemiconvulsion, hemiplegia & epilepsy (HHE) syndrome, one case of generalized tonic–clonic seizures with onset in adult age and two cases of partial epilepsy with onset in old age. Only one patient could be considered as having an idiopathic type of epilepsy. Lastly, we also identified five other relatives with febrile convulsions alone in infancy. No patient had neonatal convulsions.

Seizure onset was confirmed at ages ranging from 3 months 20 days to 7 months (Fig. 1). An almost constant characteristic was the occurrence of seizures in a cluster, with mostly brief, successive seizures, with a maximum of 8–10 per day, without reaching a true status epilepticus.

The most frequently reported semiology was: psychomotor arrest, cyanosis, head and eye deviation to one side, diffuse tonic contraction and bilateral clonic jerks. In half the cases, the side of head and eye deviation varied from one seizure to another in the same patient.

Interictal EEGs were mostly normal. When EEG was performed during a cluster of seizures, lateralized slow waves and spikes were recorded in the occipito-parietal areas and disappeared once the seizures were under control. At present we have ictal EEG recordings for about half the patients that confirm the data presented previously in detail. Follow-up of these 17 cases varied from 2 to 11 years. No child had further seizures and EEG recordings are normal. All children have normal psychomotor development, except one girl who is mildly retarded.

Discussion

Familial convulsions may be caused in the first year of life by pyridoxine dependency or deficiency. In the typical form (Bankier *et al.*, 1983), the convulsions always appear in the first days of life. Only in the atypical form (Goutières & Aicardi, 1985) does onset occur in the first months.

These seizures are resistant to treatment with common antiepileptic drugs and the clinical picture is always severe, contrasting with the evolving nature of benign seizure disorders.

Watanabe et al. (1990) have described benign partial epilepsy that appeared between 3 and 20 months of age in nine patients, four of whom had a family history of benign infantile convulsions. Some of these cases might overlap with ours. However, the seizures they described clearly had a temporal lobe onset, while those we reported had an extratemporal onset.

Some features of our patients' seizures coincide with the category of benign neonatal familial convulsions (BNFC): normal neurological state; absence of known causative factors; normal psychomotor development and family history of seizures at a similar age. Plouin (1985) and Miles & Holmes (1990) reported that the onset of seizures can occur even in the early months of life. Seizure onset later than 3 months 15 days has never been reported, either in probands or relatives, yet in none of our patients did seizures start before the age of 4 months.

Although if the age at onset is different, the two syndromes are very similar. One is the question is whether BIFC is simply a late-onset form of BNFC or a distinct form of familial convulsions.

The gene responsible for BNFC has been mapped to chromosome 20q in the close vicinity of D20S19 and D20S20 markers (Leppert et al., 1989; Ryan et al., 1991; Malafosse et al., 1992). Recently, Malafosse et al. (1994) performed a linkage analysis in eight families with BIFC and demonstrated that the BNFC gene is not responsible for BIFC.

As for the clinical aspect, it must be pointed out that ictal recordings of neonatal convulsions are very rare. By contrast, we have clinical EEG documentation for more than half of our patients with infantile convulsions, so a comparison is not possible at this time.

Nosologically, we believe that BIFC must be considered a new epileptic syndrome to be included among the idiopathic forms. The reporting of other very similar cases confirms our hypothesis (Lee et al., 1993; Lúóvígsson et al., 1993; Echenne et al., 1994). The EEG and clinical features in our patients are typical of focal seizures. The location of the ictal discharge sometimes in one hemisphere, sometimes in the other, in the same patient, is a typical feature of a very young brain.

Seizure onset in the occipito-parietal areas is probably due to the fact that, at this age, this region is more epileptogenic than the others.

Finally, it is our opinion that the term 'convulsions' is more correct. We do not know if this disorder can actually be considered a true epilepsy. Further prospective studies on probands are necessary to verify the appearance at a later age of additional seizures or EEG patterns of idiopathic epilepsies, such as rolandic spikes, spike-and-wave discharges and photoconvulsive response.

References

Bankier, A., Turner, M. & Hopkins, J. (1983): Pyridoxine dependent seizures: a wider clinical spectrum. *Arch. Dis. Child.* **58**, 415–418.

Commission on Classification and Terminology of the International League Against Epilepsy (1989): Proposal for revised classifications of epilepsies and epileptic syndromes. *Epilepsia* **30**, 389–399.

Echenne, B., Humbertclaude, V., Rivier, F., Malafosse, A. & Cheminal, R. (1994): Benign infantile epilepsy with autosomal dominant inheritance. *Brain Dev.* **16**, 108–111.

Goutières, F. & Aicardi, J. (1985): Atypical presentations of pyridoxine-dependent seizures: a treatable cause of intractable epilepsy in infants. *Ann. Neurol.* **17**, 117–120.

Lee, W.L., Low, P.S. & Rajan, U. (1993): Benign familial infantile epilepsy. *J. Pediatr.* **123**, 588–590.

Leppert, M., Anderson, V.E., Quattlebaum, T., Stauffer, D., O'Connel, P., Nakamura, Y., Lalouel, J.M. & White, R. (1989): Benign familial neonatal convulsions linked to genetic markers on chromosome 20. *Nature* **337**, 647–648.

Lúóvígsson, P., Olafsson, E., Rich, S.S., Johannesson, G. & Anderson, V.E. (1993): Benign infantile familial epilepsy: three families with multiple affected members in three generations. *Epilepsia* **34** (S2), 18.

Malafosse, A., Leboyer, M., Dulac, O., Navelet, Y., Plouin, P., Beck, C., Laklou, H., Mouchnino, G., Grandscene, P., Vallee, L., Guilloud-Bataille, M., Samolyk, D., Baldy-Moulinier, M., Feingold, J. & Mallet, J. (1992): Confirmation of linkage of benign neonatal convulsions to D20S19 and D20S20. *Hum. Genet.* **89**, 54–58.

Malafosse, A., Beck, C., Bellet, H., Di Capua, M., Dulac, O., Echenne, B., Fusco, L., Lucchini, P., Ricci, S., Sebastianelli, R., Feingold, J., Baldy-Moulinier, M. & Vigevano, F. (1994): Benign infantile familial convulsions are not an allelic form of the benign familial neonatal convulsions gene. *Ann. Neurol.* **35**, 479–482.

Miles, K.D. & Holmes, G.L. (1990): Benign neonatal seizures. *J. Clin. Neurophysiol.* **7**, 369–379.

Plouin, P. (1985): Benign neonatal convulsions (familial and non-familial). In: *Epileptic syndromes in infancy, childhood and adolescence*, eds. J. Roger, C. Dravet, M. Bureau, F.E. Dreifuss & P. Wolf, pp. 2–11. London: John Libbey.

Ryan, S.G., Wiznitger, M., Hollman, C., Torres M.C., Szekeresova, M. & Schneider, S. (1991): Benign familial neonatal convulsions: evidence for clinical and genetic heterogeneity. *Ann. Neurol.* **29**, 469–473.

Vigevano, F., Di Capua, M., Fusco, L., Ricci, S., Sebastianelli, R. & Lucchini, P. (1990): Sixth-month benign familial convulsions. *Epilepsia* **31**, 613.

Vigevano, F., Fusco, L., Di Capua, M., Ricci, S., Sebastianelli, R. & Lucchini, P. (1992): Benign infantile familial convulsions. *Eur. J. Pediatr.* **151**, 608–612.

Vigevano, F., Fusco, L., Cusmai, R., Claps, D., Ricci, S. & Milani, L. (1993): The idiopathic form of West syndrome. *Epilepsia* **34**, 743–746.

Watanabe, K., Yamamoto, N., Negoro, T., Takahashi, I., Aso, K. & Machara, M. (1990): Benign infantile epilepsy with complex partial seizures. *J. Clin. Neurophysiol.* **7**, 409–416.

Chapter 7

Developmental aspects of experimental generalized seizures induced by pentylenetetrazol, bicuculline and flurothyl

S.L. Moshé[*†‡], L. Velíšek[*†] and G.L. Holmes[§]

Departments of [*]Neurology, [†]Neuroscience and [‡]Paediatrics, Laboratory of Developmental Epilepsy, and Montefiore/Einstein Epilepsy Management Center, Albert Einstein College of Medicine, Bronx, NY 10461, USA and [§]Departments of Neurology and Paediatrics, Children's Hospital, Harvard Medical School, Boston, MA, USA

The susceptibility to and the expression of generalized seizures is modified by age. Several models of epilepsy have been used in developmental studies, including pentylenetetrazol, bicuculline and flurothyl. Based on selective EEG recordings and behavioural manifestations the seizures are assumed to be generalized. Studies of developmental changes in seizure thresholds, EEG and behavioural characteristics as well as response to various antiepileptic drugs (AEDs) suggest that, in the rat during development, there are different windows of epileptogenicity with the maximal expression of seizures during the second and third postnatal week.

Pentylenetetrazol

Pentylenetetrazol (PTZ) remains one of the most commonly used pharmacological agents for inducing seizures. As will be discussed below, pentylenetetrazol is a drug commonly used in AED screening.

Motor seizures

The behavioural and EEG manifestations of PTZ-induced seizures in rodents suggest that the drug is a model of generalized seizures (Vernadakis & Woodbury, 1969; Swinyard & Woodhead, 1982; Velíšek et al., 1992). Seizures are usually induced by a single systemic administration of pentylenetetrazol; both the dose and route of administration determine the latency to seizure onset and behavioural manifestations. The behavioural changes consist of motionless stare, myoclonic twitches, face and forelimb clonus, generalized tonic–clonic activity, and falling.

Since pentylenetetrazol is extensively used in studying epileptogenesis in both immature and mature animals, a scoring system of PTZ-induced motor seizures has been developed (Pohl & Mareš, 1987) (Table 1).

The expression of PTZ-induced motor seizures is age-dependent. Clonic motor seizures are not

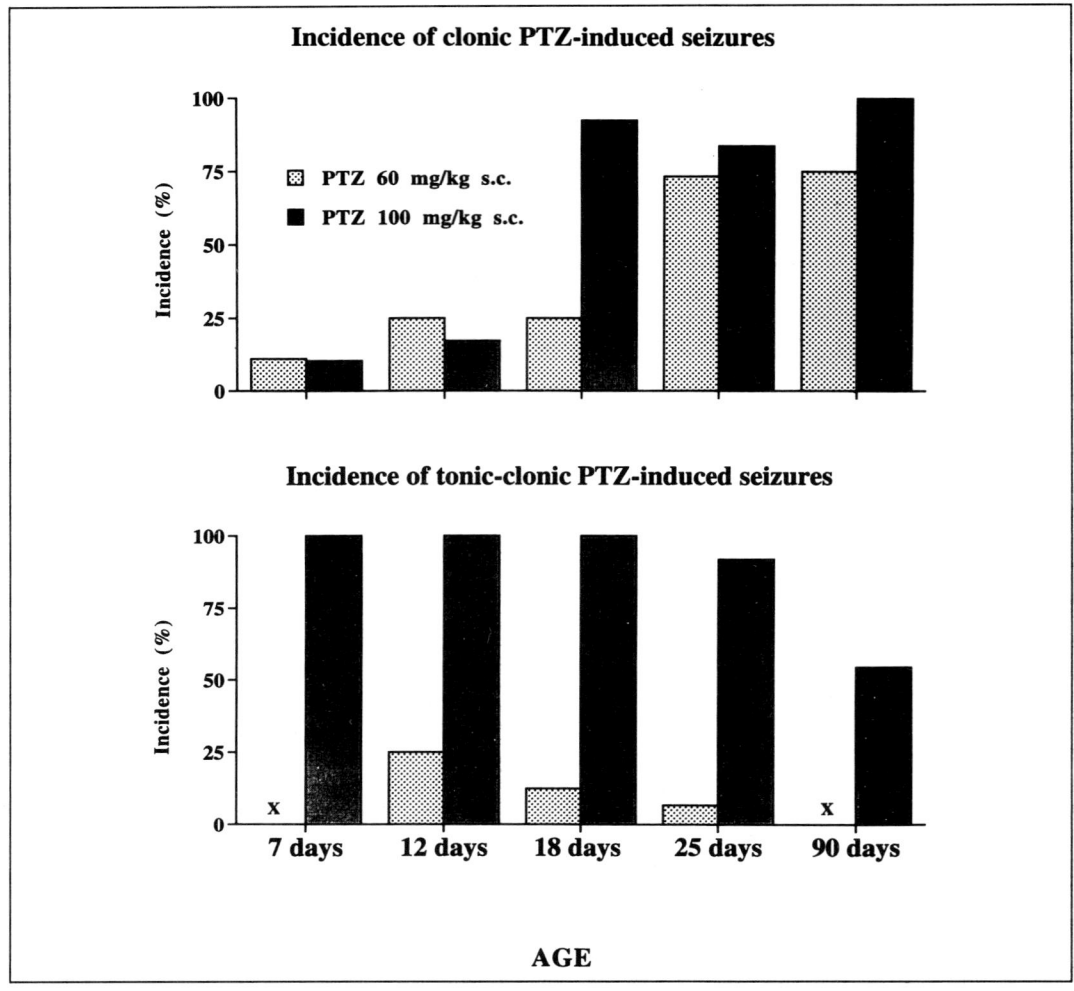

Fig. 1. The incidence of PTZ-induced clonic (top) and tonic–clonic (bottom) seizures in developing rats. x – axis: age groups 7, 12, 18, 25 and 90 days. y – axis: incidence of seizures in per cent. Clonic seizures occur regularly from the third postnatal week onwards. Tonic–clonic seizures occur at all ages tested if the dose of pentylenetetrazol is sufficiently large.

Table 1. Scoring of pentylenetetrazol seizures

0.5	Abnormal behaviour (sniffing, reorientation, rearing)
1	Isolated myoclonic twitches
2	Imperfect clonic seizures (i.e., unilateral, asynchronous, usually seen in pups)
3	Fully developed clonic seizures (preserved righting reflex, facial clonus; bilateral synchronous clonus of forelimbs, and Straub tail)
4	Incomplete tonic–clonic seizures consisting of the loss of righting reflexes and long-lasting clonus on all four limbs without the tonic stretch of the limbs
5	Fully developed tonic–clonic seizures (loss of righting reflex; short tonic phase on forelimbs and/or hindlimbs; and long-lasting clonus of all limbs)

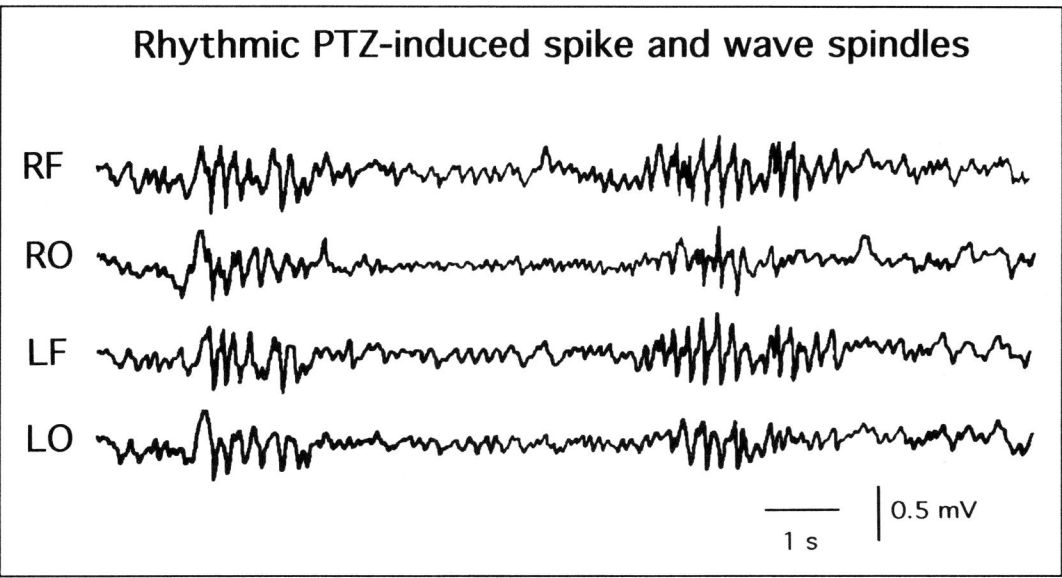

Fig. 2. Cortical EEG recordings of PTZ-induced spike-and-wave spindle activity accompanied by a motionless stare in a freely moving adult rat. Recordings from motor (RF, LF) and visual (RO, LO) cortex bilaterally.

regularly observed in rat pups before the third postnatal week and they are not fully developed until the fourth postnatal week. In contrast, myoclonic jerks and generalized tonic–clonic seizures are observed throughout development (Fig. 1). The dose needed to induce clonic seizures in 50 per cent of animals (CD_{50}) is almost constant after the third postnatal week; however, the CD_{50} for tonic–clonic seizures progressively increases with age. The latency to the onset of tonic–clonic seizure is shortest during the second and third postnatal week following a single dose of 100 mg/kg administered subcutaneously to rats, suggesting that the rats in this age group have a lower seizure threshold than other age groups (Velíšek et al., 1992).

As with a variety of other epileptogenic agents, repeated injections of pentylenetetrazol does lead to kindling with decreased seizure latency and increased seizure severity with serial injections (Diehl et al., 1984; Holmes & Weber, 1983). Kindling increases susceptibility to PTZ-induced seizures (Holmes & Weber, 1983) and kindling is facilitated after pentylenetetrazol seizures (Cain, 1981). All of these kindling-PTZ transfer studies have been performed either in adult animals, or in animals that were exposed to one seizure type in infancy and another in adulthood. There are no transfer studies performed solely in developing rats.

Metabolic studies using 2-deoxyglucose (2DG) have revealed that, in adults, metabolic activity increases during clonic seizures in the neocortex, hippocampus, globus pallidus and substantia nigra. Metabolic activity increases also in the midbrain structures during tonic–clonic seizures (Ben-Ari et al., 1981). In rat pups of postnatal (P) days 10–14, there were generalized increases in metabolic activity in limbic and motor cortex and also in brain-stem areas. In P17–P21, there were increases in metabolic activity in the brain-stem, midbrain, hypothalamus, and septum with decreases in cortex and hippocampus but not in the substantia nigra (de Vasconcelos et al., 1992).

EEG seizures

The PTZ-induced EEG phenomena are also age- and dose-dependent. Morphology or frequency of the EEG ictal discharges do not correlate with behavioural features, nor are the EEG discharges necessarily specific for a particular seizure type. Isolated sharp waves or spikes represent the first EEG sign of pentylenetetrazol seizures and they are usually accompanied by myoclonic jerks. Rhythmic spike-and-wave discharges forming a spindle (Fig. 2) may accompany the motionless stare. Clonic and tonic–clonic seizures have similar electrographic patterns consisting of rapid multiple spike-and-wave activity (Ono et al., 1990; Schickerová et al., 1984).

Maturational changes in PTZ-induced EEG discharges have been reported. In immature rats, EEG discharges can be disassociated from the behavioural seizures. The morphology of the epileptiform discharges changes with age with sharp waves becoming spikes after the second postnatal week. By P21, electrographic seizures are synchronized in all areas (Schickerová et al., 1984).

Pharmacology

The pentylenetetrazol model is widely used to screen potential antiepileptic drugs for possible efficacy in human seizure disorders. The rhythmic EEG activity accompanied by a motionless stare is considered to be a model of human absences (Marescaux et al., 1984; Velíšek et al., 1993a). Clonic seizures are considered to be a model of human myoclonic seizures, whereas tonic–clonic seizures may represent a model of primary generalized seizures of the generalized tonic–clonic type (Löscher & Schmidt, 1988; Mareš & Zouhar, 1988).

Clonic seizures are very resistant to any form of therapy. Tonic–clonic seizures, in contrast, are sensitive to the treatment with NMDA receptor antagonists (Fig. 3) (Velíšek & Mareš, 1992) and ethosuximide (Mareš & Velíšek, 1983). Several antiepileptic drugs (e.g. carbamazepine) selectively suppress only the tonic component of tonic–clonic seizures (Mareš et al., 1983). In contrast, in rat pups younger than three weeks, the administration of certain antiepileptic drugs such as phenytoin, carbamazepine, ethosuximide and flunarizine, may induce a significant increase in the incidence of clonic seizures (Kubová & Mareš, 1993; Mareš et al., 1981, 1983; Pohl & Mareš, 1987).

Although the mechanisms of action of pentylenetetrazol are still unclear, PTZ-induced seizures provide a model of epilepsy that has stood the course of time. It is useful both in immature and mature animals.

Pathology

A single pentylenetetrazol seizure does not appear to produce any pathological changes in the brain (Purpura et al., 1972) However, repeated clonic or tonic–clonic seizures may lead to loss of polymorphic neurons in the hilus of the dentate gyrus (Kock et al., 1993). Moreover, repeated tonic–clonic PTZ-induced seizures as a result of pentylenetetrazol kindling induce mossy fibre sprouting in the dentate gyrus in the adult rat (Golarai et al., 1992).

Bicuculline

Bicuculline is an alkaloid that blocks $GABA_A$ receptors (Curtis et al., 1971). Bicuculline-induced seizures are model of primary generalized seizures.

Motor seizures

The seizures can be reliably induced by systemic injection of bicuculline in the rat (de Feo et al., 1985; Zouhar et al. 1989; de Feo & Mecarelli, 1993). Myoclonic twitches and a motionless stare represent the first signs. As the seizure progresses, the rats develop clonic and tonic–clonic seizures. The seizure types clinically resemble those induced by pentylenetetrazol and the scoring system mentioned above can be easily adapted (Velíšková et al., 1990).

Behavioural and EEG changes induced by bicuculline are age-dependent. In contrast to PTZ-induced seizures, bicuculline reliably induces clonic seizures during the second postnatal week, approximately a week earlier than PTZ-induced clonic seizures occur. Tonic–clonic seizures following bicuculline occur throughout development. The CD_{50} for intraperitoneal (i.p.) bicuculline-

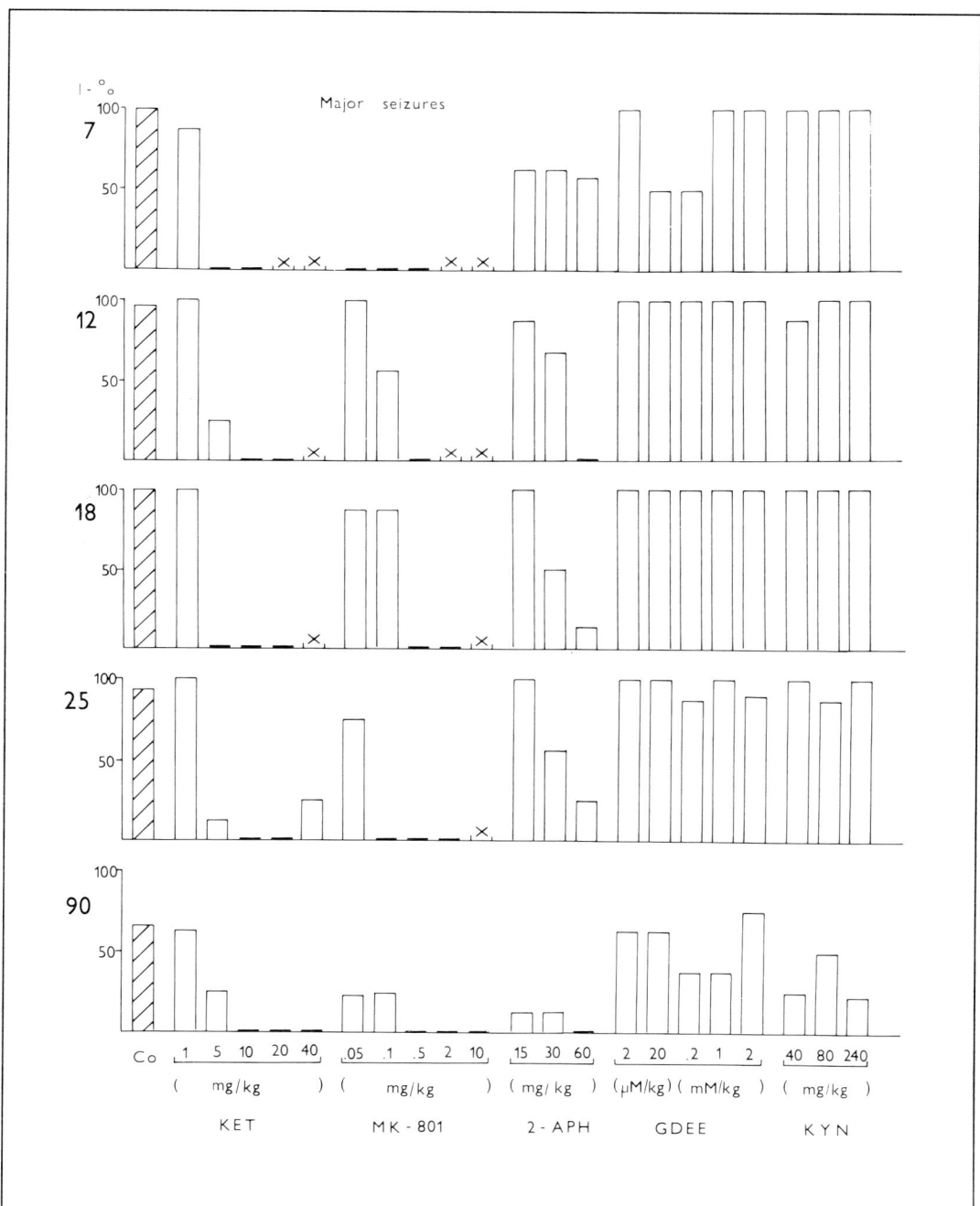

Fig. 3. Anticonvulsant effects of excitatory amino acid receptor antagonists (especially antagonists of NMDA-receptor subtype) against PTZ-induced tonic–clonic seizures in developing rats. From top to bottom: age groups 7, 15, 18, 25 and 90 days old. x-axis: drugs and doses used: Co = controls; KET = ketamine; MK-801 dizocilpine maleate; 2-APH = 2-amino-7-phosphonoheptanoic acid; GDEE = glutamic acid diethylester; and KYN = kynurenic acid. y-axis: incidence of seizures in per cent.

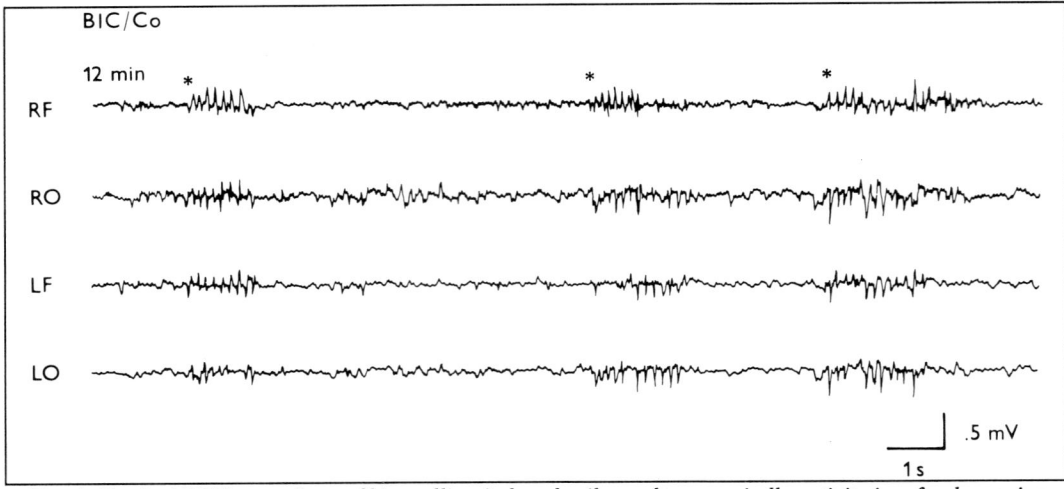

Fig. 4. Cortical EEG recordings of bicuculline-induced spike-and-wave spindle activity in a freely moving adult rat. Recordings from motor (RF, LF) and visual (RO, LO) cortex bilaterally.

induced tonic–clonic seizures is low in P7–P18 and progressively increases with age. There is not, however, a similar increase in CD_{50} for tonic–clonic seizures when bicuculline is administered intraperitoneally (i.v.). The difference between intraperitoneal and intravenous injections is due to the maturation of the liver's degradation-enzyme system (Zouhar et al., 1989).

Metabolic studies using 2DG have shown that there are almost no differences from PTZ-induced seizures. In adults, 2DG metabolic activity increases in the cortex, hippocampus, globus pallidus and substantia nigra during clonic seizures. During tonic–clonic seizures, the metabolic activity increases also in the midbrain structures (Ben-Ari et al., 1981). There are no 2DG studies in developing rats.

EEG seizures

The EEG correlates of bicuculline-induced seizures are age-dependent and similar to those observed in pentylenetetrazol seizures. In P7 and P12 rats, there are early individual sharp waves in the EEG after the bicuculline treatment. These sharp waves are usually, but not always, accompanied by myoclonic twitches (Baram & Snead, 1990). In older rats, EEG spikes occur following bicuculline administration. There is also bicuculline-induced spindle-shaped rhythmic activity recorded after low doses of bicuculline, similar to that occurring after pentylenetetrazol (Fig. 4). This activity is associated with a motionless stare and decreased reactivity of the animal (de Feo & Mecarelli, 1993). This phenomenon is also age-dependent. It can be first recorded during the second postnatal week (Zouhar et al., 1989). EEG seizures involve poorly synchronized sharp waves during the first two postnatal weeks; later in development the pattern of multiple spike-and-wave activity appears. These EEG seizures are accompanied by clonic or tonic–clonic motor seizures (Zouhar et al., 1989).

Pathology

In adolescent and adult animals, bicuculline-induced status epilepticus has been associated with a high incidence of brain damage. Meldrum and colleagues (Meldrum & Brierley, 1973; Meldrum & Horton, 1971, 1973) found that generalized bicuculline-induced seizures lasting 1.5–5.0 h resulted in selective ischaemic cell changes in the neocortex, hippocampus, and cerebellum. Bicuculline given intravenously to adolescent baboons with peripheral neuromuscular paralysis under mechanical ventilation also resulted in ischaemic cell damage in the neocortex and hippocampus but not cerebellum (Meldrum & Brierley, 1973). However, Söderfeldt and colleagues (1991) found that in neonatal marmoset monkeys bicuculline-induced status epilepticus was not associated with any intracranial pathology.

Pharmacology

There are fewer studies on the action of antiepileptic drugs on bicuculline-induced seizures than on PTZ-induced seizures, although the mechanism of action of bicuculline is well established. NMDA-receptor antagonists protect mice and rats against bicuculline-induced seizures (Turski et al., 1990; Velíšková et al., 1990) throughout development.

Flurothyl

The volatile agent hexaflurodiethyl ether is a potent and rapidly acting central nervous system stimulant that produces seizures within minutes of exposure (Truitt et al., 1960). The method of inducing seizures is easy and reliable. The rats are placed in an air-tight chamber. The liquid flurothyl is delivered via a pump at a constant rate onto a filter pad from which it evaporates. The rats remain in the chamber until they develop tonic motor seizures. Between trials, the chamber is flushed with room air and the filter changed. Because the volume of the chamber is approximately 35 times that of the rat, the oxygen content in the chamber is sufficient for the rat during the seizures.

Although the test is unaffected by temperature variation, it is likely that environmental factors such as barometric pressure and humidity might effect the rate of evaporation of the flurothyl and therefore concentration of the flurothyl. In studies comparing seizure latency we recommend that experimental and control rats be paired in the chamber to avoid the influence of these environmental factors (Velíšek et al., 1993a). The exact mechanism by which flurothyl produces seizures is not known. Woodbury (1980) has proposed that it opens sodium channels diffusely.

Motor seizures

Flurothyl-induced seizures consist of an early myoclonic jerk, followed by forelimb clonus, wild running, loss of posture, and tonic seizures. Seizure thresholds can be determined by multiplying the latency (from beginning of infusion to seizure onset) by the infusion rate and is expressed as the amount of flurothyl (μl) used to induce clonic and tonic seizures, respectively (latency × rate of infusion) (Xu et al., 1992). Continuous infusion of flurothyl can produce status epilepticus.

Truitt and colleagues (1960) administered flurothyl daily to rats. The latency of myoclonic jerks decreased with the daily injections, although there was no change in the latency to forelimb clonus. This indicates that flurothyl, like a number of other epileptogenic agents (Post et al., 1975; Vosu & Wise, 1975; Post, 1977; Cain, 1983, 1987) leads to kindling. In adult rats, there is a bidirectional transfer between flurothyl seizures and electrical kindling, i.e. repeated flurothyl-induced seizures enhance the rate of development of amygdala or cortical kindling (Wong & Moshé, 1987).

The behavioural manifestations of flurothyl-induced seizures are age-dependent. Gatt and colleagues (1993) administered flurothyl to rats at postnatal days 5, 10, 20, 30, and 70 and monitored both behavioural and EEG changes. Swimming movements were prominent in P5, followed by abrupt onset of tonus. Clonic seizures were not fully developed before P10. Behavioural features of the seizures did not change after P20 and consisted of myoclonic jerks followed by forelimb clonus, wild running, loss of posture and severe tonic posturing.

2DG studies have demonstrated that subcortical structures may be prominently involved in generalized flurothyl-induced seizures. Sperber et al. (1991) exposed P14 rats to flurothyl seizures (Sperber, 1992). After experiencing a tonic–clonic seizure, the animal was injected with 2DG and returned to the chamber. By manipulating the flow of flurothyl into the chamber these investigators elicited mild or severe seizures. Behaviours categorized as mild seizures consisted of the rats remaining quiet with little movement, periodic sniffing, chewing or head nodding. Severe seizures

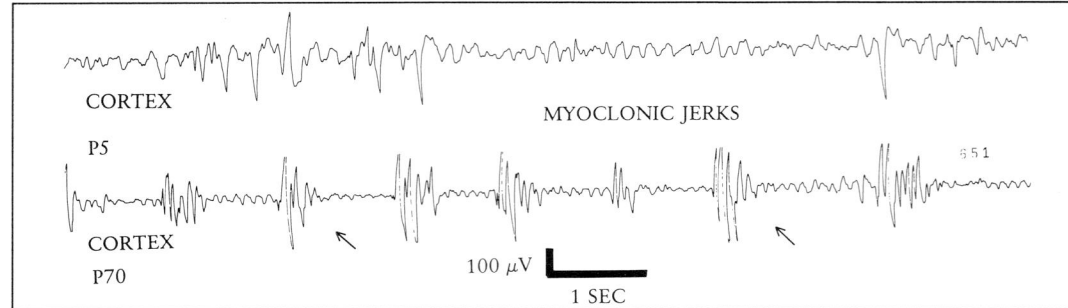

Fig. 5. Comparison of EEG-behavioural relationship following flurothyl in P5 and P70 rats. Note correlation of myoclonic jerks with multiple-spike discharges in P70 (arrows). In P5 rats, myoclonic jerks were not consistently associated with epileptiform discharges.

included having more than one tonic–clonic seizure, bouts of forelimb clonus, hindlimb extension, loss of balance and running, climbing or jumping. The pattern of 2DG mapping corresponded to the severity of the behavioural seizures. Rats in the mild seizure group demonstrated a generalized decrease in 2DG utilization. In contrast, rats in the severe seizure group demonstrated a generalized increase in 2DG utilization in the brain-stem and a corresponding decrease in the neocortex. There were no metabolic increases in the substantia nigra. These findings resemble those observed in rats experiencing pentylenetetrazol seizures (de Vasconcelos *et al.*, 1992).

EEG seizures

In a recent study, Gatt *et al.* (1993) described the EEG characteristics of flurothyl seizures in rats of various ages starting with P5 rats. Electrodes were implanted in the amygdala, hippocampus, and cortex at P5, P10, P20, P30 and P70 days and flurothyl was administered at a constant rate of 38 μl/min into the chamber where behavioural changes were monitored and the EEG recorded. In all age groups myoclonic jerks were usually associated with individual spikes. However, the correlation of the spikes with the behavioural myoclonic jerks varied as a function of age. P5 and P10 rats did not show a close correlation between spikes and myoclonic jerks while in the older rats this relationship was usually present (Fig. 5). Epileptiform discharges in the P5 and P10 rats were usually poorly formed and irregular in frequency compared to rhythmic discharges in older rats (Fig. 6).

Ictal discharges were present in all anatomical sites studied. When bilateral forelimb clonus or wild running occurred these were typically associated with long periods of spikes. In the younger rats, the spikes were better developed in the hippocampus than in the cortex while the converse was true for the older animals (Figs. 7 & 8). Ictal discharges were more irregular in the younger animals (≤ 20 days) than in the older animals. In the P5 and P10 day old rats, bursts of irregular spikes occurred while in the adults the spikes tended to be much more rhythmic and sustained. In all age groups there was waxing and waning of the spikes. As the animals went into the running and tonic

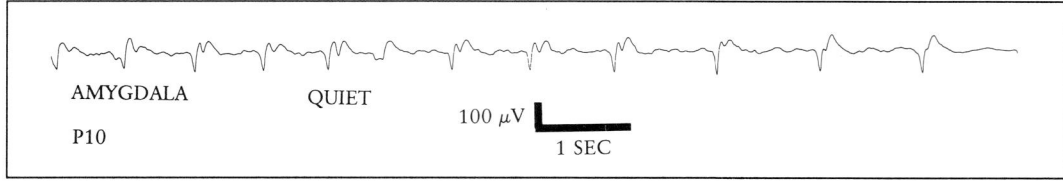

Fig. 6. Epileptiform discharges arising from the amygdala in P10 rat. These discharges rarely correlate directly with behavioural changes.

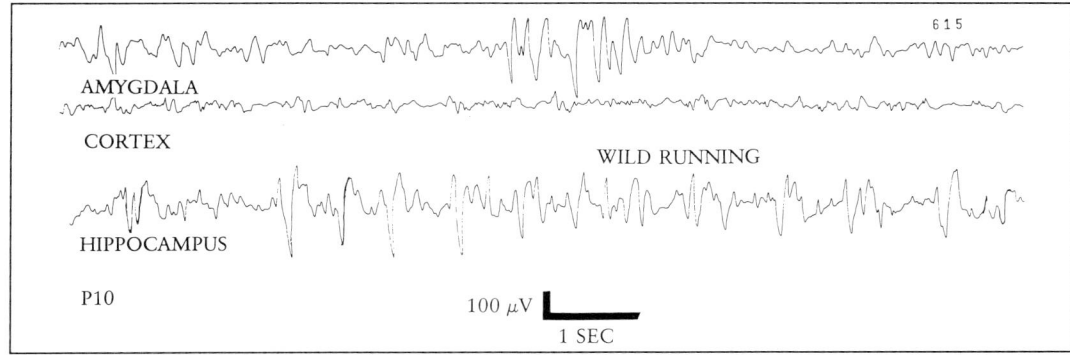

Fig. 7. Comparison of amygdala, cortex, and hippocampus recordings during wild running in P10 rats. Note that the epileptiform discharges are most prevalent in the hippocampus. Recordings are from three rats which received flurothyl together in the chamber.

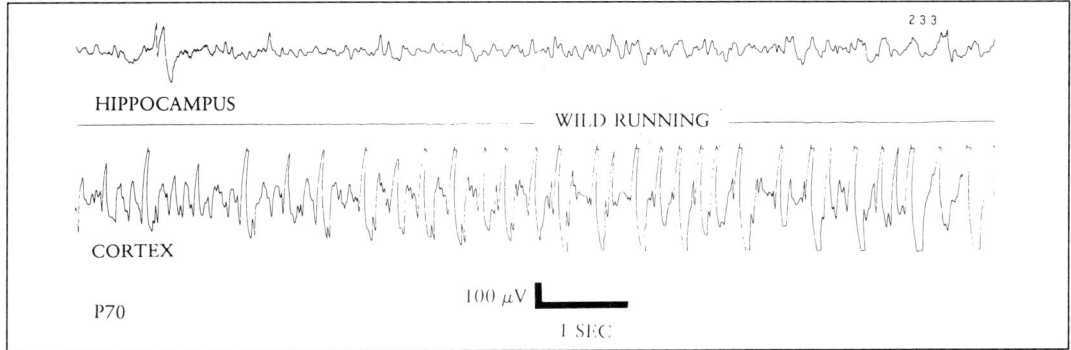

Fig. 8. Comparison of hippocampus and cortex recording in P70 rat. Note prominent involvement of cortex.

phases of the seizures, the spikes alternated with periods of suppression. Figure 9 demonstrates a sequence of EEGs from a P30 rat. The limited cortical electrographic involvement during seizures in rat pups suggests that in flurothyl seizures there is a prominent participation of subcortical structures.

Pathology

In immature animals, Wasterlain and colleagues (Wasterlain, 1976; Wasterlain & Dwyer, 1983) used flurothyl to produce status epilepticus in P4 rats. The brains of the rats were examined three days after 2 h of severe status epilepticus. The mean deficit in number of cells in the forebrain of experimental rats was 30 million. Brain RNA, DNA, protein, cholesterol, and weight were reduced to approximately the same extent, suggesting (according to the authors) a reduction in the number of brain cells without a significant change in mean cell size. Twenty-six days after the seizures, there was evidence of recuperation. No histological lesions however were noted. Mild flurothyl seizures resulted in a smaller deficit at age 7 days and complete recovery by age 30 days. The authors also found highly significant delays in the acquisition of free-fall righting and swimming ability in the flurothyl-treated animals. However, the authors did not investigate whether flurothyl seizures produce any effects in adult animals. In fact, although immature rats are more susceptible to flurothyl seizures and more prone to develop status epilepticus than adults, they also appear to be more resistant to the detrimental effects of the seizures, at least in terms of hippocampal damage. Adult rats experiencing flurothyl status epilepticus have extremely high mortality rates. In the

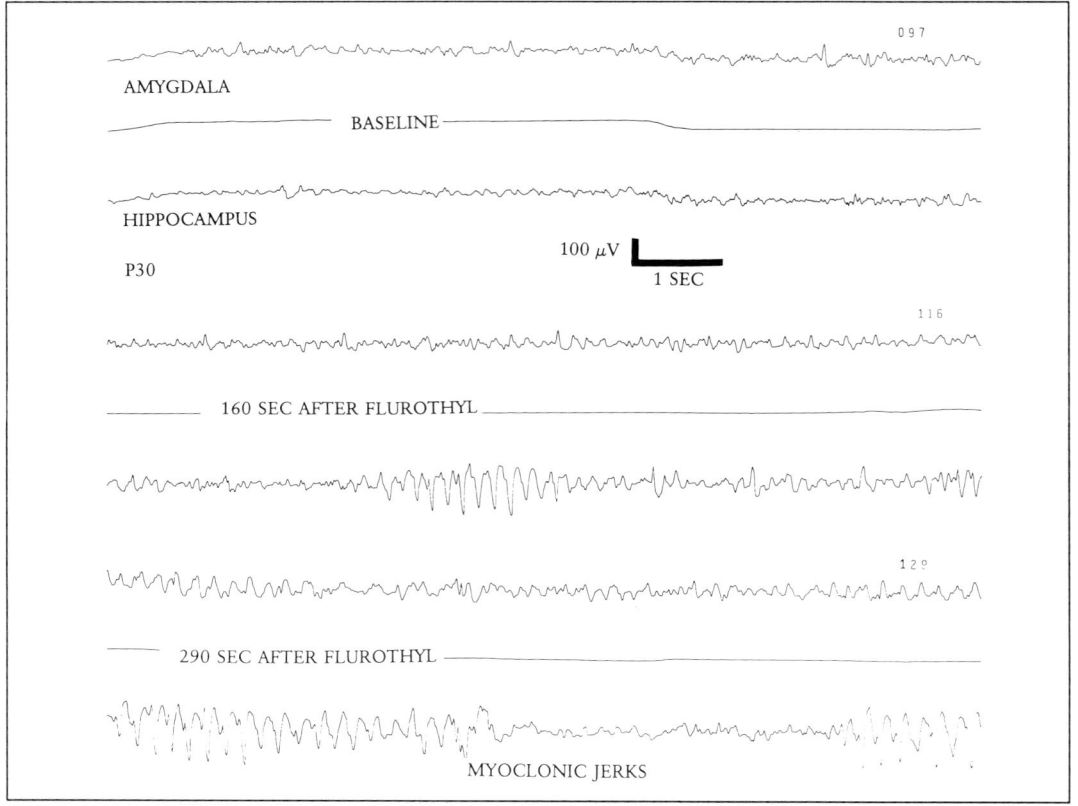

Fig. 9. Sequence of EEGs following flurothyl in P30 rat. Simultaneous recordings from the amygdala and hippocampus.

surviving rats there is a high incidence of hippocampal lesions in the CA4 area. Necrotic lesions are also present in thalamic structures and in the substantia nigra pars reticularis (Nevander et al., 1985). Developing rats have low mortality rates. Most importantly, in the surviving rats there is no evidence of hippocampal damage (Sperber et al., 1991). This may account for the relative excellent outcome of patients with benign neonatal (familial or not familial) convulsions. These infants experience severe seizures, including status epilepticus, during a narrow developmental window, and yet they do not develop partial temporal lobe seizures as they grow older (Plouin, 1985; Miles & Holmes, 1990; Plouin, 1990).

Pharmacology

The flurothyl model has been used to assess efficacy of antiepileptic drugs (Adler, 1969). Truitt and colleagues (1960) compared flurothyl with the minimal electroshock threshold (MES) and intravenous pentylenetetrazol test using the response to four antiepileptic drugs: phenobarbital, trimethadione, methocarbamol, and diphenylhydantoin sodium. The flurothyl anticonvulsant profile resembles that of the pentylenetetrazol model much more closely than that of the MES test. This finding further suggests that flurothyl-induced seizures represent a model of generalized epilepsy. It is interesting to note that the authors found that the myoclonic jerks which preceded the clonic activity were resistant to all four antiepileptic drugs.

Because there is a low variability associated with the use of flurothyl, Adler (1969) was able to study the threshold-raising ability of multiple doses of ethosuximide on flurothyl-induced seizures. Adler argued that because of the ease of administration, safety and low inter- and intra-animal variability associated with the use of flurothyl, this model is ideally suited for seizure susceptibility studies.

The seizure pathways involved in flurothyl seizures include the substantia nigra pars reticulata (SNR) (Moshé & Sperber, 1990) and the thalamus (Garant *et al.*, 1993), structures that may participate in the spontaneous cessation of the epileptic activity. These observations and subsequent experiments have led to the development of a novel way of designing putative new antiepileptic drugs. This is because the developmental changes that underlie the age-specific effects of the substantia nigra reticularis have been extensively studied in the flurothyl model. In adult rats, nigral infusions of $GABA_A$ agonists have biphasic effects on flurothyl seizures; low doses of muscimol or the $GABA_A$ agonist 4,5,6,7-tetrahydroisoxazolo[5,4-c]pyridin-3-ol (THIP) are anticonvulsant while large doses are proconvulsant. In P15 rats, $GABA_A$ agonists produce only proconvulsant effects. These phenomena may be due to site-specific developmental differences in the density, molecular composition, and function of $GABA_A$ receptors (Xu *et al.*, 1992). Studies on the molecular composition of $GABA_A$ receptors may help elucidate why the immature central nervous system is more susceptible to seizures than the adult central nervous system, and why genetically determined epileptic syndromes occur in certain strains of animals and human families.

There are also age-specific differences in the action of $GABA_B$ agonists; in adults, nigral infusions of baclofen do not have any effects on flurothyl seizures, while in P15 rats, similar infusions of baclofen are anticonvulsant. Binding studies have revealed that in the 2-week old SNR, there is an excess of $GABA_B$ receptors compared to the density of $GABA_B$ receptors in the adult SNR. The ontogenetic differences in $GABA_B$ sites may explain the age-specific action of baclofen (Garant *et al.*, 1992). After systemic administration, baclofen is proconvulsant in 9 day old rats and anticonvulsant in 15-day-old and older rats (Velíšková *et al.*, 1993).

Conclusion

The presented data suggest that development greatly influences all aspects of primary generalized seizures and that there are complex interactive effects that can not be predicted by studies in adult animals. In all three models, based on EEG data, there appears to be a delayed appearance of necortical seizure discharges. In two of the three models, 2DG studies suggest that there is limited metabolic activation of neocortical structures while there is prominent involvement of brain-stem structures, except for the substantia nigra. The data raise the hypothesis that during the early postnatal period, the substrates of seizures may involve subcortical pathways. With maturation, generalized seizures involve neocortical structures as well. Perhaps these ontogenetic difficulties may account for the differences in the behavioural and electrographic manifestations as a function of age. However, all three animal models discussed in this chapter represent models of acute (reactive seizures.) In the future, it may be desirable to perform studies in developing animals with spontaneous seizures. To date, such animal models are not available.

Acknowledgements

Supported by NIH Grant NS-20253 (S.L.M.), EFA Research Grant (L.V.) and NIH Grant NS-27984 (G.L.H.).

References

Adler, M.W. (1969): Laboratory evaluation of antiepileptic drugs. *Epilepsia* **10**, 263–280.

Baram, T.Z. & Snead III, O.C. (1990): Bicuculline induced seizures in infant rats: ontogeny of behavioral and electrocortical phenomena. *Dev. Brain Res.* **57**, 291–295.

Ben-Ari, Y., Tremblay, E., Riche, D., Ghilini, G. & Naquet, R. (1981): Electrographic, clinical and pathological alterations following systemic administration of kainic acid, bicuculline or pentetrazole: metabolic mapping using the deoxyglucose method with special reference to the pathology of epilepsy. *Neuroscience* **6,** 1361–1391.

Cain, D.P. (1981): Transfer of pentylenetetrazol sensitization to amygdaloid kindling. *Pharmacol. Biochem. Behav.* **15,** 533–536.

Cain, D.P. (1983): Bidirectional transfer of electrical and carbachol kindling. *Brain Res.* **260,** 135–138.

Cain, D.P. (1987): Kindling by repeated intraperitoneal or intracerebral injections of picrotoxin transfers to electrical kindling. *Exp. Neurol.* **97,** 243–254.

Curtis, D.R., Duggan, A.W., Felix, D. & Johnston, G.A.R. (1971): Bicuculline, an antagonist of GABA and synaptic inhibition in the spinal cord of the cat. *Brain Res.* **32,** 69–96.

de Feo, M., Mecarelli, O. & Ricci, G. (1985): Bicuculline- and allyglycine-induced epilepsy in developing rats. *Exp. Neurol.* **90,** 411–421.

de Feo, M. R. & Mecarelli, O. (1993): Ontogenetic models of epilepsy. In: *Epileptogenic and excitotoxic mechanisms*, eds. G. Avanzini, R. Fariello, U. Heinemann & R. Mutani, pp. 89–97. London: John Libbey.

de Vasconcelos, A.P., el Hamdi, G., Vert, P. & Nehlig, A. (1992): An experimental model of generalized seizures for the measurement of local cerebral glucose utilization in the immature rat. II. Mapping of brain metabolism using the quantitative [^{14}C] 2-deoxyglucose technique. *Dev. Brain Res.* **69,** 243–259.

Diehl, R.G., Smialowski, A. & Gotwo, T. (1984): Development and persistance of kindled seizures after repeated injections of pentylenetetrazol in rats and guinea pigs. *Epilepsia* **25,** 506–510.

Garant, D.S., Sperber, E.F. & Moshé, S.L. (1992): The density of GABA$_B$ binding sites in the substantia nigra is greater in rat pups than in adults. *Eur. J. Pharmacol.* **214,** 75–78.

Garant, D.S., Xu, S.G., Sperber, E.F. & Moshé, S.L. (1993): The influence of thalamic GABA transmission on the susceptibility of adult rats to flurothyl induced seizures. *Epilepsy Res.* **15,** 185–192.

Gatt, A., Velíšková, J., Liu, Z., Moshé, S.L. & Holmes, G.L. (1993): Ontogeny of flurothyl–induced seizures: a behavioral and EEG electroencephalogrpahic analysis. *Epilepsia* **34 (Suppl.6),** 63.

Golarai, G., Cavazos, J.E. & Sutula, T.P. (1992): Activation of the dentate gyrus by pentylenetetrazol evoked seizures inducesmossy fiber synaptic reorganization. *Brain Res.* **593,** 257–264.

Holmes, G.L. & Weber, D.A. (1983): Increased susceptibility to pentylenetetrazol-induced seizures in adult rats following electrical kindling during brain development. *Dev. Brain Res.* **11,** 312–314.

Kock, J., Yi, S.D., Golarai, G. & Sutula, T. (1993): Neuronal loss induced in the hilus of the dentate gyrus by repeated pentylenetetrazol-evoked seizures. *Epilepsia* **34 (Suppl 6),** 56.

Kubová, H. & Mareš, P. (1993): Anticonvulsant action of oxcarbazepine, hydroxycarbamazepine, and carbamazepine against metrazol-induced motor seizures in developing rats. *Epilepsia* **34,** 188–192.

Löscher, W. & Schmidt, D. (1988): Which animal models should be used in the search for new antiepileptic drugs? A proposal based on experimental and clinical considerations. *Epilepsy Res.* **2,** 145–181.

Mareš, P., Hlavatá, J., Lišková, K. & Mudrochová, M. (1983): Effects of carbamazepine and diphenylhydantoin on metrazol seizures during ontogenesis in rats. *Physiol. Bohemoslov.* **32,** 92–96.

Mareš, P., Marešová, D. & Schickerová, R. (1981): Effect of antiepileptic drugs on metrazol convulsions during ontogenesis in rats. *Physiol. bohemoslov.* **30,** 113–121.

Mareš, P. & Velíšek, L. (1983): Influence of ethosuximide on metrazol-induced seizures during ontogenesis in rats. *Activ. Nerv. Sup.* **25,** 295–298.

Mareš, P. & Zouhar, A. (1988): Do we possess adequate models of childhood epilepsies? *Physiol. Bohemoslov.* **37,** 1–9.

Marescaux, C., Micheletti, G., Vergnes, M., Depaulis, A., Rumbach, L. & Warter, J.M. (1984): A model of chronic spontaneous petit mal-like seizures in the rat: comparison with pentylenetetrazol-induced seizures. *Epilepsia* **25,** 326–331.

Meldrum, B.S. & Brierley, J.B. (1973): Prolonged epileptic seizures in primates: ischaemic cell change and its relation to ictal physiological events. *Arch. Neurol.* **28,** 10–17.

Meldrum, B.S. & Horton, R.W. (1971): Convulsive effects of 4-deoxypyridoxine and of bicuculline in photosensitive baboons (*Papio papio*) and in rhesus monkeys (*Maccaca mulatta*). *Brain Res.* **35,** 419–436.

Meldrum, B.S. & Horton, R.W. (1973): Physiology of status epilepticus in primates. *Arch. Neurol.* **28,** 1–9.

Miles, D.K. & Holmes, G.L. (1990): Benign neonatal seizures. *J. Clin. Neurophysiol.* **3,** 369–379.

Moshé, S.L. & Sperber, E.F. (1990): Substantia nigra-mediated control of generalized seizures. In: *Generalized epilepsy: cellular, molecular and pharmacological approaches*, eds. G. Gloor, R. Kostopoulos, M. Naquet & P. Avoli, pp. 355–367. Boston: Birkhauser Inc.

Nevander, G., Ingvar, M., Auer, R. & Siesjø, B.K. (1985): Status epilepticus in well-oxygenated rats causes neuronal necrosis. *Ann. Neurol.* **19,** 281–290.

Ono, J., Vieth, R. & Walson, P.D. (1990): Electrocorticographical observation of seizures induced by pentylenetetrazol (PTZ) injection in rats. *Funct. Neurol.* **5,** 345–352.

Plouin, P. (1985): Benign neonatal convulsions (familial and non-familial). In: *Epileptic syndromes in infancy, childhood and adolescence*, eds. J. Roger, C. Dravet, M. Bureau, F. E. Dreifus, & P. Wolf, pp. 2–11. London: John Libbey.

Plouin, P. (1990): Benign neonatal convulsions. In: *Neonatal seizures*, eds. C.G. Wasterlain & P. Pert, pp. 51–59. New York: Raven Press.

Pohl, M. & Mareš, P. (1987): Effects of flunarizine on metrazol-induced seizures in developing rats. *Epilepsy Res.* **1,** 302–305.

Post, R.M. (1977): Progressive changes in behavior and seizures following chronic cocaine administration: relationship to kindling and psychosis. *Adv. Behav. Biol.* **21,** 353–372.

Post, R.M., Kopanda, R.T. & Lee, A. (1975): Progressive behavioral changes during chronic lidocaine administration: relationship to kindling. *Life Sci.* **17,** 943–950.

Purpura, D.P., Penry, J.K., Tower, D.B., Woodbury, D.M. & Walter, R.D. (Eds.) (1972): *Experimental models of epilepsy: a manual for the laboratory worker*. New York: Raven Press.

Schickerová, R., Mareš, P. & Trojan, S. (1984): Correlation between electrocorticographic and motor phenomena induced by pentamethylenetetrazol during ontogenesis in rats. *Exp. Neurol.* **84,** 153–164.

Söderfeldt, B., Fujikawa, D.G. & Wasterlain, C.G. (1991): Neuropathology of status epilepticus in the neonatal marmoset monkey. In: *Neonatal seizures*, eds. C.G. Wasterlain & P. Vert, pp. 91–98. New York: Raven Press.

Sperber, E.F. (1992): Developmental profile of seizure-induced hippocampal damage. *Epilepsia*, **33,** 44.

Sperber, E.F., Haas, K.Z., Stanton, P.K. & Moshé, S.L. (1991): Resistance to damage of the immature hippocampus to flurothyl-induced status epilepticus. *Epilepsia* **32,** 47.

Swinyard, E.A. & Woodhead, J.H. (1982): General principles. Experimental detection, quantification and evaluation of anticonvulsants. In: *Antiepileptic drugs*, eds. D.M. Woodbury, J.K. Penry & C.E. Pippenger, pp. 111–126. New York: Raven Press.

Truitt, E.B., Ebesberg, E.M. & Ling, A.S.G. (1960): Measurement of brain excitability by use of hexaflurodiethyl ether (Indoclon). *J. Pharm. Exp. Ther.* **129,** 445–453.

Turski, W.A., Urbanska, E., Dziki, M., Parada-Turska, J. & Ikonomidou, C. (1990): Excitatory amino acid antagonists protect mice against seizures induced by bicuculline. *Brain Res.* **514,** 131–134.

Velíšek, L., Kubová, H., Pohl, M., Stanková, L., Mareš, P. & Schickerová, R. (1992): Pentylenetetrazol-induced seizures in rats: an ontogenetic study. *Naunyn-Schmiedeberg's Arch. Pharmacol.* **346,** 588–591.

Velíšek, L. & Mareš, P. (1992): Developmental aspects of the anticonvulsant action of MK-801. In: *Multiple sigma and PCP receptor ligands: mechanisms for neuromodulation and neuroprotection?*, eds. J.-M. Kamenka & E.F. Domino, pp. 779–795. Ann Arbor: NPP Books.

Velíšek, L., Moshé, S. L. & Cammer, W. (1993a): Developmental changes in seizure susceptibility in carbonic anhydrase II-deficient mice and normal littermates. *Dev. Brain Res.* **72,** 321–324.

Velíšek, L., Vondricková, R. & Mareš, P. (1993b): Models of simple partial and absence seizures in freely moving rats: action of ketamine. *Pharmacol. Biochem. Behav.* **45,** 889–896.

Velíšková, J., Velíšek, L., Mareš, P. & Rokyta, R. (1990): Ketamine suppresses both bicuculline- and picrotoxin-induced generalized tonic–clonic seizures during ontogenesis. *Pharmacol. Biochem. Behav.* **37,** 667–674.

Velíšková, J., Velíšek, L., Ptachewich, Y., Shinnar, S. & Moshé, S.L. (1993): Baclofen is anticonvulsant in 15 days old and older rats but proconvulsant in 9 day old rat pups. *Electroencephalogr. Clin. Neurophysiol.* **87,** 45.

Vernadakis, A. & Woodbury, D.M. (1969): The developing animal as a model. *Epilepsia* **10,** 163–178.

Vosu, H. & Wise, R. A. (1975): Cholinergic seizure kindling in the rat: comparison of caudate, amygdala and hippocampus. *Behav. Biol.* **13,** 491–495.

Wasterlain, C.G. (1976): Effects of neonatal status epilepticus on rat brain development. *Neurology* **26,** 975–986.

Wasterlain, C.G. & Dwyer, B.E. (1983): Brain metabolism during prolonged seizures in neonates. In: *Status epilepticus*, eds. A.V. Delgado-Escueta, C.G. Waterlain, D.M. Treiman, & R.J. Porter, pp. 241–260. New York: Raven Press.

Wong, B.Y. & Moshé, S.L. (1987): Mutual interactions between repeated flurothyl convulsions and electrical kindling. *Epilepsy Res.* **1,** 159–64.

Woodbury, D.M. (1980): Convulsants. Convulsant drugs: mechanisms of action. In: *Antiepileptic drugs: mechanisms of action*, eds. G.H. Glaser, J.K. Penry & D.M. Woodbury, pp. 249–303. New York: Raven Press.

Xu, S.G., Garant, D.S., Sperber, E.F. & Moshé, S.L. (1992): The proconvulsant effect of nigral infusion of THIP on flurothyl-induced seizures in rat pups. *Dev. Brain Res.* **68,** 275–277.

Zouhar, A., Mareš, P., Lišková-Bernášková, K. & Mudrochová, M. (1989): Motor and electrocorticographic epileptic activity induced by bicuculline in developing rats. *Epilepsia* **30,** 501–510.

Chapter 8

Gene mapping for benign familial neonatal convulsions and related syndromes

V. Elving Anderson*, Mark Leppert[†], Dick Lindhout[‡], Alain Malafosse[§] and Ortrud Steinlein[¶]

*Epilepsy Clinical Research Program, University of Minnesota, Minneapolis, Minnesota 55455, USA; [†]Department of Human Genetics, University of Utah & Howard Hughes Medical Institute, Salt Lake City, Utah 84132, USA; [‡]Department of Clinical Genetics, Faculty of Medicine, Box 1738, 3000 DR Rotterdam, The Netherlands; [§]Laboratoire de Médecine Expérimentale, INSERM U249, CNRS UPR9008, Institut de Biologie, 34060 Montpellier, France; [¶]Institut für Humangenetik und Anthropologie, Ruprechts-Karls-Universität, 69120 Heidelberg, Germany

The underlying goal of gene mapping for epilepsy is to understand the basic pathogenetic mechanisms and to develop better methods of treating those who are affected. It is now becoming apparent that each distinguishable type of epilepsy provides different opportunities (and problems) for such studies.

One useful type is known as 'benign familial neonatal convulsions', a term that was introduced 25 years ago (Bjerre & Corelius, 1968). This condition shows an autosomal dominant pattern of inheritance and has an unusual developmental history (Plouin, Ch. 5).These two interesting features merit further attention. (1) The autosomal dominant mode of inheritance is shown in the fact that the condition is transmitted from an affected person to about 40 per cent of their offspring. Thus, it is strongly genetic, but a more important point is that it develops in heterozygotes, those who have one normal and one mutant gene. This suggests that the condition may result from a 'loss of function' mutation (with the heterozygotes having only about half of the gene product that is needed for normal control of neuronal firing), or from an 'altered function' mutation (with the altered gene product interfering with usual process). (2) The developmental pattern for benign familial neonatal convulsions is such that about 80 per cent of the affected infants have a first seizure in the first week of life (most often on the third day). By 3–4 months the seizures have usually disappeared, although in about 15 per cent of the affected individuals occasional seizures develop later in life. Some alteration in gene expression may be involved, with the relevant gene being turned on (or off) too early or too late.

Presumably both of these issues will be resolved when the underlying gene has been mapped and sequenced and the basic gene product is identified. A significant step in this direction was taken when the gene for the trait was mapped to the long arm of chromosome 20 (Leppert *et al.*, 1989) by DNA linkage analysis of a family published earlier by Quattlebaum (1979). Leppert *et al.* (1993)

have more recently extended the analysis to other families. The original mapping to chromosome 20 was based on two DNA markers (RMR6 and CMM6). These markers have now been analysed in a total of six kindreds (Table 1). CMM6 has a number of size variants and is considerably more informative, but RMR6 helps to establish a haplotype (a combination of two specific alleles, one of each marker locus). It will be noted that the haplotype that segregates with the disease gene is not identical for all families, thus excluding both markers as candidate genes. Furthermore, in five of the kindreds, all affected members carried the distinctive haplotype for the respective kindred, with no exceptions.

Table 1. Linkage analysis of six benign neonatal familial convulsions (BFNC) families

Kindred	Reference	Haplotype segregating with BFNC			Logarithm of odds ratio (lod) by per cent recombination with CMM6		
		Genotype	No. aff.	No. unaff.	0.001	0.01	0.10
K1504	Quattlebaum, 1979	2,8	19	5	2.87	2.89	2.82
K1525	Zonana et al., 1984	2,5	6	3	−0.70	−0.62	−0.17
K1547	Bjerre & Corelius, 1968	2,8	11	2	2.48	2.47	2.23
K1654	Shevell et al., 1986 (Fam. B)	–	–	–	−4.15	−2.25	−0.41
K1655	Shevell et al., 1986 (Fam. A)	1,3	5	0	0.90	0.88	0.72
K1705	Ronen et al., 1993	2,10	34	6	10.53	10.51	9.62
	Total			16	11.93	13.88	14.81
	Total (excluding K1654)		75	16	16.08	16.13	15.22

In the sixth kindred (K1654) this rule was broken, and the affected members in this family did not have a common haplotype. Furthermore, the significantly negative lod scores rejected close linkage between the convulsions and the CMM6 locus. Finally, a statistical test also indicated that K1654 was different, thus providing evidence for linkage heterogeneity.

When kindred 1654 is excluded, the total lod score for the other five kindreds is extremely high, indicating odds in favor of linkage at about 10^{16}:1. Malafosse et al. (1992) confirmed this linkage assignment in a series of six French families.

Thirteen new pedigrees of benign familial neonatal convulsions have been identified in France since the initial publication by Malafosse et al. (1992). Linkage to CMM6-RMR6 has been observed in six of them, but has been rejected in three multiplex pedigrees. The four other families are not large enough to allow to classify them among 20q-linked or unlinked pedigrees. Linkage to chromosome 8q has been also rejected in the three 20q-unlinked pedigrees (Lewis). In these three pedigrees, clinical characteristics are in accordance with the criteria agreed upon during this conference. Thus, this result suggests the existence of a third locus of benign familial neonatal convulsions.

Problems encountered in linkage analysis

At this point, some of the problems encountered in linkage analysis can be identified. Errors can be introduced either by (1) false positives – cases of seizures or epilepsy that do not result from mutations at the locus for benign familial neonatal convulsion (representing phenocopies or locus heterogeneity) or (2) false negatives – unaffected individuals who do not in fact carry a mutant gene for benign familial neonatal convulsion (reflecting lack of information or lack of penetrance).

Phenocopies in this case are conditions that phenotypically resemble benign familial neonatal convulsions but have a non-genetic cause. These may be difficult to detect since the diagnosis of benign familial neonatal convulsions is mainly one of exclusion. The seizure pattern will be of little value since neonates with benign familial neonatal convulsions may display any seizure type (except myoclonic), either generalized or focal (Ronen et al., 1993), but the fact that the babies are completely normal between seizure episodes may be more helpful.

Locus heterogeneity occurs when mutations at different loci on the same or other chromosomes can produce similiar clinical pictures. This is now established for benign familial neonatal convulsions, since one family with neonatal onset maps to chromosome 8 instead of 20 (Lewis et al., 1993). The families with onset of benign familial infantile convulsions at 4–6 months (BFIC) do not map onto 20 either (Malafosse et al., 1994).

Lack of information can be suspected when informants do not have direct information about early development in families with benign familial infantile convulsions. It may be quite easy to miss a few isolated convulsions during the first week of life. For this reason we prefer to code presumed unaffected individuals as 'unknown' unless the mother (or other primary caregiver) is available.

Lack of penetrance may be an issue if a person has not yet reached the usual age at risk, but this is seldom a factor in benign familial neonatal convulsions with such an early onset. Lack of penetrance is fairly common in autosomal dominant traits, since the effect of the single mutant gene in heterozygotes may not always be expressed in the the presence of the normal allele. This observation that the gene for the trait is not always expressed suggests the possibility that appropriate intervention might further reduce the expression.

One rough approximation of degree of penetrance in benign familial neonatal convulsions can be derived from Table 1. Out of the 91 individuals who carried the haplotype which segregated with the trait there were 75 (or 82 per cent) who actually expressed the trait.

Clinical implication

The seizure manifestations are mixed, including tonic extension or clonic movements of the limbs, automatisms, ocular signs, and autonomic effects (Ronen et al., 1993). The seizures can be generalized or focal, on one side or the other (even in a single individual). This gives rise to the question as to whether benign familial neonatal convulsions should be considered a generalized or partial form of epilepsy (Aso & Watanabe, 1992).

The interictal EEGs are normal or show only minor nonspecific abnormalities. Three studies of ictal EEGs have reported similar findings – a general diffuse sudden suppression of amplitude, followed by symmetric rhythmic slow waves, interrupted by high voltage multiple spike and sharp waves (Hirsch et al., 1993; Ronen et al., 1993). Hirsch and his colleagues suggest that the seizures are 'a form of generalized tonic–clonic seizures with an asymmetric clinical expression depending on incomplete maturation of structures involved in synchronization of seizures'.

The evidence for locus heterogeneity can help to resolve these issues. The seizure and EEG patterns now can be studied separately for families which map to chromosome 20, chromosome 8, or to other defined chromosomes. If each of these group of patients shows a wide range of seizure types, representing essentially all of the seizures which can be expressed at the respective ages, then it will appear likely that the several mutations have their primary effect on mechanisms which control the age at onset. A similar comparison can be made of the EEG patterns. From this point of view, locus heterogeneity is not a devastating problem but rather a useful tool for analysis.

Questions for the future

As attention shifts to efforts for positional cloning of the genes, the emphasis changes from lod scores to obligate recombinants between markers and the disease trait in order to narrow the region for the intensive search. This may be facilitated by the important finding (Steinlein et al., 1992a) that the benign familial neonatal convulsion gene is in an area with increased recombination, so that the physical distances are markedly shorter than the recombination data would suggest.

Once the gene on chromosome 20 is sequenced and cloned, comparison with previously recognized gene sequences will help to identify the function of the gene product and the role of mutations in raising seizure susceptibility. It is tempting to hypothesize that the different genes that are responsible for the familial convulsions at different ages may belong to a family of genes with a basically similar function.

Genetic study of low-voltage EEG

The variations in human electroencephalogram (EEG) are widely genetically inherited (Vogel, 1970). However, the average EEG, like in most of the epilepsies, is influenced by several genetic and environmental factors. This makes it difficult to study the basic mechanisms behind it.

But some special EEG variants, like some of the epilepsies, follow a simple mode of Mendelian inheritance. One of them is the so-called low-voltage EEG (Vogel, 1970; Anokhin *et al.*, 1992). It is autosomal-dominantly inherited and observed in about 5 per cent of the adult population.

The main characteristic feature of the phenotype is the reduction or absence of alpha activity in the resting EEG. In the common EEG, alpha waves appear during restful awakeness, if the eyes are closed. In the low-voltage EEG, alpha waves can only be observed sometimes for a few seconds after provocation by special functional tests, such as hyperventilation or eye-opening and closing. Usually, the low-voltage EEG is combined with a low overall EEG amplitude. The records may show a certain amount of activity in the alpha frequency range, but only of diffuse waves of small amplitude without a rhythmic component. Activity in the slow delta, theta and fast beta frequency bands is often present in the low-voltage EEG. The low-voltage EEG as a trait should not be confused with alpha depression caused by tension or anxiety of the proband or transitory or permanent alpha depression which can be observed after brain trauma or in chronic neurological diseases.

The low-voltage EEG was chosen to study, by linkage analysis and positional cloning, the basic mechanism underlying the synchronization or desynchronization of brain electric activity.

A linkage study (Steinlein *et al.*, 1992b) was carried out to determine one or more genes responsible for the phenotype low-voltage EEG. EEG records and blood samples from 17 families, including a total of 190 individuals, have been collected. The families are of different size, some are small nuclear pedigrees, but families with 12, 15 or 34 members were also included. The largest family, with a total of 64 individuals investigated, was collected during an expedition to Azerbaijan.

The linkage study was based on two different approaches: without any hint of a possible localization of an EEG gene, polymorphic probes which were distributed over the whole genome, were collected and typed. For this approach classical markers, like blood group polymorphisms and serological markers as well as RFLPs and VNTRs were used. The second and at least , successful approach, was the candidate gene approach. At the beginning of the study in 1988, only a few genes could be considered as weak candidates. In 1989, Leppert *et al.* reported on the localization of a gene responsible for benign familial neonatal epilepsy, located on chromosome 20q linked to the marker CMM6 (D20S19). This gene offered the first reasonable candidate locus for the low-voltage EEG study because both loci are involved in synchronization of neuronal brain activity.

Typing the low-voltage families with the highly polymorphic markers CMM6, one part of the families showed complete linkage between this marker and the low-voltage EEG, the other part of the families showed no linkage. Results like this are very suggestive of heterogeneity.

The data were tested with an admixture test for homogeneity. The results of this test were significant for heterogeneity and linkage. Significance was obtained for the hypothesis heterogeneity versus homogeneity linkage and for heterogeneity versus homogeneity and no linkage. The proportion of linked families was estimated to be 33 per cent, with a recombination fraction of zero for the linked part of families (Steinlein *et al.*, 1992b).

Summary of the linkage study:

(1) The low voltage EEG trait appears to be genetically heterogeneous;
(2) There is significant evidence for the localization of a gene on the distal part of the chromosome 20q, linked to marker CMM6.

Future studies will have to show if this gene is identical with the gene for the benign familial neonatal epilepsy, or if there are two different genes, located in the same chromosomal region, which are both involved in the synchronization of brain electrical activity.

After localization of a gene for the low-voltage EEG the next steps will have to be taken towards cloning of this gene. First, a physical map of the distal part of chromosome 20q has been constructed (Steinlein et al., 1992a). The pulsefield map revealed some unexpected results. The physical intervals between the polymorphic probes in the candidate region are markedly shorter than the genetic distances. For example, the distance between CMM6, the marker which gave the highest lod scores, and RMR6 (D20S20) can not be more than 200 kb. Reported recombination rates are between 1 and 2 per cent. But the most important finding is clusters of rare cutter sites around CMM6. These point to at least four closely related CpG islands. Such CpG islands are often associated with genes. The most closely related CpG islands should be reasonable within a few cosmid walks.

At the time of writing, more than 400kb of the region of interest have been cloned into cosmid and P1 clones. The contigs cover at least two of the CpG islands found in the physical map. The cosmids were hybridized on a human fetal brain cDNA library and several cDNAs belonging to at least three different genes have been isolated. Two of them are mainly or exclusively expressed in brain and will be therefore further characterized.

The Rotterdam group (D. Lindhout, W.F. Arts and D.J.J. Halley)

After the assignment of a gene for benign familial neonatal convulsions to chromosome 20q (Leppert et al., 1989), the Rotterdam group sent out a questionnaire to all Dutch child neurologists, asking for the description and referral of familial cases, to investigate whether linkage to chromosome 20q could be confirmed, whether genetic heterogeneity exists, and to delineate the phenotypic spectrum of chromosome 20q-linked benign familial neonatal convulsions. Five families with apparent benign familial neonatal convulsions were referred.

The largest family consisted of three generations with seven typically affected persons, acccording to the criteria agreed upon during this conference, and one unaffected but obligate carrier. Linkage analysis with the marker RMR6 and CMM6 revealed no cross-over in seven informative meioses between affected persons or obligate carriers only (Arts et al., 1991). Four unaffected relatives had the low-risk haplotype. One of the affected persons had undiagnosed and untreated seizures during the first six months of life, and this was the only patient in whom the clinical course was complicated by mental retardation, chronic epilepsy and spastic hemiplegia. Among eight relatives at less than 50 per cent risk of being a carrier of the gene defect but who did not comply with DNA analysis, four had epilepsy with onset after the age of 1 year, of whom two also had mental retardation. Of seven other relatives with less than 25 per cent risk of being a carrier but from whom also no blood for DNA analysis could be obtained, two had a history of febrile convulsions.

The four other families were small with a low number of potentially informative meioses and with an onset of seizures at between 3 and 12 months of life. All of these four families showed at least one obligate recombination with markers RMR6 or CMM6. This suggests that a phenotype similar to benign familial infantile convulsions (BFIC) is probably not linked to chromosome 20q. These families have not yet been examined for potential linkage to chromosome 8q, the region which seems to be involved in families with benign familial neonatal convulsions not linked to chromosome 20q and which seems to represent a more pure form of benign familial neonatal convulsions with narrower phenotypic spectrum (Lewis et al., 1993).

In general, the chromosome 20q-linked families seem to have a broader phenotypic spectrum and it is remarkable that in our largest chromosome 20q-linked family a patient with complicating mental retardation and chronic epilepsy is also found. The question whether this is secondary to seizure-induced hypoxia or ischaemia or represents a pleiotropic expression of the gene defect for benign familial neonatal convulsion will probably be resolved only by identification of the gene for benign familial neonatal convulsion itself, and by a subsequent study of the function of its protein product in the central nervous system.

The mother of this severely handicapped boy considered a subsequent pregnancy and requested genetic counselling. The limitations of prenatal diagnosis and the options of early postnatal evaluation and, if necessary, treatment were discussed. Once pregnant, she decided to have neonatal cord blood examined for the presence or absence of the high-risk chromosome 20q haplotye. Immediately after birth cord blood was obtained and DNA analysis demonstrated the high-risk haplotype. On the third day after birth, the baby started to have neonatal seizures, was admitted to the hospital, and treated with antiepileptic drugs. Seizures were controlled and psychomotor development up to the age of at least 1 year has reportedly been normal. This is probably the first case of BFNC in which DNA analysis was used in prenatal counselling and postnatal treatment.

References

Anokhin, A., Steinlein, O., Fischer, C., Yping, M., Vogt, P., Schalt, E. & Vogel, F. (1992): A genetic study of the human low-voltage electroencephalogram. *Hum. Genet.* **90**, 99–112.

Arts, W.F.M., Halley, D.I.J. & Lindhout, D. (1991): Benign familial neonatal convulsions. *Clin. Neurol. Neurosurg.* **93**, 352.

Aso, K. & Watanabe, K. (1992): Benign familial neonatal convulsions generalized epilepsy? *Pediatr. Neurol.* **8**, 226–238.

Bjerre, I. & Corelius, E. (1968): Benign famililal neonatal convulsions. *Acta Pediatr. Scand.* **571**, 557–561.

Hirsch, E., Velez, A., Sellal, F., Maton, B., Grinspan, A., Malafosse, A. & Marescaux C. (1993): Electroclinical signs of benign neonatal familial convulsions. *Ann. Neurol.* **34**, 835–841.

Leppert, M., Anderson, V.E., Quattlebaum, T., Stauffer, D., O'Donnell, P., Nakamura, Y., Lalouel, J.-M. & White, R. (1989): Benign familial neonatal convulsions linked to genetic markers on chromosome 20. *Nature* **337**, 647–648.

Leppert, M., McMahon, W.M., Quattlebaum, T.G., Bjerre, I., Zonana, J., Shevell, M.I., Andermann, E., Rosales, T.O., Ronen, G.M., Connolly, M. & Anderson, V.E. (1993): Searching for human epilepsy genes. A progress report. *Brain Pathol.* **3**, 357–369.

Lewis, T.B., Leach, R.J., Ward, K., O'Connell, P. & Ryan, S.G. (1993): Genetic heterogenity in benign familial neonatal convulsions: identification of a new locus on chromosome 8q. *Am. J. Hum. Genet.* **53**, 670–675.

Malafosse, A., Beck, C., Bellet, H., Di Capua, M., Dulac, O., Echenne, B., Fusco, L., Lucchini, P., Ricci, S., Sebastianelli, R., Feingold, J., Baldy-Moulinier, M. & Vigevano, F. (1994): Benign infantile familial convulsions are not an allelic form of the benign familial neonatal convulsions gene. *Ann. Neurol.* **35**, 479–482.

Malafosse, A., Leboyer, M., Dulac, O., Navelet, Y., Plouin, P., Beck, C., Laklou, H., Mouchino, G., Grandscene, P., Vallee, L., Guilloud-Bataille, M., Samolyk, D., Baldy-Moulinier, M., Feingold, J. & Mallet, J. (1992): Confirmation of linkage of benign familial neonatal convulsions to D20S20. *Hum. Genet.* **89**, 54–58.

Quattlebaum, T.G. (1979): Benign familial convulsions in the neonatal period and early infancy. *J. Pediatr.* **95**, 257–259.

Ronen, G.M., Rosales, T.O., Connolly, M., Anderson, V.E. & Leppert, M. (1993): Seizure characteristics in chromosome 20 benign familial neonatal convulsions. *Neurology* **43**, 1355–1360.

Shevell, M.L., Sinclair, D.B. & Metrakos, K. (1986): Benign familial neonatal seizures: clinical and electroencephalographic characteristics. *Pediatr. Neurol.* **2**, 272–275.

Steinlein, O., Fischer, C., Kell, R., Smigrodzki, R. & Vogel, F. (1992a): D20S19 linked to low voltage EEG, benign neonatal convulsions and Fanconi anaemia, maps to a region of enhanced recombination and is localized between CpG islands. *Hum. Mol. Genet.* **1**, 325–329.

Steinlein, O., Anokhnin, A., Yping, M., Schalt, E. & Vogel, F. (1992b): Localization of a gene for the human low-voltage EEG on 20q and genetic heterogeneity. *Genomics* **12**, 60–73.

Vogel, F. (1962): Ergänzende Untersuchungen zur Genetik des menschlichen Niedespannungs-EEG. *Dtsch. Z. Nervenheilk.* **184**, 101–111.

Vogel, F. (1970): The genetic basis of the normal human electroencephalogram (EEG). *Hum. Genet.* **10**, 91–114.

Vogel, F., Schalt, E. & Krüger, E. (1979): The electroencephalogram (EEG) as a research tool in human behavior genetics: psychological, examination in healthy male with various inherited EEG variants. II. Results. *Hum. Genet.* **47**, 47–80.

Zonana, J., Silvey, K., & Strimling, B. (1984): Familial neonatal and infantile seizures. An autosomal-dominant disorder. *Am. J. Med. Genet.* **18**, 455–459.

Part III
Absence seizures and absence epilepsy

Chapter 9

The clinical spectrum of typical absence seizures and absence epilepsies

C.P. Panayiotopoulos

Department of Clinical Neurophysiology and Epilepsy, St Thomas' Hospital, London SE1 7EH, UK

Introduction

Typical absences are defined by the International League against Epilepsy (ILAE) (Commission, 1981) as generalized epileptic seizures clinically characterized by impairment of consciousness only (simple absences) or impairment of consciousness combined with mild clonic, atonic, tonic, and autonomic components, and automatisms (complex absences). The ictal EEG signature of an absence attack is a bilateral, usually regular and symmetrical discharge of 3 Hz (2.5–4 Hz) spike- and slow-wave complexes. Sometimes, the discharge may consist of multiple spike- and slow-wave complexes. The background activity is usually normal although paroxysmal activity (such as spikes or spike- and slow-wave complexes) may occur.

We use the term typical absences to avoid confusion with atypical absences. During atypical absences, onset and/or cessation may be less abrupt, and changes in tone may be more pronounced than in typical absences. The ictal EEG is heterogeneous and may include irregular slow spike- and slow-wave complexes, fast activity or other paroxysmal activity. Abnormalities are bilateral but often irregular and asymmetrical and the background activity is usually abnormal (Commission, 1981).

'Typical' should not be mistaken with 'classical' or 'characteristic', a common error which is demonstrated by the following extract of an expert assessor's recent review on a paper dealing with 15 patients who had various idiopathic generalized epilepsies manifested with typical absences: 'Although they suggest that they are reporting findings in typical absences, only 6 of the 15 patients have what would be regarded by most people as typical absence seizures, i.e. childhood absence epilepsy'.

More importantly, typical absences are not one symptom, but a cluster of clinical features and EEG manifestations which are syndrome-related (Panayiotopoulos *et al.*, 1989, 1992). Although, by definition, impairment of consciousness is the cardinal clinical symptom and 3 Hz spike-and-wave EEG discharge the required bioelectrical feature, other clinical and EEG manifestations are combined in a non-fortuitous manner characterizing certain epileptic syndromes. Typical absences, as

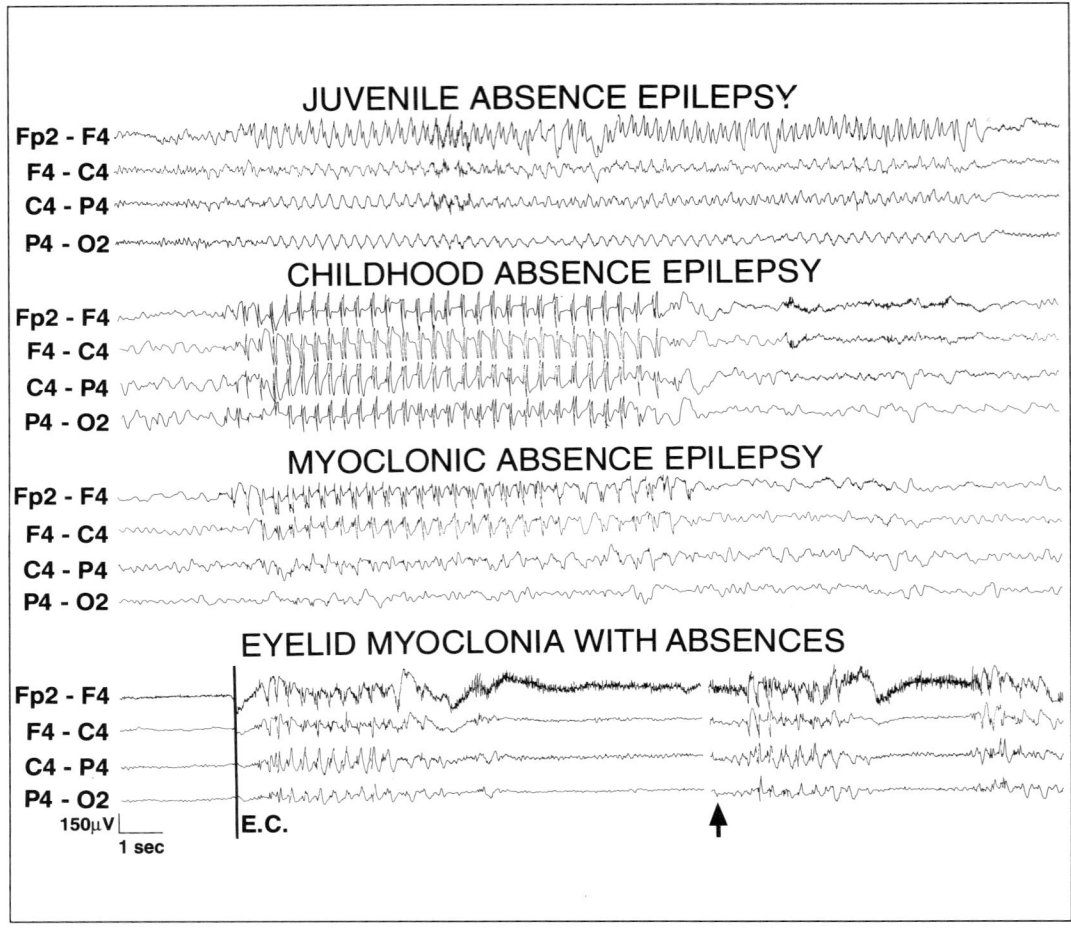

Fig. 1. From top to bottom, video-EEG of patients with juvenile absence epilepsy, childhood absence epilepsy, myoclonic absence epilepsy and eyelid myoclonia with absences (EC = eye-closure; the discharge following the arrow occurred while the eyes were closed). There are apparent EEG differences between these four epileptic syndromes but the final diagnosis has to rely also on clinical manifestations during these discharges (see text). Note the long discharges of juvenile absence epilepsy as opposed to brief ones of eyelid myoclonia with absences and the multiple spikes of myoclonic absence epilepsy and eyelid myoclonia with absences as opposed to maximum double/triple spikes of childhood absence epilepsy.

defined by ILAE, occur in many epileptic syndromes of diverse clinical manifestations, prognosis and response to treatment (Commission, 1981, 1989; Panayiotopoulos et al., 1989a, 1992, 1994).

There are four epileptic syndromes with typical absences recognized by the ILAE (Commission, 1989): childhood absence epilepsy (CAE), juvenile absence epilepsy (JAE), juvenile myoclonic epilepsy (JME), and myoclonic absence epilepsy (MAE). The first three of them (CAE, JAE, JME) are considered as idiopathic generalized epilepsies (IGE) whilst the fourth one (MAE) is categorized amongst the cryptogenic/symptomatic generalized epilepsies.

There may be more epileptic syndromes with typical absences like eyelid myoclonia with absences (Jeavons, 1977; Appleton et al., 1993), perioral myoclonia with absences (Panayiotopoulos et al., 1994), stimulus-sensitive absence epilepsy, and others awaiting further studies and confirmation.

Many of these syndromes are entirely different in presentation, severity and prognosis. Children with childhood absence epilepsy in their majority will remit, those with myoclonic absence epilepsy suffer from or may develop mental and behavioural problems and those with juvenile myoclonic epilepsy will, in their mid teens, develop lifelong myoclonic jerks and generalized tonic–clonic seizures (GTCS). Other patients may have subtle clinical manifestations during the typical 3 Hz spike-wave discharges of which they are not aware (phantom absences) (Ferner & Panayiotopoulos, 1993; Panayiotopoulos et al., 1994); they seek medical consultation only after a generalized tonic–clonic seizure develops, probably long after the onset of absences (Panayiotopoulos et al., 1992).

Recognized syndromes with typical absences

Childhood absence epilepsy (CAE)

Childhood absence epilepsy is defined by ILAE as an idiopathic generalized epileptic syndrome with onset of simple and complex absences at 4–8 years of age. They may be accompanied by upward deviation of the eyes and retropulsion of the head and trunk. Generalized tonic–clonic seizures develop in 30–40 per cent of the cases. The EEG discharge is 2.5–3.5 Hz. They are more frequent (pyknolepsy) and longer than the absences in juvenile myoclonic epilepsy (Commission, 1989; see for review Loiseau, 1992).

In accordance with this broad definition, which is inadequate to define an epileptic syndrome/disease, any child with frequent absences and 2.5–3.5 Hz spike- and slow-wave discharges should be diagnosed as having childhood absence epilepsy irrespective of severity of impairment of consciousness, ictal single or repetitive myoclonic jerks, variations of the ictal EEG discharge, occurrence of other types of seizures, prognosis and response to treatment. Studies on children and adult patients with absences indicate that the definition of childhood absence epilepsy should be revised in order to exclude patients who have absences with onset in childhood but belong to other epileptic syndromes (Panayiotopoulos et al., 1989a, 1992). For example, children with eyelid myoclonia with absences (EMA) best fulfil the ILAE definition of childhood absence epilepsy although they do not suffer from childhood absence epilepsy. Typical absences of eyelid myoclonia with absences, like those of childhood absence epilepsy, begin in childhood, occur frequently (hundreds per day) and are associated with 3–4 Hz spike- and slow-wave discharges. However, this resemblance is superficial. In eyelid myoclonia with absences, the absences are short, impairment of consciousness may be mild, eyelid myoclonia are consistent ictal clinical manifestations (fast clonic eyelid movements with probably a tonic element of contraction in eyelid myoclonia with absences as opposed to eyelid blinking-like movements occurring randomly or rhythmically in childhood absence epilepsy), patients are photosensitive, generalized tonic–clonic seizures are probably inevitable in all patients, and ictal EEGs consist mainly of brief (4–5 s) polyspike/slow-wave discharges (faster than in childhood absence epilepsy) induced by eye-closure. Furthermore, eyelid myoclonia with absences is resistant to monotherapy and does not remit in late childhood or adolescence (Appleton et al., 1993). Despite these characteristic features, eyelid myoclonia with absences is erroneously classified by many physicians as childhood absence epilepsy.

Similarly patients with juvenile myoclonic epilepsy may have onset of their disease in childhood with absence seizures: these may be frequent simple absences, with usually minor but occasionally severe impairment of consciousness (Panayiotopoulos, 1994a). A child with frequent absences, later developing myoclonic jerks and generalized tonic–clonic seizures, does not have childhood absence epilepsy evolving to juvenile myoclonic epilepsy: he has absences as the first manifestation of juvenile myoclonic epilepsy with onset in childhood.

Inclusion criteria

It has been shown that a child with childhood absence epilepsy demonstrates the following ictal symptoms (Panayiotopoulos et al., 1989a):

(a) The impairment of consciousness is very severe. There is no verbal or other response to commands and recollection of verbal ictal events is lost.

(b) The eyes open, overbreathing stops and speech discontinues within 3 s after the onset of the discharge.

(c) Automatisms occur in 2/3 of the seizures but are not stereotyped; the same patient may have simple and complex absences. Automatisms may be evoked by passive movements. Automatisms in absences indicate severe impairment of consciousness.

(d) Rhythmical blinking at 3 Hz is an infrequent, not sustained, feature. The eyes may stare but more frequently they move during the ictus, particularly if the child is loudly called by name.

(e) Retropulsive movements of the eyes and head, which characterize eyelid myoclonia with absences, are not a usual clinical feature of childhood absence epilepsy.

(f) The duration of absences in childhood absence epilepsy is shorter than in juvenile absence epilepsy.

The clinical manifestations above are associated with the following EEG features:

(a) The interictal EEG is normal or shows rhythmic posterior delta activity. Occasionally centro-temporal or occipital spikes may be seen.

(b) The ictal EEG shows generalized, spike- or double-spike (no more than three spikes are seen) and slow wave complexes at 3 Hz (no less than 2.7 Hz and no more than 4 Hz at the initial phase of the discharge; gradual, smooth decline in frequency from the initial to the terminal phase). The discharge is regular, with well-formed spikes which retain a constant relation with the slow-waves. The duration is usually around 10 s, no less than 4 s and no more than 20 s (Fig. 1).

Exclusion criteria

It is possible that one-third of patients diagnosed as childhood absence epilepsy who do not remit and may also develop generalized tonic–clonic seizures belong to other epileptic syndromes which are not childhood absence epilepsy, not recognized because of inadequate classification criteria. In view of this possibility we have introduced exclusion criteria, which at this stage of our knowledge may be as important as inclusion criteria.

Clinical exclusion criteria

(a) Absences with marked eyelid or perioral myoclonus (eyelid or perioral myoclonia with absences).

(b) Absences with marked limb and trunk rhythmic myoclonic jerks (myoclonic absence epilepsy).

(c) Absences with single ictal myoclonic jerks of the limbs, trunk or head (probably a new unrecognized syndrome of idiopathic myoclonic epilepsy).

(d) Absences with mild or not clinically detectable impairment of consciousness (juvenile myoclonic epilepsy is an example but other forms of IGE may manifest with similar absences).

(e) Other types of epileptic seizures are not part of childhood absence epilepsy. In particular, generalized tonic–clonic seizures or myoclonic jerks do not occur in childhood absence epilepsy but are common or may infrequently occur in other epileptic syndromes like juvenile myoclonic epilepsy, juvenile absence epilepsy, eyelid myoclonia with absences or perioral myoclonia with absences.

(f) Stimulus-sensitive absences: photosensitive, pattern-sensitive, self-induced pattern-sensitive or photosensitive, fixation-off sensitive or scoto-sensitive, and somato-sensory sensitive absences. All these reflex absences are often seen as part of certain epileptic syndromes (i.e. eyelid myoclonia with absences).

EEG exclusion criteria:

    (a) Discharge fragmentations and multiple spikes resembling capital Ws (more than three spikes per spike- and slow-wave complex). These are common in juvenile myoclonic epilepsy, eyelid myoclonia with absences, perioral myoclonia with absences, and absences with single ictal jerks.

    Discharge fragmentation is a transient discontinuation of a regular and rhythmical discharge, either by slower waves and/or complexes or by a true pause followed by a rapid, within 1 s, reactivation of the paroxysm.

    Ws are multiple spikes, preceding or superimposed on the slow waves of the discharge which have the appearance of compressed capital WWWs (Panayiotopoulos et al., 1989a).

    (b) Irregular, arrhythmical spike/multiple spike- and slow-wave discharges with marked variations of the intradischarge frequency.

    (c) Significant variations between the spike/multiple spike- and slow-wave relations.

    (d) Predominantly brief discharges of less than 4–5 s.

    (e) Abnormal background. However, focal abnormalities, particularly as the result of abortive discharges, are accepted. Posterior rhythmic slow activity is accepted and probably in favour of childhood absence epilepsy. Centrotemporal and occipital spikes may co-exist with childhood absence epilepsy.

Proposed definition of childhood absence epilepsy

In accordance with the above, the following definition for the disease of childhood absence epilepsy is proposed. Childhood absence epilepsy is a disease/syndrome of frequent (many per day), brief (6–14 s), typical absence seizures which occur in otherwise normal children. Age of onset is between 2 and 8 years of age, with a peak at 5 years. Remission occurs before the age of 12 years.

Clinically, there is abrupt and severe impairment (loss) of consciousness, with cessation of voluntary activity which is not restored during the ictus. The eyes spontaneously open, overbreathing, speech and other voluntary activity stop within the first 3 s from the onset of the discharge. Automatisms are frequent but have no significance in the diagnosis. The eyes stare or move slowly, random eyelid blinking (usually not sustained) may occur.

Eyelid myoclonia, perioral myoclonus, rhythmic massive limb jerking, single or arrhythmic myoclonic jerks of the head, trunk or limbs are not compatible with childhood absence epilepsy. Mild myoclonic elements of the eyes, eyebrows and eyelids may be a feature of childhood absence epilepsy but this has to be addressed in future prospective studies. Generalized tonic–clonic seizures and other types of seizures like myoclonic jerks should not be featured in childhood absence epilepsy. Visual (photic) and other sensory precipitation is most likely against a diagnosis of childhood absence epilepsy. Mild or no impairment of consciousness is not compatible with childhood absence epilepsy.

The EEG in childhood absence epilepsy has a normal background, with frequent rhythmic posterior delta activity. Ictal discharges consist of generalized high-amplitude spike and double (maximum occasional three spikes are allowed) spike- and slow-wave complexes. They are rhythmic at around 3 Hz (2.5–4 Hz) with a gradual and regular (0.5–1 Hz) slowdown from the initial to the terminal phase of the discharge. The initial phase of the discharge (1–2 s from the onset) is usually fast and unreliable for these measurements. There are no marked variations in the relation of spike to the slow wave, no fluctuations in the intradischarge frequency and certainly no fragmentations of the ictal discharges.

Juvenile absence epilepsy (JAE)

Juvenile absence epilepsy is also broadly defined by the ILAE (Commission, 1989; for review see Wolf, 1992) as follows: 'Onset around puberty. The absences are the same as in childhood absence

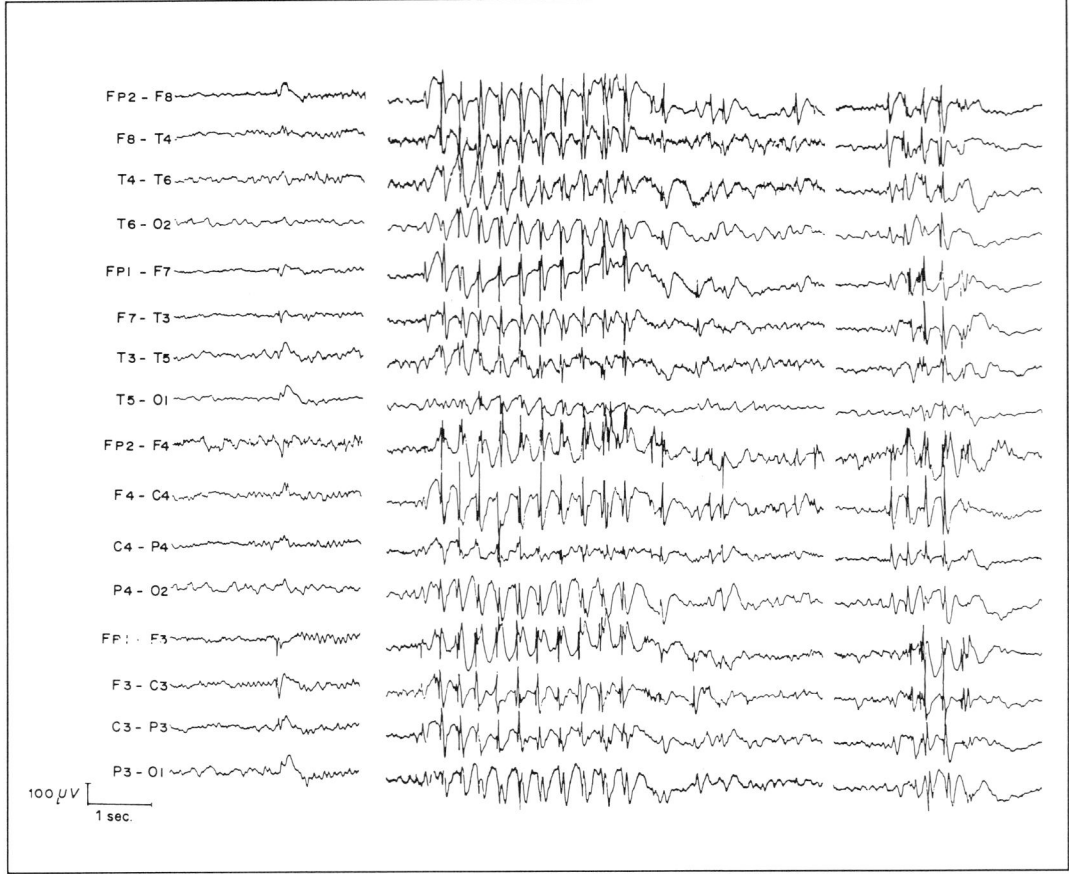

Fig. 2. EEG of a 22-year-old patient with juvenile myoclonic epilepsy. There were no apparent clinical manifestations. Note fragmentation of the discharges, multiple spike complexes (Ws), asymmetries and frequent focal abnormalities independently on right or left. (From Panayiotopoulos et al., 1994c with the permission of the Editor of Epilepsia).

epilepsy but retropulsive movements are less common. Seizure frequency is lower than in childhood absence epilepsy. Generalized tonic–clonic seizures are common, occur mainly on awakening and may precede the appearance of absences. The patients may also have myoclonic jerks. The prognosis is still unclear but appears worse than childhood absence epilepsy. The spike-wave discharge is often faster than 3 Hz'.

Juvenile absence epilepsy is the only syndrome in which the ictal manifestations of absence seizures show so many clinical and EEG similarities to those of childhood absence epilepsy (Panayiotopoulos *et al.*, 1989a). To simplify the matter, typical absences in juvenile absence epilepsy are similar but milder, less frequent and longer than those of childhood absence epilepsy.

Inclusion criteria

(a) Ictal clinical manifestations demonstrate profound impairment of consciousness which is not as severe as in childhood absence epilepsy. Awareness, perception, responsiveness, memory and recollection are deeply but not completely disturbed with marked variation in severity from seizure to seizure even in the same patient. The patient may temporarily and inadequately maintain some mild awareness and responsiveness during the absence ictus.

(b) Duration of absences is longer than in childhood absence epilepsy

(c) Typical absences is the predominant clinical feature but other seizures, rare random diurnal myoclonic jerks and generalized tonic–clonic seizures, may occur. Myoclonic jerks (which do not occur during the absence ictus) are mild and infrequent and do not show the circadian distribution of juvenile myoclonic epilepsy. Unlike juvenile myoclonic epilepsy, absences predominate over the other type of seizures in juvenile absence epilepsy.

(d) Age at onset is from 8–16 with a peak at 10–12 years. There is no justification in insisting on the arbitrary line that absences below 10 years of age is childhood absence epilepsy and above 10 years is juvenile absence epilepsy.

(e) EEG features are similar to those of childhood absence epilepsy. However, polyspikes and more rarely discharge fragmentations are seen in juvenile absence epilepsy (Fig. 1).

Exclusion criteria

Clinical exclusion criteria are similar and as significant as in childhood absence epilepsy:

(a) Absences with marked eyelid, perioral myoclonus or marked single or rhythmic limb and trunk rhythmic myoclonic jerks.

(b) Absences with mild, or not clinically detectable, impairment of consciousness.

EEG exclusion criteria:

(a) Irregular, arrhythmical spike/multiple spike- and slow-wave discharges with marked variations of the intradischarge frequency.

(b) Significant variations between the spike/multiple spike- and slow-wave relations.

(c) Predominantly brief discharges of less than 4–5 s.

(d) Abnormal background. Focal abnormalities, particularly as the result of abortive discharges, are accepted.

Proposed definition of juvenile absence epilepsy

Juvenile absence epilepsy is a syndrome of frequent (less than in childhood absence epilepsy), brief (usually longer than in childhood absence epilepsy), typical absence seizures which occur in otherwise normal older children and adolescents. Age of onset is between 8 and 16 years with a peak at 10–12 years. Remission is not expected although there is a tendency for the absences to become less severe with age.

Clinically, the typical absences are similar but less severe than those of childhood absence epilepsy. There is abrupt and severe impairment of consciousness, with cessation of voluntary activity which may be restored during the ictus. Eyelid myoclonia, perioral myoclonus, rhythmic massive limb jerking, solitary/single or arrhythmic myoclonic jerks of the head, trunk or limbs during the absence ictus are not compatible with juvenile absence epilepsy. Mild or no impairment of consciousness is not compatible with juvenile absence epilepsy. Generalized tonic–clonic seizures and myoclonia (usually random and infrequent) may occur but, unlike juvenile myoclonic epilepsy severe absences always predominate the clinical manifestations. Visual (photic) and other sensory precipitation is most likely against a diagnosis of juvenile absence epilepsy.

The EEG in juvenile absence epilepsy has a normal background. Ictal discharges are similar to those of childhood absence epilepsy but multiple spike are often manifested within the ictal generalized discharges.

Absences in juvenile myoclonic epilepsy (JMEA)

Absences in juvenile myoclonic epilepsy are also broadly described in the ILAE definition (Commission, 1989; see for review Janz, 1989): 'They occur in 30 per cent of patients with juvenile myoclonic epilepsy and are described as simple absences associated with fast 3.5–4 Hz spike/multiple spike and slow wave discharges'.

There are significant clinico-EEG differences between typical absences of juvenile myoclonic epilepsy and those of other epileptic syndromes (Panayiotopoulos, 1994b; Panayiotopoulos et al., 1989a,b):

(a) Clinical absences occur in one-third of the patients with juvenile myoclonic epilepsy. Early onset absences predate myoclonic jerks and/or generalized tonic–clonic seizures, sometimes by as long as 9 years. Absences are not antedated by myoclonic jerks or generalized tonic–clonic seizures. Thus children with typical absences of juvenile myoclonic epilepsy may erroneously be diagnosed as suffering from childhood absence epilepsy or juvenile absence epilepsy.

(b) The clinical severity of absences appears to be age-related. The earlier the onset the more severe is the disturbance of consciousness. Older children may show only subtle, mild clinical manifestations which often escape recognition (Panayiotopoulos et al., 1989b). There are not myoclonic jerks or automatisms during the absence ictus.

(c) EEG discharges are not as rhythmic and as regular as in childhood and juvenile absence epilepsy. The discharge is often interrupted (discharge fragmentation); the intradischarge frequency of the spike/multiple spike- and slow-wave complexes show great variations in frequency (6–8 Hz to 1–2 Hz); there is no constant relation between spike/multiple spike- and slow-waves; there are frequent multiple spikes which look like compressed capital Ws; the slowdown of the frequency of the discharge is irregular and not consistent (Fig. 2).

The above findings indicate that there are significant differences between typical absences of juvenile myoclonic epilepsy and those of other epileptic syndromes (Panayiotopoulos et al., 1989a). This may not be of practical significance in a patient who is seen when the full picture of juvenile myoclonic epilepsy has developed. However, they are important when one has to decide whether a child with typical absences is going to develop juvenile myoclonic epilepsy (a lifelong disease) or suffers from childhood absence epilepsy (an age-limited and age-related disease).

Myoclonic absence epilepsy (MAE)

Myoclonic absence epilepsy is a relatively recently recognized syndrome defined as follows (Commission, 1989; Tassinari et al., 1992): 'Absences with severe bilateral, rhythmical myoclonias, often associated with a tonic contraction. EEG with 3 Hz spike and slow wave discharge similar to that observed in childhood absence epilepsy (Fig. 1). The age of onset is about 7 years with poor prognosis and response to treatment'.

Marked bilateral and rhythmic myoclonic jerks during the absence ictus and mental handicaps (occurring in 50 per cent of these children) differentiate easily this syndrome from others with typical absences.

Newly individualized syndromes with typical absences

Eyelid myoclonia with absences (EMA)

Eyelid myoclonia with absences is a syndrome not yet recognized by the ILAE although vividly described by Jeavons (1977; see also Appleton et al., 1993). 'The characteristic seizure is a brief episode of marked jerking of the eyelids with upwards deviation of the eyes, associated with a generalized discharge of spike-wave, and occurring on closure of the eyes. All patients are photosensitive. The mean age of onset is 6 years. Prognosis is not as good as childhood absence epilepsy and remission is not usually expected. We have seen adult patients with this syndrome who responded well to combined treatment with sodium valproate and ethosuximide'.

In our experience and that of others (Appleton et al., 1993), eyelid myoclonia with absences is a common epileptic syndrome which is frequently misdiagnosed in children as childhood absence epilepsy despite marked differences and characteristic features. The following definition is proposed. Eyelid myoclonia with absences is manifested with frequent (pyknolepsy) typical absences with onset in early childhood (2–5 years, earlier than childhood absence epilepsy). Absences are brief (3–6 s), occur after eye-closure and demonstrate marked rhythmic eyelid myoclonias consisting of fast jerks of the eyelids (clearly different from the eyelid blinking-like, random or rare unsustained rhythmic movements of childhood absence epilepsy) and retropulsion of the eyeballs with an associated tonic component of the involved muscles. Impairment of consciousness may be mild and certainly not as severe as in childhood absence epilepsy and juvenile absence epilepsy. EEG ictal manifestations consist mainly of 3–5 Hz polyspike and slow-wave discharges (Fig. 1), which are more likely to be induced by eye-closure in an illuminated recording room (*total* darkness abolishes the eye-closure related abnormalities). All patients are highly photosensitive and self-induction may occur in some patients. Generalized tonic–clonic seizures, induced by light or spontaneous, are probably inevitable in all patients.

Furthermore, eyelid myoclonia with absences is resistant to monotherapy and does not remit in adulthood. Absences may become more infrequent with age, and eye-closure EEG abnormalities may persist without demonstrable photosensitivity.

Some patients may exhibit marked eyelid myoclonia as in eyelid myoclonia with absences but with more marked tonic components of the eyelids and the eyes which are often deviated to one side. The ictal EEG manifestations consist mainly of generalized polyspikes which are induced by eye-closure (the patients are also photosensitive) or are related to closed eyes (the patients have fixation-off sensitivity; Panayiotopoulos, 1987). The nosological categorization of these patients is uncertain.

Eyelid myoclonia with absences may be seen in patients with learning and behavioural problem which, though not belonging in the idiopathic generalized epilepsies, is again difficult to categorize.

Perioral myoclonus with absences

It has been recently reported (Panayiotopoulos et al., 1994) that absences associated with marked perioral myoclonus may constitute a new epileptic syndrome which is defined as follows: 'Perioral myoclonus with absences is a syndrome of idiopathic generalized epilepsy with onset in childhood or adolescence, characterized by frequent typical absences with variable severity of impairment of consciousness (mild or severe) and ictal localized rhythmic myoclonus of the perioral facial muscles (lip myoclonus) or occasionally of the masticatory muscles (jaw myoclonus).

Absences may be brief (2–4 s) or more prolonged (6–10 s) and patients are at high risk of absence status. Generalized tonic–clonic seizures always occur either early or many years after the onset of absences; they are usually heralded by clusters of absences or absence status. The disease is life long and often resistant to medication. There is no photosensitivity. Ictal EEG shows brief, high amplitude and frequent discharges of spikes, more often polyspike and slow wave at 3–5 Hz i.e. they are similar to those seen in eyelid myoclonia with absences, but they are not associated with eye-closure and photosensitivity.

Absences with single, non-rhythmic myoclonia

Absences manifested with moderate impairment of consciousness and single, solitary, non-rhythmic myoclonic jerks of the limbs, trunk, neck or facial muscles and EEG multiple spike and slow wave discharges at 2.5–4 Hz have not yet been studied in detail. In our own experience, there is a strong family history of similar absences, absences persist but improve with age, generalized tonic–clonic seizures are infrequent and there is usually resistance to monotherapy with sodium valproate (Panayiotopoulos et al., 1992).

Late-onset absence status and phantom absences

Absence status is considered to be seen mainly amongst female patients in their thirties, who often do not have a previous history of epilepsy (Roger *et al.*, 1974). However, we have seen cases of 'late-onset absence status' without known previous history of seizures who, on questioning had frequent mild episodes of impairment of consciousness probably since childhood (Panayiotopoulos *et al.*, 1992, 1993; Ferner & Panayiotopoulos, 1993). Their 'interictal' video-EEG showed 3–4 Hz spike and/or polyspike and slow wave discharges during which the patients demonstrated mild clinical signs mainly consisting of errors in breath-counting performance or eyelid fluttering. This indicates that they had been suffering for many years from typical absences which were not detected (phantom absences) because of their mild clinical symptomatology (Panayiotopoulos *et al.*, 1994b). A new syndrome of phantom absences and generalized tonic–clonic seizures may exist.

Reflex absences

Typical absences may be induced by flickering lights (photosensitivity), patterns (pattern sensitivity), elimination of central vision and fixation (fixation-off sensitivity), somatosensory and probably other stimuli. Self-induced absences have also been described. These reflex absences are seen either independently or within the broad framework of certain epileptic syndromes. It is beyond the purposes of this presentation to expand on them but this is another area to study and classify.

Symptomatic and secondary generalized typical absences

As opposed to atypical absences which are usually symptomatic or cryptogenic, typical absences are usually idiopathic. However, symptomatic typical absences have been described rarely mainly in patients with frontal lobe structural lesions (Ferrie *et al.*, 1994). In symptomatic typical absences there is no clinical or EEG evidence of an epileptic focus. They are generalized from the onset although one expects them to be secondarily generalized, i.e. the focal structural lesion must be responsible by generating a focus which rapidly triggers off the generalized 3 Hz spike- and slow-wave discharge (Panayiotopoulos *et al.*, 1992). We have also seen a patient with frontal lobe epilepsy who had limb and eyelid myoclonic absences which were secondary generalized. There was no demonstrable lesion.

Conclusion

In conclusion, there are significant syndrome-related clinical and EEG differences of typical absences requiring further prospective studies. Reports claiming overlapping of childhood absence epilepsy or juvenile absence epilepsy with juvenile myoclonic epilepsy, childhood absence epilepsy evolving to juvenile myoclonic epilepsy and the hypothesis of a biological continuum of absences (Bercovic *et al.*, 1987) may be theoretically attractive but should not be accepted without great reservations, because no attempt is made to classify the absence syndromes as 'clusters of symptoms and signs which occur in a non fortuitous manner' (see Commission 1989). Instead, absences are studied in a unitary fashion and patients are classified as having or not having absences with 3 Hz spike- and slow-wave discharges. This is an oversimplification which discourages diagnostic precision. Even if the various absence syndromes were phenotypic variations of the same genetic trait, existing differences in their prognosis and management makes their differentiation mandatory. Otherwise, we run the risk of regression to the old 'petit mal' attitude.

Acknowledgements

I wish to thank British Telecom Charitable Organisation and the Special Trustees of St Thomas' Hospital for their grants for my studies on the classification of epilepsies.

References

Appleton, R., Panayiotopoulos, C.P., Acomb, A.B. & Beirne, M. (1993): Eyelid myoclonia with absences: an epilepsy syndrome. *J. Neurol. Neurosurg. Psychiatry* **56**, 1312–1316.

Berkovic, S.F., Andermann, F., Andermann, E. & Gloor, P. (1987): Concepts of absence epilepsies: discrete syndromes or biological continuum? *Neurology* **37**, 993–1000.

Commission on Classification and Terminology of the International League against Epilepsy (1981): Proposed revisions of clinical and electroencephalographic classification of epileptic seizures. *Epilepsia* **22**, 480–501.

Commission on Classification and Terminology of the International League against Epilepsy (1989): Proposal for classification of epilepsies and epileptic syndromes. *Epilepsia* **30**, 389–399.

Ferner, R.E. & Panayiotopoulos, C.P. (1993): 'Phantom' typical absences, absence status and experiential phenomena. *Seizure* **2**, 253–256.

Ferrie, C.D., Giannakodimos, S., Robinson, R.O. & Panayiotopoulos, C.P. (1994): Symptomatic typical absences. In: *Typical absences and related epileptic syndromes*, eds. J.S. Duncan & C.P. Panayiotopoulos, London: Churchill Livingston (in press).

Janz, D. (1989): Juvenile myoclonic epilepsy. Epilepsy with impulsive petit mal. *Clev. Clin. J. Med.* Suppl, part I, **56**, S23–S33.

Jeavons, P.M. (1977): Nosological problems of myoclonic epilepsies in childhood and adolescence. *Dev. Med. Child. Neurol.* **19**, 3–8.

Loiseau, P. (1992): Childhood absence epilepsy. In: *Epileptic syndromes in infancy, childhood and adolescence*, eds. J. Roger, M. Bureau, C. Dravet, F.E. Dreifus, A. Perret & P. Wolf, pp. 135–150. London: John Libbey.

Panayiotopoulos, C.P. (1987): Fixation-off sensitive epilepsy in eyelid myoclonia with absence seizures. *Ann. Neurol.* **22**, 87–89.

Panayiotopoulos, C.P., Obeid, T. & Waheed, G. (1989a): Differentiation of typical absence seizures in epileptic syndromes. A video EEG study of 224 seizures in 20 patients. *Brain* **112**, 1039–1056.

Panayiotopoulos, C.P., Obeid, T. & Waheed, G. (1989b): Absences in juvenile myoclonic epilepsy: a clinical and video- electroencephalographic study. *Ann. Neurol.* **25**, 391–397.

Panayiotopoulos C.P., Chroni, E., Dascalopoulos, C., Baker, A, Rowlinson, S. & Welsh, P. (1992): Typical absences in adults: a clinical, EEG, video-EEG study and syndromic/diagnostic considerations. *J. Neurol. Neurosurg. Psychiatry* **55**, 1002–1008.

Panayiotopoulos, C.P., Baker, A., Grunewald, R., Rowlinson, S. & Welsh, P. (1993): Breath counting during 3 Hz generalised spike and wave discharges. *J. Electrophysiol. Technol.* **19**, 15–23.

Panayiotopoulos, C.P. (1994a): Fixation-off sensitive epilepsies: clinical and EEG characteristics. In: *Epileptic seizures and syndromes*, ed. P. Wolf, London: John Libbey (in press).

Panayiotopoulos, C.P. (1994b): Diagnosing juvenile myoclonic epilepsy: an underdiagnosed syndrome. In: *Epileptic seizures and syndromes*, ed. P. Wolf. London: John Libbey (in press).

Panayiotopoulos, C.P., Ferrie, C., Giannakodimos, S. & Robinson, R. (1994a): Perioral myoclonia with absences: A new syndrome? In: *Epileptic seizures and syndromes*, ed. P. Wolf. London: John Libbey (in press).

Panayiotopoulos, C.P., Roger, J., Lob, H. & Tassinari, C.A. (1974): Generalised status epilepticus expressed as a confusional state (petit mal status or absence status epilepticus) In: *Handbook of clinical neurology*, Vol. 15, eds. P.L. Vinken & G.W. Bruyn, pp. 167–196. Amsterdam: North Holland Publishing Co.

Panayiotopoulos, C.P., Giannakodimos, S. & Chroni, E. (1994B): Typical absences in adults. In: *Typical absences and related epileptic syndromes*, eds. J.S. Duncan & C.P. Panayiotopoulos. London: Churchill Livingstone (in press).

Panayiotopoulos, C.P., Obeid, T. & Tahun, A.R. (1994c): Juvenile myoclonic epilepsy: a 5-year prospective study. *Epilepsia* **35**, 285–296.

Tassinari, C.A., Bureau, M. & Thomas, P. (1992): Epilepsy with myoclonic absences. In: *Epileptic syndromes in infancy, childhood and adolescence*, eds. J. Roger, M. Bureau, C. Dravet, F.E. Dreifus, A. Perret & P. Wolf, pp. 151–160. London: John Libbey.

Wolf, P. (1992): Juvenile absence epilepsy. In: *Epileptic syndromes in infancy, childhood and adolescence*, eds. J. Roger, M. Bureau, C. Dravet, F.E. Dreifus, A. Perret & P. Wolf, pp. 307–312. London: John Libbey.

Chapter 10

What are the relevant criteria for a better classification of epileptic syndromes with typical absences?

E. Hirsch[*†], A. Blanc-Platier[†] and C. Marescaux[*†]

[*]INSERM U 398, [†]Unité d'Explorations Fonctionnelles des Epilepsies, Hôpitaux Universitaires, 1 place de l'Hôpital, 67091 Strasbourg Cedex, France

Introduction

Numerous genetic, pharmacological and semiological data suggest that epilepsies with typical absences do not constitute a homogeneous entity either in humans or in animals. Genetic characteristics of the different strains of rodents with spontaneous absences are not uniform. Bilateral and synchronous electroencephalographic (EEG) spike-and-wave discharges (SWD) can be either a recessive or dominant trait. Several mutations affecting distinct chromosomes have been reported: they appear to be correlated with phenotypical variations, frequency and duration of seizures, associated neurological symptoms, etc. (Noebels, Chapter 20; Vergnes & Marescaux, Chapter 15; Hosford et al., Chapter 18). In humans, the heterogeneity of absence epilepsies is well accepted and individualization of multiple syndromes has been proposed. Attempts of classification are based on different criteria (for review, see Panayiotopoulos, Chapter 9) related to evolution (e.g. ages of onset and offset, pharmacological reactivity, remission with treatment, with or without relapses, seizures persistence) and to symptoms (e.g. interictal state, existence of other types of seizures and, most importantly, the ictal behavioural and EEG symptoms).

Since 1987, we have regularly followed patients where typical absences had been recorded using both EEG and video. Our aim is to characterize the discriminant factors which allow us to differentiate easily different homogeneous sub-groups. This paper presents preliminary data of this study.

Patients and methods

Data were collected from 43 patients (a total of 570 absences were recorded) who have been followed for at least two years.

The only criterion for including a patient in the study was the video-EEG recording of typical absences defined by complete, or almost complete, loss of responsiveness, concomitant with bilateral and synchronous spike-and-wave discharges with a rhythmicity of 2–4 Hz (Loiseau, 1992;

Berkovic, 1993b; Panayiotopoulos, Chapter 9). The only criterion for excluding a patient from this study was the existence of cerebral lesions as evidenced by neuroradiological examination, or suspected because of major neurological and/or neuropsychological abnormalities. These criteria allowed us to avoid any selection bias and to take into account only idiopathic generalized epilepsies.

Video-EEG recordings were carried out for about 2 h: they included several hyperventilation and one intermittent light stimulation (ILS). Interictal EEG abnormalities, precipitating factors and electroclinical signs of each absence were analysed. The patient history indicated the sex, the age of onset, the possible association with other types of seizures and family history. Several video-EEG recordings performed every year allowed us to evaluate the course of the disease under treatment.

Results

Four groups of patients can be differentiated on the basis of (i) their evolution under treatment, (ii) the possible co-existence of generalized tonic–clonic seizures (GTCS) and (iii) the nature of precipitating factors (Tables 1 & 2).

Table 1. Main characteristics in four groups of patients

	Group I	Group II	Group III	Group IV
Number of patients:	23	5	4	11
Male	13	2	0	6
Female	10	3	4	5
Age of onset				
Range	2–16	9–14	3–9	1–14
< 4	2	0	1	2
4–8	17	0	2	6
> 8	4	5	1	3
Family history of IGE				
None	16	4	1	6
1st degree	1	0	3	2
2nd degree	2	1	0	1
≥ 3rd degree	4	0	0	2
Precipitating factors				
Awakening	0	2	0	0
Hyperventilation	23	3	0	10
ILS	0	0	4	1
Ictal EEG				
2.5–4 Hz only	23	5	4	11
Polyspikes preceding 2.5–4 Hz	0	0	4	4
Duration of absences				
Mean ± SE	8.0 ± 0.2	9.6 ± 0.7	4.6 ± 0.2	13.7 ± 1.0
Range	3–27	3–25	3–17	3–80
Interictal EEG				
Normal	14	5	4	8
Posterior delta	9	0	0	3

Chapter 10 What are the relevant criteria for a better classification of absence epilepsies

Table 2. Main clinical characteristics of typical complex absences in four groups of patients (several symptoms could be observed in the same patient)

	Group I	Group II	Group III	Group IV
Automatisms	20	4	4	10
Mild clonic and/or tonic components	6	5	4	6
Rhythmic eyelid blinking	6	4	0	3
Eyelid myoclonias	4	0	4	2
Eyeball myoclonias	0	0	1	1
Tonic eyeball movements	11	3	2	3
Perioral myoclonias	6	0	0	0
Sustained bilateral myoclonic jerks	3	0	0	1
Autonomic components	3	1	0	3

Group I was characterized by the existence of isolated absences, never associated with any other types of seizures and their quick remission after less than six months of treatment. This group included 23 patients (13 men and 10 women) and 313 absences were recorded. About 30 per cent of the patients had a positive family history of primary generalized epilepsy (absence or generalized tonic–clonic seizures), generally in second or third degree relatives. The age of onset was between 2 and 16 years. The absences could occur spontaneously but in all patients hyperventilation was a precipitating factor, whereas intermittent light stimulation remained without effect. One of the patients displayed only simple absences, 10 gave an association of simple and complex absences and 12 showed only complex absences. Besides the loss of responsiveness, itcal symptoms varied in a given patient from one absence to another. These symptoms were associated with automatisms, moderated clonic and/or tonic components of the limbs and different types of eyelid and eye movements (rhythmic blinking, myoclonias, tonic deviation of the eyeballs). Perioral myoclonias were observed in six patients and marked myoclonias of the limbs and body axis in three.

Ictal EEG was very uniform and showed a bilateral and synchronous spike-and-wave discharges, with a rhythmicity of 2.5 to 4 Hz, lasting between 3 and 27 s. Interictal EEG was normal or revealed, in nine out of 23 patients, delta activity at the level of the posterior derivations which disappeared upon opening of the eyes.

One patient was treated with ethosuximide (ESM) only. All the others were treated with sodium valproate (VPA). This monotherapy was effective in 15 patients. In seven patients, ethosuximide was associated 2–4 months later because absences persisted. The seven patients requiring polytherapy had 'typical' absences (n = 5) or absences with perioral myoclonias or marked myoclonias of the limbs (n = 2).

Group II was characterized by the association of a few generalized tonic–clonic seizures with absences. In this small group of five patients (two men and three women), 42 absences were recorded. A family history of absence epilepsy and/or generalized tonic–clonic seizures in second or third degree relatives was noted in one case. Absences were spontaneous or precipitated by awakening or hyperventilation. The age of onset was between 9 and 14 years. Absences preceded generalized tonic–clonic seizures in three cases and occurred afterwards in two cases. Clinical and EEG symptoms were similar to those of Group I. In this limited population, no perioral myoclonia nor any marked myoclonia were ever recorded. Both absences and generalized tonic–clonic seizures were completely controlled by VPA alone.

Group III was characterized by the association of a few generalized tonic–clonic seizures with absences and the triggering of seizures by intermittent light stimulation. This group included only four girls who had a total of 96 absence seizures during video-EEG recording. Three patients had a positive family history in first degree relatives: six relatives (five women and a man) were affected by the same syndrome. Absence seizures occurred for the first time between 3 and 9 years of age. They were rarely spontaneous and were triggered most of the time by light stimulation as encountered in everyday life (sun, flashing lights, television, video games, etc.). Conscious or unconscious self-stimulation was noted in two of the four patients and was reported in several relatives (e.g. rapid blinking of the eyelids in front of a light source or prolonged immobility with the face close to a television set). The most frequent ictal motor symptoms associated with absence seizures were eyelid myoclonias and myoclonias or tonic deviation of the eyeballs. Ictal eyelids myoclonias were in fact difficult to dissociate from the self-triggering voluntary blinking.

On the EEG recording, light-induced absences started with a short polyspike discharge followed by a typical spike-and-wave discharge. The total duration of EEG seizures was short (3–17 s).

In these patients and their relatives, a valproate monotherapy or the combination of valproate and ethosuximide controlled the seizures. However, relapses were frequent during withdrawal attempts, even when the patients were adult. In addition, compliance with the treatment was often poor, probably due to the need of self-stimulation.

Group IV was characterized by the persistence of absence seizures two years after the beginning of a treatment. In these 11 patients (six men and five women), a total of 119 absence seizures, often long lasting (3–80 s) were recorded. Family history, age of onset and ictal symptoms were quite variable among patients. The real common denominator of this group of patients was the ineffectiveness of the treatment. In five cases, a correct diagnosis had been established and the drugs prescribed appeared appropriate (valproate alone or combined with ethosuximide) but dosages were too low and treatment durations too short (less than 12 months). In six cases, erroneous diagnosis of partial seizures was made because of interictal focal abnormalities, asymmetrical onsets of spike-and-wave discharges or misleading symptoms (long lasting automatisms, lateralized myoclonias). Because of this, unadapted treatments had been prescribed (i.e. carbamazepine, phenytoin, phenobarbital or vigabatrin). In these six patients, whatever the previous time course, stopping the aggravating compounds and introducing an adapted treatment at high doses (valproate alone or combined with ethosuximide and/or lamotrigine) allowed us to totally suppress absence seizures (four cases) or to reduce them by more than 90 per cent (two cases).

Discussion

Overall, when comparing the different groups that we have characterized in the present study with the usual classification of absence epilepsies, Group I roughly corresponds to childhood absence epilepsy, Group II to juvenile absence epilepsy and Group III to eyelid myoclonia with absences (Panayiotopoulos, Chapter 9). However, there is no strict matching between the two classifications and the similarities and discrepancies require us to address several questions of terminology.

Should absence epilepsies be classified according to the age of onset? In the present study, the age of onset does not appear to be an absolute criterion because it allows much overlapping between the different syndromes. This is consistent with the literature. Some absence epilepsies starting after the age of 10–12 are described as childhood absences, whereas some others starting between 8 and 10 are considered as juvenile absences. Moreover, this type of classification does not take evolution into account: generalized tonic–clonic seizures occur in 80 per cent of absence epilepsies classified as juvenile but also in 30–40 per cent of those classified as childhood absences (Aicardi, 1986; Covanis et al., 1992; Loiseau, 1992; Wolf, 1992; Berkovic, 1993a, b; Panayiotopoulos, Chapter 9). As a matter of fact, according to data from the literature and from our own study, three conditions are generally associated with the occurrence of generalized tonic–clonic seizures in so-called childhood absences: a late onset after the age of 8, a pronounced photosensitivity and an inadequate treatment (Covanis et al., 1992; Loiseau, 1992).

Should absence epilepsies be classified according to ictal symptoms? Discrete semiological differences appear to dissociate juvenile absences from childhood absences: the intensity of loss of responsiveness, the duration and number of seizures, the EEG pattern of the discharges (Panayiotopoulos, Chapter 9). In a more demonstrative way, three symptoms have been individualized and named according to motor symptoms observed during absence seizures.

Epilepsy with myoclonic absences has been taken into account by the International Classification (Aicardi, 1986; Tassinari et al., 1992; Roger et al., 1993; Panayiotopoulos, this volume). The main characteristic of this type of absence seizures is the existence of rhythmic myoclonias of the limbs. These pronounced myoclonias may not be sufficient, however, to individualize a new form of absences. They could correspond, in some cases, to a simple exaggeration of the moderate clonic component usually described during typical absence seizures (Aicardi, 1986; Loiseau, 1992; Berkovic, 1993a, b). Epilepsy with myoclonic absences does not appear as a homogeneous entity. Some patients show mental retardation, are resistant to the treatments and sometimes evolve toward a Lennox–Gastaut syndrome. Bad prognosis appears to be correlated with personal antecedents, occurrence of generalized tonic–clonic seizures, falls during the seizures and inappropriate treatment, more than with the severity of the myoclonias (Aicardi, 1986; Tassinari et al., 1992; Roger et al., 1993). In other patients, the seizures are suppressed by a combination of valproate and ethosuximide (Tassinari et al., 1992; Roger et al., 1993). The three cases with pronounced myoclonias reported in the present study (Table 1) may correspond to this type of favourable evolution.

Absences with perioral myoclonias have been individualized by Panayiotopoulos (Chapter 9). They may not only represent a particular form of absences but define a specific syndrome with more severe evolution. However, myoclonias of moderate intensity, involving the lips and the chin, are often observed during typical childhood or juvenile absences (Loiseau, 1992; Berkovic, 1993a, b; Serratosa & Delgado-Escueta, 1993). The distinction between a moderate myoclonic component and a pronounced myoclonia appears too subjective to individualize a syndrome. In the present study, the six patients having absence seizures associated with clear perioral myoclonias, could not be distinguished from patients displaying other clinical symptoms during typical absence seizures (Table 2).

Absences with eyelid myoclonias have been individualized for many years (Binnie & Jeavons, 1992; Panayiotopoulos, this volume). By themselves, eyelids myoclonias are not specific. They may occur during childhood absences, sometimes as a slow blinking of the eyelids (Loiseau, 1992; Berkovic, 1993a, b; Serratosa & Delgado-Escueta, 1993). They are also observed during some seizures of juvenile myoclonic epilepsy (Binnie & Jeavons, 1992). In our study, several other characteristics individualize the so-called eyelid myoclonia with absences: the mode of transmission, the evolution and, most of all, the photosensitivity with self-stimulation.

What are the prognosis factors of absence epilepsies? In the present study, neither the age of onset nor the ictal symptoms are correlated with the prognosis. The only characteristics which have some influence on the evolution of the patients are (i) the type of seizures which are associated with absences, (ii) the nature of triggering factors, and (iii) the choice of treatment. All idiopathic absences are sensitive to pharmacological treatment but the probability of relapses upon treatment withdrawal is higher when absence seizures are associated with generalized tonic–clonic seizures, in particular in photosensitive patients (Covanis et al., 1992). Valproate alone or combined with ethosuximide (and/or lamotrigine) is the standard treatment. Its early and systematic use has very likely increased the number of remissions and considerably reduced the probability of secondary generalized tonic–clonic seizures (Covanis et al., 1992; Loiseau, 1992; Berkovic, 1993a, b). On the contrary, many antiepileptic compounds (carbamazepine, phenytoin, phenobarbital, vigabatrin) aggravate absence seizures and facilitate their persistence until adulthood (Snead, Chapter 14; Vergnes & Marescaux, Chapter 15).

Conclusion

A precise symptomatic approach of absence epilepsies, taking into account the age of onset and the main ictal signs, is certainly justified to select patients and families which can be included in molecular genetic studies. The results of these studies will then allow us to establish with certainty the syndromic classification of absence epilepsies and to confirm, or invalidate, the current nosological hypotheses. Up to now, in daily clinical practice, the multiplication of syndromic sub-categories does not appear relevant, either to chose a treatment, or to establish a prognosis. The only reliable clinical criteria about the course of the disease appears to be the early onset of generalized tonic–clonic seizures and the nature of the precipitating factors (hyperventilation or intermittent light stimulation). The terms 'childhood absence epilepsies', 'juvenile absence epilepsies' and 'eyelid myoclonia with absences' can be misleading and we propose to individualize three categories: (i) 'pure' absence epilepsy; (ii) generalized epilepsy with absences and tonic–clonic seizures; (iii) generalized epilepsy with photosensitive absences and tonic–clonic seizures.

Finally, the type of initial treatment is the key determinant of the prognosis. The only useful therapy is valproate alone or combined with ethosuximide (and/or lamotrigine). All the other antiepileptic compounds, besides benzodiazepines, are not only without effect but may even be aggravating.

References

Aicardi, J. (1986): Epilepsies with typical absence seizures. In: *Epilepsy in children*, ed. J. Aicardi, pp. 79–99. New York: Raven Press.

Berkovic, S.F. (1993a): Childhood absence epilepsy and juvenile absence epilepsy. In: *The treatment of epilepsy: principles and practice*, ed. E. Wyllie, pp. 547–551. Philadelphia: Lea & Febiger.

Berkovic, S.F. (1993b): Generalized absence seizures. In: *The treatment of epilepsy: principles and practice*, ed. E. Wyllie, pp. 401–410. Philadelphia: Lea & Febiger.

Binnie, C. & Jeavons, P. (1992): Photosensitive epilepsies. In: *Epileptic syndromes in infancy, childhood and adolescence*, 2nd edn, eds. J. Roger, M. Bureau, Ch. Dravet, F.E. Dreifuss, A. Perret & P. Wolf, pp. 299–305. London: John Libbey.

Covanis, A., Skiadas, K., Loli, N., Lada, C. & Theodorou, V. (1992): Absence epilepsy: early prognostic signs. *Seizure* 1, 281–289.

Hosford, D.A., Lin, F., Cao, Z., Kraemer, D.L., Huin, A., Akawie, E., Yin, Y. & Wilson, J.T. (1994): The role of $GABA_B$ receptor activation in the lethargic (*lh/lh*) mouse model of primary generalized absence seizures. In: *Idiopathic generalized epilepsies: clinical, experimental and genetic aspects*, eds. A. Malafosse, P. Genton, E. Hirsch, C. Marescaux, D. Broglin & R. Bernasconi, pp. 187–199. London: John Libbey.

Loiseau, P. (1992): Childhood absence-epilepsy. In: *Epileptic syndromes in infancy, childhood and adolescence*, 2nd edn, eds. J. Roger, M. Bureau, Ch. Dravet, F.E. Dreifuss, A. Perret & P. Wolf, pp. 135–150. London: John Libbey.

Noebels, J.L. (1994): Genetic and phenotypic heterogeneity of inherited spike-wave epilepsies. In: *Idiopathic generalized epilepsies: clinical, experimental and genetic aspects*, eds. A. Malafosse, P. Genton, E. Hirsch, C. Marescaux, D. Broglin & R. Bernasconi, pp. 215–225. London: John Libbey.

Panayiotopoulos, C.P. (1994): The clinical spectrum of typical absence seizures and absence epilepsies. In: *Idiopathic generalized epilepsies: clinical, experimental and genetic aspects*, eds. A. Malafosse, P. Genton, E. Hirsch, C. Marescaux, D. Broglin & R. Bernasconi, pp. 75–85. London: John Libbey.

Roger, J., Genton, P., Bureau, M. & Dravet, C. (1993): Less common epileptic syndromes. In: *The treatment of epilepsy: principles and practice*, ed. E. Wyllie, pp. 624–635. Philadelphia: Lea & Febiger.

Serratosa, J.M. & Delgado-Escueta, A.V. (1993): Generalized myoclonic seizures. In: *The treatment of epilepsy: principles and practice*, ed. E. Wyllie, pp. 411–424. Philadelphia: Lea & Febiger.

Snead, O.C. III (1994): Pathophysiological mechanisms of experimental generalized absence seizures in rats. In: *Idiopathic generalized epilepsies: clinical, experimental and genetic aspects*, eds. A. Malafosse, P. Genton, E. Hirsch, C. Marescaux, D. Broglin & R. Bernasconi, pp. 132–150. London: John Libbey.

Tassinari, C.A., Bureau, M. & Thomas, P. (1992): Epilepsy with myoclonic absences. In: *Epileptic syndromes in infancy, childhood and adolescence*, 2nd edn, eds. J. Roger, M. Bureau, Ch. Dravet, F.E. Dreifuss, A. Perret & P. Wolf, pp. 151–160. London: John Libbey.

Vergnes, M. & Marescaux, C. (1994): Pathophysiological mechanisms underlying genetic absence epilepsy in rats. In: *Idiopathic generalized epilepsies: clinical, experimental and genetic aspects*, eds. A. Malafosse, P. Genton, E. Hirsch, C. Marescaux, D. Broglin & R. Bernasconi, pp. 151–168. London: John Libbey.

Wolf, P. (1992): Juvenile absence epilepsy. In: *Epileptic syndromes in infancy, childhood and adolescence*, 2nd edn, eds. J. Roger, M. Bureau, Ch. Dravet, F.E. Dreifuss, A. Perret & P. Wolf, pp. 307–312. London: John Libbey.

Chapter 11

Late-onset absence status epilepticus is most often situation-related

Pierre Thomas* and Frederick Andermann[†]

*Service de neurologie, Hôpital Pasteur, 30 Voie Romaine B.P. 69, 06002 Nice Cedex, France and [†]Montreal Neurological Hospital and Institute, 3801 University St, Montreal, Quebec, Canada H3A 2B4

Summary

Absence status (AS) in elderly subjects often occurs *de novo* and satisfies many criteria of idiopathic generalized epilepsy (IGE). This study, based on the investigation of 25 patients with absence status occurring after the age of 50 years over a 12-year period, confirms that: (1) EEG shows a heterogeneous range of ictal patterns with a frequency typically below 3 Hz; (2) there is often clear focal predominance of the ictal EEG activity; (3) in some patients, there is a clear focal frontal onset of paroxysmal activity before generalization; (4) a high proportion of patients have psychiatric disturbances, are taking excessive amounts of psychotropic drugs and/or have other causative factors such as metabolic disorders or acute benzodiazepine withdrawal; (5) in patients with a remote history of generalized or focal epilepsy, triggering factors are often the same as in *de novo* cases; (6) CT scans and/or MRI often show diffuse or frontally predominant cortical–subcortical atrophy; (7) the risk of recurrence is low. In this series, absence status is most often situation-related, even in half the patients with a previous history of epilepsy. In only 15 per cent was there a previous history of focal or generalized epilepsy without obvious factors triggering the recurrence. This form of seizures illustrates well that epilepsy is a threshold phenomenon with both focal and generalized components and acquired as well as genetic factors.

Introduction

The idiopathic generalized epilepsies (IGE) are a group of age-related syndromes, each of which corresponds to strict diagnostic criteria (Commission, 1989). In 1981, Gastaut wrote that 'primary generalized epilepsy (PGE) in old age is most uncommon (1 per cent of epilepsies in this age group) and is almost exclusively represented by perimenopausal women who develop absence status (AS) with or without a prior personal history of PGE in childhood'. Absence status is one of the most frequent forms of status epilepticus in elderly subjects. In this age group, it often occurs *de novo*, without pre-existing epilepsy. Clinically, there is a fluctuating confusional state of varying severity, often associated with bilateral myoclonic jerks (Guberman *et al.*, 1986; Cascino, 1993). EEG is diagnostic, showing generalized paroxysmal activity. Thus absence status occurring in elderly patients apparently satisfies most of the cardinal features of a late-onset form of IGE syndrome. A series of 25 consecutive patients with late-onset absence status illustrates that it is commonly situation-related and rarely occurs in patients with previous history of epilepsy in the absence of triggering factors.

Patients and methods

Twenty-five consecutive cases of adult onset absence status were collected over a 12-year period in the Department of Neurology of the Nice University Hospital. Eleven were retrospectively studied, and have been published elsewhere (Thomas et al., 1992a) while the other 14 were prospectively investigated. Our inclusion criteria were: (1) age at onset over 50 years; (2) impairment of consciousness for at least 1 h; (3) EEG documentation of the status, showing generalized paroxysmal activity, and (4) disappearance of ictal EEG discharges after treatment coinciding with clear improvement in consciousness. To assess neuropsychological improvement when the impairment of consciousness was mild, a standardized neuropsychological investigation (Thomas et al., 1992b) was performed under continuous EEG video-monitoring before and after benzodiazepine (BZ) injection.

One of us (P.T.) personally evaluated 19 of these patients. The other six were studied by other neurologists and by neurophysiologists. Data on previous treatments were obtained from the patients' physicians. Twenty of the patients were regularly followed after the initial episode of absence status.

EEG tracings were obtained on a 16-channel polygraph in 21 cases, and on an 8-channel apparatus in four. Scalp electrodes were placed according to the International 10–20 system. Blood count, electrolytes, glucose, blood gases, ammonia, protein levels, enzymes and antiepileptic blood levels were measured and cranial CT or MRI were performed in all patients. Ictal and post-ictal SPECT was performed in Patients 12 and 22 and EEG mapping of ictal activity was performed in Patients 12 and 25.

Clinical and EEG data (Table 1)

The mean age was 65 years (range: 50–90). Eighteen patients were women (72 per cent). Seventeen

Table 1. Absence status of late onset in 25 consecutive patients (Thomas, Ch. 11)

Case	Sex/Age	Pre-existing epilepsy	Impairment of consciousness	EEG	Psychotropic drugs	CT/MRI	Duration (days)	Recurrence
1	F/53	No	Moderate	2/2.5 Hz PSW>L	Yes (W)	Atrophy	4	No
2	F/57	No	Mild	2.5 Hz SW	Yes (W)	Normal	5	No
3	F/49	No	Mild	0.5 Hz PSW	Yes (W)	Normal	0.5	?
4	F/56	No	Moderate	0.5 Hz SW >L	Yes (W)	Atrophy	4	No
5	F/67	No	Severe	3 Hz SW >L	Yes (W)	Atrophy	5	No
6	M/50	No	Moderate	0.5 Hz SW	Yes (W)	Normal	0.5	No
7	F/62	No	Severe	2.5 Hz SW	Yes (W)	Atrophy	2	No
8	F/48	No	Moderate	1 Hz SW/PSW >L	Yes (W)	Normal	1	No
9	F/56	No	Severe	3 Hz SW	Yes	Atrophy	1	No
10	F/66	No	Moderate	4 Hz SW	No	Normal	0.5	No
11	F/81	No	Mild	3 Hz Sharp W	No	Normal	0.3	?
12	F/81	No	Moderate	1–2 Hz PSW >R	No	Atrophy	1.5	Yes
13	F/69	No	Moderate	2.5 Hz SW >L	Yes (W)	Normal	1	No
14	M/74	No	Moderate	2 Hz Slow W >R	No	Atrophy	0.5	No
15	F/90	No	Moderate	2 Hz Sharp W	Yes (W)	Atrophy	3	No
16	F/60	Yes (IGE)	Mild	3 Hz SW	No	Normal	3	No
17	M/57	Yes (CPE)	Mild	2–3 Hz PSW >R	No	Normal	0.5	?
18	F/69	Yes (IGE)	Mild	2 Hz PSW	No	Normal	0.3	No
19	M/66	Yes (CPE)	Moderate	1–1.5 Hz PSW >L	Yes (W)	Atrophy	0.5	No
20	M/55	Yes (CPE)	Severe	1–2 Hz SW + PSW	Yes (W)	Normal	2	No
21	M/71	Yes (CPE)	Mild	3 Hz PS + PSW >L	No	Normal	1	?
22	F/82	Yes (IGE)	Severe	10 Hz PS + PSW	No	Atrophy	2	Yes
23	F/82	No	Moderate	1–3 Hz PSW	Yes	Atrophy	2	?
24	F/61	Yes (IGE)	Moderate	2 Hz PSW	No	Normal	1	No
25	M/61	No	Moderate	1.5 Hz PSW >R	No	Normal	1	Yes

(68 per cent) experienced absence status *de novo*. The remaining eight patients had a history of epilepsy: IGE in four cases, partial cryptogenic epilepsy (PCE) in four. Patient 6 had experienced a cluster of generalized tonic–clonic seizures during attempted benzodiazepine withdrawal 2 years earlier.

Impairment of consciousness varied between patients. In five cases, it was severe: the patients were bedridden, stuporous and had lost sphincter control. In 13 cases, confusion was moderate: they seemed perplexed or indifferent and were disoriented in time and space; simple orders were correctly but slowly obeyed; more complex orders could not be followed. There was with often strong perseveration on the previous task or the initial part of the order. Language output was reduced to fragments of sentences or words alternating with long periods of silence. Patient 12 had very spectacular pallidal spells. Frontal release signs (snout, palmomental and grasping reflexes) were noted in 10 patients. In the remaining seven, the mental impairment was mild, the only feature being subjective impairment of difficult actions: the patients were able to perform ordinary tasks correctly, while acts that required decision making were impaired. Bilateral myoclonic jerks predominant in cranial muscles (temporal, eyelid) were seen in 12 cases. Generalized tonic–clonic seizures initiated the absence status in three cases and occurred during the absence status in 3 others. Simple gestural automatisms were seen in eight patients.

Various types of EEG changes were found. The frequency of paroxysmal changes was between 0.5 and 4 Hz. In 19 patients, it was below 3 Hz. Four (Cases 5, 9, 10 and 16) had continuous typical, bilateral, symmetrical and synchronous spike-waves (SW) $\geq$ 3 Hz. In three (Cases 11, 14 and 15) the paroxysmal activity consisted of rhythmic/periodic sharp waves that disappeared following intravenous benzodiazepine. The remaining patients had irregular low-frequency rythmic spike-waves, polyspike-waves (PSW) or both, occurring either continuously or, more frequently, in short recurrent bursts. Case 22 had irregular bursts of 10 Hz polyspikes of 1–3 s duration, coexisting with PSW. In 11 patients (Cases 1, 4, 5, 8, 12, 13, 14, 17, 19, 21 and 25), paroxysmal activity was more or less asymmetric over anterior head regions. In Patient 12, status was organized in long recurrent seizures with a right frontal onset (see below).

Precipitating factors

De novo absence status (17 patients)

Twelve patients were receiving psychotropic drugs at the time of the absence status. These were: benzodiazepine in 10 patients, often at high daily doses and using combinations of several formulations, in association with neuroleptics (in six patients), tricyclic antidepressants (in three) or lithium carbonate (in two). In eight patients, these drugs had been taken in high doses for months to years. In four, drug abuse was associated with past or present chronic alcoholism. In nine of the 10 patients who were receiving benzodiazepine, the treatment was discontinued several hours or days prior to the onset of absence status. Three patients stopped their drugs without medical supervision, an intercurrent disease caused a reduction of treatment in two and rapid withdrawal took place in a psychiatric department in two others. In Case 1, the drugs were not resumed after a surgical procedure. In Case 8, the cause of drug withdrawal was unclear. Withdrawal was total in eight patients; only lithium carbonate was maintained in the remaining individual (Case 7). The absence status occurred at a mean of 2.7 days after discontinuation of psychotropic drugs (range: 1–4 days). In Case 13, the emergency-room physician thought that acute benzodiazepine intoxication was the most likely diagnosis, and prescribed intravenous flumazenil, a specific benzodiazepine antagonist that increased confusion and produced bilateral myoclonic jerks.

In five patients (Cases 10, 11, 12, 14, 25), there was no evidence of psychotropic drug intake or discontinuation during the weeks preceding the absence status. Theophylline, salbutamol, cimetidine, tetracosactide, cyclophosphamide, tamoxifen or spironolactone were taken by these five patients.

Laboratory investigation was normal in 15 of 17 patients. We found hypocalcaemia at 1.78 mmol/l in Patient 2 and hyponatraemia at 126 mEq/l in Patient 7. CT scan or MRI was normal in seven cases. In 10, it showed moderate, diffuse cortical and/or subcortical atrophy.

Absence status with epileptic antecedents (eight patients)

Acute withdrawal of psychotropic drugs (benzodiazepine and neuroleptics) was found in two patients (Cases 19 and 20) who had severe psychiatric antecedents in addition to focal cryptogenic epilepsy. Alcohol was thought to be the main precipitating factor in case 17 and ranitidine intoxication in Case 22. The delay between the last seizure and the absence status in the four women (Cases 16, 18, 22 and 24) who had a history of IGE was 22, 20, 22 and 32 years, respectively. No clearcut precipitating factor was found in four patients (Cases 16, 18, 21, 24).

Evolution and prognosis

EEG normalization occurred in 22 cases immediately following intravenous injection of diazepam, clonazepam or phenobarbital. Clinical normalization was delayed, occurring from 5 to 60 min after the injection, especially in older patients. In Patient 23, a loading dose (1 mg/kg) of oral clobazam stopped the status 90 min later. In Patients 5 and 6, low-dose benzodiazepine was prescribed orally and the status stopped 48 and 72 h later, respectively. Control EEGs repeatedly performed days to weeks later were consistently normal in patients with *de novo* absence status, or comparable to the pre-absence status state in those with a history of epilepsy. In the *de novo* cases, long-term antiepileptic medication was prescribed to patients who had recurrences of absence status (Cases 12 and 25 had a second attack 12 h and 5 days after the initial episode; recurrence was treated by a single injection of 18 mg/kg intravenous phenytoin) and/or to patients with a previous history of unexplained confusion (Cases 11, 12 and 25). Follow-up of 20 patients over 6 months to 10 years showed that no other epileptic phenomena occurred after absence status, even in the *de novo* patients who did not receive maintenance antiepileptic treatment.

Representative case-histories

Patient 6

A 50-year-old man abused benzodiazepines: 6 months before admission, he went from pharmacy to pharmacy with false prescriptions. He was admitted to the psychiatry department for controlled withdrawal of psychotropic drugs that included clorazepate, 200 mg/day, lorazepam, 12.5 mg/day, triazolam, 0.50 mg 4–8 times per day and clomipramine, 75 mg/day. Withdrawal was progressive for 3 weeks, and only clomipramine and lorazepam, 7.5 mg/day were maintained. The status probably began while he was being discharged: he kissed his nurse on the cheek 15 times while taking his leave. He was admitted to the neurology department the same day because he rapidly developed mental confusion with abulia and catatonic features and low-amplitude periocular myoclonias. Emergency EEG showed continuous, generalized polyspike-wave discharges. The reintroduction of oral clorazepate, 100 mg/day led to complete clinical and EEG normalization in 3 days.

Patient 22

An 83-year-old woman had IGE since age 6 and received 150 mg/day phenobarbital (PB) for 35 years. Her last seizure, a generalized tonic–clonic attack on awakening, occurred 22 years earlier. She never had absence seizures. She was admitted to the neurology department because of a confusional state probably induced by intravenous ranitidine, 300 mg day. This drug, a histamine-2 receptor antagonist, was prescribed to treat acute gastritis and is known to induce toxic encephalopathy in elderly subjects (Cantú & Korek, 1991). Phenobarbital levels were 23 mg/l. There was no hepatic or metabolic abnormality. The first EEG showed triphasic sharp waves which were not modified by intravenous clonazepam. Persistence of confusion after discontinuation of ranitidine

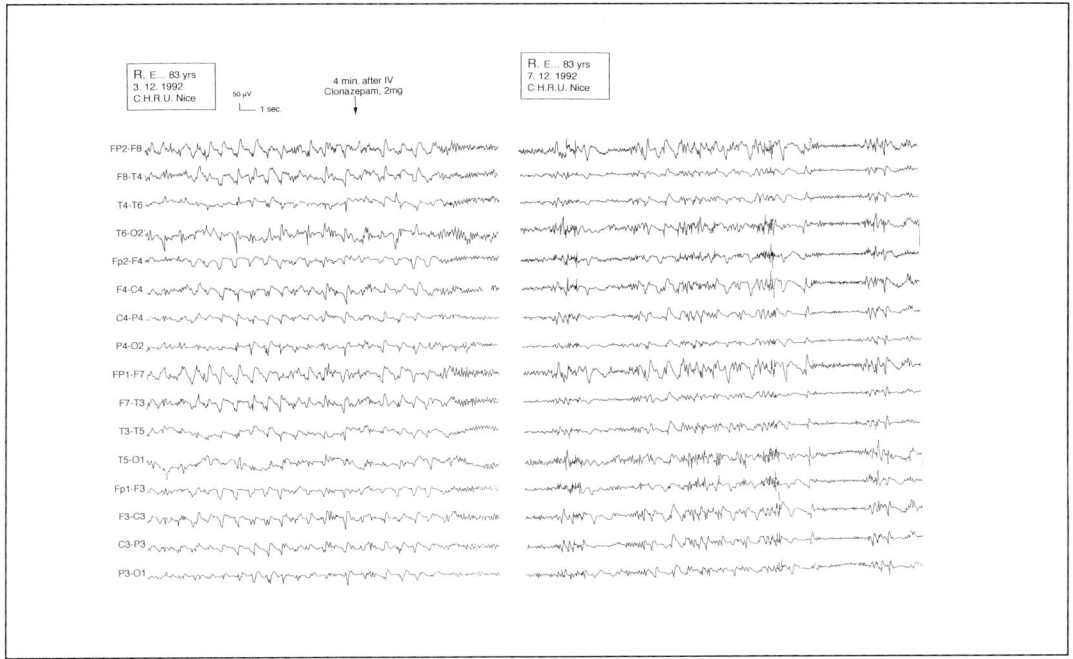

Fig. 1. Patient 22 (a) Left: first EEG (3 December, 1992): Toxic encephalopathy induced by intravenous ranitidine, 300 mg/day with triphasic sharps-waves not modified by intravenous clonazepam, 2 mg. Right: second EEG 4 days later, after immediate discontinuation of ranitidine. Paroxysmal activity. (b) EEG (8 December, 1992): typical AS. Normalization of vigilance and EEG after intravenous clonazepam, 2 mg.

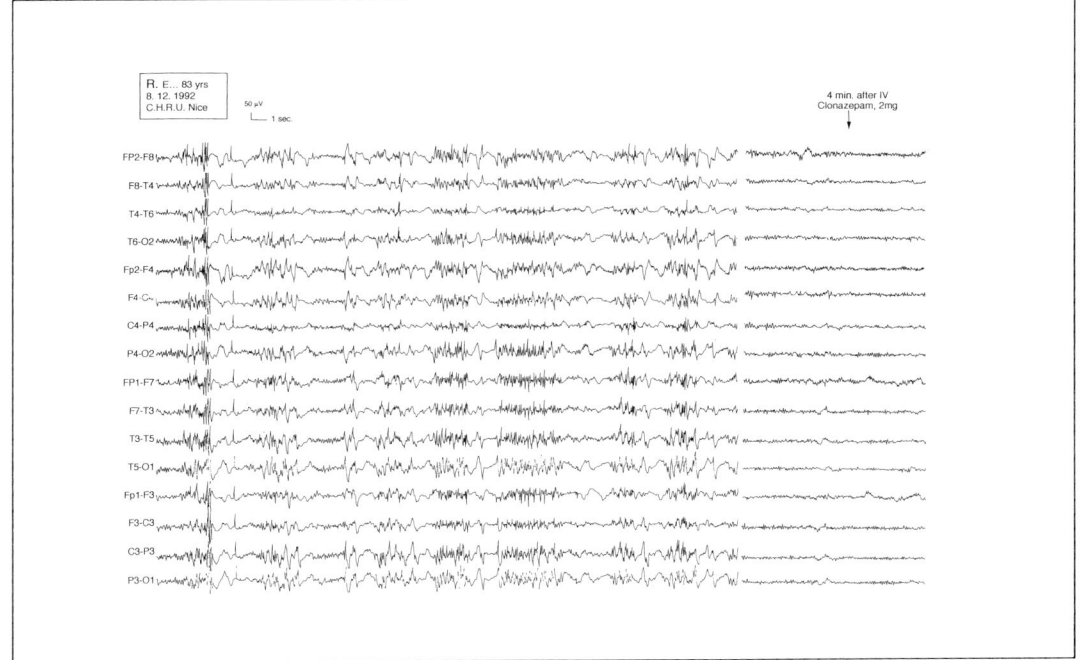

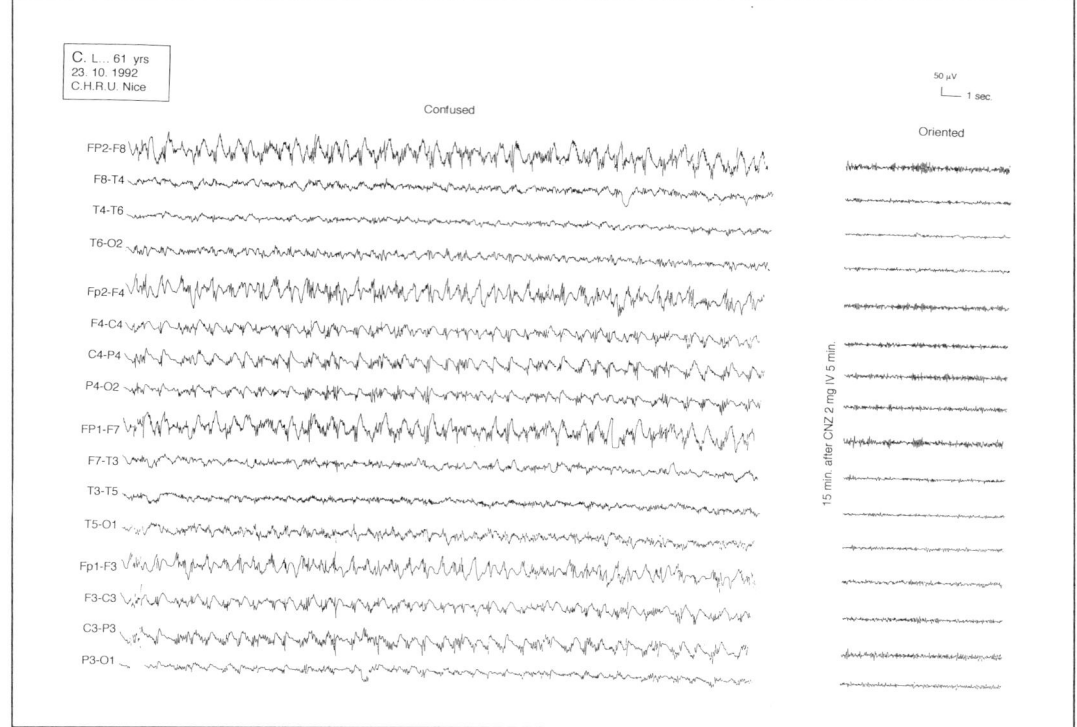

Fig. 2. (a) EEG performed during de novo *absence status in Patient 25. Continuous slow polyspike-waves, more prominent over the right frontocentral areas.*

led to a second EEG 4 days later: it showed generalized paroxysmal activity. The following day, an EEG showed generalized polyspike-waves and spike-waves discharges. Intravenous clonazepam led to complete clinical and EEG normalization (Fig. 1).

Patient 12

An 81-year-old woman without history of epilepsy was admitted to the emergency ward with the diagnosis of transient global amnesia. A few months earlier, she had had several episodes of confusion, lasting from 12 h to 2 days. Clinically, she had a mild, fluctuating confusional state with perseveration alternating with frank stupour and catatonic behaviour. Video-EEG monitoring showed evidence for a non-convulsive status epilepticus with recurrent seizures lasting 25 to 45 min, starting over the right frontal area, then proceeding to secondary bilateral synchrony (Fig. 2a & 2b). The degree of cognitive impairment was roughly proportional to the degree of spread of paroxysmal activity. Ictal and postictal SPECT (Fig. 2c) demonstrated a right frontal focus but MRI showed only marked subcortical/cortical atrophy. Intravenous benzodiazepine and valproate were ineffective but the status ceased after 15 mg/kg phenytoin were given intravenously. Seizures did not recur while she was receiving phenytoin, 250 mg/day for 2.5 years.

Discussion

Absence status, or 'petit mal status' was first described by Lennox in 1945 in children with absence epilepsy: 'rarely, however, the child may be in a state of confusion lasting for hours which the EEG proves is a petit mal status'. Further studies (Gastaut, 1967; Lob *et al.*, 1967; Gastaut, 1970) led to

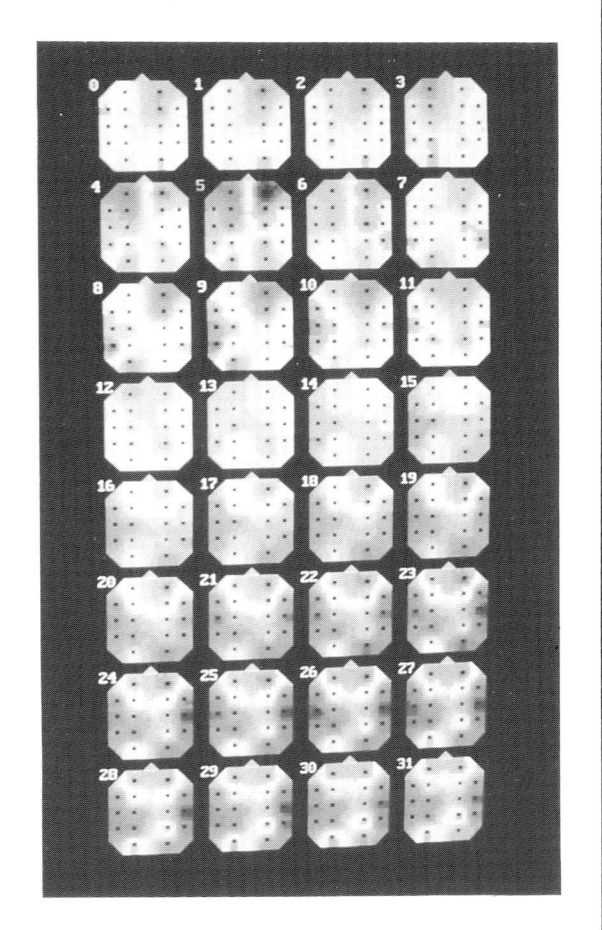

Fig. 2(b) Brain mapping of EEG activity during absence seizure in same patients. Twenty polyspike-waves have been averaged on the peak of their spiky component. Amplitude mapping was performed every 8 ms. Map no. 5 shows the distribution of potentials at the moment of maximum spike amplitude, clearly showing a dipolar distribution with maximal negativity focused over the right frontal area. The slow-wave component spreads over both anterior areas after onset over the right frontal lobe. Dark red: maximum negativity; dark blue: maximum positivity (see colour plates).

the conclusion that absence status was a heterogeneous epileptic phenomenon that can occur at all ages, usually in patients with pre-existing epilepsy. However (Table 2), the diversity of clinical presentations and the lack of precise definitions for the terms used seems responsible for the large number of different terms used to describe this condition (Andermann & Robb, 1972; Lee, 1985). In 1971, Schwartz & Scott reported four middle-aged patients with no prior history of epilepsy who had a prolonged confusional state associated with rhythmic, irregular spike-and-wave discharges; they described this entity as 'isolated petit mal status presenting *de novo* in middle age'. Seventy-nine such patients have been described between 1972 and 1992; they were around age 60 and predominantly females (63 per cent) (Table 3). Schwartz & Scott (1972) thought that *de novo* late-onset absence status was 'the extreme end of a continuum of petit mal epilepsy extending from childhood to middle age'. Others (Gibberd, 1972; Ellis & Lee, 1977; Dunne et al., 1987; Van Sweden & Mellerio, 1988) disagreed and suggested that the electroclinical presentation, precipitating factors and prognosis suggested a pathogenicity 'entirely different from absence status occurring in childhood'.

Table 2. Absence status: the various denominations used in the literature

Petit mal status (Lennox, 1945)
Prolonged epileptic twilight state with almost continuous wave-spikes* (Zappoli, 1955)
Prolonged alterations in behaviour associated with a continuous EEG spike-and-dome abnormality* (Bornstein et al., 1956)
Epilepsia minoria continua* (Friedlander & Feinstein, 1956)
Simple epileptic confusional state (Gastaut et al., 1956)
Prolonged behavioural disturbances as ictal phenomena* (Goldensohn & Gold, 1960)
Spike-wave-stupor, ictal stupor* (Niedermeyer & Kalifeh, 1965)
Minor status epilepticus (Brett, 1966)
Absence status (Gastaut, 1967; Gastaut, 1970)
Borderline petit mal status* (Hess et al., 1971)
Ictal psychosis* (Wells, 1975)
Prolonged confusion as an ictal state* (Ellis & Lee, 1977)
Senile petit mal epilepsy* (Nishiura & Oiwa, 1979)
Acute prolonged ictal confusion* (Van Zandycke et al., 1980)
Atypical absence status* (Gastaut, 1983)
Generalized nonconvulsive status epilepticus (Guberman et al., 1986)

*Term narrowed to absence status of late onset.

Clinical data in our cases were similar to those found in younger patients. There was no relevant feature allowing us to separate patients with a history of epilepsy from those with *de novo* absence status.

Diffuse slow spike-and-wave or polyspike-and-wave discharges were found in 72 per cent (18/25); a typical 3 Hz spike-and-wave pattern, identical to the one encountered in absence epilepsies, was found in only 16 per cent (4/25). Among those four patients, only one had pre-existing IGE. These data confirm the findings of Porter & Penry (1983) who stated that, in absence status, 'virtually any generalized continuous or nearly continuous (electrographic) abnormality could be a substrate for this syndrome'. In absence status of late onset, the heterogeneous range of bilaterality, frequency and symmetry of ictal patterns seems to be different from the stereotyped 3–4 Hz spike-and-wave or polyspike-and-wave pattern of childhood absence epilepsy.

The most relevant aetiological factor in this series was that more than half the patients (14/25, 56 per cent) had psychiatric disturbances and were taking excessive amounts of psychotropic drugs, a finding in 37 of the 56 reported cases (66 per cent) where one or several precipitating factors were identified (Table 3). Ten of our patients with *de novo* absence status received chronic benzodiazepine treatment: this was also found in 20 per cent (11/56) of patients described in the literature. Epileptic seizures are a frequent complication of benzodiazepine withdrawal, with an incidence of between 2.5 per cent (Tyrer & Sievewright, 1984) and 4 per cent (Schöpf, 1983). In nine of our 17 patients (53 per cent), *de novo* absence status was associated with benzodiazepine withdrawal, the delay between cessation of the drug and onset of absence status was roughly consistent with the half-life dynamics of the drug withdrawn. In Case 6, benzodiazepine withdrawal was the only clear precipitating factor. Reintroduction of the drug was effective, confirming the high probability of causative role of withdrawal. In Case 13, despite the fact that multiple psychotropic drugs were withdrawn, the aggravation caused by flumazenil suggested that benzodiazepine withdrawal was the main triggering factor (Thomas et al., 1993). Our findings indicate that *de novo* absence status may constitute a particular benzodiazepine withdrawal syndrome, characterized by non-convulsive seizures instead of convulsive attacks.

The direct effect of benzodiazepine withdrawal in triggering absence status was recognized by Dunne *et al.* in 1987 with lorazepam and oxazepam, then by Hersch & Billings (1988). In the report of Van Sweden & Mellerio (1988), ictal confusion was triggered by benzodiazepine withdrawal in half the patients in whom drug withdrawal was the triggering factor (five patients); in two other

Table 3. 'De novo' absence status of late onset: literature data (71 cases) and possible triggering factors (Thomas, Ch. 11)

Authors	No. of cases	Age
Elian, 1969	1	55
Amand, 1971	3	60,63,66
Cambier et al., 1974	2	72,74
Schwartz & Scott, 1971	4	56,62,42,54
Wells, 1975	1	62
Richard & Brenner, 1980	1	84
Van Zandycke et al., 1980	2	52,70
Weiner et al, 1980	1	30
Goldman et al., 1981	1	59
Rumpl & Hinterhuber, 1981	1	58
Vercelletto & Gastaut, 1981	1	65
Bateman et al., 1983	1	50
Pritchard & O'Neil, 1984	1	59
Lee, 1985; Ellis & Lee, 1977	11	42–72
Nishiura & Oiwa, 1979	1	74
Courjon et al., 1984	3	40,40,72
Van Sweden, 1985	4	38,39,46,57
Vollmer et al., 1985	1	70
Bourrat et al., 1986	8	80,80,78,76,76,60,70,80
Lim et al., 1986	2	55,67
Dunne et al., 1987	5	64,80,79,62,88
Hersch & Billings, 1988	1	55
Van Sweden & Mellerio, 1988	12	58,66,39,43,43,44,50,52,52,52,61,73
Vickrey & Bahls, 1989	1	64
Fagan & Lee, 1990	2	75,63
Tomson et al., 1992	8	51,61,65,66,69,74,78,81
Mean age * (62 patients)	61.7 years	
Sex ratio* (65 patients)	F = 41 (63%)	
	M = 24 (37%)	

Possible precipitating factors (79 cases)[†]

No definite precipitating factor	23
Psychotropic drugs	37
Benzodiazepine	11 (withdrawal: 8)
Others	28
Non-psychotropic drugs	7
Metabolic imbalance	15
Alcoholism	6
Miscellaneous	7

* In some cases, this information was not available; [†] in some cases, more than one possible factor was present.

patients, benzodiazepine overdosage was considered responsible for absence status, and the authors suggested the presence of a paradoxical effect. Benzodiazepine withdrawal, in our opinion, represents a major triggering factor of absence status and may easily be underestimated: in the presence of mild cognitive impairment without EEG confirmation, absence status may present as a 'simple' benzodiazepine withdrawal state or an 'amnesia and automatism syndrome' (Bismuth et al., 1980; Mellerio, 1980).

Other precipitating factors have been described alone or in combination. These include tricyclic antidepressants and/or neuroleptics (Rumpl & Hinterhuber, 1981; Van Sweden, 1985; Bourrat et

IDIOPATHIC GENERALIZED EPILEPSIES

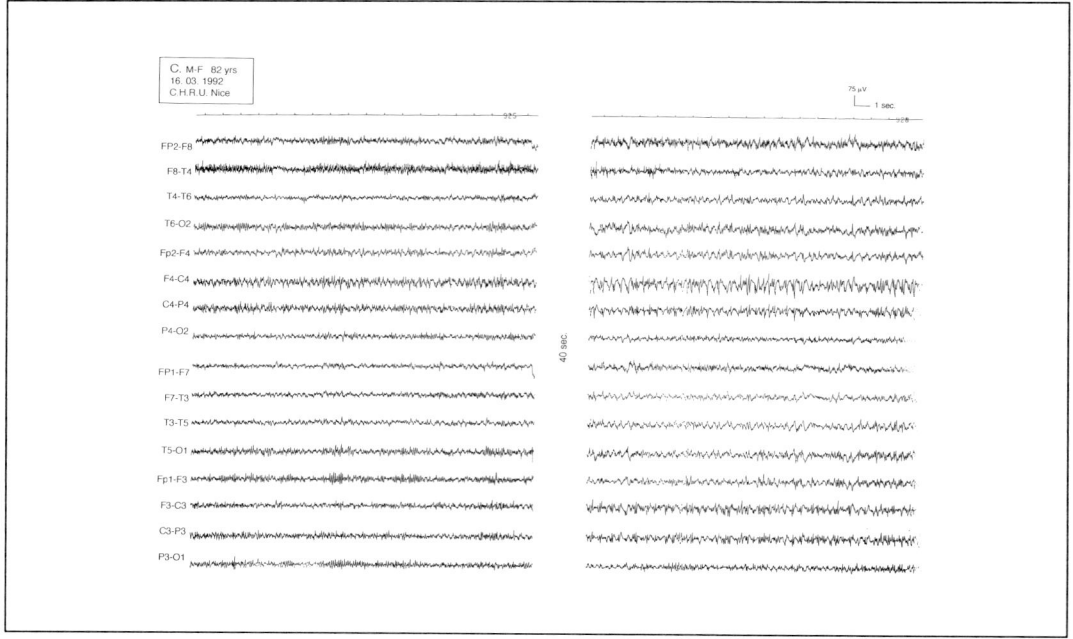

Fig. 3a. Surface EEG performed during de novo *absence status in Patient 12. Status was organized in recurrent, successive seizures lasting 25 to 45 min. (a) Onset of a seizure: paroxysmal activity is initially localized over the right frontal area.*

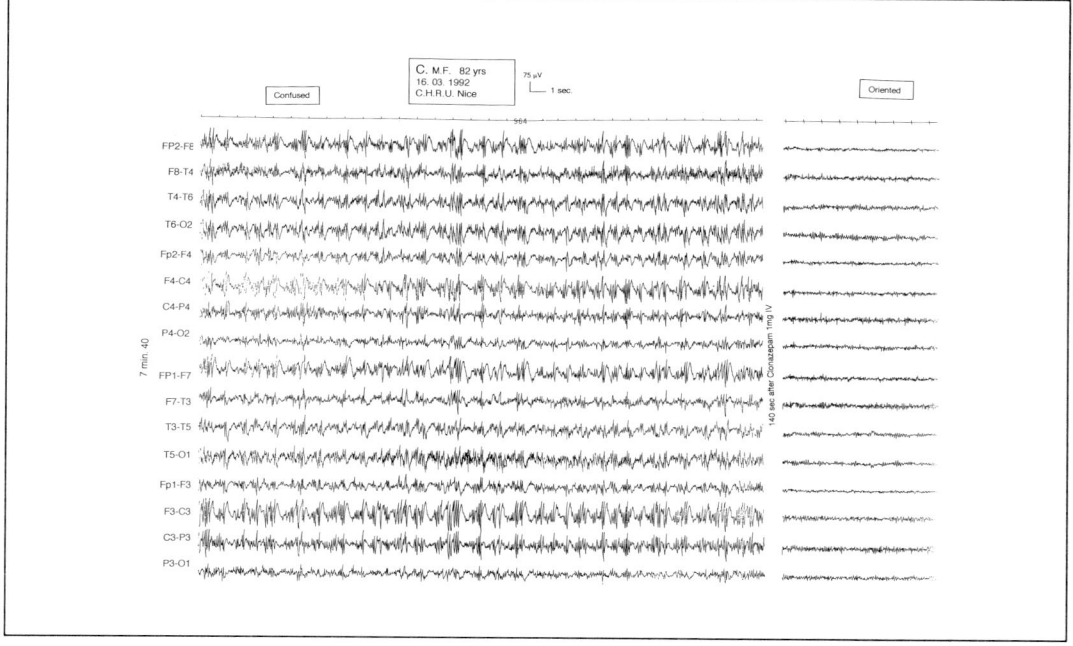

Fig. 3b. 7 min 40 s later: ictal pattern is constituted by bilateral, synchronous, perfectly symmetrical discharges. Total duration of this seizure: 32.5 min.

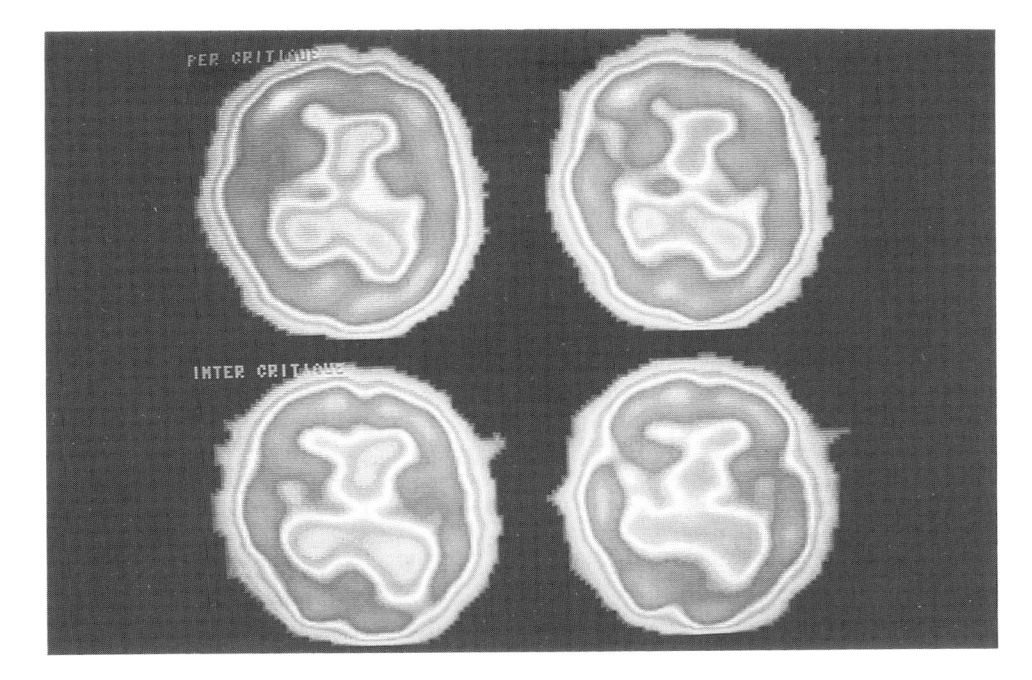

Fig. 3 (c) 99 Tc HMPAO SPECT, first performed during status, at the beginning of a seizure (top), then post-ictally (bottom). During absence status, there is a significantly increased perfusion over the right frontal area (top left of the figure) (see also colour plate).

al., 1986; Dunne *et al.*, 1987; Van Sweden & Mellerio, 1988; Tomson *et al.*, 1992), lithium carbonate (Ellis & Lee, 1977; Weiner *et al.*, 1980; Dunne *et al.*, 1987; Tomson *et al.*, 1992), theophylline (Vickrey & Bahls, 1989), cimetidine (Van Sweden, 1985), hyponatraemia (Ellis & Lee, 1977; Bourrat *et al.*, 1986; Tomson *et al.*, 1992), hypocalcaemia (Vignaendra *et al.*, 1977; Berkovic & Bladin, 1982), acute or chronic alcoholism (Ellis & Lee, 1977; Bourrat *et al.*, 1986; Van Sweden & Mellerio, 1988; Hersch & Billings, 1988; Courjon *et al.*, 1984). Such toxic or metabolic triggering factors were found in half of our absence status cases with epileptic antecedents (4/8). In Case 22, for example, both the toxic encephalopathy induced by ranitidine and the epileptic predisposition may have been responsible for the absence status (Fig. 1). Some authors (Gall *et al.*, 1978; Bourrat *et al.*, 1986; Tomson *et al.*, 1986) think that the presence of diffuse or frontally accentuated cortical-subcortical atrophy, a frequent finding on CT or MRI scans performed in these patients, may be of importance: epileptogenic factors might express themselves more easily in brains structurally damaged by vascular, degenerative and/or toxic factors.

Both by visual analysis and by EEG mapping, a clear focal predominance of ictal activity was found in 11/25 (44 per cent) patients (Fig. 2). In six patients, some degree of lateralization of ictal activity was associated with cortical atrophy. Focal changes may be transitorily apparent at the onset of absence status (Fujiwara *et al.*, 1991), after its termination (Ellis & Lee, 1977) or both (our Patient 12), suggesting that gradual organization of generalized paroxysmal activity may be caused by a mechanism of secondary bisynchrony. Similar cases with electroclinical features suggestive of a focal origin were reported by Hess *et al.* (1972), as 'borderline cases of petit mal status', then by Niedermeyer *et al.* (1979), as 'AS with focal characteristics', and by others (Aguglia *et al.*, 1983; Williamson *et al.*, 1985; Tomson *et al.*, 1986; Rey & Papy, 1987; Rohr-Le Floch *et al.*, 1988;

Thomas *et al.*, 1992a; Tomson *et al.*, 1992), who have stressed the similarity between complex partial status epilepticus of frontal origin and late-onset absence status: in some patients, the latter condition is clearly the consequence of the former, as confirmed by EEG and ictal SPECT in the case-report of Fujiwara *et al.* (1991) and in our Case 12 (Fig. 3).

We found a low risk of recurrence of *de novo* absence status compared to absence status occurring in patients with a prior history of epilepsy: only six recurrences were reported in 41 reported cases (Thomas *et al.*, 1992a), while the mean frequency of absence status attacks in 18 patients with IGE was 5.7 per year as described by Berkovic *et al.* (1989). In our personal series, absence status recurred in only 3/17 (18 per cent) of cases (11, 12 and 25). Those patients had either a history of previous unexplained confusional episodes or an immediate recurrence of the status after it was stopped by medication. In our opinion, isolated episodes of *de novo* absence status of late-onset do not justify chronic antiepileptic treatment, especially if a clear, treatable psychotropic, toxic or metabolic factor is present. Adverse effects provoked by long-term antiepileptic therapy in elderly subjects may be greater than a hypothetical risk of recurrence of absence status. In patients with epileptic antecedents, however, a renewed prescription of antiepileptic monotherapy with valproate seems justified, especially if there is no clear triggering factor.

Conclusions

This study suggests that late onset absence status is more often than not an occasional or situation-related epileptic manifestation. Epilepsy is a threshold phenomenon and the various clinical forms are considered to represent the result of interaction of acquired and genetic factors. The importance of the acquired factors is highlighted in this series with little tendency to recurrence when the major trigger can be eliminated. In patients with a previous history of epilepsy, the presence of a cryptogenic focal form in half of them is an unexpected finding. In both those with history of generalized and focal epilepsy, the previous history is significant but the late recurrence favours the importance of recent triggering factors, whether these are obvious or not. More prolonged follow-up should help identify these patients those who have a high recurrence risk from those with isolated attacks.

The present series, from a general hospital population, suggests that absence status *de novo* is more commonly a situation-related form of seizures, whereas late resurgence of idiopathic generalized epilepsy or late onset of IGE is considerably less common.

Acknowledgements

We thank Dr G. Suisse and Professor C. Dolisi who performed EEG mapping, Dr O. Migneco who performed ictal SPECT, Dr P. Genton for reviewing the manuscript and Dr A. Beaumanoir and Professor M. Chatel for their constant help and encouragement.

References

Aguglia, U., Tinuper, P. & Farnarier, G. (1983): Etat confusionnel critique à point de départ frontal chez le sujet âgé. *Rev. EEG Neuropsyiol.* **13**, 174–179.

Amand, G. (1971): Etats d'absence et états confusionnels prolongés au delà de 60 ans. *Rev. EEG Neurophysiol.* **13**, 174–179.

Andermann, F. & Robb, J.P. (1972): Absence status. A reappraisal following review of thirty-eight patients. *Epilepsia* **13**, 177–187.

Bateman, D.E., O'Grady, J.C., Willey, C.J., Longley, B.P. & Barwick, D.D. (1983): De novo minor status epilepticus of late onset presenting as stupor. *Br. Med. J.* **287**, 1673–1674.

Berkovic, S.F., Andermann, F., Gubermann, A., Hipola, D. & Bladin, P.F. (1989): Valproate prevents the recurrence of absence status. *Neurology* **39**, 1294–1297.

Berkovic, S.F. & Bladin, P.F. (1982): Absence status in adults. *Clin. Exp. Neurol.* **19**, 198–207.

Bismuth, C., Le Bellec, M., Dally, S. & Lagier, G. (1980): Dépendance physique aux benzodiazépines. 6 observations. *Nouv. Presse Med.* **9**, 1941–1945.

Bourrat, C., Garde, P., Boucher, M. & Fournet, A. (1986): Etats d'absence prolongés chez des patients âgés sans passé épileptique. *Rev. Neurol.* **142**, 696–702.

Bornstein, M., Coddon, D. & Song, S. (1956): Prolonged alterations in behaviour associated with a continuous EEG (spike and dome) abnormality. *Neurology* **6**, 444–448.

Brett, E.M. (1966): Minor epileptic status. *J. Neurol. Sci.* **3**, 52–75.

Cascino, D. (1993): Non convulsive status epilepticus in adults and children. *Epilepsia* **34(Supp. 1)**, S21–S28.

Cambier, J., Masson, M. & Dairou, R. (1974): Epilepsie tardive à forme confusionnelle. *Entretiens de Bichat – Médecine*, 585–588.

Cantú, T.G. & Korek, J.S. (1991): Central nervous system reactions to histamine-2 receptor blockers. *Ann. Intern. Med.* **114**, 1027–1034.

Courjon, J., Fournier, M.H. & Mauguière, F. (1984): Les états de mal chez les épileptiques adultes suivis dans un hôpital neurologique. *Rev. EEG Neurophysiol.* **14**, 175–179.

Commission on Classification and Terminology of the International League Against Epilepsy (1989): Proposal for revised classification of epilepsies and epileptic syndromes. *Epilepsia* **30**, 389–399.

Dunne, J.W., Summers, Q.A. & Stewart-Wynne, E.G. (1987): Non-convulsive status epilepticus: a prospective study in an adult general hospital. *Q.J. Med.* **62**, 117–126.

Elian, M. (1969): Petit-mal like discharge in the EEG of adults. *Electroencephalogr. Clin. Neurophysiol.* **27**, 216–221.

Ellis, J.M. & Lee, S.I. (1977): Acute prolonged confusion in later life as an ictal state. *Epilepsia* **19**, 119–128.

Fagan, K.J. & Lee, S.I. (1990): Prolonged confusion following convulsions due to generalized nonconvulsive status epilepticus. *Neurology* **40**, 1689–1694.

Friedlander, W.J. & Feinstein, G.H. (1956): Petit mal status. Epilepsia minoris continua. *Neurology* **6**, 357–363.

Fujiwara, T., Watanabe, M., Matsuda, K., Senbongi, M., Yagi, K. & Seino, M. (1991): Complex partial status epilepticus provoked by the ingestion of alcohol: a case report. *Epilepsia* **32**, 650–656.

Gall, M.V., Scollo-Lavizzari, G. & Becker, H. (1978): Absence status in the adult. New results including computerized transverse axial tomography. *Eur. Neurol.* **17**, 121–128.

Gastaut, H. (1967): A propos d'une classification symptomatologique des états de mal épileptiques. In: *Les états de mal épileptiques*, eds. H. Gastaut, J. Roger & H. Lob, pp. 1–8. Paris: Masson.

Gastaut, H. (1970): Clinical and electroencephalographic classification of epileptic seizures. *Epilepsia* **11**, 102–113.

Gastaut, H. (1981): Individualisation des épilepsies dites 'bénignes' ou 'fonctionnelles' aux différents âges de la vie. Appréciation des variations correspondantes de la prédisposition épileptiques à ces âges. *Rev. EEG Neurophysiol.* **11**, 346–366.

Gastaut, H. (1983): Classification of status epilepticus. In: *Status epilepticus. Advances in neurology*, Vol. 34, eds. A.V. Delgado-Escueta, C.G. Wasterlain, D.M. Treiman & R.J. Porter, pp. 15–35. New York: Raven Press.

Gastaut, H., Bernard, R., Naquet, R. & Wilson, J. (1956): Etude électroclinique quotidienne d'un état confusionnel épileptique simple ayant duré un mois. *Rev. Neurol.* **94**, 267–272.

Gibberd, F.B. (1972): Petit mal status presenting de novo in middle age [Letter]. *Lancet* **i**, 269.

Goldensohn, E.S. & Gold, A.P. (1960): Prolonged behavioral disturbances as ictal phenomena. *Neurology* **10**, 1–9.

Goldmann, J.W., Glastein, G. & Adams, A.H. (1981): Adult onset absence status, a report of six cases. *Clin. EEG* **12**, 199–204.

Guberman, A., Cantu-Reyna, G., Stuss, D. & Broughton, R. (1986): Nonconvulsive generalized status epilepticus: clinical features, neuropsychological testing, and long-term follow-up. *Neurology* **36**, 1284–1291.

Hersch, E.L. & Billings, R.F. (1988): Acute confusional state with status petit mal as a withdrawal syndrome and five year follow-up. *Can. J. Psychiatry* **33**, 157–159.

Hess, R., Scotto-Lavizzari, G. & Wyss, F.E. (1971): Borderline cases of Petit Mal Status. *Eur. Neurol.* **5**, 137–154.

Lim, J., Yagnig, P., Schraeder, P. & Wheeler, S. (1986): Ictal catatonia as a manifestation of nonconvulsive status epilepticus. *J. Neurol. Neurosurg. Psychiatry* **49,** 833–836.

Lee, S.I. (1985): Nonconvulsive status epilepticus. Ictal confusion in later life. *Arch. Neurol.* **42,** 787–781.

Lennox, W.G. (1945): The petit mal epilepsies: their treatment with tridione. *J.A.M.A.* **129,** 1069–1074.

Lob, H., Roger, J., Soulayrol, R., Régis, H. & Gastaut, H. (1967): Les états de mal généralisés à expression confusionelle. In: *Les états de mal épileptiques*, eds. H. Gastaut, J. Roger & H. Lob, pp. 91–109. Paris: Masson.

Mellerio, F. (1980): Apport de l'électroencéphalographie dans les accidents de sevrage aux tranquillisants. *Rev. EEG. Neurophysiol.* **10,** 95–103.

Niedermeyer, E., Fineyre, F., Riley, T. & Uematsu, S. (1979): Absence status (petit mal status) with focal characteristics. *Arch. Neurol.* **36,** 417–421.

Niedermeyer, E. & Khalifeh, R. (1965): Petit mal status ('spike-wave stupor'). An electro-clinical appraisal. *Epilepsia* **6,** 250–262.

Nishiura, N. & Oiwa, T. (1979): Epilepsy above 70 years of age–four cases with spike and wave complex. *Folia Psych. Neurol. Jap.* **33,** 263–268.

Porter, R.J. & Penry, J.K. (1983): Petit mal status. In: *Status epilepticus. Advances in neurology*, Vol. 34, eds. A.V. Delgado-Escueta, C.G. Wasterlain, D.M. Treiman & R.J. Porter, pp. 61–67. New-York: Raven Press.

Pritchard, P.B. & O'Neal, D.B. (1984): Non convulsive status epilepticus following metrizamide myelography. *Ann. Neurol.* **16,** 252–254.

Rey, M. & Papy, J.J. (1987): Etats d'obnubilation critique d'origine frontale: un diagnostic clinique difficile. *Rev. EEG Neurophysiol.* **17,** 377–385.

Richard, P. & Brenner, R.P. (1980): Absence status. Case reports and review of the literature. *L'Encéphale* **6,** 385–392.

Rohr-Le Floch, J., Gauthier, G. & Beaumanoir, A. (1988): Etats confusionnels d'origine épileptique. Intérêt de l'EEG fait en urgence. *Rev. Neurol.* **144,** 425–436.

Rumpl, E. & Hinterhuber, H. (1981): Unusual 'spike-wave stupor' in a patient with manic-depressive psychosis treated with amitriptyline. *J. Neurol.* **226,** 131–135.

Schöpf, J. (1983): Withdrawal phenomena after long-term administration of benzodiazepines. A review of recent investigations. *Pharmacopsychiatry* **16,** 1–8.

Schwartz, M.S. & Scott, D.F. (1971): Isolated petit mal status presenting de novo in middle age [Letter]. *Lancet* **ii,** 1399–1401.

Thomas, P., Beaumanoir, A., Genton, P., Dolisi, C. & Chatel, M. (1992a): De novo absence status. Report of 11 cases. *Neurology* **42,** 104–110.

Thomas, P., Lebrun, C. & Chatel, M. (1992b): True and false nonconvulsive confusional status epilepticus. *J. Neurol.* **239(Supp. 2),** S72.

Thomas, P., Lebrun, C. & Chatel, M. (1993): De novo absence status as a benzodiazepine withdrawal syndrome. *Epilepsia* **34,** 355–358.

Tomson, T., Svanborg, E. & Wedlund, J.E. (1986): Nonconvulsive status epilepticus: high incidence of complex partial status. *Epilepsia* **27,** 276–285.

Tomson, T., Lindbom, U. & Nilsson B.Y. (1992): Nonconvulsive status epilepticus in adults: thirty two consecutive patients from a general hospital population. *Epilepsia* **33,** 276–285.

Tyrer, P.J. & Seivewright, N. (1984): Identification and management of benzodiazepine dependence. *Postgrad. Med. J.* **60,** 41–46.

Van Sweden, B. (1985): Toxic 'ictal' confusion in middle age: treatment with benzodiazepine. *J. Neurol. Neurosurg. Psychiatry* **48,** 472–476.

Van Sweden, B. & Mellerio F. (1988): Toxic ictal confusion. *J. Epilepsy* **1,** 157–163.

Van Zandycke, M., Orban, L.C. & Van der Eecken, H. (1980): Acute prolonged ictal confusion resembling petit mal status presenting 'de novo' in later life. *Acta Neurol. Belg.* **80,** 174–179.

Vercelletto, M. & Gastaut, J.L. (1981): Les épilepsies débutant aprés soixante ans. *Rev. EEG Neurophysiol.* **11,** 537–544.

Vickrey, B.G. & Bahls, F.H. (1989): Nonconvulsive status epilepticus following cerebral angiography. *Ann. Neurol.* **25,** 199–201.

Vignaendra, V., Frank, A.O. & Lim, C.L. (1977): Absence status in a patient with hypocalcemia. *Electroencephalogr. Clin. Neurophysiol.* **43,** 429–433.

Vollmer, M.E., Weiss, H., Beanland, C. & Krumholz, A. (1985): Prolonged confusion due to absence status following metrizamide myelography. *Arch. Neurol.* **42,** 1005–1007.

Weiner, R.D., Whanger, A.D., Erwin, C.W. & Wilson, W.P. (1980): Prolonged confusional state and EEG seizure activity following concurrent ECT and lithium use. *Am. J. Psychiatry* **137,** 1452–1453.

Wells, C.E. (1975): Transient ictal psychosis. *Arch. Gen. Psychiatry* **32,** 1201–1203.

Williamson, P.D., Spencer, D.D., Spencer, S.S., Novelly, R.A. & Mattson, R.H. (1985): Complex partial status epilepticus: a depth-electrode study. *Ann. Neurol.* **18,** 647–654.

Zappoli, R. (1955): Two cases of prolonged epileptic twilight state with almost continuous 'wave-spikes'. *Electroencephalogr. Clin. Neurophysiol.* **7,** 421–423.

Chapter 12

Physiopathogenesis of feline generalized penicillin epilepsy: the role of thalamocortical mechanisms

M. Avoli & P. Gloor

Montreal Neurological Institute and Department of Neurology and Neurosurgery, McGill University, 3801 University St Montreal, QC, Canada H3A 2B4

Introduction

Generalized 3 Hz spike-and-wave (SW) discharge occurring during a clinical absence attack represents one of the most dramatic patterns seen in clinical electroencephalography. First described in epileptic patients by Gibbs *et al.* (1935) it was produced experimentally for the first time in 1946 by Jasper & Droogleever-Fortuyn by low-frequency stimulation of the midline and intralaminar nuclei of the thalamus in the cat. Much of this chapter will be devoted to a description of how thalamocortical and corticothalamic mechanisms are involved in the genesis of spike-and-wave discharge induced by the intramuscular injection of large doses of penicillin (300 000 to 500 000 IU) in the cat. This model was discovered by Prince & Farrell (1969) and was later named feline generalized penicillin epilepsy (FGPE). It has been the object of studies carried out in our laboratory over the last two decades. These studies have previously been summarized by Gloor (1988), Gloor *et al.* (1990), and by Avoli *et al.* (1990). In the present review we shall also compare the EEG patterns of generalized absence attacks and generalized convulsive seizures that can be recorded in human patients and in FGPE, and briefly describe the cellular mechanisms during such discharges in the cat cortex following penicillin administration. Finally, the mechanisms of action of some antiepileptic drugs used for absence attacks will be discussed in the context of the cellular phenomena that are responsible for the rhythmic behaviour of thalamic and cortical neurons during SW discharge.

Validity of feline generalized penicillin epilepsy (FGPE) as a model of human absence epilepsy

Feline generalized penicillin epilepsy (FGPE) is a valid model for human primary generalized epilepsy characterized clinically by absence attacks and electroencephalographically by generalized

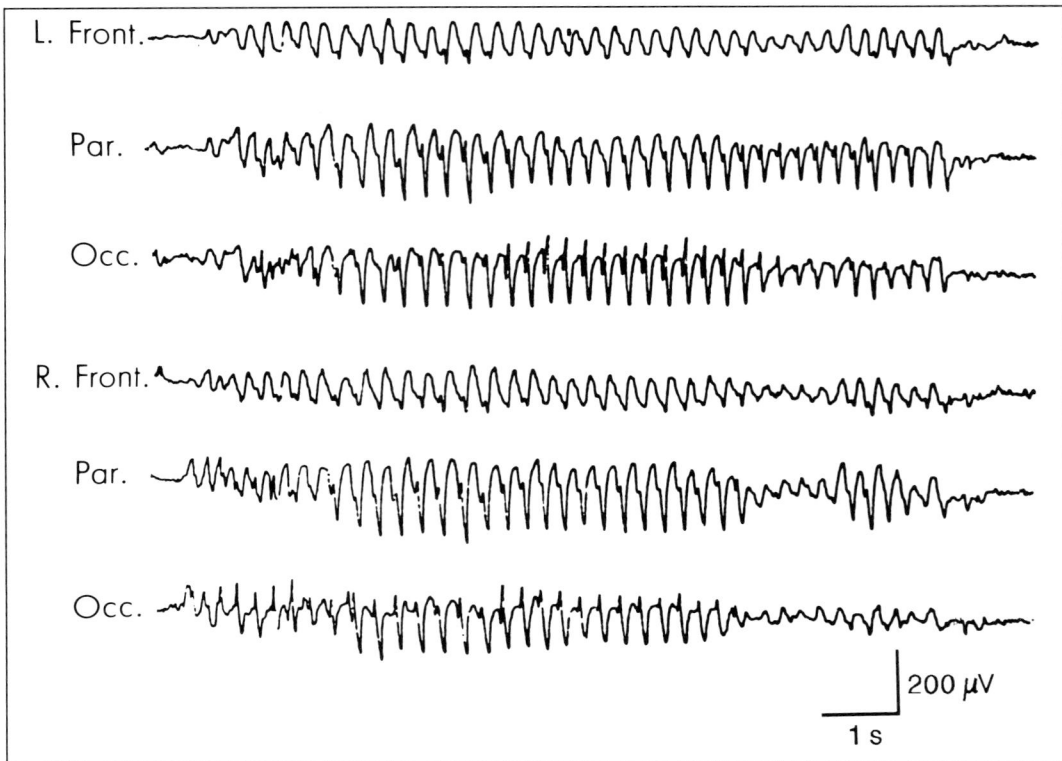

Fig. 1. EEG pattern of feline generalized penicillin epilepsy recorded with electrodes inserted chronically in the skull displays features similar to those observed in human generalized spike-and-wave discharges associated with absence attacks. Abbreviations: L, = left; R = right; Front. = frontal; Par. = parietal; Occ. = occipital. Reproduced with permission from Guberman et al. (1975).

bilaterally synchronous SW discharge. In addition to an EEG pattern that is similar to that seen in absence attacks (Fig. 1), cats exhibit behavioural manifestations that consist of rhythmic eye blinking, facial twitching, an abrupt and pronounced drop in responsiveness to stimuli presented during SW discharge in an operant conditioning procedure and arrest of self-paced motor behaviour (Taylor-Courval & Gloor, 1984). Moreover, the profile of responsiveness of the SW discharge to anticonvulsant drugs in FGPE is similar to that found in human absence epilepsy: ethosuximide and valproate are effective in reducing SW discharge, while phenytoin is not (Guberman et al., 1975; Pellegrini et al., 1978).

Spindles and spike-and-wave discharge in FGPE: a common thalamocortical mechanism

Our electrophysiological studies have indicated that spike-and-wave discharges of FGPE evolve from spindles and therefore are presumably mediated by a common thalamocortical mechanism (see for review Gloor et al., 1990). The transformation of spindles into spike-and-wave discharges in FGPE results from the penicillin-induced increased excitability of cortical neurons which is responsible for the secondary recruitment of a powerful, at least in part recurrent, intracortical inhibitory mechanism (Kostopoulos et al., 1981a,b, 1983). Hence, the 'spike' of the spike-and-wave complex represents an exaggerated spindle-wave and results from summed cortical EPSPs induced by

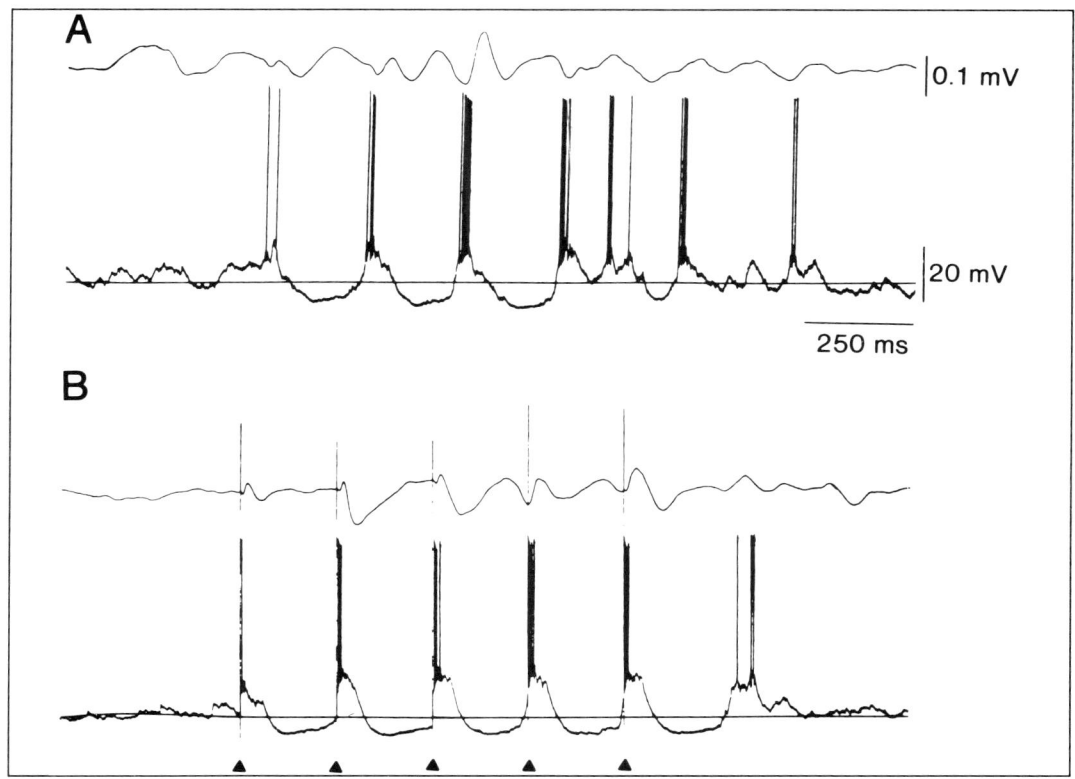

Fig. 2. Similarities in the EEG and in intracellular recordings between penicillin-induced spike-and-wave discharges (A) and thalamocortical responses (B) induced by repetitive stimuli (triangles) delivered to the nucleus ventralis lateralis of the thalamus. Reproduced with permission from Giaretta et al. (1987).

thalamocortical volleys; the 'slow-wave' component reflects the summation of intracortical IPSPs of both $GABA_A$ and $GABA_B$ type and is associated with a 200–300 ms hyperpolarization (Fig. 2) (Giaretta et al., 1987). In keeping with this type of cortical mechanism, the pattern of spike-and-wave discharge correlates at the cellular level with a striking oscillation between markedly increased firing probability of cortical neurons during the 'spike' and a reduction of this probability of firing to virtually zero during the 'slow-wave' component of the spike-and-wave complex (Fig. 5).

Both the cortex and the thalamus are required for the appearance of generalized spike-and-wave discharge in response to intramuscular penicillin. If the thalamus is transiently inactivated by an intrathalamic injection of KCl, spike-and-wave discharges in both the thalamus and cortex are abolished (Fig. 3) (Avoli & Gloor, 1981). On the other hand, when the thalamus is deprived of inputs from and outputs toward the cortex, discharge is not seen. As illustrated in Fig. 4, the thalamus of a decorticated cat does not generate spike-and-wave discharge following large doses of intramuscular penicillin (Avoli & Gloor, 1982). Under these conditions the thalamus produces spindles both before and after penicillin. Moreover, thalamic spike-and-wave in the intact brain are replaced by spindles when the cortex is inactivated bilaterally by spreading depression (Avoli & Gloor, 1982). The involvement in FGPE of a thalamocortical mechanism that is operant under normal conditions is supported by the similarities shared by incrementing cortical responses to thalamic stimuli and SW discharges induced by penicillin (Fig. 2).

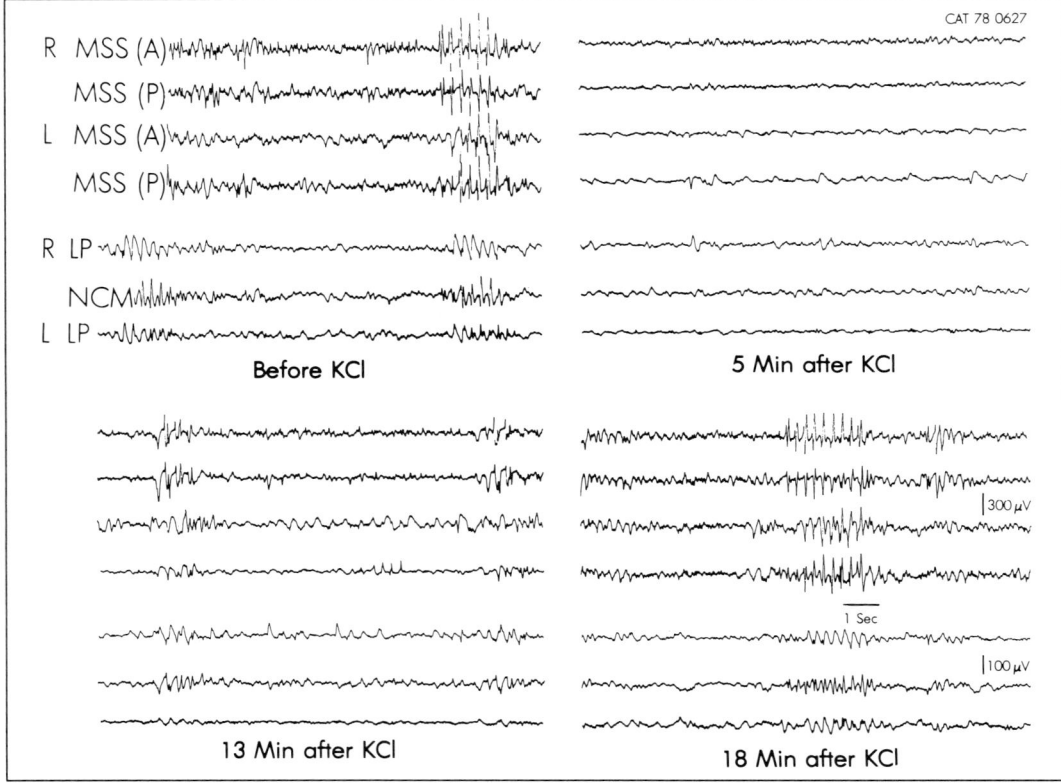

Fig. 3. Effects exerted on the spontaneous thalamic and cortical EEG activity by a thalamic microinjection of 10 μl of 25 per cent KCl into the left thalamic nucleus lateralis posterior (L LP). Note that cortical and thalamic spike-and-wave discharges disappear and recover together with the return of normal thalamic activity which is depressed most markedly at the site of the microinjection. Abbreviations: MSS = middle suprasylvian gyrus; LP = nucleus lateralis posterior; NCM = nucleus centralis medialis; R = right; L = left; (A) = anterior; (P) = posterior. Reproduced with permission from Avoli & Gloor (1981).

Respective roles of thalamus and cortex in FGPE

In the FGPE model the thalamus is secondarily, but very quickly, recruited into this oscillatory pattern via corticothalamic pathways. Accordingly, Avoli & Kostopoulos (1982) have shown that electrophysiologically identified corticothalamic neurons fire bursts of action potentials during the 'spike' of the spike-and-wave discharge. These cortical excitatory inputs impose the oscillatory modality of firing characteristics of spike-and-wave discharge on thalamic neurons; in turn, some of these are thalamocortical cells and thus project back to the neocortex.

The mechanism of interaction between thalamus and cortex in spike-and-wave discharge has been studied in detail in neurophysiological experiments in which cortical and thalamic EEGs and the firing of a pair of neurons (one in the cortex, the other in the thalamus) were studied with EEG averaging and time histogram computation techniques (Fig. 5). Two essential features were revealed by these studies (Avoli et al., 1983). First, the cortical and thalamic neurons within a thalamocortical sector fire in an oscillatory fashion in a tightly phase-locked manner. Second, the oscillatory pattern in each burst of spike-and-wave discharge appears to be initiated by the cortex

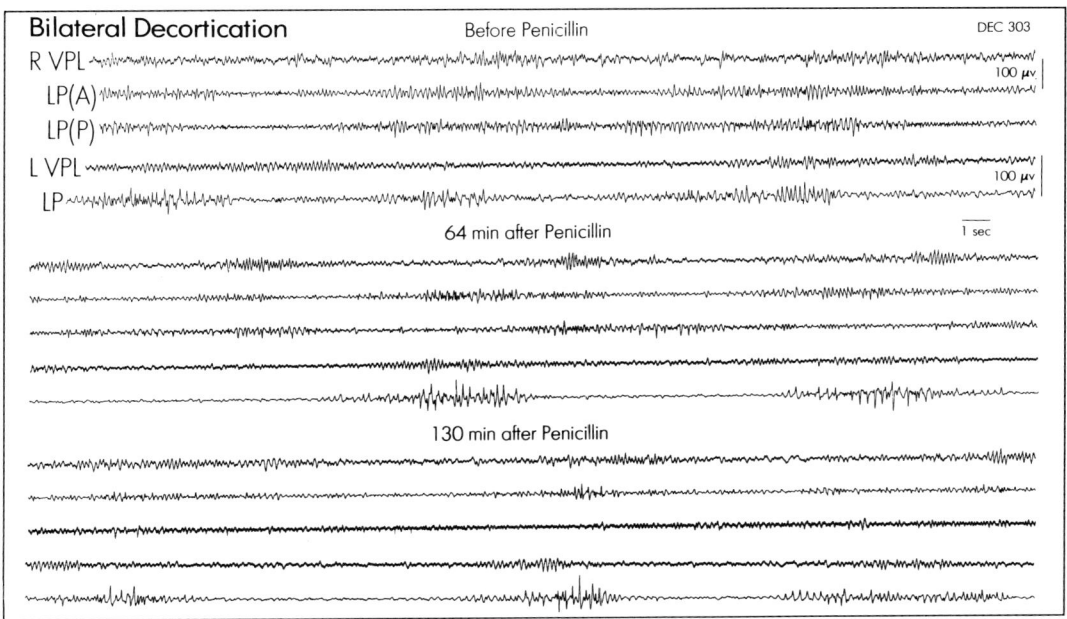

Fig. 4. EEG from the thalamus of a bilaterally decorticated cat, before and after i.m. injection of 350 000 IU/kg penicillin. Abbreviations: MSSG = middle suprasylvian gyrus; LP = nucleus lateralis posterior; VL = nucleus ventralis lateralis; VPL = nucleus ventroposterolateralis; R = right; L = Left; (A) = anterior; (P) = posterior. Reproduced with permission from Avoli & Gloor (1982b).

and entrains the thalamus secondarily. The oscillatory pattern in the thalamus is seen more clearly in neurons of the 'specific' nuclei than in those of 'nonspecific' nuclei (McLachlan et al., 1984).

Though each spike-and-wave discharge appears to be initiated from the cortex, the thalamus plays an active role in spike-and-wave discharge of FGPE. Hence, it becomes meaningless once the thalamocortical oscillation is established to ask whether the cortex or the thalamus paces the spike-and-wave rhythm. Both structures are essential and the functional and anatomical integrity of each of them is required to maintain the spike-and-wave discharge.

One important question that requires an answer is how through this corticothalamic interaction the frequency of oscillation in this thalamocortical network is reduced to about half as spindles evolve into spike-waves (Kostopoulos et al., 1981b). The explanation for this switch in frequency should presumably invoke a mechanism whereby in the thalamus the incoming corticothalamic volley engages an intrathalamic oscillatory mechanism engendering a thalamocortical volley that returns to the cortex. Our experiments did not address this problem, but it is likely that the intrathalamic oscillating mechanisms that have been described by Steriade et al. (1993) and by von Krosigk et al. (1993) are involved in this linkage between corticothalamic and thalamocortical volleys. In the spindle stage, the frequency of oscillation in thalamocortical networks is dependent upon the de-inactivation of a Ca^{2+}-conductance of thalamocortical neurons paced by rhythmic GABAergic inputs from the thalamic reticular nucleus which provide the hyperpolarization of thalamocortical neurons that is required to de-inactivate the Ca^{2+}-conductance. In FGPE all the evidence points to the fact that it is the cortex that initiates the sequence of events that switch the spindle to the spike-and-wave rhythm with the thalamus being only secondarily entrained into the oscillatory mode typical for spike-and-wave discharge. Conversely, however, the cortex on its own, without thalamic participation is not capable of sustaining the spike-and-wave rhythm.

Two possible explanations can be envisaged as to how in FGPE the thalamocortical neurons which

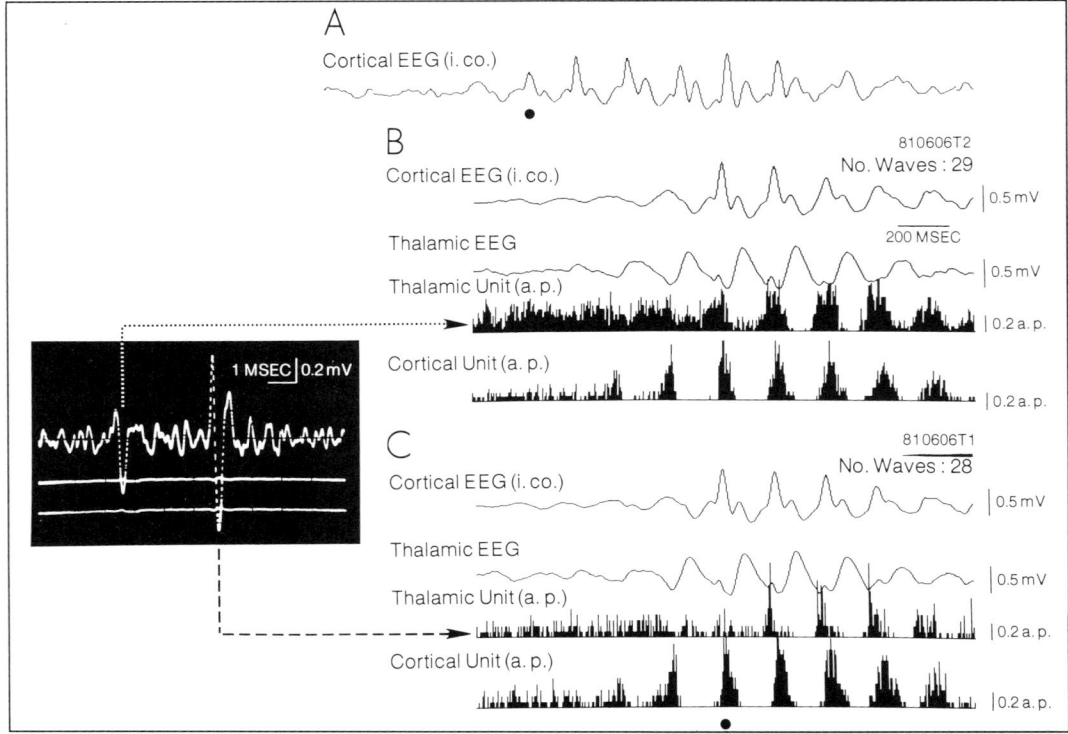

Fig. 5. EEG-unit correlation for the cortical and two thalamic neurons in generalized spike-and-wave discharge in FGPE. The first spike of a spike-and-wave burst was used to trigger the averaging of the EEG (top two channels) and the computation of unit histograms (lower two channels). Spikes of spike-and-wave complexes are associated with increased, slow waves with a decreased firing probability of both cortical and thalamic neurons. Note that the oscillatory pattern in the cortex starts one to two cycles earlier than that in the thalamus.

sustain both the spindle and the spike-and-wave rhythm, after penicillin injection respond to cortical inputs by an oscillation that has a frequency that is only half that of the spindle rhythm. The first explanation is based on the fact that penicillin is a weak $GABA_A$ antagonist. It may therefore weaken $GABA_A$-mediated inhibition provided by the reticular nucleus leaving its $GABA_B$ mechanism intact. According to von Krosigk et al. (1993), blockage of $GABA_A$ action shifts the oscillation in the network connecting the reticular nucleus to thalamic relay cells to a slower frequency that is within the range of the spike-and-wave rhythm. Apart from the fact that we found no evidence that penicillin in systemic doses required to induce FGPE weakens GABAergic inhibition, at least in the cortex (Giaretta et al., 1987; Kostopoulos et al., 1983), this explanation is unsatisfactory for another reason. If correct, one would expect the thalamus of a decorticated cat to produce a spike-and-wave rhythm instead of spindles when doses sufficient or exceeding those required to produce spike-and-wave discharge in the intact cat are injected. This is, however, not the case: the thalamus continues to produce spindles under these conditions (Fig. 4) (Avoli & Gloor, 1982). The second explanation is based on the fact that the cortical output through corticothalamic volleys becomes more powerful as spindles evolve into spike-and-waves (Kostopoulos et al., 1981a). Thus the reticular nucleus is more powerfully stimulated through corticothalamic volleys and hence produces a more powerful inhibitory output to thalamocortical neurons which therefore become more hyperpolarized. This may shift their membrane potential into the region where the

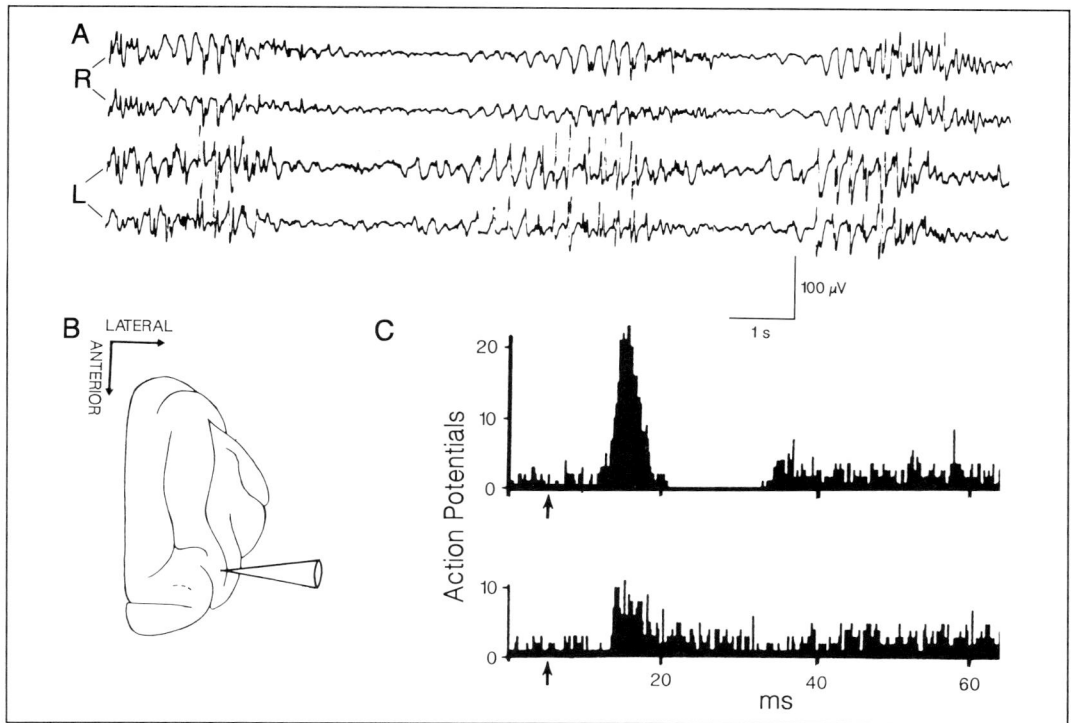

Fig. 6. Spike-and-wave discharges depress the response of a neocortical cell in the contralateral somatosensory area to electrical stimuli delivered at 2 Hz to the radial nerves. A: Spike-and-wave discharges recorded from the anterior and posterior suprasylvian gyrus of both hemispheres (R and L, right and left). B: Schematic drawing of the cat brain seen from above shows position of the recording microelectrodes. C: Upper panel shows peristimulation histogram that was constructed by selecting stimuli occurring between spike-and-wave discharges; the lower histogram was made from stimuli delivered during spike-and-wave discharge. P. White, R. Dykes, M. Avoli and P. Gloor, unpublished data.

slow delta oscillator described by Steriade *et al.* (1993) becomes activated and supersedes the spindle oscillation. The frequency of this slower oscillation is within the range of the spike-and-wave rhythm. This hypothesis is more attractive in the light of the experiments on decorticate cats mentioned above and also appears to be more readily applicable to human absence epilepsy, as it does not depend on postulating the intervention of an anti-$GABA_A$ agent like penicillin.

Both hypotheses would, however, explain the switch from the spindle to the spike-and-wave rhythm. At this slower rhythm each descending thalamocortical volley would induce a powerful and prolonged hyperpolarization of thalamocortical neurons which would trigger a rebound Ca^{2+} spike carrying a burst of action potentials initiating a powerful return projection to the cortex. In this way the spike-and-wave oscillation would be maintained through the interplay of a cortical oscillatory mechanism depending in large part upon recurrent inhibition (Kostopoulos *et al.*, 1983), and a thalamic oscillatory mechanism depending upon the interplay of membrane hyperpolarization and de-inactivation of a Ca^{2+}-conductance in thalamocortical neurons.

Comparison with other models of absence attacks

Spike-and-wave discharges in other experimental models of generalized epilepsy (e.g. some rodent models) appear to be initiated from thalamic structures rather than the cortex. However, this conclusion is based solely on EEG recordings and there has not been any study at the cellular level in these models. For instance, at the EEG level, spike-and-wave discharges in the Strasbourg Wistar model often start in the thalamus and then seem to entrain the cortex (Vergnes *et al.*, 1987). However, a tightly interlocked thalamocortical mechanism is also seen in the Strasbourg Wistar model. Moreover, in these experiments, as well as in two other pharmacological rodent models (low doses of pentylenetetrazol and γ-hydroxybutyric acid), both the thalamus and cortex are required for absence seizure activity, since neither structure alone can sustain bilateral spike-and-wave discharge (Snead, 1988). Hence, in different models the spike-and-wave rhythm may be initiated either from the cortex or the thalamus, but this point is relatively trivial compared with the importance of the role of the oscillation in thalamocorticothalamic loop in the elaboration and maintenance of generalized spike-and-wave discharges.

Thalamocortical mechanisms in spike-and-wave (SW) discharge and information processing

Thalamocortical projections represent an important link in the final processing of sensory information coming from the periphery. The tight synchronization that occurs during spike-and-wave discharge between thalamus and cortex might interfere with this processing of peripheral inputs and thus account for the marked impairment of such processing during an absence attack. To test this hypothesis, somatosensory responses were recorded with an extracellular recording microelectrode positioned in the somatosensory area of the neocortex while stimulating with electrical shocks (2 Hz) the contralateral radial nerve during spike-and-wave discharges induced by penicillin. As illustrated in Fig. 6, when stimuli occurred between one spike-and-wave burst and the next, the somatosensory neocortical cell discharge showed a prominent response to electrical radial nerve stimulation. By contrast, this response was greatly reduced when the stimuli occurred during the spike-and-wave discharge. This markedly reduced response to a sensory stimulus during spike-and-wave discharge coupled with its preservation in inter-spike-and-wave-burst interval, dovetails with the marked reduction of behavioural responsiveness during spike-and-wave discharge in the cat subject to FGPE that contrasts with its full preservation between spike-and-wave bursts (Taylor-Courval & Gloor, 1984). This situation perfectly mimics that seen in human absence attacks. These experiments also underscore the fact that the pattern of cortical neuronal discharge during spike-and-wave activity is highly disruptive of integrated cortical function and explains the deficit in cognitive functioning that characterizes absence attacks (Gloor, 1979).

Intracortical inhibition and transition from spike-and-wave discharge to generalized tonic–clonic seizure activity

A hallmark of generalized spike-and-wave discharges of FGPE is the 'preservation' of $GABA_A$- and $GABA_B$-mediated intracortical inhibitory mechanisms. They underlie the slow-wave component of the spike-and-wave complex (Giaretta *et al.*, 1987). However, cortical IPSPs disappear shortly before the onset of, as well as during, the EEG pattern that is commonly associated with generalized tonic–clonic convulsions (Kostopoulos *et al.*, 1983). EEG tonic–clonic convulsions are commonly seen in cats with reticular-formation lesions or after several hours of spike-and-wave discharge. Therefore the transition from spike-and-wave discharges of absence attack to generalized convulsive seizures is accompanied and possibly caused by the breakdown of one or more hyperpolarizing inhibitory potentials in the cortex. The preservation of GABA-mediated mechanisms in pure absence epilepsy might explain the differences in prognostic outlook that characterize that form of epilepsy from seizures in which GABAergic mechanisms break down, as is the case in generalized convulsive and partial seizures (Avoli & Gloor, 1994; Gloor, 1989).

Thalamocortical mechanisms and mechanisms of action of antiepileptic drugs

An important role in the oscillatory behaviour seen during spike-and-wave discharge is played by ionic mechanisms that are intrinsic to neurons in the cortex and the thalamus. One of these, the so-called low-threshold Ca^{2+} conductance, is de-inactivated by membrane hyperpolarization and is particularly prominent in the thalamic structures. Therefore it might play a role in the rhythmic behaviour of neurons located in the thalamus which participates in spike-and-wave discharge (Deschênes et al., 1982; Jahnsen & Llinás, 1984; Steriade, 1990; Steriade et al., 1993; von Krosigk et al., 1993). This type of ionic conductance is diminished and eventually blocked by the anti-absence drug ethosuximide (Coulter et al., 1989, 1990). On the other hand, as the membrane hyperpolarization seen during the 'slow wave' of spike-and-wave discharge is necessary for de-inactivating the Ca^{2+}-current, drugs that antagonize the synaptic mechanism responsible for this hyperpolarization might be effective as anti-absence agents (Marescaux et al., 1992). This is the case for the $GABA_B$ antagonist CGP35348 which is capable of decreasing spike-and-wave discharge in the Strasbourg Wistar rat model (Marescaux et al., 1992). Similar findings have been obtained in the lethargic mouse which represents a model of primary generalized absence seizures (Hosford et al., 1992).

A different mechanism of action should be considered for valproate which is effective in controlling absence attacks as well as generalized tonic–clonic seizures. Valproate is able to reduce voltage-gated Na^+ currents in cortical cells (Zona & Avoli, 1990), a mechanism that is of obvious relevance for reducing the sustained depolarizations and action-potential discharges that are seen in generalized tonic–clonic activity. However, the site of action of valproate for controlling absence attacks remains unknown. A clue for this latter mechanism might come from recent data obtained in subicular neurons that have indicated that a Na^+ current might be responsible for the brief bursts generated by these cells (Mattia et al., 1993). This burst shares some similarities with the bursts generated by thalamic neurons, including the occurrence at the end of a hyperpolarizing pulse (the so-called post-anodal exaltation). However, whether this Na^+ mechanism is present in neocortical cells still remains to be elucidated.

Acknowledgement

This work was supported by MRC of Canada grant MT-8109 to Dr Avoli.

References

Avoli, M. & Gloor, P. (1981): The effects of transient functional depression of the thalamus on spindles and on bilateral synchronous discharges of feline generalized penicillin epilepsy. *Epilepsia* **22**, 443–452.

Avoli, M. & Gloor, P. (1982): Interaction of cortex and thalamus in spike-and-wave discharges of feline generalized penicillin epilepsy. *Exp. Neurol.* **76**, 196–217.

Avoli, M. & Gloor, P. (1994): Physiopathology of focal and generalized *vs* that of generalized non-convulsive seizures. In: *Epileptic seizures and syndromes*, ed. P. Wolf, pp. 553–567. London: John Libbey.

Avoli, M., Gloor, P. & Kostopoulos, G. (1990): Focal and generalized epileptiform activity in the cortex: in search of differences in synaptic mechanisms, ionic movements, and long-lasting changes in neuronal excitability. In: *Generalized epilepsy: neurobiological approaches*, eds. M. Avoli, P. Gloor, G. Kostopoulos & R. Naquet, pp. 213–231. Boston, Basel, Berlin: Birkhäuser.

Avoli, M., Gloor, P., Kostopoulos, G. & Gotman, J. (1983): An analysis of penicillin-induced generalized spike-and-wave discharges using simultaneous recording of cortical and thalamic single units. *J. Neurophysiol.* **50**, 819–837.

Avoli, M. & Kostopoulos, G. (1982): Participation of corticothalamic cells in penicillin induced spike-and-wave discharges. *Brain Res.* **247**, 159–163.

Coulter, D.A., Huguenard, J.R. & Prince, D.A. (1989): Specific petit mal anticonvulsants reduce calcium currents in thalamic neurons. *Neurosci. Lett.* **98**, 74–78.

Coulter, D.A., Huguenard, J.R. & Prince, D.A. (1990): Cellular actions of petit mal anticonvulsants: implication of thalamic low-threshold calcium current in generation of spike-wave discharge. In: *Generalized epilepsy: neurobiological approaches*, eds. M. Avoli, P. Gloor, G. Kostopoulos & R. Naquet, pp. 425–435. Boston, Basel, Berlin: Birkhäuser.

Deschênes, M., Roy, J.P. & Steriade, M. (1982): Thalamic bursting mechanism: an inward slow current revealed by membrane hyperpolarization. *Brain Res.* **239**, 289–293.

Giaretta, D., Avoli, M. & Gloor, P. (1987): Intracellular recordings in pericruciate neurons during spike-and-wave discharges of feline generalized penicillin epilepsy. *Brain Res.* **405**, 68–79.

Gibbs, F.A., Davis, H. & Lennox, W.G. (1935): The electroencephalogram in epilepsy and in conditions of impaired consciousness. *Arch. Neurol. Psychiat.* **34**, 1133–1148.

Gloor, P. (1979): Generalized epilepsy with spike-and-wave discharge: a reinterpretation of its electrographic and clinical manifestations. *Epilepsia* **20**, 571–588.

Gloor, P. (1988): Neurophysiological mechanism of generalized spike-and-wave discharge and its implications for understanding absence seizures. In: *Elements of petit mal epilepsy*, eds. M.S. Myslobodsky & A.F. Mirsky, pp. 159–209. New York, Bern, Frankfurt, Paris: Peter Lang.

Gloor, P. (1989): Epilepsy: relationships between electrophysiology and intracellular mechanisms involving second messengers and gene expression. *Can. J. Neurol. Sci.* **16**, 8–21.

Gloor, P., Avoli, M. & Kostopoulos, G. (1990): Thalamocortical relationships in generalized epilepsy with bilaterally synchronous spike-and-wave discharge. In: *Generalized epilepsy: neurobiological approaches*, eds. M. Avoli, P. Gloor, G. Kostopoulos & R. Naquet, pp. 190–212. Boston, Basel, Berlin: Birkhäuser.

Guberman, A., Gloor, P. & Sherwin, A.L. (1975): Response of generalized penicillin epilepsy in the cat to ethosuximide and diphenylhydantoin. *Neurology* **25**, 758–764.

Hosford, D.A., Clark, S., Cao, F., Wilson, W.A., Liu, F.H., Morrisett, R.A. & Huin, A. (1992): The role of $GABA_B$ receptor activation in absence seizures of lethargic (*lh/lh*) mice. *Science* **257**, 398–401.

Jahnsen, H. & Llinás, R. (1984): Electrophysiological properties of guinea-pig thalamic neurones: an *in vitro* study. *J. Physiol. (Lond.)* **349**, 205–226.

Jasper, H.H. & Droogleever-Fortuyn, J. (1946): Experimental studies on the functional anatomy of petit mal epilepsy. *Res. Publ. Assoc. Nerv. Ment. Dis.* **26**, 272–298.

Kostopoulos, G., Avoli, M. & Gloor, P. (1983): Participation of cortical recurrent inhibition in the genesis of the spike-and-wave discharges in feline generalized penicillin epilepsy. *Brain Res.* **267**, 101–112.

Kostopoulos, G., Gloor, P., Pellegrini, A. & Gotman, J. (1981a): A study of the transition from spindles to spike-and-wave discharge in feline generalized penicillin epilepsy: microphysiological features. *Exp. Neurol.* **73**, 55–77.

Kostopoulos, G., Gloor, P., Pellegrini, A. & Siatitsas, I. (1981b): A study of the transition from spindles to spike-and-wave discharge in feline generalized penicillin epilepsy: EEG features. *Exp. Neurol.* **73**, 43–54.

Marescaux, C., Vergnes, M. & Bernasconi, R. (1992): Generalized nonconvulsive epilepsy: focus on $GABA_B$ receptors. *J. Neural Transm.* **35** (Suppl.) 1–198.

Mattia, D., Hwa, G.G.C. & Avoli, M. (1993): Membrane properties of rat subicular neurons *in vitro*. *J. Neurophysiol.* **70**, 1244–1248.

McLachlan, R.S., Gloor, P. & Avoli, M. (1984): Differential participation of some 'specific' and 'non-specific' thalamic nuclei in generalized spike-and-wave discharges of feline generalized penicillin epilepsy. *Brain Res.* **307**, 277–287.

Pellegrini, A., Gloor, P. & Sherwin, A.L. (1978): Effect of valproate sodium on generalized penicillin epilepsy in the cat. *Epilepsia* **19**, 351–360.

Prince, D.A. & Farrell, D. (1969): 'Centrencephalic' spike-wave discharges following parenteral penicillin injection in the cat. *Neurology* **19**, 309–310.

Snead, O.C. (1988): γ-Hydroxybutyrate model of generalized absence seizures: further characterization and comparison with other absence models. *Epilepsia* **29**, 361–368.

Steriade, M. (1990): Spindling, incremental thalamocortical responses, and spike-wave epilepsy. In: *Generalized epilepsy: neurobiological approaches*, eds. M. Avoli, P. Gloor, G. Kostopoulos & R. Naquet, pp. 161–180. Boston, Basel, Berlin: Birkhäuser.

Steriade, M., McCormick, D.A. & Sejnowski, T.J. (1993): Thalamocortical oscillations in the sleeping and aroused brain. *Science* **262**, 679–685.

Taylor-Courval, D. & Gloor, P. (1984): Behavioral alterations associated with generalized spike-and-wave discharges in the EEG of the cat. *Exp. Neurol.* **83**, 167–186.

Vergnes, M., Marescaux, C., Depaulis, A., Micheletti, G. & Warter, J.M. (1987): Spontaneous spike-and-wave discharges in thalamus and cortex in a rat model of genetic petit mal-like seizures. *Exp. Neurol.* **96**, 127–146.

von Krosigk, M., Bal, T. & McCormick, D.A. (1993): Cellular mechanisms of a synchronized oscillation in the thalamus. *Science* **261**, 361–364.

Zona, C. & Avoli, M. (1990): Effects induced by the antiepileptic drug valproic acid upon the ionic currents recorded in rat neocortical neurons in cell culture. *Exp. Brain Res.* **81**, 313–317.

Chapter 13

Thalamocortical rhythm generation *in vitro*: physiological mechanisms, pharmacological control, and relevance to generalized absence epilepsy

Douglas A. Coulter and Yun-fu Zhang

Department of Neurology, Medical College of Virginia and the MCV Comprehensive Epilepsy Institute of Virginia, Commonwealth University, Richmond, Virginia 23298–0599, USA

Introduction

In the thalamocortical system, a combination of the tight reciprocally connected synaptic circuitry and ensemble of oscillatory voltage-dependent ionic conductances within neurons comprising the circuit predisposes the system to support phasic bursting activity as one of two main behavioural states (reviewed in Steriade and Llinás (1988)). This bursting activity consists of 7–14 Hz spindle activity during periods of slow-wave sleep, and of pathological 3–4 Hz generalized spike-and-wave discharges (SWDs) in patients with generalized absence (GA) epilepsy (reviewed in Gloor & Fariello (1991)). The basic synaptic circuitry of the thalamocortical system is well characterized (for review, see Jones (1985)). Each principle thalamic sensory nucleus sends an ordered projection to the appropriate area of the neocortex, and receives a prominent feedback projection from the same cortical area. Both the thalamocortical and corticothalamic axons, in addition to innervating their main targets, send a collateral projection to nucleus reticularis thalami (NRT), a nucleus comprised exclusively of GABAergic neurons (Houser *et al.*, 1984). This nucleus sends a large inhibitory feedforward (and feedback) projection onto the thalamic neurons from which it receives collaterals (this circuitry is summarized in Fig. 1). This thalamocortical network is particularly simplified in rodents, which are essentially devoid of GABAergic interneurons in thalamic somatosensory nuclei (Jones, 1985; Harris & Hendrickson, 1987).

Although much is known about rhythm generation in the thalamocortical system due to intensive investigation of the anatomical and physiological processes generating sleep spindles (reviewed in

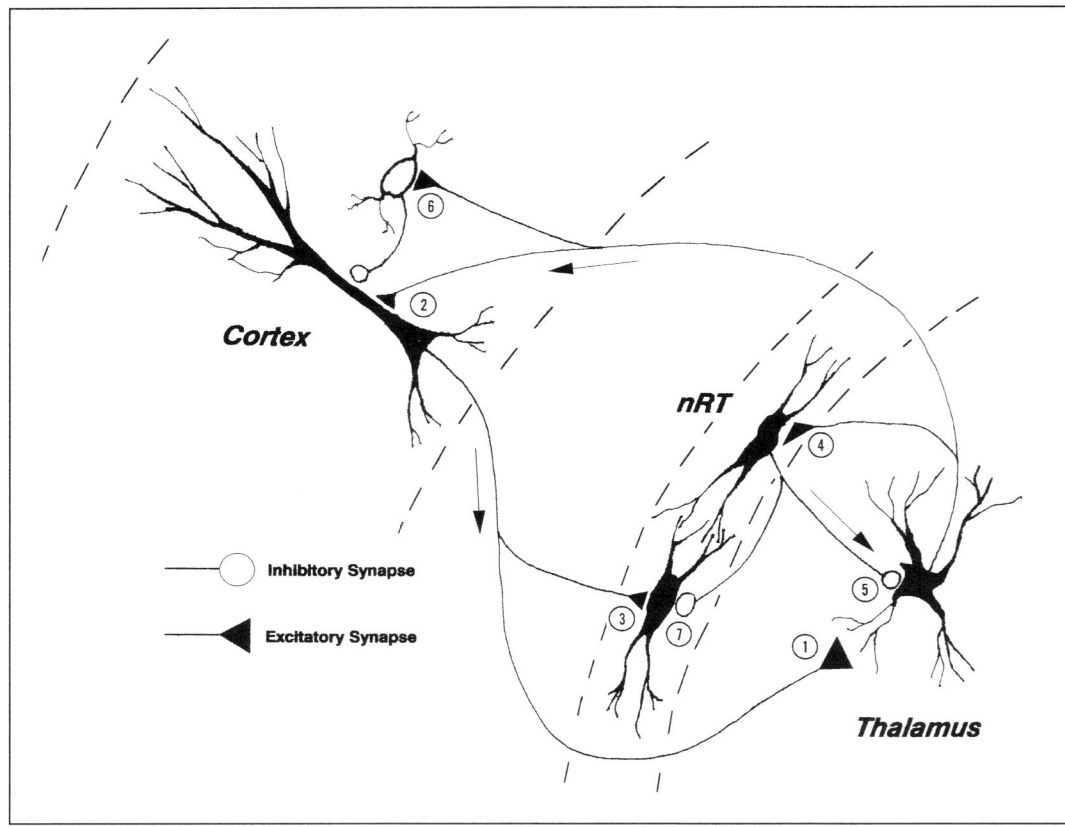

Fig. 1. Schematic of synapses important in thalamocortical rhythm generation. The thalamus receives a large excitatory feedback projection from cortex (synapse #1), and sends a large excitatory projection to cortex, which activates both pyramidal neurons (#2), and intrinsic GABAergic interneurons (#6). Each of these pathways (thalamocortical and corticothalamic) sends an excitatory collateral projection to nucleus reticularis thalami (nRT; synapses #3 and 4). nRT in turn provides a large inhibitory projection onto thalamic neurons (synapse #5), as well as reciprocal inhibitory synapses within nRT (#7).

Steriade and Llinás (1988)), understanding of normal and pathological thalamocortical oscillatory mechanisms could benefit from development of an *in vitro* system which supports these rhythms, where more direct study of critical factors is possible using higher resolution neurophysiological recording techniques. Such a system has several requirements to function as an effective *in vitro* model of thalamocortical rhythmicity. First, the basic neuronal elements and synaptic circuits supporting rhythm generation must be preserved *in vitro*; second, rhythms similar to those seen *in vivo* must be generated by the *in vitro* preparation; and third, the rhythms generated by the *in vitro* system must be pharmacologically similar to those seen *in vivo*. This chapter describes the development of a system which preserves the basic synaptic connections between somatosensory thalamus, NRT, and somatosensory cortex; generates spontaneous thalamocortical rhythms of appropriate frequency, duration, and anatomical distribution when perfused with low Mg^{2+} medium; and supports thalamocortical rhythms which physiologically parallel *in vivo* rhythms, in that they are generated by an interaction between inhibition impinging onto thalamic neurons, triggering activation of a large, regenerative low-threshold calcium conductance, which amplifies and drives further activity. These rhythms also pharmacologically parallel *in vivo* rhythms, in that they are blocked by GA anticonvulsants, unaffected by anticonvulsants ineffective in controlling generalized absence epilepsy, and potentiated by convulsants.

Methods

Slice preparation

Mouse or rat thalamocortical slices (400–450 µm thick) were prepared from both juvenile (10–13 days postnatal) and adult animals employing the slicing angle developed by Agmon & Connors (1991), using conventional techniques. Animals were anaesthetized and decapitated, and the brain removed and placed on a 10° ramp, rostral side down. The brain was then rotated 55° from a parasagittal plane, and blocked at this angle, glued to the stage of a vibratome, and sliced. Usually 1–2 mouse, and 2–3 rat slices maintained reciprocal connections between thalamus and cortex, as well as connections with nucleus reticularis. Thalamocortical connections were verified by microscopic examination of slices, and through physiological studies (see below). Once cut and examined, slices were transferred to an incubator, where they were kept submerged in warmed (35 °C) oxygenated medium until use. The slice medium (ACSF) was composed of (in mM): NaCl, 130; KCl, 3; NaH_2PO_4, 1.25; $MgCl_2$, 0 or 2; $CaCl_2$, 2; $NaHCO_3$, 26; and dextrose, 10. A separate incubator allowed pre-exposure of individual slices to low Mg^{2+} medium prior to recording. Slices were incubated at least 1 h after dissection, and 1 h or more in low Mg^{2+} medium before recording.

Prior to recording, slices were transferred to an interface type recording chamber, where they were maintained at 35 ± 1 °C. Differential AC-coupled extracellular recordings were conducted using 2 MΩ insulated tungsten electrodes (bandpass filtered at 10–3000 Hz). Extracellular stimulation was conducted using bipolar insulated tungsten electrodes, glued together with their tips approximately 100 µm apart. Brief (100 µs) 20–800 µA constant current pulses were delivered to the slice at a frequency of 0.1 to 10 Hz.

Intracellular recordings: conventional sharp electrode and slice patch recording

Intracellular recordings from thalamic neurons in thalamocortical slices were conducted using either conventional sharp ('impalement') electrodes, or patch electrodes and the 'blind slice patch' whole-cell current-clamp recording mode, as described by Blanton *et al.* (1991). Sharp electrodes, 100–150 MΩ in resistance, were pulled on a Brown-Flaming microelectrode puller, and filled with 4 M K^+ acetate. Patch electrodes were fabricated using thick-walled borosilicate capillary glass and a two-stage pull. Patch electrodes were filled with a solution containing (in mM): 130 K^+ gluconate, 1 $MgCl_2$, 1.1 EGTA, 10 HEPES, pH 7.4, with the osmolarity adjusted to 10 per cent lower than the ACSF bathing the slice. This osmolarity difference facilitated seal formation. A patch electrode is lowered into the slice, with positive pressure on the electrode, to prevent the tip from getting dirty in the dead outer layer of the slice. Positive pressure is then taken off, and the electrode is advanced in small steps, with current pulses monitoring the resistance of the electrode. When a cell is encountered, the resistance of the electrode increases, suction is applied, and, in about 25 per cent of attempts, a high resistance (5–20 GΩ) seal is formed. A further pulse of suction breaks the membrane inside the electrode, instituting the whole-cell mode of recording. Cells are usually stable in this recording mode for about 1 h. Patch recordings were usually conducted from slices from younger animals (10–30-day-old rats), since this seemed to aid seal formation and facilitated recordings. Sharp electrode recordings were conducted from slices prepared from adult animals. In both cases, signals were amplified and recorded with an Axoclamp 2A amplifier.

Results

When cut using the slice angle described by Agmon & Connors (1991), both rat and mouse thalamocortical slices preserve the main synaptic interconnections responsible for generation of thalamocortical rhythms (Fig. 1). This is most evident in physiological recordings of spontaneous

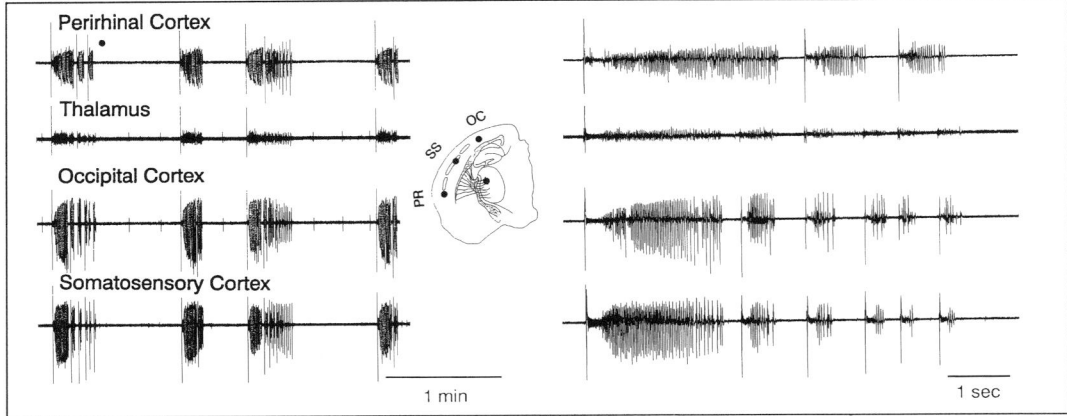

Fig. 2. Perfusion of rat thalamocortical slices with a medium containing no added Mg^{2+} elicits spontaneous generalized thalamocortical bursting. Multiple channel extracellular field potential recordings in a rat thalamocortical slice from a 45-day-old animal illustrate the tightly coupled, generalized activity evident in these slices. Spontaneous rhythms occurred every 30–40 s, and were 15–30 s in duration, and 10–15 Hz in frequency. The position of the recording electrodes is illustrated in the inset cartoon of a thalamocortical slice.

and evoked activity recorded in these slices, but also has been verified using various dyes in fixed thalamocortical slices (Agmon & Connors, 1991). The feedback connection from cortex is preserved (synapse # 1 in Fig. 1), as is evident in paired recordings from thalamus and cortex (Figs. 2, 3; Coulter & Lee, 1993). The thalamocortical projection is also preserved (synapses #2 and 6 in Fig. 1; Agmon & Connors (1991), Coulter & Lee (1993)), as are the axon collaterals innervating NRT (synapses #3 and 4 in Fig. 1; see Figs. 3, 4; Coulter & Lee (1993)).

Thalamocortical slices are not spontaneously active in normal medium. When slices were perfused with a medium containing no added Mg^{2+}, they cycled through a series of excitability stages, which culminated after 40–80 min in slices from adult animals in the appearance of spontaneous thalamocortical rhythms, which then persisted stably for the life of the slice. This activity consisted in many slices of burst complexes 5–10 s long, which reoccurred every 20–40 s (Fig. 2). In cortical extracellular and intracellular recordings, single burst complexes were triggered by a paroxysmal depolarizing shift (PDS), which was then followed by a series of smaller bursts, firing at anything from 4 to 15 Hz, but most often in the frequency range of 8–10 Hz (Fig. 2; Coulter & Lee (1993)). This type of activity was seen in 60–70 per cent of slices from adult animals, but rarely in slices of young juvenile (10–13 days postnatal) animals, which only exhibited recurrent single PDSs, or PDSs followed by brief periods of activity in medium containing no added Mg^{2+} (Fig. 3). As animals developed, the tendency to see rhythmic thalamocortical bursting gradually increased (e.g. Fig. 4, from a 30 day-old animal). Preliminary experiments indicate that the difference in activity between adult and juvenile thalamocortical slices may be due to immaturity of corticocortical connections since thalamic/NRT connections appear functionally mature in juvenile slices (e.g. Figs. 3 and 4, and additional data not shown). In many recordings from juvenile animals, but rarely in adults, the thalamus appears to drive the thalamocortical rhythms triggered in low-Mg^{2+} medium (e.g. Fig. 3a).

Extra- and intracellular recording in thalamic neurons from adult animals following perfusion with low Mg^{2+} medium also revealed spontaneous activity consisting of 2–10 s long burst complexes, which reoccurred every 20–40 s (Fig. 2; Coulter & Lee (1993)). Again, as in the cortex, single burst complexes were triggered by a PDS-like event, which was followed by a series of smaller bursts, firing at 4–15 Hz (Fig. 2). Thalamic intracellular recordings of burst complexes in adult animals

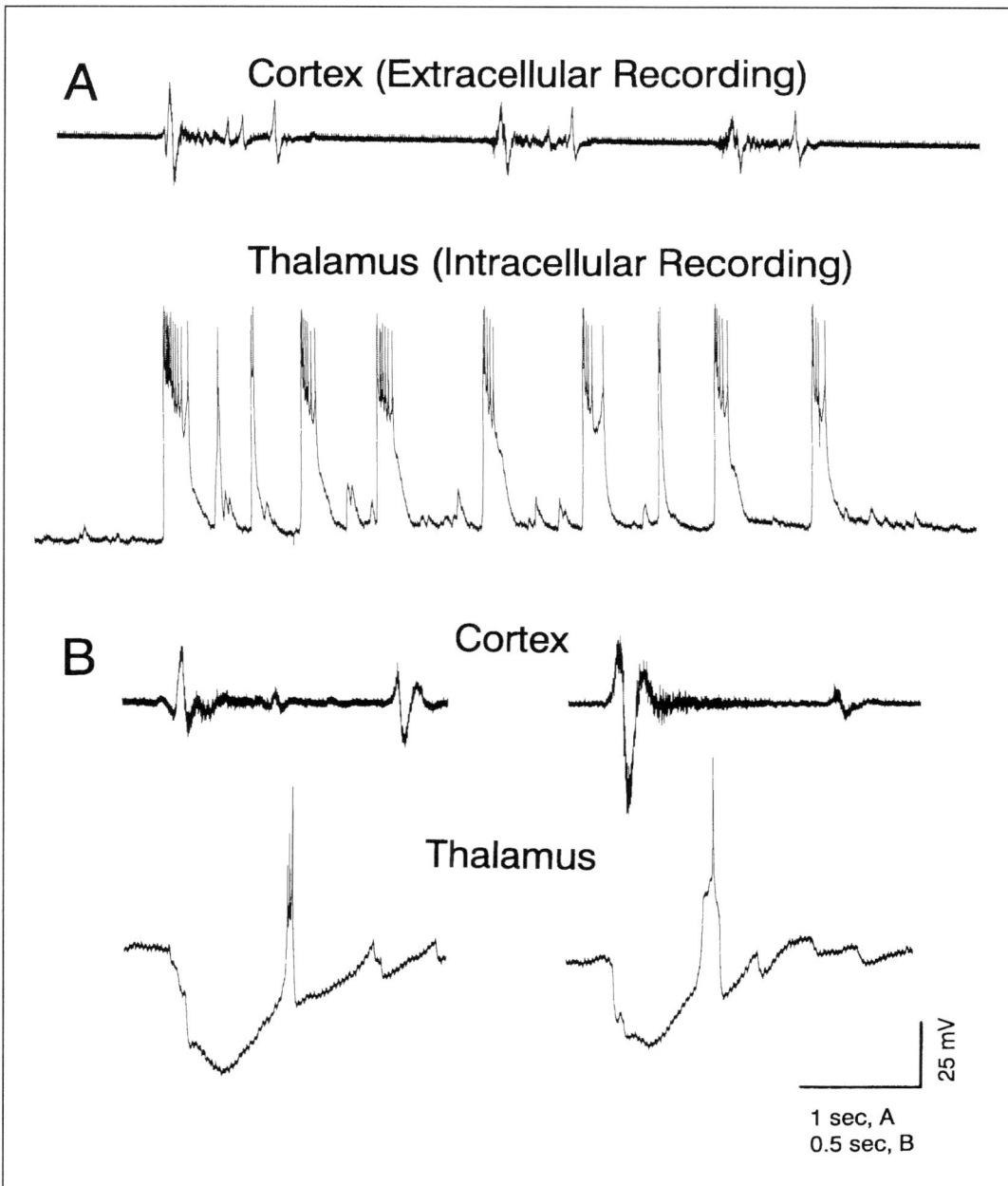

Fig. 3. Simultaneous extracellular and slice patch intracellular recordings from somatosensory cortex and thalamus (respectively) in thalamocortical slice from an 11-day old (A) and a 13-day-old rat (B) during low-Mg^{2+} activity. In A, the activity in the thalamic neuron appeared to lead activity in the cortex, and IPSPs were less prominent. In B (a different neuron, and a different animal than A), two examples are shown where the activity in the cortex led activity in the thalamic neuron, and the activity in the thalamus consisted of an initial, very large two-component IPSP, on the decay phase of which a large low-threshold calcium burst was triggered. $V_M = -73$ mV (A), -75 mV (B).

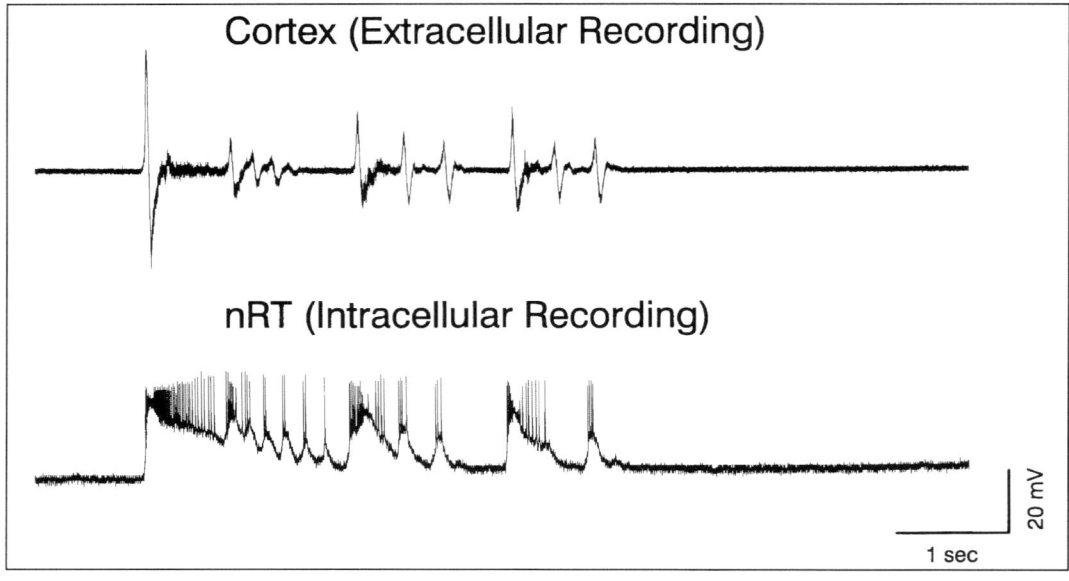

Fig. 4. Simultaneous extracellular and slice patch intracellular recordings from somatosensory cortex and nucleus reticularis thalami (respectively) in a thalamocortical slice from a 30-day-old rat. Note the tightly coupled cortical and NRT activity, and the tonic depolarization occurring during the 5–6 Hz thalamocortical burst discharges. $V_M = -42$ mV.

could be seen to be riding on an underlying wave of hyperpolarization (Coulter & Lee, 1993). One component contributing to this underlying hyperpolarization is evident in many slice patch recordings from thalamic neurons, in which cortical burst activity triggered large biphasic IPSPs in thalamic neurons, presumably due to feedforward activation of the NRT/thalamus GABAergic synapse (synapse #5 in Fig. 1) through activation of NRT via a collateral projection of corticothalamic axons (synapse # 3 in Fig. 1). These large, NRT-triggered IPSPs frequently activated large bursts of action potentials on the rebound of the IPSP (Fig. 3b), which could presumably reactivate the thalamocortical circuitry and prolong the oscillation in slices from older animals. Intracellular recordings from NRT neurons during spontaneous thalamocortical bursting revealed a quite different pattern of activity to that seen in thalamic relay neurons during thalamocortical activity. NRT neurons tonically depolarized during thalamocortical oscillatory activity, with bursts of activity riding a large depolarization (Fig. 4), unlike thalamic neurons, where either a long, slow hyperpolarization (Fig. 3b, Coulter & Lee (1993)) or no change in membrane potential (Fig. 3a) were evident during thalamocortical oscillations. This suggested that inhibitory synapses within NRT (synapse #7 in Fig. 1) were not playing a major role in synchronization of thalamocortical oscillations.

In order to explore the dependence of rhythm-generating mechanisms on intact thalamocortical circuitry, lesioning experiments were conducted. Expression of thalamocortical burst activity, but not the cortical PDS, was dependent on preservation of intact thalamocortical connections. Severing thalamocortical connections traversing the striatum abolished all spontaneous activity in the thalamus, and reduced burst complexes in the cortex to a single PDS, with occasional late small arrhythmic bursts (Coulter and Lee, 1993). To characterize further the spontaneous rhythmic burst activity recorded in thalamocortical slices, the anticonvulsant and convulsant pharmacology of these rhythms was characterized. Bath application of ethosuximide (200 µM–1 mM) or the active metabolite of trimethadione (dimethadione, 1–10 mM) reduced or blocked spontaneous burst activity, while bath application of phenytoin (10 μM) or carbamazepine (10 μM) had no effect on spontaneous rhythms (Coulter, 1992a). Thus, the anticonvulsant pharmacology of spontaneous burst activity was very similar to the spike-and-wave discharges of generalized absence epilepsy, in that this activity was reduced by GA anticonvulsants, and not by anticonvulsants ineffective in controlling generalized absence epilepsy. Pentylenetetrazol (PTZ) potentiates thalamocortical spike-and-wave discharges and elicits generalized convulsions when administered to rodents (Marescaux et al., 1984), and PTZ-induced seizures are employed as an assay to test drugs for potential efficacy as GA anticonvulsants. When perfused onto active thalamocortical slices in low Mg^{2+} medium, pentylenetetrazol (1–10 mM) increased the amplitude of extracellular fields recorded in cortex and thalamus, and increased the duration of burst complexes 2–3-fold (Coulter & Lee, 1993).

Discussion

Rat and mouse thalamocortical slices retain the ability to generate spontaneous thalamocortical rhythms *in vitro*. These rhythms appear to share similar physiological generating mechanisms to those described *in vivo*, in that NRT-mediated inhibition is important in synchronizing the thalamocortical rhythms (Fig. 3, 4), while low threshold calcium spikes, triggered on the rebound of the NRT-mediated IPSPs, serve to amplify and drive thalamocortical rhythmicity (Fig. 3b), as is seen *in vivo*. In addition to similar mechanisms important in generation of rhythms, the *in vitro* thalamocortical rhythms share a similar pharmacology to those seen *in vivo*, in that they are potentiated by convulsant agents which can trigger or exacerbate *in vivo* thalamocortical rhythms (Coulter, 1992b; Coulter & Lee, 1993), and are blocked by agents which can block or reduce thalamocortical rhythms *in vivo*, such as the anticonvulsants ethosuximide and dimethadione (Coulter & Zhang, 1993), but not by anticonvulsants ineffective in control of generalized absence epilepsy (Coulter, 1992a; Zhang & Coulter, manuscript in preparation). Ethosuximide and dimethadione, when applied in clinically relevant concentrations (achieved as free serum levels in medicated patients) have previously been shown to specifically block the low threshold ('T'-type) calcium current responsible for generation of low-threshold calcium spikes in thalamic neurons, which in turn are responsible for amplifying and driving thalamocortical oscillations (Coulter et al., 1989a, b; Coulter et al., 1990). This cellular mechanism could certainly be viewed as potentially an anticonvulsant effect both *in vivo*, and in the presently discussed *in vitro* preparation, given our current understanding of factors important in generation of thalamocortical oscillations.

Thalamocortical rhythms in rodents span a range of frequencies, with sleep spindles usually reported as being 2–4 s in duration, and 10–15 Hz in frequency (Buzsaki et al., 1990), while spike-and-wave discharges are 5–10 Hz in frequency and 1–10 s in duration in genetic models of generalized absence (Buzsaki et al., 1990; Hosford, this volume; Noebels, this volume; Vergnes, this volume; Vergnes et al., 1987). Low Mg^{2+} thalamocortical bursting is 4–15 Hz in frequency (Figs. 2, 3, 4; Coulter & Lee (1993)), and individual burst complexes are 2–15 s long (Figs. 2, 3, 4), resembling either spindles or spike-and-wave discharge rhythms. In addition, the anatomic distribution of low Mg^{2+} thalamocortical bursting resembles spindles and spike-and-wave discharges in that large portions of cortex and thalamus participate in synchronized, high voltage bursting (Fig. 2), as is seen *in vivo* (Buzsaki et al., 1990; Hosford, this volume; Noebels, this volume; Vergnes, this volume). However, low Mg^{2+} thalamocortical bursting differs from spindle and spike-and-wave discharges in that individual low Mg^{2+} burst complexes are triggered by a PDS, unlike spindles or spike-and-wave discharges (Figs. 2, 3, 4), and require reduced extracellular divalent cation levels for expression.

In thalamic slices, perfusion with low Mg^{2+} medium elicits non-synchronized rhythmic activity in individual relay neurons (Soltesz et al., 1991), due to reductions in divalent cation concentrations producing 'depolarizing' screening charge effects (e.g. Frankenhaeuser & Hodgkin, 1957); direct effects of altered divalent concentrations on calcium currents; and unblocking of the NMDA receptor pore by removal of Mg^{2+}, causing release of excitatory neurotransmitters and activation of excitatory amino acid receptors. Similar effects occur in cortex, where perfusion of medium containing no added Mg^{2+} can trigger large synchronized PDSs and ictiform discharges (Thomson & West, 1986). However, in neither thalamic nor cortical slices alone are discharges produced which activate both thalamus and cortex (Fig. 2, 3, 4), which depend on intact thalamocortical connections for expression (Coulter & Lee, 1993), and which exhibit similar pharmacology to thalamocortical rhythms *in vivo* (Coulter, 1992a, b; Coulter & Lee, 1993; Coulter & Zhang, 1993; Zhang & Coulter manuscript in preparation).

The results from experiments employing the rodent thalamocortical slice are the first to demonstrate that thalamocortical rhythm generation can be preserved *in vitro*. Thalamocortical burst activity in these slices appears similar in physiological mechanism, morphology, anatomical distribution, and pharmacology to thalamocortical spindle activity recorded *in vivo* during slow-wave sleep (Steriade & Llinás, 1988), and during seizure activity in patients with generalized absence epilepsy (Gloor & Fariello, 1988). Future studies using this system, exploiting the advantages of *in vitro* preparations, could prove invaluable in investigation of physiological and pharmacological mechanisms important in generation of both normal and pathological thalamocortical rhythms.

Acknowledgement

We thank George P. Nanos III for technical assistance. Supported by Grants from the NIH-NINDS (R29 NS 31000), the Epilepsy Foundation of America, a Milken Family Award from the American Epilepsy Society, and by the Sophie and Nathan Gumenick Foundation Neuroscience and Alzheimer's Research Fund.

References

Agmon, A. & Connors, B.W. (1991): Thalamocortical responses of mouse somatosensory (barrel) cortex *in vitro*. *Neuroscience* **41**, 365–379.

Blanton, M. G., LoTurco, J.J. & Kriegstein, A.R. (1989): Whole cell recordings from neurons in slices of reptilian and mammalian cerebral cortex. *J. Neurosci. Methods* **30**, 203–210.

Buzsáki, G., Laszlovszky, I., Lajtha, A. & Vadász, C. (1990): Spike-and-wave neocortical patterns in rats: genetic and aminergic control. *Neuroscience* **38**, 323–333.

Coulter, D.A. (1992a): Physiological studies of thalamocortical rhythms, recorded *in vitro* in a brain slice preparation. *Soc. Neurosci. Abs.* **18**, 1391.

Coulter, D.A. (1992b): Pentylenetetrazol effects on mouse thalamocortical rhythms and synaptic potentials *in vitro*. *Epilepsia* **33**, (Supplement 3): 21 (Abstract).

Coulter, D.A. & Lee, C.-J. (1993): Thalamocortical rhythm generation *in vitro*: extra-and intracellular recordings in mouse thalamocortical slices perfused with low-Mg^{2+} medium. *Brain Res.* **631**, 137–142.

Coulter, D.A. & Zhang, Y.-F. (1993): Development of spontaneous generalized activity in rat thalamocortical slices in low Mg^{2+} medium. *Soc. Neurosci. Abs.* **19**, 1565.

Coulter, D.A., Huguenard, J.R. & Prince, D.A. (1989a): Calcium currents in rat thalamocortical relay neurones: kinetic properties of the transient, low-threshold current. *J. Physiol. (Lond.)* **414**, 587–604.

Coulter, D.A., Huguenard, J.R. & Prince, D.A. (1989b): Characterization of ethosuximide reduction of low-threshold calcium current in thalamic neurons. *Ann. Neurol.* **25**, 582–593.

Coulter, D.A., Huguenard, J.R. & Prince, D.A. (1990): Differential effects of petit mal anticonvulsants and convulsants on thalamic neurones. I. Calcium current reduction. *Br. J. Pharmacol.* **100**, 800–806.

Frankenhaeuser, B. & Hodgkin, A.L. (1957): The action of calcium on electrical properties of squid axons. *J. Physiol. (Lond.)* **137**, 218–244.

Gloor, P. & Fariello, R.G. (1988): Generalized epilepsy: some of its cellular mechanisms differ from those of focal epilepsy. *Trends Neurosci.* **11**, 63–68.

Harris, R.M. & Hendrickson, A.E. (1987): Local circuit neurons in the rat ventrobasal thalamus-a GABA immunohistochemical study. *Neuroscience* **21**, 229–236.

Houser, C.R., Vaughn, J.E., Barber, R.P. & Roberts, E. (1980): GABA neurons are the major cell type of nucleus reticularis thalami. *Brain Res.* **200**, 341–354.

Jones, E.G. (1985): *The thalamus*. New York: Plenum Press.

Marescaux, C., Micheletti, G., Vergnes, M., Depaulis, A., Rumbach, L. & Warter, J.M. (1984): A model of chronic spontaneous petit mal-like seizures in the rat: comparison with pentylenetetrazol-induced seizures. *Epilepsia* **25,** 326–331.

Soltesz, I., Lightowler, S., Leresche, N., Jassik-Gerschenfeld, D., Pollard, C. & Crunelli, V. (1991): Two inward currents and the transformation of low-frequency oscillations of rat and cat thalamocortical cells. *J. Physiol. (Lond.)* **441,** 175–197.

Steriade, M. & Llinás, R.R. (1988): The functional states of the thalamus and the associated neuronal interplay. *Physiol. Rev.* **68,** 649–742.

Thomson, A.M. & West, D.C. (1986): *N*-Methylaspartate receptors mediate epileptiform activity evoked in some, but not all, conditions in rat neocortical slices. *Neuroscience* **19,** 1161–1177.

Vergnes, M., Marescaux, C., Depaulis, A., Micheletti, G. & Warter, J.M. (1987): Spontaneous spike-and-wave discharges in thalamus and cortex in a rat model of genetic petit mal-like seizure. *Exp. Neurol.* **96,** 127–186.

Chapter 14

Pathophysiological mechanisms of experimental generalized absence seizures in rats

O. Carter Snead III

Department of Neurology, University of Southern California School of Medicine, Children's Hospital Los Angeles, Los Angeles, California 90027, USA

Introduction

Generalized absence seizures may be defined as a paroxysmal loss of consciousness, without aura or postictal state, associated with bursts of bilaterally synchronous spike-and-wave discharges which usually occur at a frequency of three cycles per s. This disorder is seen primarily in children between the ages of 4 years and adolescence, although it may occur at either ends of that age spectrum (Penry *et al.*, 1975; Aicardi, 1986; Holmes, 1987; Lockman, 1989; Murphy & Dehkharghani, 1994). The seizures are pharmacologically unique responding only to ethosuximide (Sherwin, 1989), trimethadione (Booker, 1989), valproic acid (Bourgeois, 1989), or benzodiazepines (Sato, 1989) and being resistant to, or made worse by phenytoin (Roseman, 1961), barbiturates, or carbamazepine (Snead & Hosey, 1985).

Generalized absence seizures arise from aberrant thalamocortical rhythms (Gloor, 1984; Steriade & Llinas, 1988; Gloor *et al.*, 1990). Therefore, to discuss proposed hypotheses of the pathogenesis of this disorder, it is first necessary to review synaptic circuitry and neurotransmission of intrinsic thalamic, thalamocortical, and corticothalamic pathways, the unique oscillatory thalamocortical rhythms generated by that circuitry, the cellular mechanisms underlying these neuronal oscillations, the ascending pathways, extrinsic to thalamus and cortex, which modulate the function of those structures, and, in the final analysis, the relation of all of these pathways, neurotransmitters, and ionic mechanisms to consciousness.

Because the electrical activity of mammalian forebrain as recorded on the electroencephalogram (EEG) varies with the behavioural alertness of the animal, the EEG is state dependent. A state of alertness is associated with desynchronization of the EEG which is defined as a replacement of synchronized rhythms by lower amplitude and faster wave forms. Alternatively, certain altered states of consciousness (e.g. slow-wave sleep) are associated with synchronous EEG activity defined as high-amplitude oscillations with relatively slow frequencies (Steriade *et al.*, 1990). These state-related alterations in EEG are a reflection of fundamental and dynamic underlying changes in the activity of forebrain neurons in response to both the action of ascending neurotransmitter

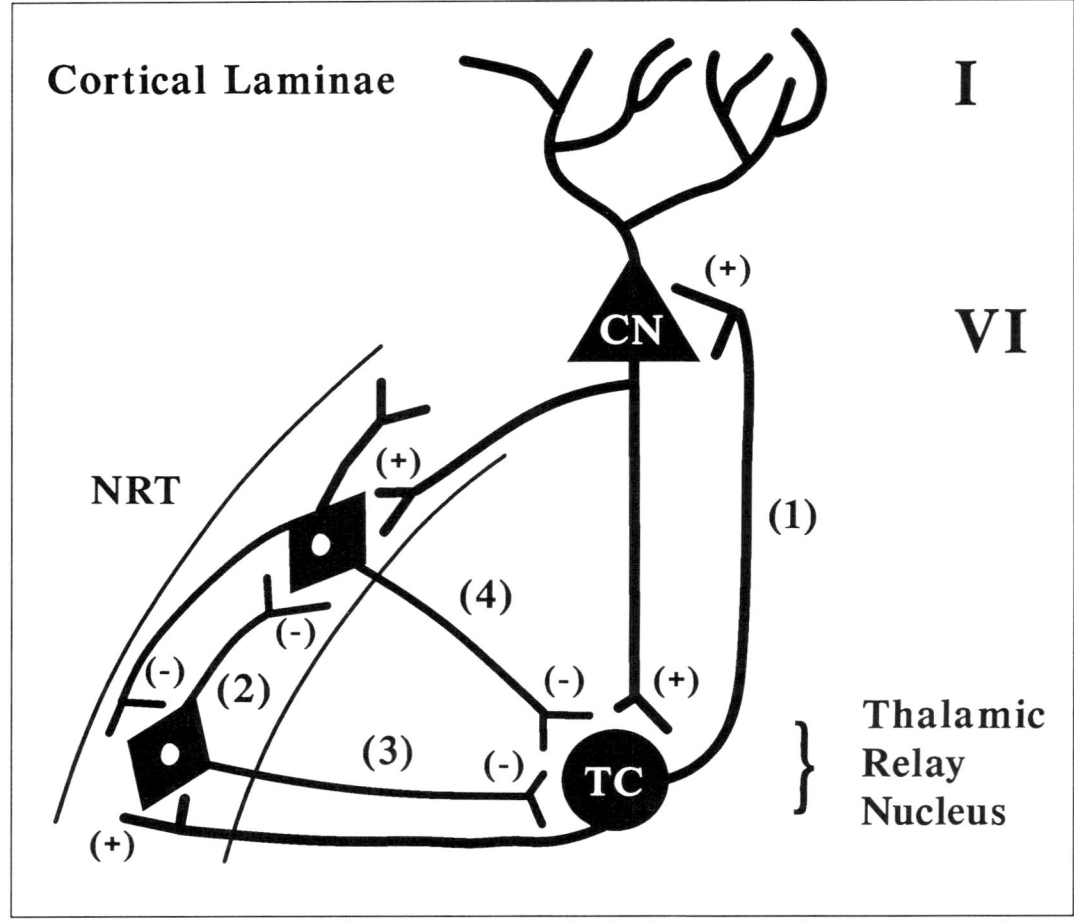

Fig. 1. Schematic diagram of thalamocortical circuitry showing the relationship between neurons in the nucleus reticularis thalami (NRT), thalamic relay nucleus (TC), and corticothalamic neurons (CN) in layer VI of the cerebral cortex. This diagram is illustrative of reciprocal excitation between thalamocortical and cortical neurons (1), reciprocal inhibition between NRT neurons (2), recurrent inhibition between thalamocortical and NRT neurons (3), and parallel excitation between corticothalamic neurons and NRT and thalamocortical relay neurons (4). The neurotransmitter at all inhibitory neurons (−) within this circuit is thought to be GABA while the neurotransmitter at the exictatory synapses (+) between thalamocortical and corticothalamic neurons and corticothalamic neurons and NRT neurons is probably glutamate.

systems upon thalamocortical circuitry as well as the intrinsic activity of the thalamocortical circuitry itself.

Thalamocortical circuitry: functional aspects

Thalamic neurons have the unique ability to shift between the oscillatory and tonic firing mode. In this way the traffic of extrinsic stimuli to the cortex via the thalamus is regulated. The alert behavioural state with desynchronized EEG is associated with tonic firing of thalamocortical neurons which allows for faithful signal transmission from the external environment of the organism to cortex via the thalamus; on the other hand, the non-alert state is associated with a shift of the pattern of these neurons to an oscillatory, rhythmic, burst firing which raises the threshold in thalamus for EPSPs and dampens signal transmission from the exterior world to the cortex (Steriade & Llinas, 1988; Steriade et al., 1990, 1993a; McCormick, 1992).

Oscillatory neuronal behaviour within thalamocortical circuits relies upon an intrinsic ability of a group of thalamic neurons within the nucleus reticularis thalami (NRT) to impose their oscillatory behaviour upon thalamocortical circuitry (Fig. 1). The NRT forms a shell which surrounds much of the dorsal and lateral extent of the dorsal thalamus (Jones, 1985) and is composed of GABAergic neurons which project heavily to one another and to almost all thalamic relay nuclei. NRT neurons receive excitatory, glutamatergic inputs from axon collaterals of thalamocortical fibres that traverse the NRT on their way from thalamic relay nuclei to cortex and of corticothalamic fibres that project back from lamina VI of cerebral cortex to thalamic relay nuclei (Steriade et al., 1984; Yen et al., 1985; Cornwall et al., 1990; Spreafico et al., 1991; McCormick & von Krosigk, 1992; Bal & McCormick, 1993). In higher animals, such as non-human primates and presumably humans, there is also a network of GABAergic interneurons within the thalamus (Yi et al., 1993). In addition, there is some evidence that NRT neurons may also project to contralateral dorsal thalamus in the intrathalamic commissure thus influencing the cerebral cortex and basal ganglia of both hemispheres (Raos & Bentivoglio, 1993; Pare & Steriade, 1993). That the NRT is uniquely situated to influence the flow of information between the thalamus and cerebral cortex is demonstrated by the fact that NRT cells show rhythmic burst firing during periods of synchronized EEG activity and tonic, single-spike firing during wakefulness. The transition from slow-wave sleep to the waking state is associated with an abolition of rhythmic burst firing and the appearance of tonic single spike activity in NRT neurons (Mulle et al., 1986; Steriade et al., 1986, 1993a,b,c,d; Steriade & Llinas, 1988; Buzsaki, 1991; Bal & McCormick, 1993; Contreras et al., 1993).

The cellular event which underlies the ability of NRT neurons to shift between an oscillatory and firing mode and therefore dictate EEG synchronization/desynchronization and ultimately consciousness is the low threshold Ca^{2+} spike. This event is triggered via $GABA_B$-mediated late IPSPs which, in turn, gives rise to a rebound burst of high-frequency action potentials (von Krosigk et al., 1993). These low threshold Ca^{2+} potentials represent a key membrane property involved in burst firing excitation and are associated with the oscillatory activity observed in thalamocortical cells during synchronized sleep (Steriade & Llinas, 1988; Crunelli & Leresche, 1991). There is evidence that the antiepileptic drugs ethosuximide and trimethadione may owe their anti-absence activity to their ability to decrease low threshold calcium currents (Coulter et al., 1989a,b, 1990).

Thalamocortical function in experimental generalized absence seizures

Generalized absence seizures represent a perturbation of neocortical rhythmicity in favour of the rhythmic burst-firing mode with a resultant pathological alteration in consciousness during the bilaterally synchronous spike-and-wave discharges (SWD) as recorded on the EEG. Therefore, the clinical and pharmacological uniqueness of experimental and clinical absence (Berkovic et al., 1987; Snead, 1992a) may be attributed to the special neurophysiological and neurochemical properties of intrinsically bursting neurons in thalamus and cortex and to their synaptic circuitry not only with one other but also with ascending pathways in the brain.

The cell bodies of those ascending pathways which project to the thalamus and cortex and which influence rhythmic thalamocortical activity can be found in the brain-stem, hypothalamus, and basal forebrain (McCormick, 1992; Bal & McCormick, 1993) and involve multiple neurotransmitter systems including GABAergic neurons from basal forebrain (Asanuma & Porter, 1990), substantia nigra pars reticulata (Di Chiara et al., 1979; Pare et al., 1990), the globus pallidus, and the superior colliculus (Di Chiara et al., 1979; Yamasaki & Kruathamer, 1990); cholinergic neurons from the basal forebrain, pedunculopontine, and lateral dorsal tegmental nuclei of brain-stem (Bigl et al., 1982; Steriade et al., 1987; Hallanager et al., 1987; Levey et al., 1987; Eckenstein et al., 1988;

Lysakowski et al., 1989; Asanuma, 1989; McCormick, 1990, 1992); noradrenergic neurons from the locus ceruleus (Ahlsen & Lo, 1982; Foote et al., 1983; Hughes & Mullikin, 1984; Foote & Morrison, 1986; Asanuma, 1992); and serotonergic neurons from the dorsal raphe nucleus (Cropper et al., 1984; Morrison & Foote, 1986; Kosofsky & Molliver, 1987; Berger et al., 1988; Wilson & Hendrickson, 1988; Tork, 1990; Lavoie & Parent, 1991). In addition, thalamocortical activity is modulated by GABAergic interneurons within the cerebral cortex (Jones, 1993; McCormick et al., 1993).

Much of the information available which concerns basic synaptic circuitry, and neurotransmitter pathways in the thalamus and cortex and their relation to normal behavioural states has been obtained by using basic electrophysiological techniques *in vitro* in rodents and cats (Gloor, 1984; Steriade & Llinas, 1988; Steriade et al., 1990; McCormick, 1992; McCormick et al., 1993). However, most of the data concerning the effect of perturbation of various neurotransmitter systems on the phenomenon of generalized absence seizures in rats has been generated using *in vivo* studies in experimental models of absence in this species. Therefore, formulation of any hypothesis that will explain the pathogenesis of generalized absence seizures must entail a synthesis of *in vitro* electrophysiological data with the results of *in vivo* whole animal experiments.

Animal models of generalized absence seizures should, in addition to reflecting the clinical and pharmacological characteristics of this disorder (Penry et al., 1975; Aicardi, 1986; Holmes, 1987; Lockman, 1989; Murphy & Dehkharghani, 1994), meet other criteria as well (Mirski et al., 1986; Fariello & Golden, 1987; Snead, 1988). These criteria (Table 1) include reproducibility and predictability as well the ability to standardize and quantify the model. In addition, animal models of absence should reflect the fact that both clinical and experimental absence seizures are exacerbated by both direct and indirect GABA agonists (Myslobodsky et al., 1979; van der Linden et al., 1981; Vergnes et al., 1984; Snead, 1984, 1990; Gloor & Fariello, 1988; Peeters et al., 1989a). Finally, involvement of thalamocortical circuitry and specific *noninvolvement of hippocampal circuitry* must be demonstrated for an animal model of absence seizures to be valid (Gloor, 1984; Vergnes et al., 1987, 1990a,b; Gloor & Fariello, 1988; Steriade et al., 1990; Steriade & Llinas, 1988; Bannerjee et al., 1993). The rat models meeting these criteria which have been used to generate the data reviewed below are both pharmacological and genetic. The pharmacological animal models include those which utilize either low dose (20 mg/kg) pentylenetetrazole or γ-hydroxybutyric acid (Snead, 1992a). Genetic models include the genetic absence epilepsy rat of Strasbourg (GAERS) (Marescaux et al., 1992a), and the WAG/Rij strain of rat (Van Luijtelaar & Coenen, 1986; Coenen et al., 1992).

Table 1. Criteria for experimental absence seizures

1. Bilaterally synchronous spike-and-wave discharges associated with behavioural arrest ± facial twitching, head drops, and eye movements;
2. Reproducibility, predictability;
3. Ability to standardize and quantify;
4. Attenuated or blocked by ethosuximide, valproic acid, trimethadione, and benzodiazepines;
5. Appropriate ontogeny;
6. Exacerbated by GABAergic drugs;
7. Blocked by GABA$_B$ antagonists;
8. Spike-and-wave discharges originate in thalamus and/or cortex;
9. Hippocampus is silent during seizure activity

In the rat both the thalamus and cortex seem to be required for absence seizure activity since neither structure alone can sustain bilaterally synchronous spike-and-wave discharge in any model studied in this species (Vergnes et al., 1987, 1990a,b). Although the rat seems unable to generate the classical 3/s spike-and-wave discharge usually observed in human absence seizures (McQueen & Woodbury, 1975), the frequency and morphology of the wave forms of the spike-and-wave discharge in the pharmacological and genetic models are identical as are their pharmacological profiles (Snead 1992a; Marescaux et al., 1992a).

The role of thalamocortical pathways in the genesis of spike-and-wave discharge has been demonstrated clearly in the GAERS, γ-hydroxybutyric acid, and PTZ models of absence seizures in rat. However, the pharmacological models differ from the GAERS in that spike-and-wave discharge may be recorded from ventrolateral thalamus and cortex in the genetic model (Vergnes et al., 1990b) while in the pharmacological models, spike-and-wave discharges are recorded from layer I–III of cortex, with deeper layers being silent during spike-and-wave discharge bursts, and from medial thalamic nuclei (Bannerjee et al., 1993). The hippocampus and amygdala are silent during spike-and-wave discharges in all models of absence seizures in rat (Vergnes et al., 1987, 1990a,b; Banerjee et al., 1993).

Existing experimental evidence which addresses the role of various neurotransmitter systems in the pathophysiology of generalized absence seizures in rat focuses primarily upon GABA- and excitatory amino acid-mediated mechanisms although there are some available data concerning noradrenergic and dopaminergic mechanisms. There is no information concerning involvement of histaminergic pathways (McCormick, 1992) and little or no evidence that serotonergic pathways play a role in experimental absence seizures in rats.

GABA-mediated mechanisms in absence seizures

Enhancement of GABAergic inhibition in the brain potentiates clinical (Myslobodsky, 1976; van der Linden et al., 1981) and all experimental forms of generalized absence (Snead 1984, 1990; Vergnes et al., 1984; Fariello & Golden, 1987; Gloor & Fariello, 1988; Peeters et al., 1989a; Smith & Bierkamper, 1990) and may even be sufficient to produce it under certain conditions (Fariello & Golden, 1987; Gloor & Fariello, 1988; Fariello, 1990). This effect is opposite to that seen in animal models of generalized convulsive and partial seizures where GABAergic inhibition is anticonvulsant (Snead, 1983). While it should be remembered that GABAergic neurons in extrathalamocortical structures, e.g. the pars reticulata of the substantia nigra (Depaulis et al., 1988a, 1989, 1990), superior colliculus (Depaulis, 1990), and the interneurons of cerebral cortex (Jones, 1993; McCormick et al., 1993), may be intimately involved in controlling cerebral excitability and therefore absence seizures, most of the attention devoted to investigation of GABAergic pathways in experimental absence seizures has focused upon the thalamus.

During spike-and-wave discharges recorded from thalamus and cortex in experimental absence seizures there is preservation of GABAergic function, sparing of classical IPSPs, and the absence of typical paroxysmal depolarizing shifts seen in focal epileptogenesis (Gloor, 1984; Gloor & Fariello, 1988; Kostopoulos, 1986; Avoli et al., 1990). Preservation of GABAergic inhibition contributes to synchronization of spike-and-wave discharges because the pacing of spike-and-wave discharges and bursts of action potentials are dependent upon rhythmically recurring inhibition in both cortex and thalamus (Gloor & Fariello, 1988) which is driven by NRT GABAergic neurons (Bal & McCormick, 1993; Steriade et al., 1993a; von Krosnigk et al., 1993)

There is evidence that both $GABA_A$ and $GABA_B$-mediated inhibition play a role in the pathogenesis of experimental absence seizures in rodent. Systemic administration of $GABA_A$ agonists results in a marked exacerbation of spike-and-wave discharge duration in both pharmacological (Snead, 1984, 1990; Smith & Bierkamper, 1990) and genetic models (Vergnes et al., 1984; Micheletti et al., 1985; Peeters et al., 1989a). Microinjection studies in GAERS have shown that administration of γ-vinyl GABA (GVG), an irreversible GABA transaminase inhibitor, into the thalamic relay nuclei resulted in an exacerbation of absence seizures, while administration of GVG into the NRT resulted in inhibition of spike-and-wave discharges. These data were interpreted to mean that GABAergic neurons in the NRT and their projections to the specific relay nuclei of the thalamus were involved in the elicitation and control of absence seizures. Thus, if NRT neurons were directly inhibited by application of GVG, the spike-and-wave discharge duration decreased. However if NRT inhibition of the relay neurons were enhanced by application of GVG directly to the thalamic relay neurons, spike-and-wave discharge duration in the GAERS was increased (Liu et al., 1991a).

The therapeutic efficacy of benzodiazepines in generalized absence seizures has been difficult to reconcile with the consistent finding that $GABA_A$ agonists make absence seizures worse since benzodiazepines are known to augment GABAergic function in brain (Haefely, 1990; Stephenson, 1990) and therefore would be predicted to exacerbate absence seizures. Recently, Huguenard & Prince (1993) have shed light upon this question by demonstrating in vivo, that benzodiazepines enhance $GABA_A$-mediated inhibition within the NRT and thereby suppress $GABA_B$-mediated inhibition in relay neurons; hence in the context of the experiments of Liu et al. (1991a) reviewed above, this action of benzodiazepines on the NRT would be predicted to decrease spike-and-wave discharge duration in generalized absence seizures.

In spite of the fact that enhancement of $GABA_A$-mediated inhibition uniformly exacerbates absence seizures, the $GABA_A$ receptor complex appears not to be altered in either pharmacological (Snead & Liu, 1993) or genetic models of absence in rat (Snead et al., 1992a; Knight & Bowery, 1992). However, enhancement of [^{3}H]flunitrazepam binding and abundance of β_2-β_3 subunits of $GABA_A$ receptor were both reported to be decreased in the sensorimotor cortex and anterior thalamus of the GAERS vs. control animals (Spreafico et al., 1993).

While experimental absence seizures have been shown to be potentiated by $GABA_A$ agonists, they are not blocked by $GABA_A$ antagonists such as bicuculline (Snead, 1984) suggesting that this disorder is not a simple $GABA_A$-mediated event. The discovery that the late, long-lasting, potassium-dependent IPSP was mediated by the $GABA_B$ receptor and that $GABA_B$ receptor-mediated IPSPs in thalamus activated low-threshold calcium potential which led to burst firing and oscillatory behaviour in thalamic neurons gave rise to the hypothesis that $GABA_B$-receptor-mediated mechanisms might be operative in the pathogenesis of generalized absence seizures (Crunelli & Leresche, 1991). This hypothesis was given further credence by three separate groups of experiments. A specific $GABA_B$ antagonist, CGP 35348, was shown to either attenuate or block spike-and-wave discharges in the GAERS (Liu et al., 1992; Marescaux et al., 1992b); the γ-hydroxybutyric acid and PTZ models in rat (Snead, 1992b), and the lh/lh mouse, a proposed model of absence (Hosford et al., 1992), in a dose-dependent fashion. Moreover, there is evidence that pretreatment with the $GABA_B$ agonist, baclofen, exacerbated the spike-and-wave discharges in the γ-hydroxybutyric acid and PTZ models of absence much more potently than the $GABA_A$ agonist, muscimol (Snead, 1992b). These experiments, taken in conjunction with the in vivo data demonstrating the role of $GABA_B$-mediated IPSP in regulating thalamocortical oscillatory behaviour via low threshold calcium currents (Bal & McCormick, 1993; von Krosigk et al., 1993; Steriade et al., 1993a), strongly suggest that $GABA_B$-mediated mechanisms might be involved in the pathogenesis of absence seizures. Indeed, the animal model data suggest that the $GABA_B$ receptor may be the final common pathway in absence seizures. However, there is no evidence that $GABA_B$-receptor activity as measured by autoradiographic binding techniques is altered in the GAERS (Knight & Bowery, 1992). Moreover, in spite of the fact that Cd^{2+}, known to block Ca^{2+} and Ca^{2+}-dependent K^+ conductances, reversibly suppressed spike-and-wave discharges when given into NRT of GAERS (Avanzini et al., 1993), the voltage dependence and kinetics of the low threshold calcium current in thalamo-cortical neurons in GAERS did not differ from that of control animals (Guyon et al., 1993).

Excitatory amino acid mediated mechanisms in absence seizures

Although an integral part of the modulation and regulation of thalamocortical rhthymicity is effected through glutamate receptor-mediated, recurrent excitation between thalamocortical and corticothalamic pathways both of which project excitatory axon collaterals to the NRT (Fig. 1) (McCormick, 1992; McCormick & von Krosigk, 1992; McCormick et al., 1993), there is little information concerning excitatory neurotransmission in experimental absence seizures. However, recent data demonstrate that pharmacological manipulation of NMDA-mediated excitation results in a profound effect on spike wave discharge duration in a number of experimental models of generalized absence seizures. In the γ-hydroxybutyric acid model of absence seizures (Banerjee & Snead, 1992, 1993) as well as in the GAERS (Marescaux et al., 1992a) administration of either NMDA agonists or antagonists resulted in attenuation of spike-and-wave discharge duration. In the WAG/Rij genetic model of absence seizures the non-competitive NMDA receptor antagonist MK-801 also reduced spike wave discharge duration (Peeters et al., 1989b). NMDA had the opposite effect, but the increase in spike-and-wave discharges was not observed until 4 h after the intracerebroventricular (i.c.v.) administration of NMDA (Peeters et al., 1990) making the significance of this observation uncertain, particularly in view of the fact that in both the pharmacological models (Bannerjee & Snead, 1992) and the GAERS (Marescaux et al., 1992b) NMDA produced a non-specific suppression of spike wave discharge after i.c.v. administration of doses below 40 ng, but led to convulsions at doses in excess of 40 ng. Pretreatment of the WAG/Rij model with CNQX, a non-NMDA receptor antagonist, led to decreased spike wave discharge duration, an effect antagonized both by NMDA and AMPA agonists (Ramakers et al., 1991).

Recently, the regional distribution of radioactive ligand binding for three components of the N-methyl-D-aspartate (NMDA) receptor complex was measured on tissue sections by autoradiography in brains taken from GAERS and a control colony (Snead et al., 1992b). The ligands employed included [^{3}H]glutamate for NMDA-sensitive glutamate-binding sites; [^{3}H]glycine for strychnine-insensitive glycine-binding sites; and [^{3}H]MK-801 for the NMDA receptor gated channel site. There was significantly increased strychnine-insensitive [^{3}H]glycine binding in layers IV–VI of parietal cortex in the GAERS. Although not significant, there was an overall trend toward increased [^{3}H]MK-801 binding in deeper layers of cortex in the GAERS. There were no other significant changes noted between GAERs and control animals. Those data are in keeping with recent neurophysiological observations by Pumain et al. (1992) showing enhanced expression of NMDA-mediated excitation in the middle and deep cortical layers of the GAERS. Also, glycine has been shown to enhance the aggravating effects of GVG on absence seizures in the GAERS (Liu et al., 1990). Since glycine enhances NMDA-receptor mediated synaptic activity in neocortical slices (Johnson & Ascher, 1987; Thompson et al., 1989; Thompson, 1990) the increased strychnine-insensitive [^{3}H]glycine binding shown by Snead et al. (1992b) might reflect increased activity of strychnine-insensitive glycine-binding sites in the middle and deep cortical layers which may explain the neurophysiological findings. However, whether the observed increase in strychnine-insensitive [^{3}H]glycine binding in the GAERS is related to the pathogenesis of absence seizures in this model or caused by them is unclear.

Monoaminergic mechanisms in generalized absence seizures

There is some evidence that noradrenergic neurotransmission may participate in the control of generalized absence seizure activity. Drugs which decrease α-noradrenergic neurotransmission such as the $α_1$-antagonist, prazosin, or the $α_2$-agonist, clonidine, exacerbate experimental absence seizures while pharmacological manipulation which increases α-noradrenergic neurotransmission, i.e. $α_1$-agonists or $α_2$-antagonists, reduce spike-and-wave discharge duration in experimental models of absence seizures. Drugs which influence β-noradrenergic neurotransmission seem to be ineffective in experimental absence seizures (Micheletti et al., 1987; Kleinlogel, 1985; Frey & Voits, 1991; King & Burhman, 1982). There is less unanimity of opinion concerning studies of experimental absence seizures in which the noradrenergic system was lesioned. Lannes et al. (1991) showed no long-term effect on absence seizures in the GAERS in animals with either neonatal 6-hydroxydopamine (6-OHDA) lesions or locus ceruleus (LC) lesions. Others have shown that electrical stimulation of the LC suppressed spike-and-wave discharges in the low dose PTZ model (Libet et al., 1977). In the γ-hydroxybutyric acid model of absence seizures neonatal 6-OHDA lesions of noradrenergic pathways resulted in a change from bilaterally synchronous spike-and-wave discharges to burst suppression (Snead, 1987a), an effect identical to that seen in the γ-hydroxybutyric acid model in which animals were treated with NMDA agonists or antagonists prior to induction of spike-and-wave discharges with γ-hydroxybutyric acid (Banerjee & Snead, 1992). In the *tg/tg* totterer, a mouse model of absence which also expresses other neurological abnormalities as well as other types of seizures in addition to absence seizures (Noebels & Sidman, 1979), neonatal 6-OHDA treatment blocked the development of spike-and-wave discharges as did lesioning of the LC (Noebels, 1984).These animals appear to have an abnormal increase in LC axons without a corresponding increase in the number of cell somata in the LC (Levitt & Noebels, 1981).

Dopaminergic pathways may also be operative in the control of generalized absence seizures. Mixed dopaminergic D_1/D_2 agonists such as L-Dopa, apomorphine, or amphetamine result in a dose-dependent reduction of spike-and-wave discharge duration in experimental absence seizures while mixed dopaminergic D_1/D_2 antagonists, e.g. haloperidol, flupentixol, and pimozide, exacerbate experimental absence seizures (Snead, 1978; Warter *et al.*, 1988; Frey & Voits, 1991; Cools & Peeters, 1992). It should be noted that dextroamphetamine has some therapeutic efficacy in clinical absence seizures (Livingston, 1966). The mechanism by which dopaminergic pathways interact with thalamocortical pathways is not clear. The effect of pars reticulata neurons upon generalized absence seizures appears to be mediated solely by GABAergic nigro-collicular pathways since it remains intact in the face of lesioning of dopaminergic pars compacta neurons (Depaulis *et al.*, 1990).

Serotonergic neurons do not appear to be involved in the pathogenesis of generalized absence seizures. Neither 5-hydroxytryptophan (5-HT), inhibitors of serotonin synthesis, or uptake, nor 5-HT receptor agonists or antagonists have any effect on spike-and-wave discharge duration in the GAERS (Marescaux *et al.*, 1992a). There are no published studies of the effect of lesioning the dosal raphe nucleus on experimental absence.

Cholinergic mechanisms in experimental absence seizures

Cholinergic projections from the nucleus basalis to the cerebral cortex exert a profound influence upon the activity of the thalamocortical system in terms of arousal (Buzsaki *et al.*, 1988; McCormick, 1989; Steriade & Deschenes, 1988). Because both clinical and experimental generalized absence seizures are tightly related to level of arousal, being suppressed during activity and sleep (Lannes *et al.*, 1988; Coenen *et al.*, 1991), cholinergic mechanisms have been thought to play a role in the pathogenesis of this disorder. Anticholinesterases, muscarinic cholinergic agonists, and nicotonic cholinergic agonists have been shown to decrease experimental absence seizures while muscarinic antagonists appear to have a biphasic effect on spike-and-wave discharges in absence models (Guberman & Gloor, 1974; Frey & Voits, 1991; Riekkinen *et al.*, 1991; Danober *et al.*, 1993). These effects of cholinergic agonists and antagonists may be related to their action on arousal rather than a direct effect on thalamocortical mechanisms at play in generalized absence seizures.

γ-Hydroxybutyric acid (GHB) mediated mechanisms in experimental absence seizures

γ-Hydroxybutyric acid is a short-chain fatty acid which is synthesized from GABA (Snead *et al.*, 1989) and occurs naturally in mammalian brain (Snead, 1987b). This compound is significant in the pathogenesis of absence seizures for a number of reasons. First, γ-hydroxybutyric acid has many properties which suggest a role as a neurotransmitter or neuromodulator (Vayer *et al.*, 1987) including the presence of specific, high-affinity binding sites for γ-hydroxybutyric acid with an anatomical distribution that correlates with γ-hydroxybutyric acid turnover (Vayer *et al.*, 1988; Hechler *et al.*, 1987). Second, γ-hydroxybutyric acid has the ability to induce absence-like seizures in a number of species as well as exacerbate absence in other models (Snead, 1988; Depaulis *et al.*,

1988b) apparently by a γ-hydroxybutyric acid-mediated mechanism (Liu *et al.*, 1991b; Maitre *et al.*, 1990; Snead, 1992c). Third, the density of [^{3}H]γ-hydroxybutyric acid binding sites in the ventrobasal thalamus of GAERS is higher than in control animals (Snead *et al.*, 1990) and [^{3}H]γ-hydroxybutyric acid binding sites in thalamus and cortex are upregulated during the onset and duration of spike-and-wave discharges induced by γ-hydroxybutyric acid (Banerjee *et al.*, 1993). Fourth, the specific γ-hydroxybutyric acid antagonist, NCS 382, decreases spike-and-wave discharge duration in both GAERS (Maitre *et al.*, 1990) and pharmacological models of absence (Snead, 1992c). Fifth, there is an exact concordance between the ontogeny of γ-hydroxybutyric acid-induced absence seizures and that of [^{3}H]γ-hydroxybutyric acid binding sites in frontal cortex in the rat with both appearing at the 18th postnatal day (Snead, 1992d).

Although γ-hydroxybutyric acid is metabolically derived from GABA and is structurally similar to that compound, γ-hydroxybutyric acid is not a GABA agonist because it fails to compete for binding at the GABA$_A$ (Enna & Maggi, 1979; Lloyd & Dreksler, 1979) or GABA$_B$ (Snead, 1992c) site, nor do GABA$_A$ or GABA$_B$ agonists or antagonists compete for binding at the γ-hydroxybutyric acid site (Benavides *et al.*, 1982; Snead *et al.*, 1992c; Snead, 1992c). Furthermore, although there are some neurophysiological similarities between γ-hydroxybutyric acid and baclofen in regard to their post-synaptic action (Engberg & Nissbrandt, 1993; Xie & Smart, 1992; Williams *et al.*, 1993), γ-hydroxybutyric acid and GABA$_B$ receptor binding sites have very different ontogenic profiles (Snead, 1992d) and the regional anatomical distribution in brain of [^{3}H]γ-hydroxybutyric acid and [^{3}H]GABA$_B$ binding sites is decidedly different (Bowery *et al.*, 1987; Chu *et al.*, 1990; Hechler *et al.*, 1987; 1992), the only site of colocalization being the superficial laminae of cerebral cortex. Therefore, in many respects γ-hydroxybutyric acid and GABA$_B$ receptor sites seem to be separate from one another, yet both appear to be involved in the pathogenesis of experimental absence seizures since γ-hydroxybutyric acid induces and GABA$_B$ agonists exacerbate absence seizures while specific γ-hydroxybutyric acid and GABA$_B$ receptor antagonists block the occurrence of spike-and-wave discharges in experimental absence models.

One way to reconcile the GHB/GABA$_B$ data is to hypothesize a pre- rather than post-synaptic interaction between the two systems. Both γ-hydroxybutyric acid (Hechler *et al.*, 1989, 1991) and GABA$_B$ (Bourdelais & Kalivas, 1990) receptor sites are known to mediate presynaptic events. Since GABA$_B$ receptor sites converge upon ion channels with other non-GABA$_B$ neurotransmitter sites (e.g. 5-HT, μ, D$_1$) via a G protein-mediated coupling mechanism (Andrade *et al.*, 1986; Hill *et al.*, 1984), a similar coupling mechanism might allow presynaptic GABA$_B$ and γ-hydroxybutyric acid receptors to converge upon Ca^{2+} activated K$^+$ channels (Neer & Clapham, 1988) and thus control thalamocortical excitability by presynaptic modulation of neurotransmitter release. Indirect evidence of a G-protein mediated mechanism in the pathogenesis of generalized absence seizures may be found in experiments showing that i.c.v. pre-treatment with pertussis toxin, a compound known to inhibit G-proteins by ADP-ribosylation, resulted in a significant decrease in the duration of seizure in both the PTZ and γ-hydroxybutyric acid model of absence (Snead, 1992e).

In conclusion, there are a number of common pharmacologicAL denominators in experimental absence in rats which may provide clues to the basic pathophysiology of this disorder (Table 2). (1) By definition, all experimental rat models of absence respond to pretreatment with anti-absence drugs such as ethosuximide, valproic acid, and trimethadione and are exacerbated by phenytoin and carbamazepine; (2) experimental seizures are exacerbated by mixed D$_1$/D$_2$ dopaminergic blockers and alleviated by mixed D$_1$/D$_2$ agonists; (3) spike-and-wave discharge duration in both the genetic and pharmacologicAL models is decreased by both NMDA agonists and antagonists; (4) absence seizures are enhanced by increasing and exacerbated by decreasing α-noradrenergic neurotransmission; (5) experimental absence seizures are enhanced by γ-hydroxybutyric acid and blocked by γ-hydroxybutyric acid antagonists; (6) apparently absence seizures are attenuated by cholinergic agonists; (7) most importantly, enhancement of GABAergic activity potentiates experimental generalized absence seizures in all these models and may even be sufficient to produce it under certain conditions. Moreover, while both GABA$_A$ and GABA$_B$ agonists prolong experimental absence seizures, only GABA$_B$ antagonists have the universal ability to block these seizures.

Table 2. Pharmacology of experimental absence seizures

Attenuated by:	Exacerbated by:
GABA$_B$ antagonists	GABA$_B$ agonists >> GABA$_A$ agonists
Mixed D$_1$/D$_2$ agonists	Mixed D$_1$/D$_2$ antagonists
α_1-Noradrenergic agonists	α_1-Noradrenergic antagonists
α_2-Noradrenergic antagonists	α_2-Noradrenergic agonists
GHB antagonist	γ-hydroxybutyric acid
Ethosuximide, valproic acid, trimethadione, benzodiazepines	Phenytoin, carbamazepine
NMDA agonists/antagonists	
?Cholinergic agonist	

One could explain much of the available pharmacologic data by postulating that the paroxysmal discharges which characterize generalized absence seizures result from low threshold calcium currents in NRT neurons. The low threshold calcium spike is mediated directly by GABA$_B$ receptors via slow IPSPs and indirectly by NMDA receptors since initial excitation is required ultimately to generate the low threshold calcium current (von Krosigk et al., 1993; Steriade et al., 1993a). Hence, administration of NMDA would be expected to produce tonic firing and prevent low threshold calcium currents from ever developing while NMDA antagonists would be predicted to block the initial EPSPs which are required to trigger the fast and slow IPSP which lead to the low threshold calcium current. Similarly, ethosuximide and valproate may owe their anti-absence activity to their ability to block or reduce low threshold calcium current (Coulter et al., 1989a,b, 1990). Benzodiazepines may act by decreasing GABA$_B$-mediated inhibition and therefore low threshold calcium currents via increasing GABA$_A$-mediated inhibition in the NRT (Huguenard et al., 1993).

Thalamocortical rhythmicity, although driven by the NRT, may be significantly modulated by ascending cholinergic pathways which project to thalamus and cortex. An additional modulatory effect could be exerted indirectly by dopaminergic pathways via their effect on nigrothalamic and nigrotectal GABAergic pathways. Moreover, noradrenergic and dopaminergic neurons also have the potential to exert a modulatory effect on the cortical end of the thalamocortical loop (McCormick et al., 1993) by influencing bursting cells in layer V as well as upon layer I where dendrodendritic connections are to be found between thalamocortical projections from the medial thalamic nuclei and projections from bursting pyramidal cells in layer V (Sylva et al., 1991; Chagnac-Amitai et al., 1990; Chagnac-Amatai & Conners, 1989; Conners & Gutnick, 1990). Alternatively, keeping the same synaptic circuitry and neurotransmitters in mind, one could also postulate a scenario whereby *presynaptic* GABA$_B$ and γ-hydroxybutyric acid receptors might contribute to the regulation of thalamocortical rhythmicity by precise control of excitation and inhibition through modulation of excitatory and inhibitory neurotransmitter release (Snead, 1992c).

Acknowledgements

This work was supported in part by grant No. NS-17117 from the NINDS.

References

Ahlsen, G. & Lo, F.-S. (1982): Projection of brain-stem neurons to the perigeniculate nucleus and the lateral geniculate nucleus in the cat. *Brain Res.* **238**, 433–438.

Andrade, R., Malenka, R.C. & Nicoll, R. (1986): A G protein couples serotonin and GABA$_B$ receptors to the same channels in hippocampus. *Science* **234**, 1261–1265.

Aicardi, J. (1986): In: *Epilepsy in children*, pp. 79–99. New York: Raven Press.

Asanuma, C. (1989): Axonal arborizations of a magnocellular basal nucleus input and their relation to the neurons in the thalamic nucleus of rats. *Proc. Natl. Acad. Sci. (USA)* **86,** 4746–4750.

Asanuma, C. (1992): Noradrenergic innervation of the thalamic reticular nucleus. A light and electron microscopic immunohistochemical study in rats. *J. Comp. Neurol.* **319,** 299–311.

Asanuma, C. & Porter, L.L. (1990): Light and electron microscopic evidence for a GABAergic projection from the caudal basal forebrain to the thalamic nucleus in rats. *J. Comp. Neurol.* **302,** 159–172.

Avanzini, G., Vergnes, M., Spreafico, R. & Marescaux, C. (1993): Calcium-dependent regulation of genetically determined spike-and-waves by the reticular thalamic nucleus of rats. *Epilepsia* **34,** 1–7.

Avoli, M., Gloor, P. & Kostopoulos, G. (1990): Focal and generalized epileptiform activity in the cortex: in search of differences in synaptic mechanisms, ionic movements, and long lasting changes in neuronal excitability. In: *Generalized epilepsy: neurobiological approaches*, eds. M. Avoli, P. Gloor, G. Kostopoulos & R. Naquet, pp. 213–231. Boston: Birkhauser.

Bal, T. & McCormick, D.A. (1993): Mechanisms of oscillatory activity in guinea pig nucleus reticularis thalami *in vitro*: a mammalian pacemaker. *J. Physiol.* **468,** 669–691.

Banerjee, P.K. & Snead, O.C. (1992): Excitatory amino acid-mediated mechanisms in the γ-hydroxybutyrate model of absence. *Neuropharmacology* **31,** 1009–1019.

Banerjee, P.K. & Snead, O.C. (1993): Intrathalamic infusions of both NMDA and its antagonist, MK-801 suppress γ-hydroxybutyrate induced generalized absence-like seizures in rats. *Soc. Neurosci. Abs.* **19,** 1468.

Banerjee, P.K., Hirsch, E. & Snead, O.C. (1993): γ-Hydroxybutyric acid induced spike-and-wave discharges in rats: relation to high affinity [^{3}H]-γ-hydroxybutyric acid binding sites in the thalamus and cortex. *Neuroscience* **56,** 11–21.

Benavides, J., Rumigny, J.F., Bourguignon, J.J., Cash, C., Wermuth, C.G., Mandel, P., Vincendon, G. & Maitre, M. (1982): High affinity binding site for γ-hydroxybutyric acid in rat brain. *Life Sci.* **30,** 953–961.

Berger, B., Trottier, S., Virney, C., Gaspar, P. & Alvarez, C. (1988): Regional and laminar distribution of the dopamine and serotonin innervation in the macaque cerebral cortex: an autoradiographic study. *J. Comp. Neurol.* **273,** 99–119.

Berkovic, S.F., Andermann, F., Andermann, E. & Gloor, P. (1992): Concepts of absence epilepsies: discrete syndromes or biological continuum? *Neurology* **37,** 993–1000.

Bigl, V., Woolfe, N.J. & Butcher, L.L. (1982): Cholinergic projections form the basal forebrain to frontal, parietal, temporal, occipital, and cingulate cortices: a combined fluorescent tracer and acetyl cholinesterase analysis. *Brain Res. Bull.* **8,** 727–749.

Booker, H.E. (1989): Trimethadione. In: *Antiepileptic drugs*, 3rd edn., eds. R. Levy, R. Mattson, B. Meldrum, J.K. Penry & F.E. Dreifuss, pp. 715–720. New York: Raven Press.

Bonanno, G. & Raiteri, M. (1993): Multiple GABA$_B$ receptors. *Trends Pharmacol. Sci.* **14,** 259–261.

Bourdelais, A.J. & Kalivas, P.W. (1992): Modulation of extracellular gamma-amino butyric acid in the ventral pallidum using *in vivo* microdialysis. *J. Neurochem.* **5F,** 2311–2320.

Bourgeois, B.F.D. (1989): Valproate: clinical use. In: *Antieipleptic drugs*, 3rd edn., R. Levy, R. Mattson, B. Meldrum, J.K. Penry & F.E. Dreifuss, pp. 633–642. New York: Raven Press.

Bowery, N.G., Hudson, A.L. & Price, G.W. (1987): GABA$_A$ and GABA$_B$ receptor site distribution in the rat central nervous system. *Neuroscience* **20,** 365–383.

Buzsaki, G., Bickford, R.G., Ponomareff, G., Thal, L.J., Mandel, R.J. & Gage, F.H. (1988): Nucleus basalis and thalamic control of neocortical activity in the freely moving rat. *J. Neurosci.* **8,** 4007–4026.

Buzsaki, G. (1991): The thalamic clock: emergent network properties. *Neuroscience* **41,** 351–364.

Chagnac–Amitai, Y. & Conners, B.W. (1989): Synchronized excitation and inhibition driven by intrinsically bursting neurons in neocortex. *J. Neurophysiol.* **62,** 1149–1162.

Chagnac-Amitai, Y., Luhmann, H.J. & Prince, D.A. (1990): Burst generating and regular spiking layer 5 pyramidal neurons of rat neocortex have different morphological features. *J. Comp. Neurol.* **296,** 598–613.

Chu, D.C.M., Albin, R.L., Young, A.B. & Penney, J.B. (1990): Distribution and kinetics of GABA$_B$ binding sites in rat central nervous system: a quantitative autoradiographic study. *Neuroscience* **34,** 341–357.

Coenen, A.M., Drinkenburg, W.H., Peeters, B.W.M.M., Vossen, J.M.H. & van Luijtelaar, E.L.J.M. (1991): Absence epilepsy and the level of vigilance in rats of the WAG/Rij strain. *Neurosci. Biobehav. Rev.* **15,** 259–276.

Coenen, A.M., Drinkenburg, W.H., Inoue, M. & van Luijtelaar, E.L. (1992): Genetic models of absence epilepsy, with emphasis on the WAG/Rij strain of rats. *Epilepsy Res.* **12,** 75–86.

Conners, B.W. & Gutnick, M.J. (1990): Intrinsic firing patterns of diverse neocortical neurons. *Trends Neurosci.* **13,** 99–104.

Contreras, D., Dossi, R.C. & Steriade, M. (1993): Electrophysiological properties of cat reticular thalamic neurones *in vivo*. *J. Physiol.* **470,** 273–294.

Cools, A.R. & Peeters, B.W.M.M. (1992): Differences in spike wave discharges in two rat selection lines characterized by opposite dopaminergic activities. *Neurosci. Lett.* **134,** 253–256.

Cornwall, J., Cooper, J.D. & Phillipson, O.T. (1990): Projections to the rostral reticular thalamic nucleus in the rat. *Exp. Brain Res.* **80,** 157–171.

Coulter, D.A., Huguenard, J.R. & Prince, D.A. (1989a): Specific petit mal anticonvulsants reduce calcium currents in thalamic neurons. *Neurosci. Lett.* **98,** 74–78.

Coulter, D.A., Huguenard, J.R. & Prince, D.A. (1989b): Characterization of ethosuximide reduction of low-threshold calcium current in thalamic neurons. *Ann. Neurol.* **25,** 582–593.

Coulter, D.A., Huguenard, J.R. & Prince, D.A. (1990): Differential effects of petit mal anticonvulsants and convulsants on thalamic neurones: calcium current reduction. *Br. J. Pharmacol.* **100,** 800–805.

Cropper, E.C., Eisenman, J.S. & Azmitia, E.C. (1984): An immunocytochemical study of the serotonergic innervation of the thalamus of the rat. *J. Comp. Neurol.* **224,** 38–50.

Crunelli, V. & Leresche, N. (1991): A role for $GABA_B$ receptors in excitation and inhibition of thalamocortical cells. *Trends Neurosci.* **14,** 16–21.

Danober, L., Depaulis, A., Marescaux, C. & Vergnes, M. (1993): Effects of cholinergic drugs on genetic absence seizures in rats. *Eur. J. Pharmacol.* **234,** 263–268.

Depaulis, A., Vergnes, M., Marescaux, C., Lannes, B. & Warter, J.-M. (1988a): Evidence that activation of GABA receptors in the substantia nigra suppresses spontaneous spike-and-wave discharges in the rat. *Brain Res.* **448,** 20–29.

Depaulis, A., Bourguignon, J. Marescaux, C., Vergnes, M., Schmitt, M., Micheletti, G. & Warter, J.-M. (1988b): Effect of γ-hydroxybutyrate and γ-butyrolactone derivatives on spontaneous generalized non-convulsive seizures in the rat. *Neuropharmacology* **27,** 6863–6869.

Depaulis, A., Snead, O.C., Marescaux, C. & Vergnes, M. (1989): Suppressive effects of intranigral injection of muscimol in three models of generalized non-convulsive epilepsy induced by chemical agents. *Brain Res.* **498,** 64–72.

Depaulis, A., Vergnes, M., Liu, Z., Kempf, E. & Marescaux, C. (1990): Involvement of the nigral oputput pathways in the inhibitory control of the substantia nigra over generalized non-convulsive seizures in the rat. *Neuroscience* **39,** 339–349.

Di Chiara, G., Porceddu, M.L., Morelli, M. & Gessa, G.L. (1979): Evidence for a GABAergic projection from the substantia nigra to the ventromedial thalamus and to the superior colliculus of the rat. *Brain Res.* **176,** 273–284.

Eckenstein, F.P., Baughman, R.W. & Quinn, J. (1988): An anatomical study of cholinergic innervation in rat cerebral cortex. *Neuroscience* **25,** 457–474.

Engberg, G. & Nissbrandt, H. (1993): γ-Hydroxybutyric acid (GHBA) induces pacemaker activity and inhibition of substantia nigra dopamine neurons by activating $GABA_B$-receptors. *Nauyn-Schmiedeberg's Arch. Pharmacol.* **348,** 491–497.

Enna, S.J. & Maggi, A. (1979): Biochemical pharmacology of GABAergic agonists. *Life Sci.* **34,** 1727–1736.

Fariello, R.G. & Golden, G.T. (1987): The THIP induced model of bilateral synchronous spike-and-wave in rodents. *Neuropharmacology* **26,** 161–165.

Fariello, R.G. (1990): Pharmacology of the inhibitory systems in primary generalized epilepsy of 'petit mal' type. In: *Generalized epilepsy: neurobiological approaches*, eds. M. Avoli, P. Gloor, G. Kostopoulos & R. Naquet, pp. 232–237. Boston: Birkhauser.

Foote, S.L. & Morrison, J.H. (1986): Extrathalamic modulation of cortical function. *Rev. Neurosci.* **10,** 67–95.

Foote, S.L., Bloom, F.E. & Aston-Jones, G. (1983): Nucleus locus coeruleus: new evidence of anatomical and physiological specificity. *Physiol. Rev.* **63,** 844–914.

Frey, H.-H. & Voits, M. (1991): Effect of psychotropic agents on a model of absence epilepsy in rats. *Neuropharmacology* **30,** 651–656.

Gloor, P. (1984): Electrophysiology of generalized epilepsy. In: *Electrophysiology of epilepsy*, eds. P.A. Schwartzkroin & H. Wheal, pp. 107–136. New York: Academic Press.

Gloor, P. & Fariello, R.G. (1988): Generalized epilepsy: some of its cellular mechanisms differ from those of focal epilepsy. *Trends Neurosci.* **11,** 63–68.

Gloor, P., Avoli, M. & Kostopoulos, G. (1990): Thalamo-cortical relationships in generalized epilepsy with bilateraly synchronous spike-and-wave discharge. In: *Generalized epilepsy: neurobiological approaches*, eds. M. Avoli, P. Gloor, G. Kostopoulos & R. Naquet, pp. 190-212. Boston: Birkhauser.

Guberman, A. & Gloor, P. (1974): Cholinergic drug studies of generalized penicillin epilepsy in the cat. *Brain Res.* **78,** 203–208.

Guyon, A., Vergnes, M. & Leresche, N. (1993): Thalamic low threshold calcium current in a genetic model of absence epilepsy. *Neuro Rep.* **4,** 1231–1234.

Haefely, W. (1990): The GABA-benzodiazepine interaction fifteen years later. *Neurochem. Res.* **15,** 169–174.

Hallanager, A.E., Levey, A.I., Lee, J.J., Rye, D.B. & Wainer, B.H. (1987): The origins of cholinergic and other subcortical afferents to the thalamus in the rat. *J. Comp. Neurol.* **262,** 105–124.

Hechler, V., Weissman, D., Mach, E., Pujol, J.-F. & Maitre, M. (1987): Regional distribution of high affinity γ-[^{3}H]hydroxybutyrate binding sites as determined by quantitative autoradiography. *J. Neurochem.* **49,** 1025–1032.

Hechler, V., Gobaille, S. & Maitre, M. (1989): Localization studies of γ-hydroxybutyrate receptors in rat striatum and hippocampus. *Brain Res. Bull.* **23,** 129–135.

Hechler, V., Gobaille, S., Bourguignon, J.-J. & Maitre, M. (1991): Extracellular events induced by γ-hydroxybutyrate in striatum: a microdialysis study. *J. Neurochem.* **56,** 938–944.

Hechler, V., Gobaille, S. & Maitre, M. (1992): Selective distribution pattern of γ-hydroxybutyrate receptors in the rat forebrain and midbrain as revealed by quantitative autoradiography. *Brain Res.* **572,** 345–348.

Hill, D.R., Bowery, N.G. & Hudson, A.L. (1984): Inhibition of GABA$_B$ receptor binding by guanyl nucleotides. *J. Neurochem.* **42,** 652–657.

Holmes, G.L. (1987): *Diagnosis and management of seizures in children*. pp. 173–186. Philadelphia: W.B. Saunders.

Hosford, D.A., Clark, S., Cao, Z., Wilson, W.A., Lin, F.-H., Morrisett, R.A. & Huin, A. (1992): The role of GABA$_B$ receptor activation in absence seizures of lethargic (lh/lh) mice. *Science* **257,** 398–401.

Hughes, H.C. & Mullikin, W.H. (1984): Brain-stem afferents to the geniculate nucleus of the cat. *Exp. Brain Res.* **54,** 253–258.

Huguenard, J.R. & Prince, D.A. (1993): Clonazepam suppresses GABA$_B$ inhibition in relay cells through actions in the reticular nucleus. *Soc. Neurosci. Abs.* **19,** 1704.

Johnson, J.W. & Ascher, P. (1987): Glycine potentiates the NMDA response in cultured mouse brain neurons. *Nature* **325,** 529–531.

Jones, E.G. (1985): *The thalamus*. Plenum Press, New York.

Jones, E.G. (1993): GABAergic neurons and their role in cortical plasticity in primates. *Cerebral Cortex* **3,** 361–372.

King, G.A. & Burnham, W.M. (1982): α_2-Adrenergic antagonists suppress epileptiform EEG activity in a petit mal seizure model. *Life Sci.* **30,** 293–299.

Kleinlogel, H. (1985): Spontaneous EEG paroxysms in the rat: effects of psychotropic and α-adrenergic agents. *Neuropsychobiology* **13,** 206–213.

Knight, A.R. & Bowery, N.G. (1992): GABA receptors in rats with spontaneous generalized nonconvulsive epilepsy. *J. Neural Trans. Suppl.* **35,** 189–196.

Kosofsky, B.E. & Molliver, M.E. (1987): The serotonergic innervation of cerebral cortex: different classes of axon terminals arise from dorsal and median raphe nuclei. *Synapse* **1,** 153–168.

Kostopoulos, G. (1986): Neuronal sensitivity to GABA and glutamate in generalized epilepsy with spike-and-wave discharges. *Exp. Neurol.* **92,** 20–36.

Lannes, B., Micheletti, G., Vergnes, M., Marescaux, C., Depaulis, A. & Warter, J.-M. (1988): Relationship between spike-wave discharges and vigilance levels in rats with spontaneous petit mal-like seizures. *Epilepsy Res.* **9,** 79–85.

Lannes, B., Vergnes, M., Marescaux, C., Depaulis, A., Micheletti, G., Warter, J.-M. & Kempf, E. (1991): Lesions of noradrenergic neurons in rats with spontaneous generalized non-convulsive epilepsy. *Epilepsy Res.* **9**, 79–85.

Lavoie, B. & Parent, A. (1991): Serotonergic innervation of the thalamus in primate: an immunohistochemical study. *J. Comp. Neurol.* **312**, 1–18.

Levitt, P. & Noebels, J.L. (1981): Mutant mouse tottering: selective increase of locus coeruleus in a defined single-locus mutation. *Proc. Natl. Acad. Sci. (USA)* **78**, 4630–4634.

Levey, A.I., Hallanger, A.E. & Wainer, B.H. (1987): Cholinergic nucleus basalis neurons may influence the cortex via the thalamus. *Neurosci. Lett.* **10**, 7–13.

Libet, B., Gleason, C.A., Wright, E.W. & Feinstein, B. (1977): Supression of an epileptiform type of electrocortical activity in the rat by stimulation in the vicinity of locus coeruleus. *Epilepsia* **18**, 451–462.

Liu, Z., Seiler, N., Marescaux, C., Depaulis, A. & Vergnes, M. (1990): Potentiation of γ-vinyl GABA (vigabatrin) effects by glycine. *Eur. J. Pharmacol.* **182**, 109–115.

Liu, Z., Vergnes, M., Depaulis, A. & Marescaux, C. (1991a): Evidence for a critical role of GABAergic transmission within the thalamus in the genesis and control of absence seizures in the rat. *Brain Res.* **545**, 1–7.

Liu, Z., Snead, O.C., Vergnes, M., Depaulis, A. & Marescaux, C. (1991b): Intrathalamic injections of γ-hydroxybutyric acid increase genetic absence seizures in rats. *Neurosci. Lett.* **125**, 19–21.

Liu, Z., Vergnes, M., Depaulis, A. & Marescaux C. (1992): Involvement of intrathalamic $GABA_B$ neurotransmission in the control of absence seizures in the rat. *Neuroscience* **48**, 87–93.

Livingston, S. (1966): *Drug therapy for epilepsy*. Springfield, IL: C.C. Thomas.

Lloyd, K.G. & Dreksler S. (1979): An analysis of [^{3}H]γ-aminobutyric acid (GABA) binding in the human brain. *Brain Res.* **163**, 77–87.

Lockman, L.A. (1989): Absence, myoclonic, and atonic seizures. *Pediatr. Clin. North Am.* **36**, 331–343.

Lysakowski, A., Wainer, B.H., Bruce, G. & Hersh, L.B. (1989): An atlas of the regional and laminar distribution of choline acetyltransferase immunoreactivity in rat cerebral cortex. *Neuroscience* **28**, 291–336.

Maitre, M., Hechler, V., Vayer, P., Gobaille, S., Cash, C.D., Schmidtt, M. & Bourguignon, J.-J. (1990): A specific γ-hydroxybutyrate receptor ligand possesses both antagonistic and anticonvulsant properties. *J. Pharmacol. Exp. Ther.* **255**, 657–663.

Marescaux, C., Vergnes, M. & Depaulis, A. (1992a): Genetic absence epilepsy in rats from Strasbourg – a review. *J. Neural Trans.* **Suppl. 35**, 37–70.

Marescaux, C., Vergnes, M., Depaulis, A. & Bernasconi, R. (1992b): $GABA_B$ receptor involvement in the control of genetic absence in rats. *Epilepsy Res. Supp.* **9**, 121–138.

McCormick, D.A. (1989): Cholinergic and noradrenergic modulation of thalamocortical processing. *Trends Neurosci.* **12**, 215–221.

McCormick, D.A. (1990): Cellular mechanisms of cholinergic control of neocortical and thalamic neuronal excitability. In: *Brain cholinergic systems*, eds. M. Steriade & D. Biesold, pp. 236–264. New York: Oxford University Press.

McCormick, D.A. (1992): Neurotransmitter actions in the thalamus and cerebral cortex and their role in neuromodulation of thalamocortical activity. *Progr. Neurobiol.* **39**, 337–388.

McCormick, D.A. & von Krosigk, M. (1992): Corticothalamic activation modulates thalamic firing through activation of glutamate metabotropic receptors. *Proc. Natl. Acad. Sci. (USA)* **89**, 2774–2778.

McCormick, D.A., Wang, Z. & Huguenard, J. (1993): Neurotransmitter control of neocortical neuronal activity and excitability. *Cerebral Cortex* **3**, 387–398.

McQueen, J.K. & Woodbury, D.M. (1975): Attempts to produce spike wave complexes in the electrocorticogram of the rat. *Epilepsia* **16**, 295–299.

Micheletti, G., Marescaux, C., Vergnes, M., Rumbach, L. & Warter, J.M. (1985): Effects of GABA mimetics and GABA antagonists on spontaneous nonconvulsive seizures in Wistar rats. In: *L.E.R.S. Monograph Series*, Vol 3., eds. G. Bartholini, L. Bossi, K.G. Lloyd & M.L. Morselli, pp. 129–137. New York: Raven Press.

Micheletti, G., Warter, J.-M., Marescaux, C., Depaulis, A., Tranchant, C., Rumbach, L. & Vergnes, M. (1987): Effects of drugs affecting noradrenergic neurotransmission in rats with spontaneous petit-mal seizures. *Eur. J. Pharmacol.* **135**, 397–402.

Mirsky, A.F., Duncan, C.C. & Myslobodsky, M.S. (1986): Petit mal epilepsy: a review and integration of recent information. *J. Clin. Neurophysiol.* **3,** 179–208.

Morrison, J.H. & Foote, S.L. (1986): Noradrenergic and serotonergic innervation of cortical, thalamic, and tectal visual structures in old and new world monkeys. *J. Comp. Neurol.* **243,** 117–138.

Mulle, C., Madariga, A. & Deschenes, M. (1986): Morphology and electrophysiological properties of reticularis thalami neurons in cat: *in vivo* study of a thalamic pacemaker. *J. Neurosci.* **6,** 2134–2145.

Murphy, J. & Dehkharghani, F. (1994): Diagnosis of childhood seizure disorders. *Epilepsia* **35 (Suppl. 2),** S7–S17.

Myslobodsky, M. (1976): *Petit mal epilepsy.* New York: Academic Press.

Myslobodsky, M.S., Ackermann, R.F. & Engel, J. (1979): Effects of γ-acetylenic GABA and γ-vinyl GABA on metrazol activated and kindled seizures. *Pharmacol. Biochem. Behav.* **11,** 265–271.

Neer, E.J. & Clapham, D.E. (1988): Roles of G protein subunits in transmembrane signalling. *Nature* **333,** 129–134.

Noebels, J.L. (1984): A single gene error of noradrenergic axon growth synchronizes central neurons. *Nature* **310,** 409–411.

Noebels, J.L. & Sidman, R.M. (1979): Inherited epilepsy: spike-wave and focal motor seizures in the mutant mouse tottering. *Science* **204,** 1334–1336.

Pare, D., Hazrati, L.-N., Parent, A. & Steriade, M. (1990): Substantia nigra pars reticulata projects to the reticular thalamic nucleus of the cat: a morphological and electrophysiological study. *Brain Res.* **535,** 139–146.

Pare, D. & Steriade, M. (1993): The reticular nucleus projects to the contralateral dorsal thalamus in macaque monkey. *Neurosci. Lett.* **154,** 96–100.

Peeters, B.W.M.M., van Rijn, C.M., Vossen, J.M.H. & Coenen, A.M.L. (1989a): Effects of GABAergic agents on spontaneous non-convulsive epilepsy, EEG, and behavior, in the WAG/Rij inbred strain of rats. *Life Sci.* **45,** 1171–1176.

Peeters, B.W.M.M., van Rijn, C.M., van Luijtelaar, E.L.J.M. & Coenen, A.M.L. (1989b): Antiepileptic and behavioral actions of MK-801 in an animal model of spontaneous absence epilepsy. *Epilepsy Res.* **3,** 178–181.

Peeters, B.W.M.M., van Rijn, C.M., Vossen, J.M.H. & Coenen, A.M.L. (1990): Involvement of NMDA receptors in non-convulsive epilepsy in WAG/Rij rats. *Life Sci.* **47,** 523–529.

Penry, J.K., Porter, R.J. & Dreifuss, F.E. (1975): Simultaneous recording of absence seizures with videotape and electroencephalography. A study of 374 seizures in 48 patients. *Brain* **98,** 427–440.

Pumain, R., Louvel, J., Gastard, M., Kurcewicz, I. & Vergnes, M. (1992): Responses to N-methyl-D-aspartate are enhanced in rats with petit mal-like seizures. *J. Neural Trans. Suppl.* **35,** 97–108.

Ramakers, G.M.J., Peeters, B.W.M.M., Vossen, J.M.H. & Coenen, A.M.L. (1991): CNQX, a new non-NMDA receptor antagonist, reduces spike wave discharges in the WAG/Rij rat model of absence epilepsy. *Epilepsy Res.* **9,** 127–131.

Raos, V. & Bentivoglio, M. (1993): Crosstalk between the two sides of the thalamus through the reticular nucleus: a retrograde and anterograde tracing study in the rat. *J. Comp. Neurol.* **332,** 145–154.

Riekkinen, Jr, P., Riekkinen, M., Jakala, P., Sirvio, J., Lammintausta, R. & Riekkinen, P. (1991): Combination of atipamezol and tetrahydroaminoacridine/pilocarpine treatment suppresses high voltage spindle activity in aged rats. *Brain Res. Bull.* **27,** 237–245.

Roseman, E. (1961): Dilantin toxicity: a clinical and EEG study. *Neurology* **11,** 912–917.

Sato, S. (1989): Benzodiazepines: clonazepam. In: *Antiepileptic drugs,* 3rd edn., eds. R. Levy, R. Mattson, B. Meldrum, J.K. Penry & F.E. Dreifuss, pp. 675–684. New York: Raven Press.

Sherwin, A.L. (1989): Ethosuximide: clinical use. In: *Antiepileptic drugs,* 3rd edn., eds. R. Levy, R. Mattson, B. Meldrum, J.K. Penry & F.E. Dreifuss, pp. 685–698. New York: Raven Press.

Smith, K.A. & Bierkamper, G.G. (1990): Paradoxical role of GABA in a chronic model of petit mal (absence)-like epilepsy in the rat. *Eur. J. Pharmacol.* **176,** 46–45–55.

Snead, O.C. (1978): γ-Hydroxybutyrate in monkey IV: dopaminergic mechanisms. *Neurology* **28,** 1179–1182.

Snead, O.C. (1983): On the sacred disease: the neurochemistry of epilepsy. *Int. Rev. Neurobiol.* **24,** 93–190.

Snead, O.C. (1984): γ-Hydroxybutyric acid, γ-aminobutyric acid, and petit mal epilepsy. In: *Neurotransmitters, seizures, and epilepsy II*, eds. R.G. Fariello, P.L. Morseli, K.G. Lloyd, L.F. Quesney & J. Engel, pp. 37–47. New York: Raven Press.

Snead, O.C. (1987a): Noradrenergic mechanisms in γ-hydroxybutyrate-induced seizure activity. *Eur. J. Pharmacol.* **136,** 103–108.

Snead, O.C. (1987b): γ-Hydroxybutyric acid in subcellular fractions of rat brain. *J. Neurochem.* **48,** 196–201.

Snead, O.C. (1988): The γ-hydroxybutyrate model of generalized absence seizures: further characterization and comparison to other absence models. *Epilepsia* **29,** 361–368.

Snead, O.C. (1990): The ontogeny of GABAergic enhancement of the γ-hydroxybutyrate model of generalized absence seizures. *Epilepsia* **31,** 253–258.

Snead, O.C. (1992a): Pharmacologic models of absence seizures. *J. Neural Trans. Suppl.* **35,** 7–20.

Snead, O.C. (1992b): Evidence for GABA$_B$-mediated mechanisms in experimental absence seizures. *Eur. J. Pharmacol.* **213,** 343–349.

Snead, O.C. (1992c): GABA$_B$ receptor mediated mechanisms in experimental absence seizures in rat. *Pharmacol. Commun.* **2,** 63–69.

Snead, O.C. (1992d): GABA$_B$-mediated mechanisms in the γ-hydroxybutyric acid model of absence seizures: ontogeny studies. *Epilepsia* **33 (Suppl. 3),** 41.

Snead, O.C. (1992e): Evidence for G-protein modulation of experimental generalized absence seizures in the rat. *Neurosci. Lett.* **148,** 15–18.

Snead, O.C. & Hosey, L.C. (1985): Exacerbation of seizures in children by carbamazepine. *N. Engl. J. Med.* **313,** 916–921.

Snead, O.C., Furner, R. & Liu, C.C. (1989): In vivo conversion of γ-aminobutyric acid and 1,4 butanediol to γ-hydroxybutyric acid in rat brain: studies using stable isotopes. *Biochem. Pharmacol.* **38,** 4375–4380.

Snead, O.C., Hechler, V., Vergnes, M., Marescaux, C. & Maitre, M. (1990): Increased γ-hydroxybutyric acid receptors in thalamus of a genetic animal model of petit mal epilepsy. *Epilepsy Res.* **7,** 121–128.

Snead, O.C., Depaulis, A., Banerjee, P.K., Hechler, V. & Vergnes, M. (1992a): The GABA$_A$ receptor complex in experimental absence seizures in rat: an autoradiographic study. *Neurosci. Lett.* **140,** 9–12.

Snead, O.C., Banerjee, P.K., Depaulis, A. & Vergnes, M. (1992b): NMDA receptor complex in experimental absence seizures: an autoradiographic study. *Epilepsia* **33 (Suppl 3),** 32.

Snead, O.C., Nichols, A.C. & Liu, C.C. (1992c): γ-Hydroxybutyrate binding sites: interaction with the GABA-benzodiazepine-picrotoxinin receptor complex. *Neurochem. Res.* **17,** 201–204.

Snead, O.C. & Liu, C.C. (1993): GABA$_A$ receptor function in the γ-hydroxybutyrate model of generalized absence seizures. *Neuropharmacology* **32,** 401–409.

Spreafico, R., Battaglia, G. & Frassoni, C. (1991): The reticular thalamic nucleus (RTN) of the rat: cytoarchitectural, Golgi, immunocytochemical, and horseradish peroxidase study. *J. Comp. Neurol.* **304,** 478–490.

Spreafico, R., Mennini, T., Danober, L., Cagnotto, A., Regondi, M.C., Miari, A., DeBlas, A., Vergnes, M. & Avanzini, G. (1993): GABA$_A$ receptor impairment in the genetic absence epilepsy rats from Strasbourg (GAERS): an immunocytochemical and receptor binding autoradiographic study. *Epilepsy Res.* **15,** 229–238.

Stephenson, F.A. (1988): Understanding the GABA$_A$ receptor: a chemically gated ion channel. *Biochem. J.* **249,** 21–32.

Steriade, M., Parent, A. & Hada, J. (1984): Thalamic projections of nucleus reticularis thalami of cat: a study using retrograde transport of horseradish peroxidase and fluorescent tracers. *J. Comp. Neurol.* **229,** 531–547.

Steriade, M., Domich, L. & Oakson, G. (1986): Reticularis thalami neurons revisited: activity changes during shifts in states of vigilance. *J. Neurosci.* **6,** 68–81.

Steriade, M., Domich, L. & Oakson, G. (1987): The deafferented reticular thalamic nucleus generates spindle rhythmicity. *J. Neurophysiol.* **57,** 260–273.

Steriade, M. & Dechenes, M. (1988): Intrathalamic and brain-stem–thalamic networks involved in resting and alert states. In: *Cellular thalamic mechanisms*, eds. M. Bentivoglio & R. Spreafico, pp. 37–47. Amsterdam: Elsevier.

Steriade, M. & Llinas, R.R. (1988): The functional states of the thalamus and the associated neuronal interplay. *Physiol. Rev.* **68**, 649–742.

Steriade, M., Gloor, P., Llinas, R.R., Lopes da Silva, F.H. & Mesulam, M.-M. (1990): Basic mechanisms of cerebral rhythmic activites. *Electroencephalogr. Clin. Neurophysiol.* **76**, 481–508.

Steriade, M., McCormick, D.A. & Sejnowski, T.J. (1993a): Thalamocortical oscillations in the sleeping and aroused brain. *Science* **262**, 679–685.

Steriade, M., Nunez, A. & Amzica, F. (1993b): A novel slow (Hz) oscillation of neocortical neurons *in vivo*: depolarizing and huperpolarizing components. *J. Neurosci.* **13**, 3252–3265.

Steriade, M., Nunez, A. & Amzica, F. (1993c): Intracellular analysis of relations between the slow (Hz) neocortical oscillation and other sleep rhythms of the electroencephalogram. *J. Neurosci.* **13**, 3266–3283.

Steriade, M., Contreras, D., Curro Dossi, R. & Nunez, A. (1993d): The slow (<1Hz) oscillation in reticular thalamic and thalamocortical neurons: scenario of sleep rhythm generation in interacting thalamic and neocortical networks. *J. Neurosci.* **13**, 3284–3290.

Sylva, L.R., Amitai, Y. & Conners, B.W. (1991): Intrisinic oscillations of neocortex generated by layer 5 pyramidal neurons. *Science* **251**, 432–435.

Thompson, A.M., Walker, V.E. & Flynn, D.M. (1989): Glycine enhances NMDA-receptor mediated synaptic potentials in neocortical slices. *Nature* **338**, 422–424.

Thompson, A.M. (1990): Glycine is a co-agonist at the NMDA receptor channel complex. *Prog. Neurobiol.* **35**, 53–74.

Tork, I. (1990): Anatomy of the serotonergic system. *Ann. N.Y. Acad. Sci.* **600**, 9–24.

van der Linden, G.J., Meinardi, H., Meijer, S.W.A., Bossi, L. & Gomeni, C.A. (1981): A double blind crossover trial with Progabide (SL76002) against placebo in patients with secondary generalized epilepsy. In: *Advances in epileptology: XIIth International Epilepsy Symposium*, eds. M. Dam, L. Gram & J.K. Penry, pp. 141–144. New York: Raven Press.

van Luijtelaar, E.L.J.M. & Coenen, A.M.L. (1986): Two types of electrocortical paroxysms in an inbred strain of rats. *Neurosci. Lett.* **70**, 393–397.

Vayer, P., Mandel, P. & Maitre, M. (1987): γ-Hydroxybutyrate, a possible neurotransmitter. *Life Sci.* **41**, 1547–1557.

Vayer, P., Ehrhardt, J.D., Gobaille, S., Mandel, P. & Maitre, M. (1988): γ-Hydroxybutyrate distribution and turnover rates in discrete brain regions of the rat. *Neurochem. Int.* **12**, 53–59.

Vergnes, M., Marescaux, C. Micheletti, G., Depaulis, A., Rumbach, L. & Warter, J.-M. (1984): Enhancement of spike-and-wave discharges by GABA-mimetic drugs in rat with spontaneous petit mal-like epilepsy. *Neurosci. Lett.* **44**, 91–94.

Vergnes, M., Marescaux, C., Depaulis, A., Micheletti, G. & Warter, J.-M. (1987): Spontaneous spike-and-wave discharges in thalamus and cortex in a rat model of genetic petit mal-like seizures. *Exp. Neurol.* **96**, 127–136.

Vergnes, M., Marescaux, C., Depaulis, A., Micheletti, G. & Warter, J.-M. (1990a): The spontaneous spike-and-wave discharges in Wistar rats: a model of genetic generalized non convulsive epilepsy. In: *Generalized epilepsy: neurobiological approaches*, eds. M. Avoli, P. Gloor, G. Kostopoulos, & R. Naquet, pp. 238–253. Boston: Birkhauser.

Vergnes, M., Marescaux, C. & Depaulis, A. (1990b): Mapping of spontaneous spike-and-wave discharges in Wistar rats with genetic generalized non-convulsive epilepsy. *Brain Res.* **523**, 87–91.

von Krosigk, M., Bal, T. & McCormick, D.A. (1993): Cellular mechanisms of a synchronized oscillation in the thalamus. *Science* **261**, 361–364.

Warter, J.-M., Vergnes, M., Depaulis, A., Tranchant, C., Rumbach, L., Micheletti, G. & Marescaux, C. (1988): Effects of drugs affecting dopaminergic neurotransmission in rats with spontaneous petit mal-like seizures. *Neuropharmacology* **27**, 269–274.

Williams, S.R., Turner, J.P. & Crunelli, V. (1993): γ-Hydroxybutyrate hyperpolarizes rat thalamocortical cells by a direct action on GABA$_B$ receptors. *Soc. Neurosci. Abs.* **19**, 527.

Wilson, J.R. & Henrickson, A.E. (1988): Serotonergic axons in the monkey's lateral geniculate nucleus. *Vis. Neurosci.* **1**, 125–133.

Xie, X. & Smart, T.G. (1992): γ-Hydroxybutyrate hyperpolarizes hippocampal neurones by activating GABA$_B$ receptors. *Eur. J. Pharmacol.* **212**, 291–294.

Yamasaki, D.S.G. & Krauthamer, G.M. (1990): Somatosensory neurons projecting from the superior colliculus to the intralaminar thalamus in the rat. *Brain Res.* **523,** 188–194.

Yen, C.T., Conley, M., Hendry, S.H.C. & Jones, E.G. (1985): The morphology of physiologically identified GABAergic neurons in the somatic sensory part of the thalamic reticular nucleus in the cat. *J. Neurosci.* **5,** 2254–2268.

Yi, H., Ilinsky, I. & Kultas-Ilinsky, K. (1993): Reticular thalamic nucleus input to the nuclei of the monkey thalamus: light and electron-microscopic study. *Soc. Neurosci. Abs.* **19,** 1436.

Chapter 15

Pathophysiological mechanisms underlying genetic absence epilepsy in rats

M. Vergnes and C. Marescaux

INSERM U 398, Clinique Neurologique, Hôpitaux Universitaires, 1 place de l'Hôpital, 67091 Strasbourg Cedex, France

Introduction

The spontaneous occurrence of rhythmic spike-and-wave discharges on the cortical electroencephalogram (EEG) of laboratory rats has been described by many authors. Libouban & Oswaldo-Cruz (1958) first described such patterns, which they related to facial twitching. Klingberg & Pickenhain (1968) found that 20 per cent of their rats presented with large 'spindle' discharges predominant in the frontal cortex and occurring in awake, but quiet animals. Since these first descriptions, several dozen papers have mentioned similar paroxystic EEG patterns in various strains of rodents (for review see Marescaux *et al.*, 1992b). Their significance is controversial: they have been considered to correspond either to a physiological state, typical of rodent's brain, or to a manifestation of epilepsy (for review, see Kaplan, 1985; Marescaux *et al.*, 1992b).

While searching in the 1980s for a model of partial epilepsy in rats, we recorded EEG in control rats without any lesion. We found then, that about 30 per cent of the Wistar rats from our breeding colony presented spontaneous spike-and-wave discharges (SWD) which were bilateral and synchronous all over the cortex. During the spike-and-wave discharges, the rats were immobile. These episodes appeared similar to the generalized non-convulsive seizures of absence, or petit mal, epilepsy in humans. To demonstrate the validity of this hypothesis, we have undertaken a systematic analysis of this phenomenon. As only a small proportion of the animals were affected, we tried to increase their numbers by selecting breeders with spike-and-wave discharges. A strain in which all animals had spike-and-wave discharges was obtained in a few generations. This strain was named 'Genetic Absence Epilepsy Rats from Strasbourg' (GAERS) and has now been inbred through 25 generations. Similarly, a control strain free of any spontaneous spike-and-wave discharges was outbred over 20 generations.

According to the degree of similarity with human diseases, three categories of animal models may be distinguished: isomorphic models with similar symptoms and occurrence; predictive models with a similar therapeutic profile; and homologous models with a similar aetiology to the considered pathology (Kornetsky, 1977). The results obtained over the past years in neurophysiological, beha-

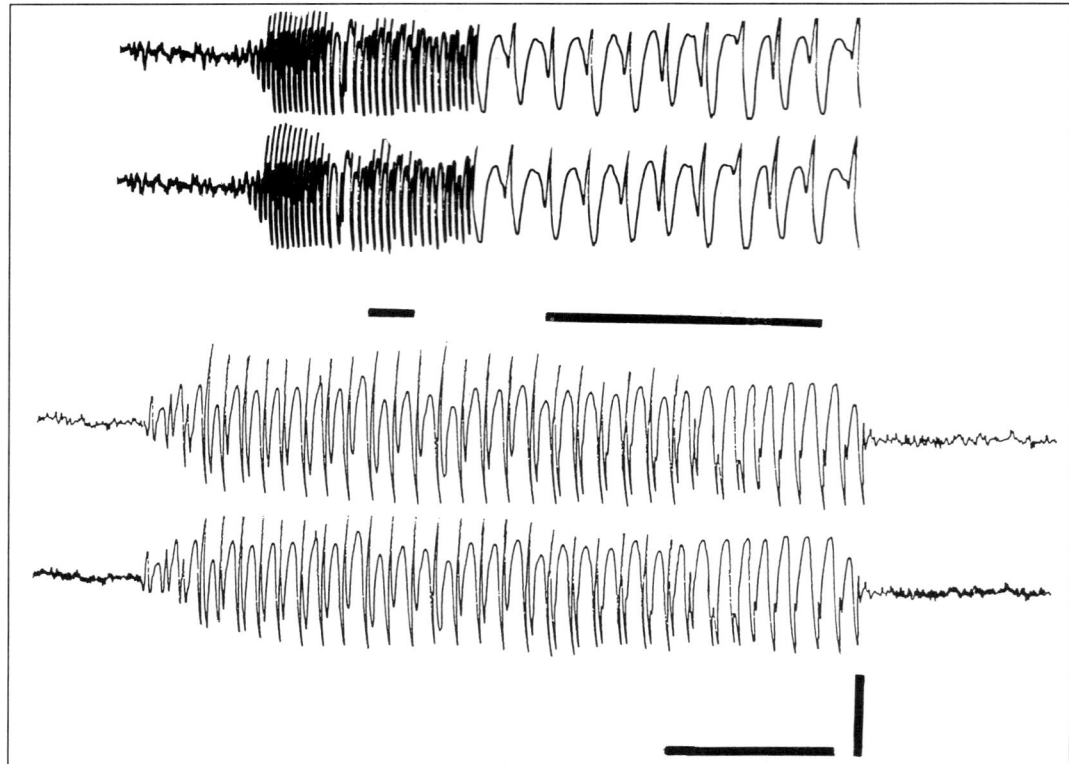

Fig. 1. Spontaneous bilateral cortical spike-and-wave discharges recorded at various speeds in two different GAERS. Calibration 1 s, 400 µV.

vioural and pharmacological studies demonstrate that spike-and-wave discharges in GAERS fulfil all the requirements for an isomorphic and predictive model of petit mal seizures (Marescaux et al., 1992b). These requirements are: (1) EEG and (2) behavioural similarities with human absences, i.e. spike-and-wave discharges of 5 to 15 s duration on a normal background EEG, associated with arrest of movement and reduced responsiveness; (3) an increased occurrence of spike-and-wave discharges by decreased arousal and a decreased occurrence of spike-and-wave discharges by increased arousal; (4) a pharmacological profile that reflects the results obtained in clinical practice; (5) an age-related developmental profile; and (6) potentiation of the spike-and-wave discharges by drugs inducing petit mal-like seizures. Pathophysiological mechanisms underlying absence seizures in humans are still unknown. Thus, analysis of networks, neuromediators and genetic factors involved in GAERS may be fruitful in investigations of the pathogenesis of generalized absence epilepsy.

EEG and behavioural characteristics of GAERS

Cortical EEG

Several hundreds of adult GAERS were implanted with single contact electrodes over the cortex. During the recording session, which lasted 1 to 12 h, the rats placed in a Plexiglass box, were freely moving under permanent observation. The spike-and-wave discharges started and ended abruptly on a normal background EEG. The mean frequency of spike-and-wave complexes within a discharge was 9 ± 0.5 cps (range 7–11 cps); their voltage, which varied from 300 to 1000 µV, was always three- to tenfold over baseline activity (Fig. 1). Sometimes, the discharge began with a monophasic activity at the same frequency as spike-and-wave complexes but with a lower amplitude. The mean duration of spike-and-wave discharges was 17 ± 10 s (range 0.5–75 s). When the animals were maintained in a state of quiet wakefulness, the mean number of spike-and-wave discharges was 1.3 per minute, and the mean cumulative duration of spike-and-wave discharges was 25 ± 8 s/min (Vergnes et al., 1982, 1990b; Marescaux et al., 1992b).

Behaviour during spike-and-wave discharges

Spike-and-wave discharges were usually observed when the animals were motionless in a state of quiet wakefulness. During the discharges, the animals wore a fixed stare and were completely inert. Frequently rhythmic twitching of the vibrissae and of the facial muscles was observed. Muscle tone in the neck was sometimes diminished, inducing a gradual and slight drop of the head. At the end of the spike-and-wave discharge, a sudden extension of the head preceded the recovery of the previous position. In some instances, spike-and-wave discharges appeared when the rat was moving: the movement was suddenly interrupted and resumed as soon as the discharge stopped (Vergnes et al., 1982, 1990b; Marescaux et al., 1984, 1992b).

During spike-and-wave discharge responsiveness to non-significant or mild sensory stimuli was abolished. However, spike-and-wave discharges were immediately interrupted by strong and unexpected stimulations. Analysis of behavioural parameters showed that GAERS were not impaired in spontaneous activity, exploration, feeding, social interactions or learning of positively or negatively reinforced tasks. Sexual and reproductive behaviours also appear normal. Spike-and-wave discharges did not interfere with active behaviours, as they only occurred when attention and activity were already reduced: during the performance of various tasks, EEG did not record any spike-and-wave discharges as long as the animal was motivated to obtain a reward. Spike-and-wave discharges reappeared as soon as the animal became inactive, either because the reward was withdrawn, or because the motivation to get it had vanished (Vergnes et al., 1991).

Relationship between spike-and-wave discharges and wakefulness

To analyse the relationship between spike-and-wave discharges and wakefulness, GAERS fitted with cortical, hippocampal and myographic electrodes were recorded during 12 h-periods. The number and duration of spike-and-wave discharges were determined during the various vigilance states. Sixty-six per cent of the spike-and-wave discharges started and then ended during wakefulness. During the periods preceding sleep, spike-and-wave discharges were more frequent and longer. They were seldom seen during active behaviour. Twenty per cent of the spike-and-wave discharges appeared during transition from wakefulness to slow-wave sleep, and 7 per cent during transition from slow-wave sleep to arousal. Less than 7 per cent started and ended in slow-wave sleep, and then usually during the first minute of a sleep episode. Spike-and-wave discharges were exceptional in paradoxical sleep (Lannes et al., 1988).

Ontogenic development of spike-and-wave discharges

In order to determine the developmental profile of spike-and-wave discharges, GAERS were recorded every week, during several months, since the age of 30 days. At 30 days, none of the animals had spike-and-wave discharges. At 40 days, 30 per cent were affected. The number of rats with spike-and-wave discharges then increased regularly with age and reached 100 per cent at 4 months. The first spike-and-wave discharges were rare (1 or 2/h) and short-lasting (1–3 s), with a low frequency (4–5 cps). With age, the number and duration of spike-and-wave discharges, and the frequency of spike-and-wave complexes, increased. The number of spike-and-wave discharges reached its maximum around the age of 6 months. Spike-and-wave discharges could be recorded over months, and never disappeared spontaneously (Vergnes et al., 1986).

GAERS: an isomorphic model of absence seizures

GAERS share many common characteristics with other genetic models in rodents (Noebels, Ch. 20; Hosford et al., Ch. 18; Chocholova, 1983; Van Luijtelaar & Coenen, 1986) and with typical absences in humans. Human absences are concomitant with unresponsiveness to environmental stimuli and cessation of activity. They start and end abruptly, and may be associated with mild clonic components. They may occur as frequently as several hundred times per day, mainly during quiet wakefulness, inattention, and in the transitions between sleep and waking; they are interrupted by attention and unexpected sensory stimulations (Jung, 1962; Guey et al., 1969; Loiseau, 1992). The behavioural symptomatology of GAERS during a spike-and-wave discharge is quite identical. Despite spike-and-wave discharges, the ability to perform spontaneous and learned behavioural activities is unimpaired in GAERS. Similarly, in childhood absence epilepsy, intelligence is considered to be normal (Loiseau, 1992).

The EEG pattern of the rat spike-and-wave discharges is similar to that observed in humans during absence seizures. However the frequency of spike-and-wave complexes during spike-and-wave discharges in humans and rats differs. The spike-and-wave frequency in human is classically 3 cps, whereas in GAERS the frequency varies from 7 to 11 cps. In fact, it is impossible to elicit spike-and-wave discharges at a frequency of 3 cps during absence seizures in rodents (MacQueen & Woodbury, 1975; Avoli, 1980). In penicillin-induced absences in cats, the mean frequency is 4.5 cps (Avoli & Gloor, Ch. 12). Only in primates can 3 cps spike-and-wave discharges be elicited during absences (Snead, 1978). The frequency of spike-and-wave discharges during generalized non-convulsive seizures seems to be dependent on species.

The second way in which absences in humans and rats differ is the age of onset. In humans, pure absence epilepsy is a disease of childhood which tends to disappear with adulthood (Loiseau, 1992). In rats, the spike-and-wave discharges appear after full maturation of cortical electrogenesis, by 4 to 5 weeks of age for spontaneous spike-and-wave discharges (Chocholova, 1983; Vergnes et al., 1986; Marescaux et al., 1992b), at 3 weeks for pentylenetetrazol-induced spike-and-wave discharges (Schickerova et al., 1984), and at 4 weeks for γ-hydroxybutyrate-induced spike-and-wave discharges (Snead, 1988). Spontaneous spike-and-wave discharges persist until death. Since the process and degree of maturation of the human and the rat brain differ profoundly, it is not surprising that the ontogenetic development of petit mal epilepsy is quite different in the two species.

Pharmacological characteristics of spike-and-wave discharges in GAERS

Antiepileptic drugs and epileptogenic drugs were tested for their effects on spike-and-wave discharges. Each experiment was performed on adult rats under EEG control. After the freely moving animals were adapted to the recording environment, a reference EEG was recorded for 20 min. The drug was then injected (usually intra-peritoneally) and the EEG recorded for three to six consecutive 20 min periods. The high number of spontaneous spike-and-wave discharges permit a clear evaluation of the kinetics of action of acutely administered drugs.

Antiepileptic drugs

ethosuximide, trimethadione, valproic acid and benzodiazepines suppressed spike-and-wave discharges in a dose-dependent manner. A mean efficacy exceeding 90 per cent was observed for ethosuximide 100 mg/kg, trimethadione 200 mg/kg, valproic acid 200 mg/kg and diazepam 2 mg/kg. Carbamazepine was ineffective at 10 mg/kg, whereas spike-and-wave discharges were aggravated at doses above 20 mg/kg. Phenytoin was ineffective at 10 to 40 mg/kg and increased spike-and-wave discharges at doses above 80 mg/kg. Phenobarbital evoked biphasic effects: it was effective at 2.5 to 10 mg/kg, but no more at 20 mg/kg (Marescaux et al., 1984).

New drugs were also tested. γ-Vinyl-GABA, tiagabine and gabapentin aggravated spike-and-wave discharges. Felbamate and progabide were ineffective. UCB Lo59, 2-en-valproate and partial agonists of benzodiazepine receptors suppressed spike-and-wave discharges (Marescaux et al., 1992a,b and unpublished results).

Epileptogenic drugs

The spike-and-wave discharges were increased by pentylenetetrazol (10–20 mg/kg); γ-hydroxybutyrate (250–500 mg/kg); THIP (4–12 mg/kg) and penicillin (1.25–2.5 × 10^6 iu/kg) (Marescaux et al., 1984, 1992b).

GAERS: a predictive model of absence seizures

The therapeutic profile of GAERS and of other genetic models in rodents are identical (Peeters et al., 1988; Marescaux et al., 1992b; Hosford et al., Ch. 18). Moreover, the pharmacological reactivity of genetic spike-and-wave discharges in rodents is similar to that of absence epilepsy in humans. In GAERS, spike-and-wave discharges are suppressed by the four main antiepileptics which are effective against human absences and worsened by the two drugs which are ineffective or aggravating in humans (Loiseau, 1992). The results obtained in GAERS with new potential antiepileptics are, up to now, predictive of their effects in human absences. Finally, spike-and-wave discharges in GAERS are increased by drugs that are commonly used to induce petit mal-like seizures (Marescaux et al., 1992b; Snead, Ch. 14).

Networks involved in the genesis of spike-and-wave discharges in GAERS

Mapping of spike-and-wave discharges

To determine which brain structures are involved in spike-and-wave discharges, chronic and acute EEG recordings were performed with cortical and depth electrodes (Fig. 2). The largest spike-and-wave discharges were recorded from the lateral frontoparietal cortex and the posterolateral thalamus. The cortical initiation of spike-and-wave discharges might vary from one discharge to another in the same rat. Usually spike-and-wave discharges appeared simultaneously all over the cortex. Sometimes they started over the frontoparietal areas, and very rarely over the occipital ones. In some rats, the beginning of the lateral thalamic spike-and-wave discharges occasionally preceded that of the cortical spike-and-wave discharges. Small-amplitude or delayed spike-and-wave discharges were present in the striatum, lateral hypothalamus and ventral tegmentum. Spike-and-wave discharges were absent or considerably reduced in the anterior and midline nuclei of the thalamus. No spike-and-wave discharges were recorded from the limbic structures: hippocampus, septum, amygdala, cingular and piriform cortex (Vergnes et al., 1987, 1990a,b; Marescaux et al., 1992b).

Effects of cortical and thalamic lesions

Cortical spreading depression

Cortical spreading depression was produced by a local injection of KCl through a permanently implanted cannula. The EEG was recorded bilaterally from the cortex and from lateral thalamic areas. To avoid propagation of the spike-and-wave discharges from one hemisphere to the other, the corpus callosum and the medial thalamus had been previously transected (see below). In GAERS, unilateral injection of KCl into the superficial layers of the cortex immediately suppressed cortical and thalamic spike-and-wave discharges for several minutes. However, the ipsilateral thalamus had an apparently normal EEG. The injected cortex recovered progressively. After normalization of the background cortical EEG, the first spike-and-wave discharges was recorded 30 to 50 min after the KCl injection, simultaneously in the cortex and the thalamus, on the injected side. Contralaterally the EEG and spike-and-wave discharges were unchanged, in the cortex and in the thalamus, throughout the experiment (Vergnes & Marescaux, 1992).

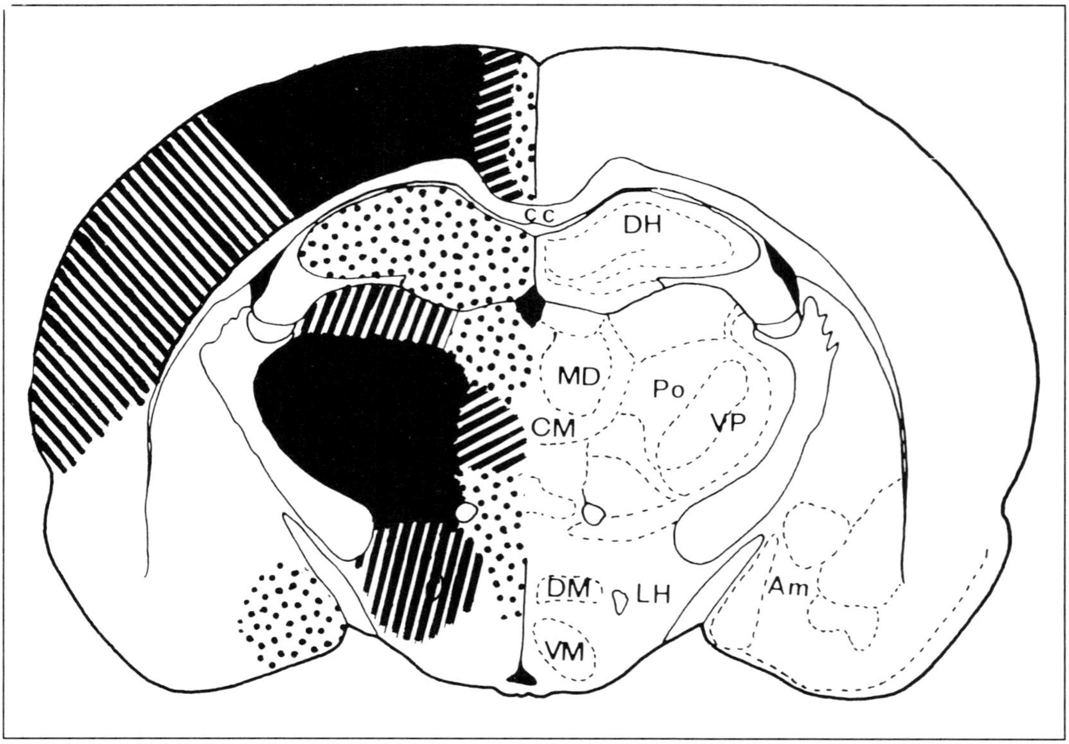

Fig. 2. Schematic mapping of spike-and-wave discharges on a coronal section of a rat brain (according to the Atlas of Paxinos & Watson, 1982). Am, amygdala; DH, dorsal hippocampus; LH, lateral hypothalamus; DM, dorsomedial nucleus of the hypothalamus; VM, ventromedial nucleus of the hypothalamus; CM, centromedial; MD, mediodorsal; Po, posterior; VP, ventroposterior nucleus of the thalamus. Black areas, sustained and large spike-and-wave discharges; stripes, small and irregular spike-and-wave discharges; dots, no spike-and-wave discharges recorded.

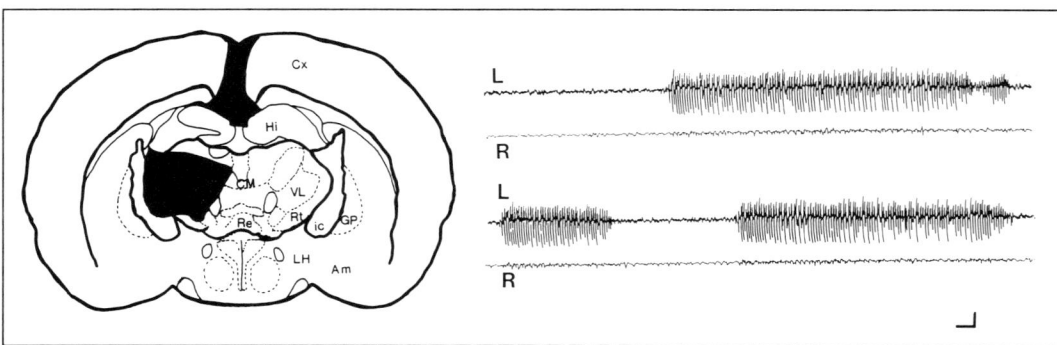

Fig. 3. Left panel: coronal section showing a unilateral lesion of the right lateral thalamus, with a transection of the corpus callosum. Am, amygdala; CM, central medial; Cx, cortex; GP, globus pallidus; Hi, hippocampus; Ic, internal capsule; LH, lateral hypothalamus; Re, reuniens n; Rt, reticular n; VL, ventrolateral n (according to the Atlas of Paxinos & Watson, 1982).
Right panel: EEG recordings in the same rat. Spike-and-wave discharges are suppressed on the cortex ipsilateral to the thalamic lesion. L, left cortex; R, right cortex. Calibration 1 s, 200 μV.

Thalamic lesions

Electrolytic lesions were made at various sites in the thalamus. Bilateral lesions of the anterior thalamus, of the ventromedial thalamus and of the medial thalamus did not affect spike-and-wave discharges which appeared bilateral and synchronous (Vergnes & Marescaux, 1992).

Large bilateral lesions of the lateral thalamus suppressed spike-and-wave discharges. However animals lost weight and usually died after one to three weeks. For this reason, the lateral thalamus was lesioned unilaterally in GAERS, with a prior transection of the corpus callosum (see below). In this latter preparation, no spike-and-wave discharges was recorded from the cortex ipsilateral to the thalamic lesion, which had a slow baseline EEG (Fig. 3). On the unlesioned side, the cortical EEG was normal with many spike-and-wave discharges. In these animals, THIP, γ-hydroxybutyrate and pentylenetetrazol consistently produced a significant increase of spike-and-wave discharges on the unlesioned side; however, no spike-and-wave discharges ever occurred in the cortex ipsilateral to the thalamic lesion (Vergnes et al., 1990b; Vergnes & Marescaux, 1992).

After the reticular nucleus was lesioned by the excitotoxic agent ibotenic acid, spike-and-wave discharges were completely suppressed on the ipsilateral hemisphere during the first 3 days. From the fourth day, low frequency (3–5 cps) sharp waves appeared on the lesioned side and persisted throughout the observation period (Avanzini et al., 1993).

Thalamo-cortical mechanisms in absence seizures

In GAERS, EEG recordings from various brain regions suggest that the frontoparietal cortex and the relay nuclei of the lateral thalamus play a predominant role in the development of spike-and-wave discharges. Discharges involving the cortex and the thalamus are also observed in other strains of rats with spontaneous spike-and-wave discharges (Klingberg & Pickenhain, 1968; Chocholova, 1983; Semba & Komisaruk, 1984; Buzsaki et al. 1990), and in generalized absences induced by penicillin in the cat (Avoli & Gloor, Ch. 12). In humans, spike-and-wave discharges are similarly recorded over the cortex and in the thalamus (Williams, 1953). In some rodent models of absence seizures, spike-and-wave discharges are recorded from the dorsal hippocampus (Noebels, 1984; Fariello & Golden, 1987). In our experiments, as well as in others (Marescaux et al., 1992b; Snead, Ch. 14), no spike-and-wave discharges were recorded with a bipolar electrode located within the hippocampus or any limbic structure. Differences between strains, or artifacts due to monopolar recording in small animals may account for this discrepancy.

When a functional cortical lesion is produced in GAERS by a spreading depression, the spike-and-wave discharges are transiently suppressed not only in the injected cortex, but also in the ipsilateral thalamus. Only after full recovery of the cortical activity does the spike-and-wave discharge reappear simultaneously in the ipsilateral thalamus and cortex. These data demonstrate that spike-and-wave discharges cannot occur in an 'isolated' thalamus. In cats, penicillin-induced thalamic spike-and-wave discharges are also suppressed by cortical spreading depression (Gloor & Fariello, 1988; Avoli & Gloor, Ch. 12). Reciprocally, the cortical spike-and-wave discharges are definitely suppressed in GAERS after extensive lesioning of the lateral thalamus, including the relay and the reticular nuclei. Drugs which induce spike-and-wave discharges in non-epileptic rats and potentiate spike-and-wave discharges in GAERS never produce spike-and-wave discharges on the lesioned side, whereas the spike-and-wave discharges on the unlesioned side are markedly increased. These results clearly show that spike-and-wave discharges cannot develop from a cortex deprived of its thalamic afferents. On the contrary, none of the anterior, ventromedial or midline nuclei of the thalamus appear necessary to the occurrence of spike-and-wave discharges in GAERS; however in the cat, spike-and-wave discharges may be elicited by electrical stimulation of the intralaminar and medial nuclei (Hunter & Jasper, 1949). Similar results were obtained in different models of bilateral spike-and-wave discharges. Buzsaki et al. (1988) showed that lesions of the nucleus reticularis suppress cortical high-voltage spike-and-wave discharges in old rats. Pentylenetetrazol-induced cortical spike-and-wave discharges in rats are also abolished by blocking thalamic activity by spreading depression (Pohl & Mares, 1983). In the model of generalized penicillin epilepsy in the cat, large lesions of the lateral thalamus abolish cortical spike-and-wave discharges, whereas lesions of the anterior nuclei, the massa intermedia or the ventromedial thalamus are ineffective (Gloor & Fariello, 1988; Avoli & Gloor, Ch. 12).

Thus, the thalamic relay nuclei are necessary for spike-and-wave discharges to occur. These nuclei are characterized by their reciprocal connectivity with the cortex: from every cortical area, cortico-thalamic connections return to the thalamic nuclei providing input to that same cortical area (Jones, 1985). This organization in a closed loop may furnish the substrate allowing an oscillatory activity, which can be amplified and expressed as spike-and-wave discharges. The cortico-thalamic fibres give collaterals to the reticular nucleus, which, in turn projects GABAergic efferents on most of the thalamic neurons, thus modulating their activity and possibly controlling their ability to discharge with rhythmic bursts (Steriade & Deschenes, 1984). The function of the thalamic reticular nucleus in the control of spike-and-wave discharges has to be further investigated.

These results demonstrate that the cortex and the thalamus are both intimately involved in the genesis of spike-and-wave discharges in GAERS. Whether the generation of spike-and-wave discharges is the result of an excessive cortical excitability, as was proposed in feline generalized penicillin epilepsy (Avoli & Gloor, Ch. 12), or of an excessive thalamic synchronization, possibly under the control of inhibitory GABAergic mechanisms (Crunelli *et al.*, Ch. 19), remains debatable.

The thalamo-cortical loop is under the control of several inhibitory or excitatory systems. Absence seizures can be suppressed by 'remote' endogenous circuits involving several brain structures, such as the pars reticulata of substantia nigra (Depaulis, Ch. 42), and dopaminergic, noradrenergic and cholinergic pathways (see below).

Bilateralization and synchronization of spike-and-wave discharges in GAERS: role of callosal and thalamic pathways

In unlesioned GAERS, the spike-and-wave discharges are always bilateral and synchronous. The corpus callosum is the major interhemispheric commissure, connecting preferentially homotopic cortical areas (Innocenti, 1986), and it is the most likely pathway underlying bilateral spread and synchronization of cortical paroxystic activities and especially of spike-and-wave discharges. However subcortical pathways, such as intrathalamic connections, may contribute to bilateral synchronization of the thalamo-cortical spike-and-wave discharges. In order to examine these questions, three kinds of lesions were performed in GAERS: section of the corpus callosum alone; section of both the corpus callosum and the midline thalamus; and lesion of the midline thalamus alone (Vergnes *et al.*, 1989, 1990b, 1992; Marescaux *et al.*, 1992b).

The corpus callosum was transected through a midline slit in the skull with a surgical blade fixed in a stereotaxic holder and moved anteriorily along the midline of the brain from 2 to 12 mm anterior, and 4 to 4.5 mm ventral to the lambda. The midline thalamus was sectioned in addition to the corpus callosum by lowering the blade 7 mm ventral to the lambda from 4.5 to 7 mm anterior to the lambda. Lesions of the midline thalamic nuclei alone were performed electrolytically by a 2 mA current applied at different sites for 15 s (AP = 4–7 mm; DV = 6–7mm). Electrodes were implanted bilaterally over the frontoparietal cortex for EEG control. The animals recovered rapidly and survived without any apparent deficit. EEG was recorded repeatedly for several weeks in freely moving animals. Bilateral synchronization was appreciated visually on EEG and confirmed on oscilloscope.

After transection of the corpus callosum, the bilateral synchronism was abolished and three patterns emerged: (a) the spike-and-wave discharges occurred unilaterally and independently on each hemisphere, and sometimes alternated from one side to the other (50 per cent of the spike-and-wave discharges); (b) spike-and-wave discharges started on one side and then continued bilaterally after delays varying from 0.5 to several seconds (40 per cent of the spike-and-wave discharges); (c) some

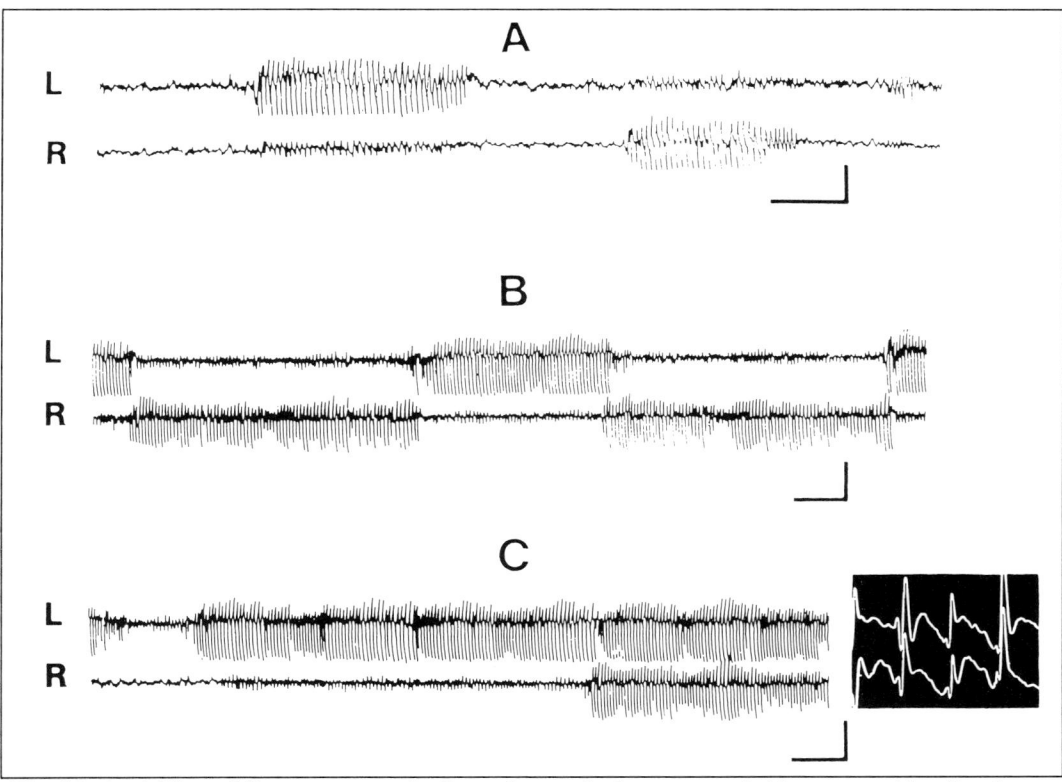

Fig. 4 (a, b, c). Three different patterns of spike-and-wave discharges recorded in one rat with callosal transection. When they are bilateral, each single spike-and-wave complex occurs synchronously on both sides (C, see oscilloscopic recording). Calibrations 400 µV, 2 s.

bilateral synchronous spike-and-wave discharges still occurred in most animals (10 per cent of the spike-and-wave discharges). When the spike-and-wave discharges were present bilaterally, each single spike-and-wave complex was synchronous on both hemispheres (Fig. 4). Lesion of the midline thalamic nuclei alone separating the thalamus in two lateral parts did not affect spike-and-wave discharges. They occurred in the same amount as in intact animals and synchronously on both hemispheres (Fig. 5a). However, when the transection of the corpus callosum was associated with a midline cut through the thalamus, the interhemispheric desynchronization was more complete: during a bilateral spike-and-wave discharge, the single spike-and-wave complexes occurred independently on each hemisphere. In spite of the desynchronization of spike-and-wave discharges, the total amount of seizures, measured on both hemispheres, was comparable to the values found in intact rats (Fig. 5b).

In other animal models with bilateral and synchronous spike-and-wave discharges, the corpus callosum appears to be the main structure ensuring bilateral synchronization. Section of the corpus callosum in rats, cats or primates abolished bilateral synchronization of discharges induced by epileptogenic substances (Marcus et al., 1969; Musgrave & Gloor, 1980), or by intermittent light stimulation (Naquet et al., 1975). Taken together, all these data show that initiation of thalamo-cortical spike-and-wave discharges in absence seizures may occur independently in both hemispheres. The corpus callosum is the major pathway involved in bilateralization of spontaneous spike-and-wave discharges in GAERS. However the transection of the corpus callosum does not totally

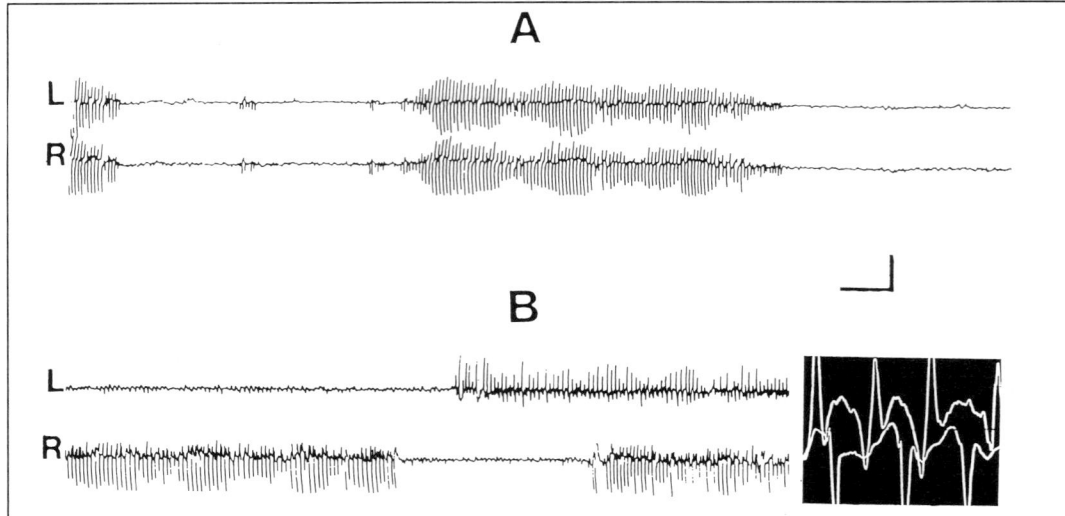

Fig. 5 (a) Spike-and-wave discharges recorded in a rat with medial thalamic lesions: spike-and-wave discharges are bilateral and synchronous; (b) spike-and-wave discharges recorded in a rat with both corpus callosum and medial thalamus sections. Spike-and-wave discharges are completely desynchronized: when bilateral spike-and-wave discharges occur, each spike-and-wave complex appears independently on each side (see oscilloscopic recording). Calibrations 400 µV, 2 s.

abolish bilateral synchronism of the spike-and-wave discharges, suggesting that additional pathways are also involved. According to our results, the midline thalamus is likely to fulfil this role: full interhemispheric dissociation of spike-and-wave discharges is only achieved when the midline thalamus is sectioned in addition to the corpus callosum. However the midline thalamus plays a minor role in bilateral transfer, as isolated destruction of this area does not affect occurrence of bilateral and synchronous spike-and-wave discharges.

Neurotransmitters involved in the genesis and/or control of spike-and-wave discharges

Noradrenaline, dopamine, serotonin and acetylcholine

Drugs that decrease α-noradrenaline or dopamine transmission, increased spike-and-wave discharges. Conversely, potentiation of dopamine or α-noradrenaline transmission decreased spike-and-wave discharges. However, these discharges were never induced in rats from the control strain by antagonists of α-noradrenaline or dopamine receptors. Similarly, bilateral lesions of the locus coeruleus (noradrenaline neurons), or of the substantia nigra (dopamine neurons) which transiently aggravated spontaneous spike-and-wave discharges in GAERS, never induced spike-and-wave discharges in control rats. β-Noradrenaline agonists or antagonists were ineffective. Thus, catecholamines are involved in the control of spike-and-wave discharges but not in their genesis (Marescaux et al., 1992a,b).

Drugs interacting with serotonin neurotansmission, or lesion of serotoninergic neurons of the nucleus raphae magnus did not modify spike-and-wave discharges (Marescaux et al., 1992a,b).

Drugs which potentiate acetylcholine transmission, as well as acetylcholine antagonists, suppressed spike-and-wave discharges. Lesions of the cholinergic neurons of the nucleus basalis reduced spike-and-wave discharges. These data suggest that cholinergic activity accounts for the preferential occurrence of absence seizures in states of reduced arousal and for their disappearance during sleep or active behaviour (Danober et al., 1993, 1994).

Glutamate

Intraperitoneal (i.p.) or intracerebroventicular (i.c.v.) administration of low doses of NMDA decreased spike-and-wave discharges in GAERS. At high doses, NMDA produced convulsions within a few minutes, but never aggravated spike-and-wave discharges. NMDA did not induce spike-and-wave discharges in control non-epileptic rats (Marescaux et al., 1992a,b). Competitive and non-competitive antagonists of NMDA, as well as antagonists of the glycine site, suppressed spike-and-wave discharges. Major behavioural and EEG side-effects were induced by these drugs: continuous sniffing up and down, horizontal movements of the head, rotations, ataxia associated with slow and paroxysmal high-amplitude waves on the EEG (Marescaux et al., 1992a,b).

Thus, NMDA receptors are implicated in the control of absences in GAERS. The thalamo-cortical and cortico-thalamic pathways underlying spike-and-wave discharges involve glutamatergic synapses. Their dysregulation at NMDA-receptor sites by NMDA agonists or antagonists may interrupt the thalamo-cortical loop. Moreover, NMDA antagonists and NMDA itself provoke motor activation and increased arousal respectively, states that are incompatible with the appearance of spike-and-wave discharges.

GABA

The effects of GABA are mediated by $GABA_A$ (GABA/benzodiazepine complex) and $GABA_B$ receptors, which differ in terms of pharmacological profile, mechanism of action and regional distributions.

$GABA_A$ receptors

In GAERS, activation of the $GABA_A$ receptors (administration of $GABA_A$ agonists, GABA transaminase inhibitors, or GABA reuptake inhibitors) induced a dose-dependent increase in the duration of spike-and-wave discharges, whether the drugs are administered systematically or into the relay nuclei of the thalamus (Liu et al., 1991; Marescaux et al., 1992a,b). At high doses, GABA-mimetics induced permanent spike-and-wave discharges with a reduced frequency (5–6 cps) or isolated spikes on a flat background. No doses of $GABA_A$ antagonists picrotoxin or bicucullin ever exerted a significant effect on the spike-and-wave discharges; at high doses, convulsive seizures appeared (Marescaux et al., 1992a,b). GABA-mimetics aggravate the seizures in all models of generalized non-convulsive epilepsy in rodents, as well as in cats (Fariello et al., 1980; Marescaux et al., 1992b). They also aggravate the bilateral spike-and-wave discharges induced by light flashes in the baboon, *Papio papio* (Meldrum & Horton, 1980). Moreover, administration of GABA-mimetics in non-epileptic animals induces bilateral spike-and-wave discharges that resemble generalized non-convulsive seizures (Fariello & Golden, 1987; Marescaux et al., 1992a).

These results suggest that an increased $GABA_A$ neuromediation may be involved in the genesis of spontaneous spike-and-wave discharges. However, $GABA_A$ antagonists are unable to suppress spike-and-wave discharges and no difference in $GABA_A$ receptors have been found between GAERS and rats from the control strain (Snead et al., 1992).

$GABA_B$ receptors

In order to study the role of $GABA_B$ transmission in absence seizures, systemic and intrathalamic administration were performed in GAERS using Baclofen, an agonist, and CGP 35 348, an antagonist of $GABA_B$ receptors. Baclofen injected i.p. increased spike-and-wave discharges in GAERS; it also induced paroxysmal oscillatory activity which resemble spike-and-wave discharges in control rats free of spontaneous spike-and-wave discharges. By contrast, i.p. or p.o. administration of CGP 35 348 suppressed spike-and-wave discharges in GAERS without apparent side effects. $GABA_B$ antagonists also suppressed spike-and-wave discharges induced in non-epileptic rats by γ-hydroxybutyrate or pentylenetetrazol (Marescaux et al., 1992c). Similar results were obtained after intrathalamic micro-injections of $GABA_B$ agonists and antagonists. R-Baclofen injected into the specific relay nuclei or the reticular nucleus of the thalamus increased duration of spike-and-wave discharges in GAERS and elicited rhythmic oscillations on the cortical EEG in non-epileptic control rats. Intrathalamic injections of CGP 35 348 into the same nuclei suppressed spontaneous spike-and-wave discharges (Liu *et al.*, 1992).

These results demonstrate the involvement of $GABA_B$-mediated neurotransmission in the development of spike-and-wave discharges in generalized non-convulsive epilepsy. $GABA_B$ receptors within the thalamus were shown to participate in an oscillatory activity which most probably underlies the rhythmic spike-and-wave discharges recorded during absence seizures. The capacity of thalamic neurons to generate repeated bursts of action potentials is related to the occurrence of rhythmic low-threshold calcium currents, which are de-inactivated when the cell membrane is hyperpolarized. Low-threshold calcium currents were shown to underlie episodes of sleep spindles, and possibly also of spike-and-wave discharges. $GABA_B$ receptor activation mediates a late and long-lasting inhibitory post-synaptic potential (IPSP), which produces the hyperpolarization necessary to elicit these low-threshold calcium currents (for review, see Crunelli *et al.*, Ch. 19).

The aggravating effect obtained by micro-injections of $GABA_B$ agonists into the relay nuclei, as well as the suppression of spike-and-wave discharges induced by administration of $GABA_B$ antagonists into the same sites are in agreement with these cellular mechanisms and suggest that the $GABA_B$-mediated late inhibitory post-synaptic potential in thalamic neurons is critical for the development of spike-and-wave discharges. However, the density and affinity of $GABA_B$ receptors is similar in GAERS and in control non-epileptic rats (Mathivet *et al.*, Ch. 17). The absence of abnormality in these characteristics does not exclude the possibility that the coupling of these receptors to the second messenger is modified in GAERS.

Genetic transmission of spike-and-wave discharges in GAERS

In our initial colony of Wistar rats, 30 per cent of the animals showed spontaneous spike-and-wave discharges. Inbreeding of selected parents over a few generations produced a strain in which 100 per cent of the rats were affected. Similarly, we selected a control strain apparently free of spike-

Table 1. *Genetic transmission of spike-and-wave discharges in GAERS, controls and F_1*

	Crossing	Age (months)	SWD duration (s per min)				
			0 non-affected	< 5	5–10	10–15	> 15
	Controls × Controls	4	177/177 (100%)	–	–	–	–
		12	134/143 (94%)	9/143 (6%)	–	–	–
		30	16/19 (84%)	1/19 (5%)	2/19 (11%)	–	–
	GAERS × GAERS	4	–	1/62 (2%)	9/62 (15%)	15/62 (24%)	37/62 (60%)
		12	–	–	1/55 (2%)	7/55 (13%)	47/55 (85%)
F_1	Controls × GAERS	4	31/82 (38%)	29/82 (35%)	10/82 (12%)	7/82 (9%)	5/82 (6%)
		12	3/82 (4%)	13/82 (16%)	27/82 (33%)	13/82 (16%)	26/82 (32%)

Number (and percentage) of offsprings from different kinds of crossing showing spike-and-wave discharges at different ages. Non-affected rats: 0 s of spike-and-wave discharges per minute. Affected rats are classified in four groups according to the mean duration of spike-and-wave discharges per minute of EEG recording.

and-wave discharges. These data demonstrated that spike-and-wave discharges were genetically controlled.

We analysed the mode of inheritance of spike-and-wave discharges in GAERS by performing a classical Mendelian cross-breeding study. Six-hundred and fifty-one offspring from different kinds of crossing were used. At 4 months of age, the rats were fitted with standard EEG electrodes. EEG's were recorded for 40 min every month, between 4 and 12 months (579 rats were still alive and recorded at 12 months). When it was possible, rats from the control non-epileptic strain were recorded until the age of 30 months. For each rat, the mean duration of spike-and-wave discharges per minute was measured during each 40-min recording. Results are summarized in Tables 1, 2 and 3.

Table 2. Genetic transmission of spike-and-wave discharges in F_2

	Age (months)	SWD duration (s per min)				
		0 non-affected	< 5	5–10	10–15	> 15
All F1 × All F1	4	100/226 (44%)	78/226 (35%)	19/226 (8%)	20/226 (9%)	9/226 (4%)
	12	9/196 (5%)	44/196 (22%)	64/196 (33%)	25/196 (13%)	54/196 (28%)
Low SWD F1 × Low SWD F1	4	17/19 (89%)	2/19 (11%)	–	–	–
	12	3/18 (17%)	11/18 (61%)	2/18 (11%)	2/18 (11%)	–
High SWD F1 × High SWD F1	4	4/31 (13%)	8/31 (26%)	4/31 (13%)	6/31 (19%)	9/31 (29%)
	12	–	1/29 (3%)	3/29 (10%)	7/29 (24%)	18/29 (62%)

Symbols and conventions as in Table 1. Low-spike-and-wave discharge F1 display less than 5 s spike-and-wave discharges per minute. High-spike-and-wave discharge F1 display more than 15 s spike-and-wave discharges per minute.

Table 3. Genetic transmission of spike-and-wave discharges in back-crosses

	Age (months)	SWD duration (s per min)				
		0 non-affected	< 5	5–10	10–15	> 15
All F1 × Controls	4	85/104 (82%)	15/104 (14%)	1/104 (1%)	2/104 (2%)	1/104 (1%)
	12	36/103 (35%)	39/103 (38%)	13/103 (13%)	6/103 (6%)	9/103 (9%)
Low-SWD F1 × Controls	4	23/23 (100%)	–	–	–	–
	12	12/23 (52%)	7/23 (30%)	2/23 (9%)	2/23 (9%)	–
High-SWD F1 × Controls	4	13/23 (56%)	7/23 (30%)	–	2/23 (9%)	1/23 (4%)
	12	3/22 (14%)	7/22 (32%)	3/22 (14%)	2/22 (9%)	7/22 (32%)

Symbols and conventions as in Tables 1 and 2.

Inheritance of spike-and-wave discharges in GAERS

One-hundred and seventy-seven offspring of parents from the 10th to the 19th generation of the control non-epileptic strain were recorded. All had a normal EEG, without spike-and-wave discharges, up to 8 months. At 12 months, 6 per cent (nine of the 143 remaining rats) and at 30 months, 16 per cent (three of the 19 remaining rats) showed short (<5 s/min), low-amplitude, irregular discharges.

All 62 offspring of parents from the 14th to the 21st generation of the GAERS strain displayed spike-and-wave discharges on the first EEG at 4 months. At 12 months, the mean duration of the high-amplitude regular spike-and-wave discharges was between 15 and 30 s/min.

Sixty-two per cent (51 of 82) of F_1 offspring from control × GAERS reciprocal crosses showed spike-and-wave discharges at 4 months, and 96 per cent (79 of 82) at 12 months. Crossing of male or female GAERS with controls produced a similar distribution of spike-and-wave discharges among F_1 offspring. Male and female F_1 were identically affected. Inter-individual variability of spike-and-wave discharges was extremely high for age of appearance (between 4 and 12 months) and duration (between 1 and 25 s/min).

Two-hundred and twenty-six F_2 offspring were obtained from F1 × F1 crosses. Spike-and-wave discharges were recorded in 56 per cent (126 of 226) of F_2 offsprings at 4 months and in 95 per cent (187 of 196) at 12 months. As in F_1, inter-individual variability for age of onset and duration was high. The characteristics of spike-and-wave discharges in F_2 offspring were correlated to that of F_1 parents. F_2 were obtained by crossing low-seizing F_1 (spike-and-wave discharges < 5 s/min), and high-seizing ones (spike-and-wave discharges > 15 sec/min). At 12 months, 83 per cent (15 of 18) of F_2 from low-spike-and-wave discharges F_1 had spike-and-wave discharges (mean discharge duration in affected rats: 3.5 s/min), and 100 per cent (29 of 29) of F_2 from high-spike-and-wave discharges F_1 (mean discharge duration: 19 s/min).

F_1 were back-crossed with control rats from the non-epileptic strain. Nineteen of their 104 offsprings (18 per cent) showed spike-and-wave discharges at 4 months, and 67 of 103 (65 per cent) at 12 months. As for F_2, duration and age of onset of spike-and-wave discharges in back-crosses were correlated to that of the F_1 parent. At 12 months, 48 per cent (11 of 23) back-crosses from low-spike-and-wave discharges F_1 had spike-and-wave discharges (mean discharge duration in affected rats: 5 s/min), and 86 per cent (19 of 22) back-crosses from high-spike-and-wave discharges F_1 (mean discharge duration in affected rats: 12 s/min).

Genetic heterogeneity of spike-and-wave discharges in rodents

Our results confirm that all GAERS showed spike-and-wave discharges in their EEG and that none of the control rats did so before 12 months of age. However, in the control non-epileptic strain, up to 16 per cent of old rats displayed short spike-and-wave discharges. These observations, which demonstrate that the breeding of a pure non-epileptic control strain is uneasy, are in agreement with data from the literature reporting that spike-and-wave discharges may be recorded in 10 to 90 per cent of rats in almost all laboratory colonies. The 96 per cent spike-and-wave discharge rats in the F1 generation suggest that there is a dominant transmission. Similar spike-and-wave discharges in males and females in the F1 generation indicate that the transmission is autosomal.

The high variability for duration and age of onset in F_1, F_2 and back-crosses suggests that the inheritance of spike-and-wave discharges is probably not due to a single gene locus. Moreover, at 12 months, 95 per cent and 65 per cent of the rats showed spike-and-wave discharges in the F_2 and back-cross generations respectively. These scores are higher than one would expect if the occurrence was determined by one gene only. The fact that the control strain is not completely devoid of spike-and-wave discharges may also contribute to the over-representation of the spike-and-wave discharge phenotype in F_2 and back-crosses. Data obtained with F2 and back-crosses from low- and high-spike-and-wave discharges F_1 suggest that the mode of transmission can be differentiated according to the severity (duration and age of onset) of spike-and-wave discharges. The high variability of spike-and-wave discharge duration in F_1 is not related to a variable penetrance. 'Short' and 'long' spike-and-wave discharges in F_1 are genetically determined and are inherited by F_2 and back-crosses. 'Short' spike-and-wave discharges appear to depend on a single autosomal dominant gene, whereas 'long' spike-and-wave discharges may depend on one or several additional genes.

Similar data have been obtained in WAG/Rij rats. Their spike-and-wave discharges are apparently controlled by several genes: one dominant gene determines the occurrence of spike-and-wave discharges, while other genes modulate their number and duration (Peeters et al., 1990). However, the inheritance of spike-and-wave discharges in rodents may vary from one strain to another. Spike-and-wave discharges are transmitted in a recessive way in mice, moreover, they may result from several different mutations that provoke the same phenotype (Qiao & Noebels, 1991; Noebels, 1984, Ch. 20).

The cause of human absence epilepsies is regarded as genetic. In monozygotic twins, concordance rates of 84 per cent for EEG discharges, and of 75 per cent for absence seizures were found, while dizygotic twins showed no concordance (Lennox & Lennox, 1960). The high incidence of the presence of 3 cps spike-and-waves in first-degree relatives best fits an irregular autosomal dominant mode of inheritance, the gene having its highest penetrance in childhood and early adolescence (Gloor et al., 1982). Alternatively, several genetic factors have been suggested as being responsible for petit mal epilepsy (Doose et al., 1973).

Conclusion

Absence epilepsy remains one of the most enigmatic of neurological disorders and there is no widely accepted theory of its aetiology. No structural lesion of any kind – anatomical or biochemical – has ever been identified as its substrate (Berkovic et al., 1987; Gloor & Fariello, 1988). Its cause is increasingly regarded as genetic. It seems to be provoked by an abnormal oscillatory pattern of discharges that involve a thalamo-cortical loop. These thalamo-cortical circuits may normally sustain the physiological spindles. The study of absence epilepsy is dependent upon use of models, as ethical considerations rule out use of the neuroscientist's modern tools in intact children brains.

Many species of animals develop spontaneous absence seizures. We have selected a strain of rats (Genetic Absence Epilepsy Rats from Strasbourg, GAERS), in which 100 per cent of the animals present recurrent generalized non-convulsive seizures characterized by bilateral and synchronous spike-and-wave discharges accompanied with behavioural arrest, staring and sometimes twitching of the vibrissae. Spontaneous spike-and-wave discharges (7–11 cps, 300–1000 µV, 0.5–75 s) start and end abruptly on a normal background EEG. They usually occur at a mean frequency of 1.3 per min when the animals are in a state of quiet wakefulness. Drugs effective against absence seizures in humans (ethosuximide, trimethadione, valproate, benzodiazepines) suppress the spike-and-wave discharges dose-dependently, whereas drugs specific for convulsive or focal seizures (carbamazepine, phenytoin) are ineffective. Spike-and-wave discharges are increased by epileptogenic drugs inducing petit mal-like seizures, such as pentylenetetrazol, γ-hydroxybutyrate, THIP and penicillin.

Cortical and depth EEG recordings and lesion experiments show that spike-and-wave discharges in GAERS depend on cortical and thalamic structures with a possible rhythmic triggering by the lateral thalamus. This thalamo-cortical loop is under the inhibitory control of several 'remote' endogenous circuits. Most neurotransmitters are involved in the control of spike-and-wave discharges (dopamine, noradrenaline, NMDA, acetylcholine), but GABA seems to play a critical role. Spike-and-wave discharges are genetically determined with an autosomal dominant inheritance. The variable expression of spike-and-wave discharges in offsprings from GAERS and control reciprocal crosses may be due to the existence of multiple genes.

Neurophysiological, behavioural, pharmacological and genetic studies demonstrate that spontaneous spike-and-wave discharges in GAERS fulfil all the requirements for an experimental model of absence epilepsy. The analysis of the genetic thalamo-cortical dysfunction in GAERS may be fruitful in investigations of the pathogenesis of generalized non-convulsive seizures.

Acknowledgements

Special thanks are given to A. Boehrer for excellent technical assistance.

References

Avanzini, G., Vergnes, M., Spreafico, R. & Marescaux, C. (1993): Calcium-dependent regulation of genetically determined spike and waves by the reticular thalamic nucleus of rats. *Epilepsia* **34**, 1–7.

Avoli, M. (1980): Electroencephalographic and pathophysiologic features of rat parenteral penicillin epilepsy. *Exp. Neuropharmacol.* **69**, 373–382.

Avoli, M. & Gloor, P. (1994): Physiopathogenesis of feline generalized penicillin epilepsy: the role of thalamocortical mechanisms. In: *Idiopathic generalized epilepsies: clinical, experimental and genetic aspects*, eds. A. Malafosse, P. Genton, E. Hirsch, C. Marescaux, D. Broglin & R. Bernasconi, pp. 111–121. London: John Libbey.

Berkovic, S.F., Andermann, F., Andermann, E. & Gloor, P. (1987): Concepts of absence epilepsies: discrete syndrome or biological continuum? *Neurology* **37**, 993–1000.

Buzsaki, G., Bickford, R.G., Ponomareff, G., Thal, L.J., Mandel, R.J. & Gage, F.H. (1988): Nucleus basalis and thalamic control of neocortical activity in the freely moving rat. *J. Neurosci.* **8**, 4007–4026.

Buzsaki, G., Smith, A., Berger, S., Fisher, L.J. & Gage, F.H. (1990): Petit mal epilepsy and parkinsonian tremor: hypothesis of a common pacemaker. *Neuroscience* **36**, 1–14.

Chocholova, L. (1983): Incidence and development of rhythmic episodic activity in the electroencephalogram of a large rat population under chronic conditions. *Physiol. Bohemoslov.* **32**, 10–18.

Crunelli, V., Turner, J.P., Williams, S.R., Guyon, A. & Leresche, N. (1994): Potential role of intrinsic and $GABA_B$ IPSP-mediated oscillations of thalamic neurones in absence epilepsy. In: *Idiopathic generalized epilepsies: clinical, experimental and genetic aspects*, eds. A. Malafosse, P. Genton, E. Hirsch, C. Marescaux, D. Broglin & R. Bernasconi, pp. 201–213. London: John Libbey.

Danober, L., Depaulis, A., Marescaux, C. & Vergnes, M. (1993): Effects of cholinergic drugs on genetic absence seizures in rats. *Eur. J. Pharmacol.* **234**, 263–268.

Danober, L., Vergnes, M., Depaulis, A. & Marescaux, C. (1994): Nucleus basalis lesions suppress spike and wave discharges in rats with spontaneous absence-epilepsy. *Neuroscience* **59**, 531–539.

Depaulis, A. (1994): Relevance of the nigral control of seizures in the treatment of generalized epilepsies. In: *Idiopathic generalized epilepsies: clinical, experimental and genetic aspects*, eds. A. Malafosse, P. Genton, E. Hirsch, C. Marescaux, D. Broglin & R. Bernasconi, pp. 497–510. London: John Libbey.

Doose, H., Gerken, H., Horstmann, T. & Völzke, E. (1973): Genetic factors in spike-and-wave absences. *Epilepsia* **14**, 57–75.

Fariello, R.G. & Golden, G.T. (1987): The THIP-induced model of bilateral synchronous spike and wave in rodents. *Neuropharmacology* **26**, 161–165.

Fariello, R.G., Golden, G.T. & Black, J.A. (1980): Potentiation of a feline model of corticoreticular epilepsy by systematically administered inhibitory amino acids. In: *Advances in epileptology*, XIth Epilepsy International Symposium, eds. R. Canger, F. Angeleri & J.K. Penry, pp. 339–342. New York: Raven Press.

Gloor, P., Metrakos, J., Metrakos, K., Andermann, E. & Van Gelder, N. (1982): Neurophysiological, genetic and biochemical nature of the epileptic diathesis. In: *Henri Gastaut and the Marseille School's contribution to the neurosciences*, ed. R.J. Broughton, pp. 45–56, EEG suppl. 35. Amsterdam: Elsevier Biomedical Press.

Gloor, P. & Fariello, R.G. (1988): Generalized epilepsy: Some of its cellular mechanisms differ from those of focal epilepsy. *TINS* **11**, 63–68.

Guey, J., Bureau, M., Dravet, C. & Roger, J. (1979): A study of the rhythm of petit mal absences in children in relation to prevailing situations. The use of EEG telemetry during psychological examinations, school exercices and periods of inactivity. *Epilepsia* **10**, 441–451.

Hosford, D.A., Lin, F., Cao, Z., Kraemer, D.L., Huin, A., Akawie, E., Yin, Y. & Wilson, J.T. (1994): The role of GABA$_B$ receptor activation in the lethargic (*lh/lh*) mouse model of primary generalized absence seizures. In: *Idiopathic generalized epilepsies: clinical, experimental and genetic aspects*, eds. A. Malafosse, P. Genton, E. Hirsch, C. Marescaux, D. Broglin & R. Bernasconi, pp. 187–199. London: John Libbey.

Hunter, J. & Jasper, H.H. (1949): Effects of thalamic stimulation in unanesthetized animals. *EEG Clin. Neurophysiol.* **1**, 305–324.

Innocenti, G. (1986): General organization of callosal connections in the cerebral cortex. In: *Cerebral cortex*, Vol. 5, eds. E.G. Jones & A. Peters, pp. 291–353. New York: Plenum Press.

Jones, E.G. (1985): *The thalamus*, p. 935. New York: Plenum Press.

Jung, R. (1962): Blocking of petit-mal attacks by sensory arousal and inhibition of attacks by an active change in attention during the epileptic aura. *Epilepsia* **3**, 435–437.

Kaplan, B.J. (1985): The epileptic nature of rodent electrocortical polyspiking is still unproven. *Exp. Neurol.* **88**, 425–436.

Klingberg, F. & Pickenhain, L. (1968): Das Auftreten von 'Spindelentladungen' bei der Ratte in Beziehung zum Verhalten. *Acta Biol. Med. Gem.* **20**, 45–54.

Kornetsky, C. (1977): Animal models: promises and problems. In: *Animal models in psychiatry and neurology*, eds. I. Hanin & E. Udsin, pp. 1–7. Oxford: Pergamon Press.

Lannes, B., Micheletti, G., Vergnes, M., Marescaux, C., Depaulis, A. & Warter, J.M. (1988): Relationship between spike-wave discharges and vigilance levels in rats with spontaneous petit mal-like epilepsy. *Neurosci. Lett.* **94**, 187–191.

Lennox, W.G. & Lennox, M.A. (1960): *Epilepsy and related disorders 1*. Boston: Little, Brown & Co.

Libouban, S. & Oswaldo-Cruz, E. (1958): Quelques observations relatives aux activités évoquées et spontanées du cerveau du rat blanc. *J. Physiol. (Paris)* **50**, 380–383.

Liu, Z., Vergnes, M., Depaulis, A. & Marescaux, C. (1991): Evidence for a critical role of GABAergic transmission within the thalamus in the genesis and control of absence seizures in the rat. *Brain Res.* **545**, 1–7.

Liu, Z., Vergnes, M., Depaulis, A. & Marescaux, C. (1992): Involvement of intrathalamic GABA$_B$ neurotransmission in the control of absence seizures in the rat. *Neuroscience* **48**, 87–93.

Loiseau, P. (1992): Childhood absence-epilepsy. In: *Epileptic syndromes in infancy, childhood and adolescence*, 2nd edn., eds. J. Roger, M. Bureau, Ch. Dravet, F.E. Dreifuss, A. Perret & P. Wolf, pp. 135–150. London: John Libbey.

McQueen, J.K. & Woddbury, D.M. (1975): Attempts to produce spike-and-wave complexes in the electro-corticogram of the rat. *Epilepsia* **16**, 295–299.

Marcus, E.M., Watson, C.W. & Jacobson, S. (1969): Role of the corpus callosum in bilateral synchronous discharges induced by intravenous pentylenetetrazol. *Neurology* **19**, 309.

Marescaux, C., Micheletti, G., Vergnes, M., Depaulis, A., Rumbach, L. & Warter, J.M. (1984): A model of chronic spontaneous petit mal-like seizures in the rat: comparison with pentylenetetrazol-induced seizures. *Epilepsia* **25**, 326–331.

Marescaux, C., Vergnes, M., Depaulis, A., Micheletti, G. & Warter, J.M. (1992a): Neurotransmission in rats' spontaneous generalized nonconvulsive epilepsy. In: *Neurotransmistters in epilepsy*, eds. G. Avanzini, J. Engel, R. Fariello & U. Heinemann. *Epilepsy Res. Suppl.* **8**, 335–343.

Marescaux, C., Vergnes, M. & Depaulis, A. (1992b): Genetic absence epilepsy in rats from Strasbourg. A review. *J. Neural Transm.* **35**, Suppl. 37–69.

Marescaux, C., Vergnes, M. & Bernasconi, R. (1992c): GABA$_B$ receptor antagonists: potential new anti-absence drugs. *J. Neural Transm.* **35**, Suppl. 179–188.

Mathivet, P., Bernasconi, R., de Barry, J., Mickel, S., Froestl, W. & Bittiger, H. (1994): Characteristics of GABA$_B$ receptor binding sites in genetic absence epilepsy rats from Strasbourg (GAERS) and in non-epileptic rats. In: *Idiopathic generalized epilepsies: clinical, experimental and genetic aspects*, eds. A. Malafosse, P. Genton, E. Hirsch, C. Marescaux, D. Broglin & R. Bernasconi, pp. 177–185. London: John Libbey.

Meldrum, B. & Horton, R. (1980): Effects of the bicyclic GABA agonist, THIP, on myoclonic and seizure responses in mice and baboons with reflex epilepsy. *Eur. J. Pharmacol.* **61**, 231–237.

Musgrave, J. & Gloor, P. (1980): The role of the corpus callosum in bilateral interhemispheric synchrony of spike and wave discharge in feline generalized penicillin epilepsy. *Epilepsia* **21**, 369–378.

Naquet, R., Catier, J. & Menini, C. (1975): Neurophysiology of photically induced epilepsy in *Papio papio*. In: *Advances in neurology*, Vol. 10, eds. B.S. Meldrum & C.D. Marsden, pp. 107–118. New York: Raven Press.

Noebels, J.L. (1984): A single gene error of noradrenergic axon growth synchronizes central neurones. *Nature* **310**, 409–411.

Noebels, J.L. (1994): Genetic and phenotypic heterogeneity of inherited spike-wave epilepsies. In: *Idiopathic generalized epilepsies: clinical, experimental and genetic aspects*, eds. A. Malafosse, P. Genton, E. Hirsch, C. Marescaux, D. Broglin & R. Bernasconi, pp. 215–225. London: John Libbey.

Paxinos, G. & Watson, C. (1982): *The rat brain in stereotaxic coordinates*. New York: Academic Press.

Peeters, B.W.M.M., Sporen, W.P.J.M., van Luijtelaar, E.L.J.M. & Coenen, A.M.L. (1988): The WAG/Rij rat model for absence epilepsy: anticonvulsant drug evaluation. *Neurosci. Res. Commun.* **2**, 93–97.

Peeters, B.W.M.M., Kerbusch, J.M.L., van Luijtelaar, E.L.J.M., Vossen, J.M.H. & Coenen, A.M.L. (1990): Genetics of absence epilepsy in rats. *Behav. Genet.* **20**, 453–460.

Pohl, M. & Mares, P. (1983): Localization of the origin of metrazol-induced rhythmic electrocorticographic activity in rats. *Physiol. Bohemoslov.* **32**, 162–170.

Qiao, X. & Noebels, J.L. (1991): Genetic and phenotypic heterogeneity of inherited spike-wave epilepsy: two mutant gene loci with independent cerebral excitability defects. *Brain Res.* **555**, 43–50.

Schickerova, R., Mares, P. & Trojan, S. (1984): Correlation between electro-corticographic and motor phenomena induced by pentamethylenetetrazol during ontogenesis in rats. *Exp. Neurol.* **84**, 153–164.

Semba, K. & Komisaruk, B.R. (1984): Neural substrates of two different rhythmical vibrissal movements in the rat. *Neuroscience* **12**, 761–774.

Snead, O.C. III (1978): Gamma-hydroxybutyrate in the monkey. *Neurology* **28**, 636–642.

Snead, O.C. III (1988): Gamma-hydroxybutyrate model of generalized absence seizures: further characterization and comparison with other absence models. *Epilepsia* **29**, 361–368.

Snead, O.C. III, Depaulis, A., Banerjee, P.K., Hechler, V. & Vergnes, M. (1992): The $GABA_A$ receptor complex in experimental absence seizures in rat: an autoradiographic study. *Neurosci. Lett.* **140**, 9–12.

Snead, O.C. III. (1994): Pathophysiological mechanisms of experimental generalized absence seizures in rats. In: *Idiopathic generalized epilepsies: clinical, experimental and genetic aspects*, eds. A. Malafosse, P. Genton, E. Hirsch, C. Marescaux, D. Broglin & R. Bernasconi. London: John Libbey.

Steriade, M. & Deschenes, M. (1984): The thalamus as a neuronal oscillator. *Brain Res. Rev.* **8**, 1–63.

Van Luijtelaar, E.L.J.M. & Coenen, A.M.L. (1986): Two types of electrocortical paroxysms in an inbred strain of rats. *Neurosci. Lett.* **70**, 393–397.

Vergnes, M., Marescaux, C., Micheletti, G., Reis, J., Depaulis, A., Rumbach, L. & Warter, J.M. (1982): Spontaneous paroxysmal electroclinical patterns in rat: a model of generalized non-convulsive epilepsy. *Neurosci. Lett.* **33**, 97–101.

Vergnes, M., Marescaux, C., Depaulis, A., Micheletti, G. & Warter, J.M. (1986): Ontogeny of spontaneous petit mal-like seizures in Wistar rats. *Develop. Brain Res.* **30**, 85–87.

Vergnes, M., Marescaux, C., Depaulis, A., Micheletti, G. & Warter, J.M. (1987): Spontaneous spike and wave discharges in thalamus and cortex in a rat model of genetic petit mal-like seizures. *Exp. Neurol.* **96**, 127–136.

Vergnes, M., Marescaux, C., Lannes, B., Depaulis, A., Micheletti, G. & Warter, J.M. (1989): Interhemispheric desynchronization of spontaneous spike-wave discharges by corpus callosum transection in rats with petit mal-like epilepsy. *Epilepsy Res.* **4**, 8–13.

Vergnes, M., Marescaux, C. & Depaulis, A. (1990a): Mapping of spontaneous spike and wave discharges in Wistar rats with genetic generalized non-convulsive epilepsy. *Brain Res.* **523**, 87–91.

Vergnes, M., Marescaux, C., Depaulis, A., Micheletti, G. & Warter, J.M. (1990b): Spontaneous spike-and-wave discharges in Wistar rats: a model of genetic generalized nonconvulsive epilepsy. In: *Generalized epilepsy*, eds. M. Avoli, P. Gloor, G. Kostopoulos & R. Naquet, pp. 238–253. London: Birkhäuser.

Vergnes, M., Marescaux, C., Boehrer, A. & Depaulis, A. (1991): Are rats with genetic absence epilepsy behaviorally impaired? *Epilepsy Res.* **9**, 97–104.

Vergnes, M. & Marescaux, C. (1992): Cortical and thalamic lesions in rats with genetic absence epilepsy. *J. Neural Transm.* **35**, Suppl., 71–83.

Williams, D. (1953): A study of thalamic and cortical rhythms in petit mal. *Brain* **76**, 50–69.

Chapter 16

Brain metabolism and blood flow in models of generalized idiopathic epilepsies in rodents

A. Nehlig, M. Vergnes, E. Hirsch and C. Marescaux

INSERM U398, Faculté de Médecine, rue Humann, 67000 Strasbourg, France

Introduction

Quantitative autoradiographic methods have been developed to measure the local rates of glucose utilization (Sokoloff *et al.*, 1977) or blood flow (Sakurada *et al.*, 1978) simultaneously in all regions of the brain in conscious animals. These methods are also currently used now in men with a high spatial resolution (Phelps *et al.*, 1979; Reivich *et al.*, 1979). In the present paper, we will document the usefulness and the limits of these techniques for the measurement of cerebral functional activity, both glucose utilization and blood flow, in two models of idiopathic generalized epilepsy in rodents.

Quantitative autoradiographic methods for the measurement of cerebral glucose utilization and blood flow

Local cerebral glucose utilization

Local cerebral metabolic rates for glucose (LCMRglc) can be determined by using [^{14}C]2-deoxyglucose (2DG) method described by Sokoloff *et al.* (1977). The 2DG is transported bidirectionally between blood and brain by the same carrier that transports glucose across the blood–brain barrier. In the brain, 2DG is phosphorylated to 2DG-6P by hexokinase. 2DG and glucose are therefore competitive substrates for both blood–brain transport and phosphorylation by hexokinase. Unlike glucose-6P which is metabolized further to CO_2 and H_2O, 2DG-6P cannot be converted to fructose-6P, and is not a substrate for glucose-6P dehydrogenase. 2DG-6P, once formed, remains therefore essentially trapped in cerebral tissues, at least for the duration of the experimental period. The amount of 2DG-6P accumulated in brain tissues is directly proportional to their levels of glucose utilization which can be calculated by means of the operational equation of the method (Sokoloff *et al.*, 1977).

However, the 2DG method can only be applied when glucose metabolism, both plasma glucose level and the rate of glucose consumption, remain in a steady state throughout the experimental period, i.e. 45 min. These conditions cannot always be achieved, especially during epileptic events and alternative methods must be used, such as cerebral blood flow measurement which can be performed over very short periods.

Local cerebral blood flow

To measure quite short-lasting changes in cerebral functional activity, the quantitative autoradiographic [^{14}C]iodoantipyrine (IAP) technique of Sakurada *et al.* (1978) can alternatively be used to determine local cerebral blood flow (LCBF). Indeed, in most situations, local cerebral blood flow and LCMRglcs are closely coupled in all cerebral regions, so that modifications in cerebral activity elicit parallel changes in LCMRglc and LCBF (Kuschinsky, 1983). [^{14}C]Iodoantipyrine is a freely diffusible molecule which rapidly distributes between blood and tissues. When the steady state of blood saturation is reached, usually within about 1 min, the intracerebral concentration of tracer is proportional to cerebral blood flow.

For very short events, even the IAP technique for which the time of measurement can be reduced to about 20 s, may still be a limitation to the approach of subtle and rapid fluctuations of cerebral functional activity. Recently, laser-Doppler flowmetry (LDF) has been applied to the measurement of cerebral blood flow. This technique is based on the fact that the Doppler shift of a backscattered laser beam from a moving red blood cell is related to its velocity. In laser-Doppler flowmetry, the output signal reflects not only red blood cell velocity, as does the Doppler ultrasound method, but also red blood cell concentration in a given volume, and hence blood flow (Wadhwani & Rapoport, 1990). Laser-Doppler flowmetry allows reliable, noninvasive, and continuous recordings of the actual time course of cerebral blood flow. The needle probe can be placed either on the external surface of a cranial plastic window or on the skull which has been previously made thinner until becoming completely transparent. The readings represent the flow in the cerebral cortex. Compared to the IAP technique, laser-Doppler flowmetry is continuous, but measures blood flow only in a single area of the cerebral cortex, whereas IAP is multiregional but represents only one time point. Furthermore, laser-Doppler flowmetry gives only a flow signal and not an absolute value of cerebral blood flow. However, the signal has been standardized against cerebral blood flow measured with other techniques (Wadhwani & Rapoport, 1990).

In the following part of this paper, the application of these techniques to the measurement of cerebral functional activity in animal models of generalized idiopathic epilepsies will be described.

Cerebral glucose utilization and blood flow in rats with spontaneous genetic absence epilepsy

Local cerebral glucose utilization changes with absences

LCMRglcs were measured by means of the 2DG method in a selected strain of Genetic Absence Epilepsy Rats from Strasbourg (GAERS) and compared to those of a control nonepileptic strain (NE) whose EEG pattern was normal. The EEG, behavioural and pharmacological characteristics of this model have been recently reviewed in detail (Marescaux *et al.*, 1992; Vergnes *et al.*, 1990). Briefly, bilateral and synchronous spike-and-wave discharges (SWD) are mainly recorded all over the cortex as well as in the lateral thalamic nuclei, whereas they do not occur in limbic structures. These generalized, nonconvulsive seizures occur in the calm awake state and are accompanied by immobility and sometimes clonus of the facial and cervical muscles. They are suppressed by antiepileptic drugs effective in the treatment of human childhood absence epilepsy, while they are unresponsive to pharmacological agents specific for focal or convulsive seizures.

During the 2DG procedure, the epileptic rats exhibited spike-and-wave discharges, 7–10 cycles/s, 250–800 µV in amplitude recorded on the frontoparietal cortex. Their number was 61 ± 10 (mean ± SEM of five rats) over the 45 min experimental period and their duration was 16.6 ± 1.7 s per min of recording. The EEG of the control strain was normal. An overall consistent increase in LCMRglcs was recorded in epileptic rats compared to controls (Figs. 1 and 2). This increase was statistically significant in 52 out of the 59 regions studied, ranged from 16 to 50 per cent over levels

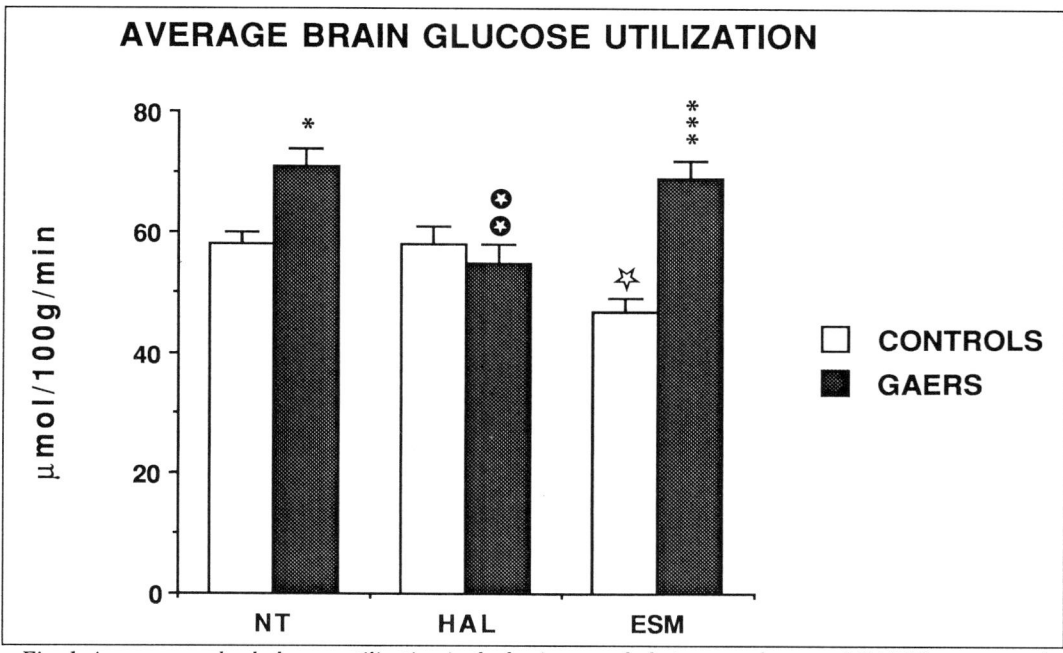

Fig. 1. Average cerebral glucose utilization in the brain as a whole in control rats and GAERS, not treated (NT, left colums), exposed to haloperidol (HAL, middle columns) or ethosuximide (ESM, right columns). *$P < 0.05$, ***$P < 0.001$, statistically significant differences between GAERS and their corresponding controls; ☆$P < 0.05$, statistically significant difference between treated and not treated controls. ✪✪$P < 0.01$, statistically significant difference between treated and not treated GAERS.

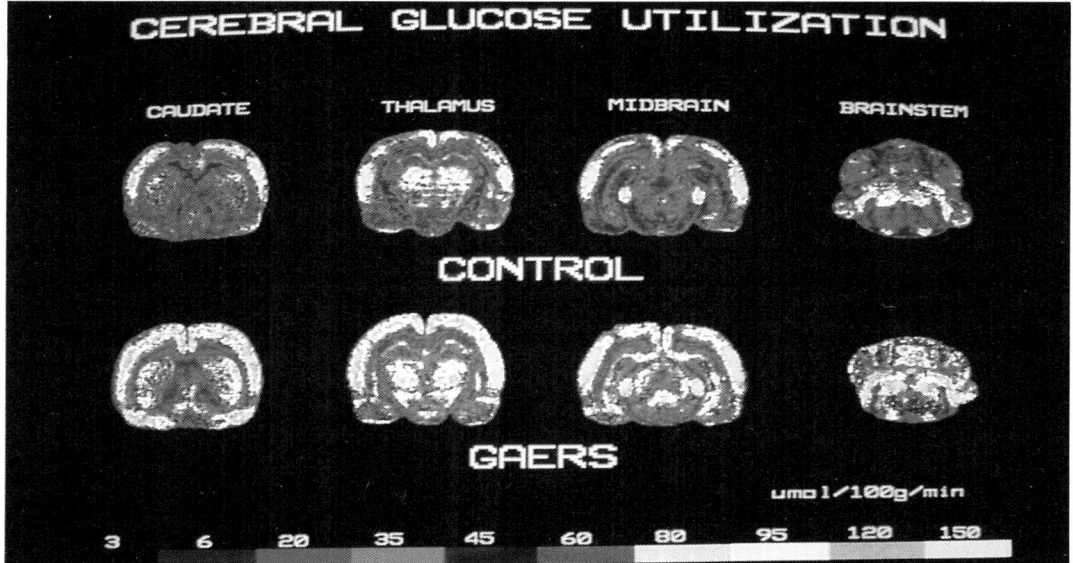

Fig. 2. Colour-coded autoradiographs of GAERS and control rat brain sections taken at the level of the caudate nucleus, thalamus, midbrain and brain-stem. By reference to the colour scale located at the bottom, the diffuse metabolic increase in epileptic rats compared to controls is striking in all cerebral regions (see also colour plates).

in control rats and concerned all cerebral functional systems, whether they exhibit spike-and-wave discharges (neocortex and thalamus) or not (limbic and motor systems) (Fig. 2). These results are also in good accordance with the marked diffuse increase recorded during positron emission tomography measurements of LCMRglc in humans with typical childhood absence epilepsy (Engel et al., 1985). There is a lack of anatomical correlation between the areas exhibiting hypermetabolism and those where spike-and-wave discharges are recorded, showing that the diffuse increase in LCMRglcs in the epileptic rats over control levels is not directly related to the occurrence of spike-and-wave discharges (Nehlig et al., 1991, 1992).

In order to characterize further the pathophysiological mechanisms underlying the metabolic responses of epileptic rats, we measured the cerebral metabolic effects of one drug aggravating petit mal absences, a dopaminergic antagonist, haloperidol (2 mg/kg) and of one antiepileptic specific for the treatment of absences, ethosuximide (200 mg/kg). The two drugs were injected intraperitoneally 10 min before the initiation of the 2DG procedure to both epileptic and control rats.

In the presence of haloperidol, the epileptic rats exhibited almost continuous spike-and-wave discharges which were lasting 44.2 ± 4.9 s per min of recording (mean ± SEM of six rats) over the 45 min 2DG experimental period whereas the EEG of the controls was unaffected by haloperidol. However, despite these striking EEG changes, the difference in the levels of cerebral energy metabolism between the epileptic rats and the controls exposed to haloperidol was abolished and LCMRglcs were similar in all structures of both groups of animals, as can be seen in Fig. 1 for the average rate of cerebral glucose utilization.

The administration of ethosuximide totally suppressed spike-and-wave discharges in GAERS rats and did not affect the EEG of controls. Conversely, rates of cerebral energy metabolism were decreased by ethosuximide in controls but remained higher by 31 to 72 per cent in all areas for epileptic rats compared to their corresponding controls (Fig. 1). These data demonstrate further the lack of correlation between the occurrence of spike-and-wave discharges and the levels of cerebral energy metabolism. They are also in favour of a normal or decreased ictal metabolism and of an increased interictal glucose utilization by the brain in absence seizures (Nehlig et al., 1992, 1993). However, since the quantitative measurement of LCMRglc can only be performed accurately over a long time, i.e. 45 min, the rates of energy metabolism recorded in the epileptic rats not exposed to any drug are a mixture of epileptic and non-epileptic events. It is therefore impossible to discriminate the exact part of each of these phases to the final result. Therefore, to record the continuous changes occurring in cerebral functional activity during absence seizures and transition phases between ictal and interictal periods, we measured cerebral blood flow by the non-invasive laser-Doppler flowmetry technique allowing continuous recording of cerebral blood flow.

Local cerebral blood flow changes with absences

In the epileptic rats, the occurrence of spike-and-wave discharges was accompanied by a decrease in the level of cerebral blood flow. The onset of the decrease was usually delayed by 3–7 s compared to the beginning of the spike-and-wave discharges recorded on the other side of the cortex (Fig. 3). The decrease in cerebral blood flow lasted as long as the spike-and-wave discharges and at the end of them, cerebral blood flow instantaneously returned to a level either equal to or higher than the one recorded before their onset. The administration of haloperidol (2 mg/kg) induced the appearance of continuous spike-and-wave discharges which translated into a decreased level of cerebral blood flow remaining at a constantly low level as long as the discharges were continuous. When spike-and-wave discharges became intermittent, the oscillations of cerebral blood flow appeared again with high rates in the interictal period and low rates during the discharges (Fig. 4). The decrease in cerebral blood flow recorded during absences was not related to an abnormal vascular reactivity since a normal vasodilatory response to CO_2 could be recorded in the epileptic rats.

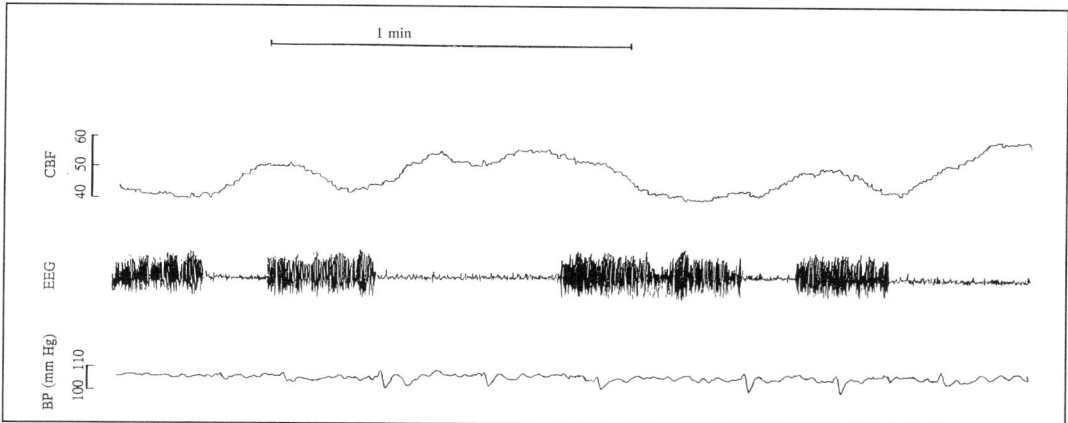

Fig. 3. Laser-Doppler flowmetry recording of cortical blood flow in GAERS during the course of spontaneously occurring absences. The decrease of cerebral blood flow starts with a latency of 6 s after the onset of the spike-and-wave discharges. Cortical blood flow is given in arbitrary units.

In conclusion, taken together, our data demonstrate that in this genetic model of absence seizures, cerebral functional activity changes are not correlated to electrical events. Morereover, in contrast to convulsive seizures, in nonconvulsive absence epilepsy the levels of cerebral functional activity are reduced during the ictal period and increased in the interictal period.

Cerebral blood flow during audiogenic seizures

Cerebral blood flow was measured by means of the [^{14}C]IAP technique in a strain of rats inbred in the Centre de Neurochimie (Strasbourg, France) for their susceptibility to sound. In that strain, a prolonged high-intensity acoustic stimulus induces audiogenic seizures characterized by one or two running episodes, followed by a tonic phase with dorsal hyperextension and extension of the head and forepaws. The tonic phase is associated with a short flattening of the EEG preceding a regular low-voltage theta-like activity. The absence of cortical spikes or spike-and-waves discharges is

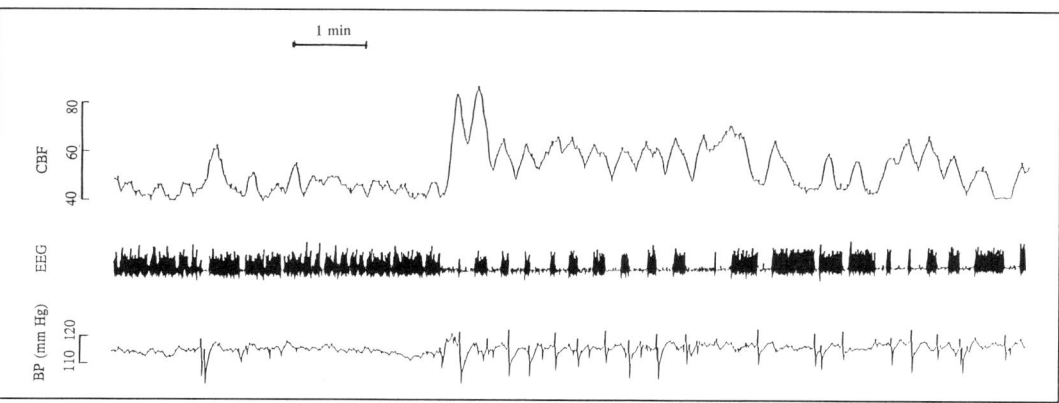

Fig. 4. Laser-Doppler flowmetry recording of cortical blood flow in GAERS after the intraperitoneal administration of haloperidol. When spike-and-wave discharges are intermittent, as can be seen at the beginning of the recording, cerebral blood flow is fluctuating. When spike-and-wave discharges become permanent, cortical blood flow is remaining at a low stable value. As soon as spike-and-wave discharges become intermittent again, cerebral blood flow starts to fluctuate. Cortical blood flow is given in arbitrary units.

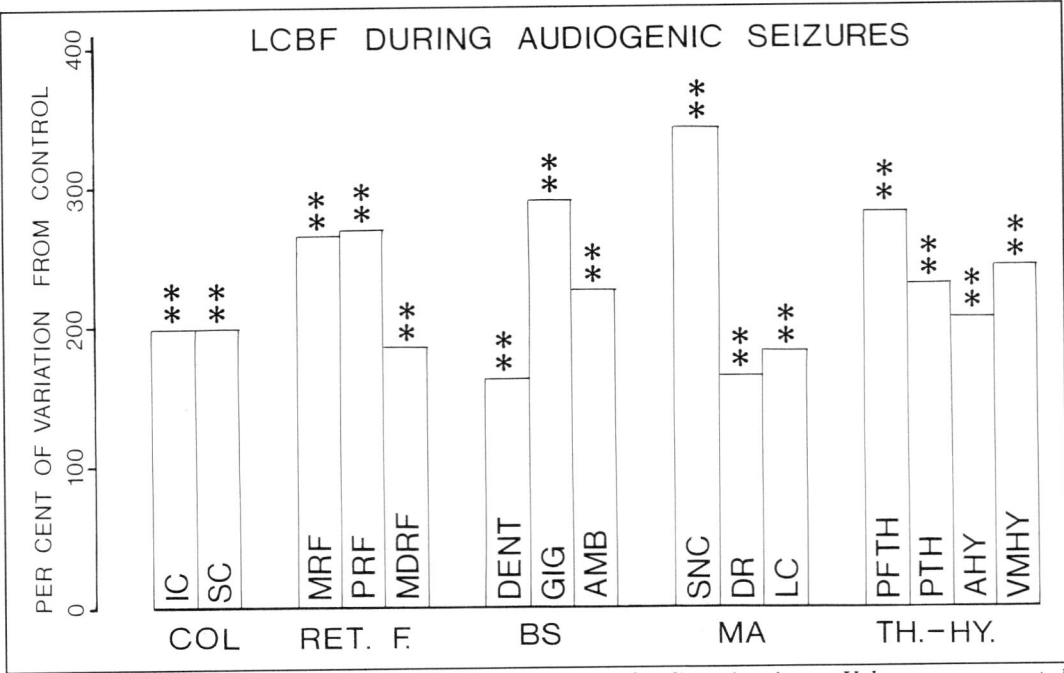

Fig. 5. Changes in local cerebral blood flow during the course of audiogenic seizures. Values are represented as percent of variation from control. COL, colliculi; RET. F., reticular formation; BS, brain-stem; MA, monoaminergic cell groupings; TH.-HYP., thalamus–hypothalamus, IC, inferior colliculus; SC, superior colliculus; MRF, mesencephalic reticular formation; PRF, pontine reticular formation; MDRF, medullary reticular formation; DENT, dentate nucleus; GIG, gigantocellularis nucleus; AMB, ambiguus nucleus; SNC, substantia nigra pars compacta; DR, dorsal raphe; LC, locus coeruleus; PFTH, parafascicular thalamus; PTH, posterior thalamus; AHY, anterior hypothalamus; VMHY, ventromedian hypothalamus.
$**P < 0.0005$, statistically significant differences from control.

explained by the fact that audiogenic seizures originate in brain-stem structures such as inferior colliculus and reticular formation (Browning, 1986; Faingold & Boersma Anderson, 1991). The propagation of these seizures is limited to the brain-stem and does not involve forebrain structures as hippocampus or cerebral cortex (Faingold, 1988; Marescaux et al., 1987).

Because of the short duration of the audiogenic seizure, usually 60–90 s, LCMRglcs cannot be measured and the mapping of cerebral functional activity can only been performed by the IAP technique measuring cerebral blood flow in less than 1 min. Compared to basal levels of local cerebral blood flow measured in a control strain of rats not sensitive to sound and exposed to the same acoustic stimulus, local cerebral blood flow largely increased in almost all brain areas during audiogenic seizures. Highest increases (>150 per cent) were recorded in the structures directly involved in the generation of these seizures, such as inferior colliculus, medullary, pontine and mesencephalic reticular formation and substantia nigra. Such large increases in local cerebral blood flow rates were also recorded in other brain-stem areas, like monoaminergic cell groupings, brain-stem auditory relay nuclei, posterior vegetative areas and some hypothalamic and thalamic regions (Figs. 5 & 6). The lowest increases in local cerebral blood flow (<50 per cent) were recorded in many cortical areas, piriform, entorhinal, prefrontal, parietal, motor and auditory cortices, all hippocampal regions, some anterior limbic regions and genu of the corpus callosum (Figs. 6 & 7). Thus, during audiogenic seizures, there appears to be a good correlation between the structures

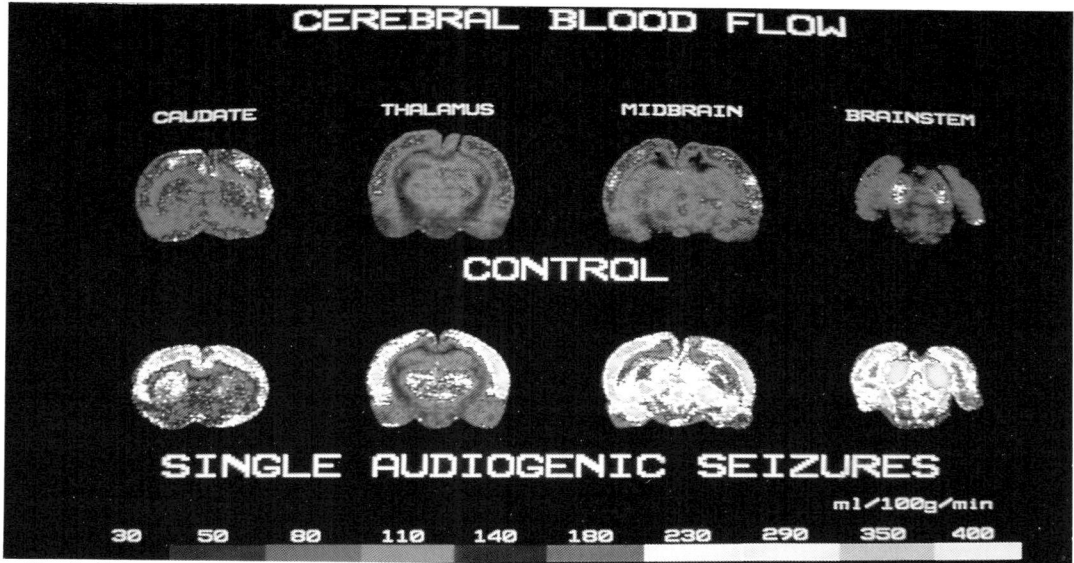

Fig. 6. Colour-coded autoradiographs of audiogenic and control rat brain sections taken at the level of the caudate nucleus, thalamus, midbrain and brain-stem. By reference to the colour scale located at the bottom, the generalized metabolic increase in audiogenic rats compared to controls is striking in all cerebral areas and of markedly higher amplitude in posterior than in anterior regions (see also colour plates).

involved in the generation of the convulsive events and those where rates of local cerebral blood flow are mostly increased.

In conclusion, the quantitative autoradiographic techniques and laser-Doppler flowmetry allowing the continuous noninvasive recording of cortical blood flow represent powerful tools for the assess-

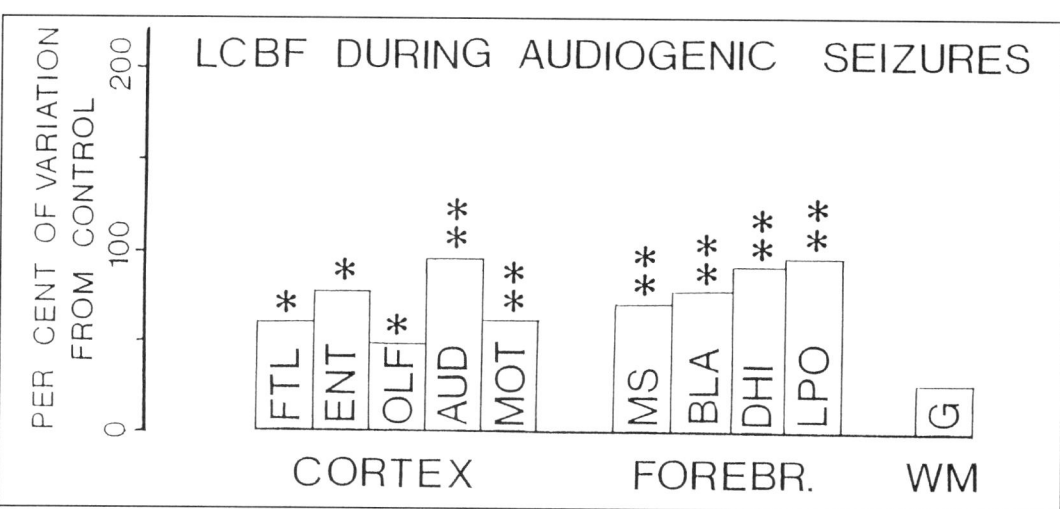

Fig. 7. Changes in local cerebral blood flow during the course of audiogenic seizures. Values are represented as percent of variation from control.; Abbreviations: FOREBR., forebrain; WM, white matter; FTL, frontal cortex; ENT, entorhinal cortex; OLF, olfactory cortex; AUD, auditory cortex; MOT, motor cortex; MS, medial septum; BLA, basolateral amygdala; DHI, dorsal hippocampus; LPO, lateral preoptic area; G, genu of the corpus callosum. *$P < 0.005$, **$P < 0.0005$, statistically significant differences from control.

ment of cerebral functional activity in discrete events such as epileptic seizures. However, the quite long temporal resolution of the 2DG method limits the study of short events such as absences or audiogenic seizures. In those cases, a quantitative measurement of functional activity during ictal and interictal phases, respectively, can only been assessed by cerebral blood flow techniques.

Reference

Browning, R.A. (1986): Neurobiology of seizure disposition – the genetically epilepsy-prone rat. VII. Neuroanatomical localization of structures responsible for seizures in the GEPR: lesion studies. *Life Sci.* **39**, 857–867.

Engel, J. Jr., Lubens, P., Kuhl, D.E. & Phelps, M.E. (1985): Local cerebral metabolic rate for glucose during petit mal absences. *Ann. Neurol.* **17**, 121–128.

Faingold, C.L. (1988): The genetically epilepsy-prone rat. *Gen. Pharmacol.* **19**, 331–338.

Faingold, C.L. & Boersma Anderson C.A. (1991): Loss of intensity-induced inhibition in inferior colliculus neurons leads to audiogenic seizure susceptibility in behaving genetically epilepsy-prone rats. *Exp. Neurol.* **113**, 354–363.

Kuschinsky, W. (1983): Coupling between functional metabolism and blood flow in the brain: state of the art. *Microcirculation* **2**, 357–378.

Marescaux, C., Vergnes, M. & Depaulis, A. (1992): Genetic absence epilepsy in rats from Strasbourg – a review. *J. Neurol. Transm.* **35[Suppl.]**, 37–69.

Marescaux, C., Vergnes, M., Kiesmann, M., Depaulis, A., Micheletti, G. & Warter J.M. (1987): Kindling of audiogenic seizures in Wistar rats: an EEG study. *Exp. Neurol.* **97**, 160–168.

Nehlig, A., Vergnes, M., Marescaux, C., Boyet, S. & Lannes, B. (1991): Local cerebral glucose utilization in rats with petit mal-like seizures. *Ann. Neurol.* **29**, 72–77.

Nehlig, A., Vergnes, M., Marescaux, C. & Boyet, S. (1992): Mapping of cerebral energy metabolism in rats with genetic generalized nonconvulsive epilepsy. *J. Neural Transm.* **35[Suppl.]**, 141–153.

Nehlig, A., Vergnes, M., Marescaux, C. & Boyet, S. (1993): Cerebral energy metabolism in rats with genetic absence epilepsy is not correlated with the pharmacological increase or suppression of spike-wave discharges. *Brain Res.* **618**, 1–8.

Phelps, M.E., Huang, S.C., Hoffman, E.J., Selin, C., Sokoloff, L. & Kuhl, D.E. (1979): Tomographic measurement of local cerebral glucose metabolic rate in humans with (F-18)2-fluoro-2-deoxy-d-glucose: validation of method. *Ann. Neurol.* **6**, 371–388.

Reivich, M., Kuhl, D., Wolf, A. Greenberg, J., Phelps, M., Ido, T., Cassella, V., Fowler, J., Hoffman, E., Alavi, A., Som, P. & Sokoloff, L. (1979): The [^{18}F]fluorodeoxyglucose method for the measurement of local cerebral glucose utilization in man. *Circ. Res.* **44**, 127–137.

Sakurada, O., Kennedy, C., Jehle, J., Brown, J.D., Carbin, G.L. & Sokoloff, L. (1978): Measurement of local cerebral blood flow with [^{14}C]iodoantipyrine. *Am. J. Physiol.* **234**, H59–H66.

Sokoloff, L., Reivich, M., Kennedy, C., Des Rosiers, M.H., Patlak, C.S., Pettigrew, K.D., Sakurada, O. & Shinohara, M. (1977): The [^{14}C]deoxyglucose method for the measurement of local cerebral glucose utilization: theory, procedure and normal values in the conscious and anesthetized albino rat. *J. Neurochem.* **28**, 897–916.

Vergnes, M., Marescaux, C., Depaulis, A., Micheletti, G. & Warter, J.M. (1990): Spontaneous spike-and-wave discharges in Wistar rats: a model of genetic generalized nonconvulsive epilepsy. In: *Generalized epilepsy. Neurobiological approaches*, eds. M. Avoli, P. Gloor, G. Kostopoulos & R. Naquet, pp. 238–253. Boston: Birkhäuser.

Wadhwani, K.C. & Rapoport, S.I. (1990): Blood flow in the central and peripheral nervous systems. In: *Laser-doppler flowmetry*, eds. A.P. Shepherd & P.A. Oberg, pp. 265–288. Boston: Kluwer Academic.

Chapter 17

Characteristics of $GABA_B$-receptor binding sites in genetic absence epilepsy rats from Strasbourg (GAERS) and in non-epileptic control rats

Pascal Mathivet[*], Raymond Bernasconi[*], Jean de Barry[†], Stuart Mickel[‡], Wolfgang Froestl[‡] and Helmut Bittiger[‡]

[*]INSERM Unité 398, Neurobiologie et Neuropharmacologie des Epilepsies Généralisées, 67084 Strasbourg Cedex, France, [†]Laboratoire de Neurobiologie Cellulaire, UPR 9009, CNRS, Strasbourg, France and [‡]Research and Development Department, Pharmaceuticals Division, Ciba-Geigy, Basel, Switzerland

Introduction

One of the most important characteristics of generalized absence seizures is the aggravation of their symptoms by increased GABAergic activity in the brain (King, 1979). Enhancement of GABAergic activity potentiates all clinical and experimental forms of generalized non-convulsive seizure activity and under certain conditions may even be sufficient to induce bilaterally synchronous spike-and-wave discharges (SWD) (Gloor & Fariello, 1988). Although GABA agonists exacerbate experimental absence seizures, $GABA_A$ antagonists do not block experimental absence epilepsy. The macromolecular $GABA_A$-receptor complex does not appear to be involved in the development and control of bilaterally synchronous spike-and-wave discharges (Knight & Bowery, 1992; Snead et al., 1992). Recently, we reported that $GABA_B$-receptor agonists such as R-(−)-baclofen or 3-aminopropylmethylphosphinic acid dose-dependently increase the total duration of spike-and-wave discharges in the Genetic Absence Epilepsy Rat from Strasbourg (GAERS), a genetic model of absence seizures (Marescaux et al., 1992a,b). Conversely, $GABA_B$ receptor antagonists induced a dose-dependent and progressive suppression of spike-and-wave discharges in GAERS. Administration of R-(−)-baclofen to GAERS produced petit mal status in these rats, but did not affect rats from the control strain. These results may indicate that $GABA_B$ receptors in GAERS are qualitatively different from those of their non-epileptic littermates.

In lethargic (*lh/lh*) mice, another genetic model of absence epilepsy, Hosford et al. (1992a,b) reported similar observations demonstrating a central role of $GABA_B$ receptors in the genesis and control of generalized non-convulsive epilepsy. Using this model, Lin et al. (1993) were able to demonstrate that the number (B_{max}) of $GABA_B$ receptors in neocortical membranes was significantly greater (30 per cent) in *lh/lh* than in wild +/+ age-matched control mice. The equilibrium dissociation constant (K_d) was of the same order of magnitude in both strains. These data suggest that an excessive density of $GABA_B$ receptors in the neocortex seems to favour the expression of absence seizures in *lh/lh* mice. In contrast, Knight & Bowery (1992) have not found significant differences in [^{3}H]GABA-binding sites in brain slices of GAERS by autoradiography. The reasons for this apparent discrepancy may lie in the different animal species used (*lh/lh* mice *vs.* Wistar rats) or experimental paradigm employed (displaceable radioligand binding to isolated plasma membranes versus tissue slices).

A reevaluation of the role of $GABA_B$ receptors in the development and control of absence seizures in GAERS appears pertinent.

To test this hypothesis, we assessed the kinetics of $GABA_B$-binding sites in cortical, thalamic, hippocampal and cerebellar membranes prepared from GAERS and age-matched control rats. By using saturation curves with the $GABA_B$-antagonist radioligand [^{3}H]CGP 54626 we determined two parameters of these receptors: K_d and B_{max}. We also examined the regulation of $GABA_B$ binding by 5'-guanylimidodiphosphate [Gpp(NH)p] as an index of the coupling of $GABA_B$ receptors to guanine nucleotide-binding proteins (G proteins). These experiments have revealed several $GABA_B$-binding sites, and we compared the populations of these binding sites in both strains.

Experimental procedures

Materials

The potent and selective tritiated $GABA_B$-receptor agonist [^{3}H]CGP 27492 (15.0 Ci/mmol) was synthesized by Ciba-Geigy (Horsham, UK). The very potent and selective tritiated $GABA_B$ receptor antagonist, [^{3}H]CGP 54626 specific activity 60 Ci/mmol, was synthesized by Anawa (Wangen/ZH, Switzerland). All $GABA_B$-receptor agonists (R-(–)-baclofen) and antagonists were synthesized in the chemistry laboratories of Ciba-Geigy Ltd. Unless specified, the term baclofen indicates the pure stereoisomer R-(–)- baclofen. Gpp(NH)p was purchased from Boehringer Mannheim and ethylene imine polymer (PEI) was obtained from Fluka (Buchs).The purity of the custom-made radioligand was determined by high-pressure liquid chromatography (HPLC). All other reagents were obtained from commercial sources and were of the highest available purity.

Animals

Adult male rats (300–450 g) were used. Epileptic rats were chosen from a strain of Wistar rats selected from the breeding colony at the Unité INSERM in Strasbourg and called GAERS (Marescaux *et al.*, 1992c; Vergnes & Marescaux, Ch. 15). They were chosen from the 22th and the 24th generations. Controls were from the same generations of a strain which never displayed bilateral spike-and-wave discharges. Epileptic and non-epileptic rats were of the same age. They were kept in groups of four to six per cage under a 12/12 h normal light/dark cycle, with food and water *ad libitum*.

Method for the $GABA_B$-receptor assay using [^{3}H]CGP 54626 and [^{3}H]CGP 27492 as radioligands

Crude membrane fractions from rat cerebral cortex, thalamus, hippocampus and cerebellum were prepared from GAERS and controls by the method of Bittiger *et al.* (1990). The $GABA_B$ radioreceptor assay, using the antagonist radioligand [^{3}H]CGP 54626, was performed according to Bittiger *et al.* (1992). Briefly, 200–300 µg membrane proteins were incubated in 1 ml Krebs–Henseleit buffer pH 7.40, containing 20 mM Tris, 1 nM [^{3}H]CGP 54626 and in some experiments 10^{-9} to 10^{-3} M of R-(–)-baclofen and/or 300 µM Gpp(NH)p. Incubation was performed at 20°C for 20 min and

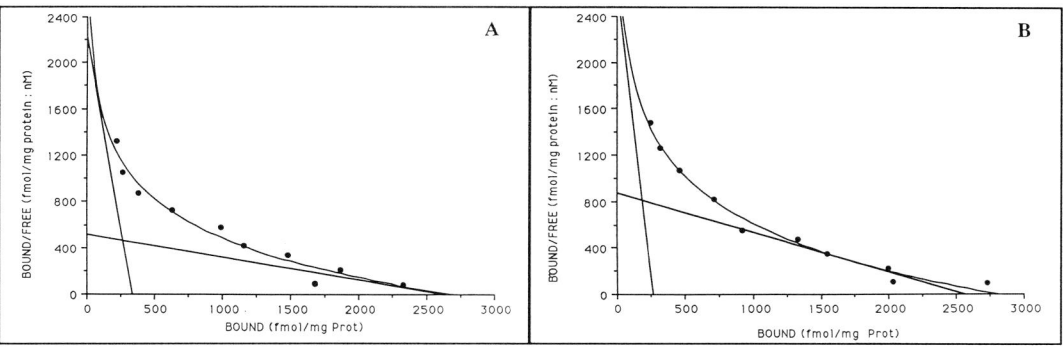

Fig. 1. Comparative Scatchard analysis of the saturable binding of [³H]CGP 54626 to cortical membranes prepared from (a) GAERS and (b) non-epileptic rats. Crude membranes were incubated with varying concentrations of [³H]CGP 54626 (0.1 to 27.5 nM) to determine total binding. The results shown in this figure are taken from a representative single experiment performed in triplicate, which has been repeated seven times. Standard errors of the means were less than 5 per cent and have been omitted for clarity. The curvilinear Scatchard plots have been resolved into two components by computer analysis and the parameters used to determine the lines shown on the graph are given together with those observed in cerebellum, hippocampus and thalamus in Table 1.

terminated by rapid filtration through Whatman GF/B glass filters, which had been treated with 0.2 per cent PEI in 60 per cent isopropanol. The membranes were washed on the filter four times with 5 ml cold buffer. Incubations were performed in triplicate and the non-specific binding was determined in the presence of 10 µM CGP 54626.

The [³H]CGP 27492 agonist radioligand assay was performed in a total volume of 2 ml Krebs-Henseleit buffer with 1 nM radioligand as previously described by Bittiger et al. (1988 & 1990). Incubations were performed at 20 °C for 40 min, and membranes were washed on the filter twice with 5 ml cold buffer. Non-specific binding was determined in the presence of 10 µM R-(–)-baclofen. The use of filtration assays with radioligand concentrations of 1 nM [³H]CGP 54626 or 1nM [³H]CGP 27492 gave about 80 per cent specific binding.

Protein determinations were performed using the method of Lowry et al. (1951) with bovine serum albumin as a standard.

Data analysis

To define two types of parameters, the equilibrium dissociation constants (K_d) and the apparent maximum number of binding sites (B_{max}), Scatchard analyses were performed by transformation of saturation experiments using 10–12 different concentrations in triplicate of [³H]CGP 54626, ranging from 0.1 nM to 30 nM. These two parameters were pre-calculated with the EBDA programme and the values obtained were subjected to nonlinear least-squares regression analysis with the LIGAND programme (Munson & Rodbard, 1980). For determination of IC_{50} values, binding assays were performed with 20–24 different concentrations of each displacing drug.

The calculated B_{max}, K_d and apparent Hill coefficient (nH) and IC_{50} values were obtained by computer-aided curve fitting, according to a one- or two-site model. Comparisons between GAERS and the non-epileptic control rats were calculated using two-tailed independent Student's t-test.

Results

Saturation analysis of antagonist [³H]CGP 54626 binding in GAERS and in non-epileptic rats

Scatchard plots of specifically bound [³H]CGP 54626 to cortical membranes of GAERS and non-epileptic control rats were curvilinear (Fig. 1a,b). Analyses of the data were performed using

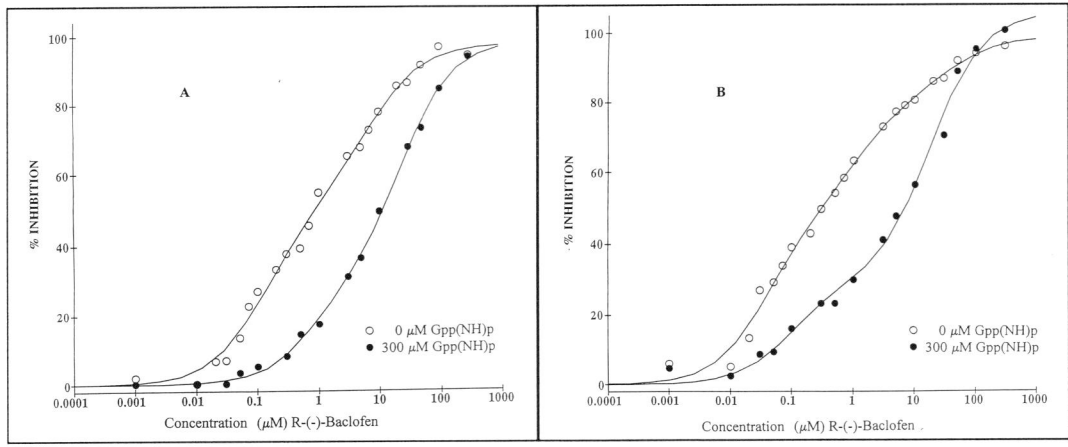

Fig. 2. Displacement of specifically bound [^{3}H] CGP 54626 by R-(−)-baclofen to cortical membranes prepared from (a) GAERS or from (b) non-epileptic rats. 1 nM [^{3}H]CGP 54626 was incubated with unlabelled R-(−)-baclofen in concentrations ranging from 1 nM to 300 μM in the presence of 300 μM Gpp(NH)p or in its absence. The data shown in this figure are from a single representative experiment, which was repeated twice. Standard errors of the means were less than 5 per cent and not plotted for the sake of clarity. The number of binding sites, the IC$_{50}$ values and Hill coefficients were calculated with the LIGAND programme and the data are shown in Table 2.

the LIGAND program, a non-linear least-squares optimization technique by fitting them to a one- or two-site model. The two-site model provided the best approximation to the observed data; the probability that [^{3}H]CGP 54626 binds specifically to two different affinity states of GABA$_B$ receptors was higher than 99 per cent. The high-affinity sites with a K_d between 0.12 and 0.15 nM represented a small population (10 to 11 per cent) of the total number of cortical receptors. The larger part of the binding sites (approximately 90 per cent) showed an affinity for [^{3}H]CGP 54626 between 1.7 and 2.3 nM (Table 1). These parameters were similar in GAERS and in non-epileptic control rats ($P > 0.10$, Student's t-test).

Table 1. Comparison of B_{max} and K_d for two GABA$_B$-binding sites in cortical, cerebellar, hippocampal and thalamic membranes of GAERS and non-epileptic rats

	% Site 1	B_{max} Site 1 (fmol/mg protein)	K_d Site 1 (nM)	B_{max} Site 2 (fmol/mg protein)	K_d Site 2 (nM)
Controls					
Cortex	11.3	321 ± 88	0.15 ± 0.06	2510 ± 1041	2.3 ± 0.3
Cerebellum	11.2	794 ± 693	0.46 ± 0.17	6316 ± 1947	13.0 ± 4.8
Thalamus	8.3	236 ± 188	0.19 ± 0.06	2606 ± 1251	13.1 ± 4.3
Hippocampus	10.4	68 ± 60	0.50 ± 0.18	588 ± 100	9.3 ± 5.6
GAERS					
Cortex	10.3	322 ± 163	0.12 ± 0.07	2797 ± 137	1.7 ± 0.2
Cerebellum	20.0	1777 ± 1170	0.78 ± 0.48	7092 ± 3900	10.0 ± 7.5
Thalamus	5.8	70 ± 42	0.43 ± 0.28	1127 ± 293	19.3 ± 10.8
Hippocampus	4.9	82 ± 47	0.37 ± 0.27	1670 ± 700	26.3 ± 18.4

Values for cortical membranes represent mean ± SEM of eight experiments (n) performed in triplicate. n was equal to 3 for cerebellar, hippocampal and thalamic membranes. The values obtained with epileptic brains did not differ significantly from the values obtained in control brains ($P > 0.10$, Student's t-test).

Similarly, two different binding sites were observed in cerebellar, hippocampal and thalamic membranes. K_d and B_{max} were of the same order of magnitude as those measured in the cortex and were not different in GAERS and controls (Table 1).

Inhibition by R-(−)-baclofen of antagonist [^{3}H]CGP 54626 specific binding to cortical membranes in GAERS and non-epileptic rats in presence and in absence of Gpp(NH)p

The slopes of the displacement curves of [^{3}H]CGP 54626 specifically bound to cortical membranes by R-(−)-baclofen were flat with Hill coefficients for GAERS and non-epileptic control rats of 0.53 ± 0.02 and 0.50 ± 0.09, respectively (Fig. 2a,b, Table 2). The curves shown in Fig. 2a,b provide the best mathematical approximation of the observed data. In contrast to Fig. 1 we were unable to calculate the probability for two, three or four binding sites.

Table 2. Competition of [^{3}H]CGP 54626 binding by R-(−)-baclofen in cortical membranes of GAERS and non-epileptic rats

Gpp(NH)p 0 μM	nH	B_{max} Site 1 %	B_{max} Site 2 %	B_{max} Site 3 %	IC$_{50}$ Site 1 (nM)	IC$_{50}$ Site 2 (nM)	IC$_{50}$ Site 3 (nM)
Controls	0.50 ± 0.09	12.9 ± 1.9	50.3 ± 5.9	36.8 ± 0.7	10.3 ± 4.9	104 ± 27	5670 ± 630
GAERS	0.53 ± 0.02	11.4 ± 4.1	50.3 ± 1.1	38.3 ± 4.6	4.5 ± 1.0	198 ± 15	7060 ± 100

Gpp(NH)p 300 μM	nH	B_{max} Site A %	B_{max} Site B %	IC$_{50}$ Site A (nM)	IC$_{50}$ Site B (nM)
Controls	0.55 ± 0.02	30.9 ± 2.1	69.1 ± 2.1	340 ± 170	18900 ± 410
GAERS	0.59 ± 0.06	37.7 ± 4.6	62.3 ± 4.6	720 ± 120	26340 ± 920

Data were obtained by LIGAND analysis of [^{3}H]CGP 54626 displacement experiments. Values are the mean ± SEM of two experiments performed in triplicate. The percentage of binding sites, the IC$_{50}$ values and the Hill coefficients obtained in GAERS were not different from those observed in non-epileptic rats ($P > 0.10$, Student's t-test).

If one assumes there are three sites, the calculated IC$_{50}$ values in GAERS for the high-affinity site was 4.5 ± 1.0 nM (11.4 ± 4.1 per cent), for the medium site 198 ± 15 nM (50.3 ± 1.1 per cent) and for the low affinity site 7060 ± 100 nM (38.3 ± 4.6 per cent). The corresponding IC$_{50}$ values in the non-epileptic control rats were 10.3 ± 4.9 nM (12.9 ± 1.9 per cent), 104 ± 27 nM (50.3 ± 5.9 per cent) and 5670 ± 630 nM (36.8 ± 0.7 per cent), respectively (Table 2). The number of binding sites, IC$_{50}$ values and Hill coefficients in GAERS did not differ from those of control rats ($P > 0.10$, Student's t-test).

Agonist binding to GABA$_B$ receptors is inhibited by GTP and by its metabolically stable analogue Gpp(NH)p through interaction with a G-protein (Hill et al., 1984; Dolphin & Scott, 1987). Gpp(NH)p decreased the affinity of GABA$_B$ receptors to agonists by transforming the high-affinity conformation to a conformation with lower affinity (Hill et al., 1984).

We investigated the effect of 300 μM Gpp(NH)p on the inhibition of [^{3}H]CGP 54626 binding by R-(−)-baclofen. The addition of Gpp(NH)p to the assay caused a shift to the right of the competition curves. The concentration of Gpp(NH)p is sufficient to transform all high-affinity conformations into low-affinity ones (see section on *Inhibition of Agonist [^{3}H]CGP 27492 binding by Gpp(NH)p in GAERS and in control rats*, next page). Analyses using the LIGAND program of the inhibition by baclofen of [^{3}H]CGP 54626 binding fitted to a two-site model with a probability of 99 per cent.

Similar binding parameters and Gpp(NH)p shifts were observed in GAERS and in control rats ($P > 0.10$), suggesting that the interaction between GABA$_B$ receptors and G proteins in GAERS does not differ from the interaction observed in the non-epileptic control rats. Inhibition by baclofen of the specific binding of [^{3}H]CGP 54626 to frozen and thawed crude membranes prepared from the cerebelli of GAERS and controls rats gave similar results (results not shown).

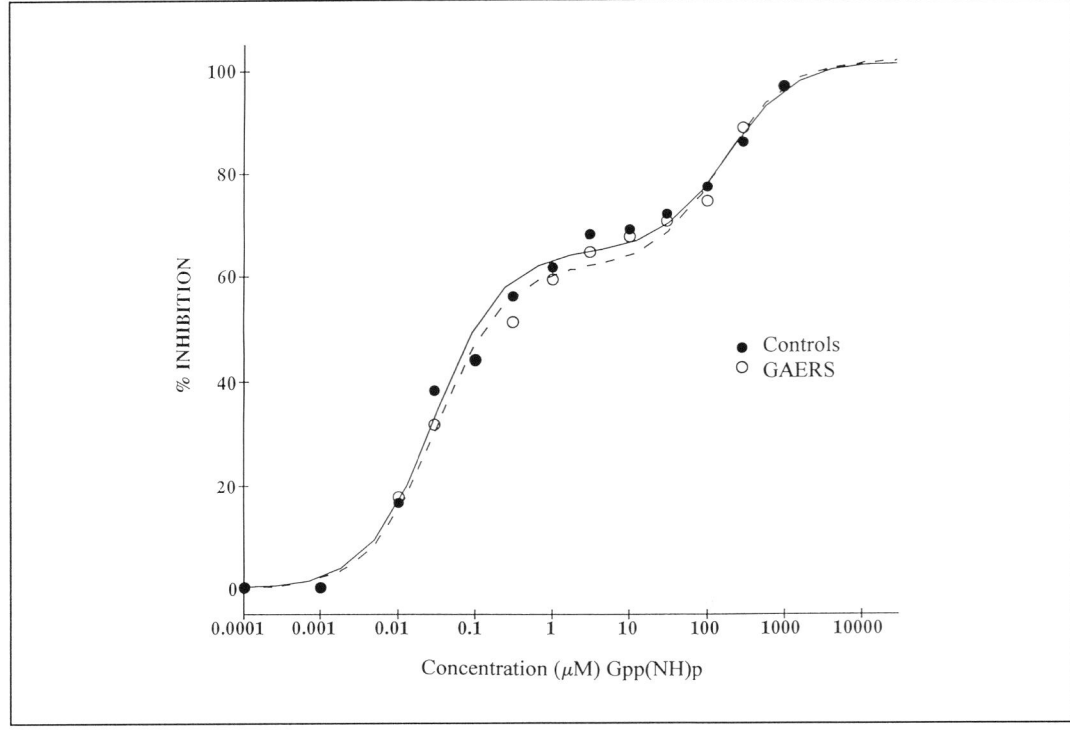

Fig. 3. Inhibition by Gpp(NH)p of specific [³H]CGP 27492 binding to GABA$_B$ receptors in cortical membranes from GAERS and from non-epileptic rats. Membranes were incubated in the presence of 1 nM [³H]CGP 27492 with increasing concentrations of Gpp(NH)p (from 0.1 nM to 1 mM). Total binding was measured in the absence of Gpp(NH)p. Standard errors of the means were less than 5 per cent and not shown. The binding parameters calculated by computer analysis (LIGAND) are shown in Table 3.

Inhibition of agonist [³H]CGP 27492 binding by Gpp(NH)p in GAERS and in control rats

We examined the regulation of GABA$_B$ binding by Gpp(NH)p as an index of the coupling of GABA$_B$ receptors to G proteins. We utilized this effect to test whether this coupling is altered in GAERS as compared to non-epileptic control rats. Concentrations of Gpp(NH)p from 0.1 nM to 1 mM inhibited [³H]CGP 27492 binding in GAERS and controls in a concentration-dependent manner (Fig. 3 & Table 3). Analyses of the displacement curves revealed two IC$_{50}$ values, which may be taken as an indication for two different interactions between GABA$_B$ receptors and G proteins.

Table 3. Binding parameters of the inhibition of [³H]CGP 27492 binding by Gpp(NH)p in cortical membranes of GAERS and non-epileptic rats

	n_H	B_{max} Site A %	B_{max} Site B %	IC$_{50}$ Site A (nM)	IC$_{50}$ Site B (μM)
Controls	0.31 ± 0.02	60.5 ± 0.9	39.5 ± 2.3	29.1 ± 2.5	184.2 ± 50.5
GAERS	0.31 ± 0.02	63.6 ± 1.0	36.4 ± 2.9	31.9 ± 2.5	161.0 ± 33.8

Data for cortical membranes represent the mean ± SEM of four experiments performed in triplicate. Similar results were observed in the cerebellum (n = 2) and in the hippocampus (n = 1). The values for the binding parameters obtained in GAERS did not differ from those observed in non-epileptic control rats ($P > 0.10$, Student's t-test).

The high affinity IC_{50} values in GAERS and controls were 31.9 ± 2.5 nM and 29.1 ± 2.5 nM, respectively. The low affinity IC_{50} value in GAERS was 161.0 ± 33.8 μM as compared to 184.2 ± 50.5 μM in non-epileptic Wistar rats. The binding parameters analysed in this displacement experiment were similar in GAERS and in controls ($P < 0.10$, Student's t-test).

Discussion

Affinity states of antagonist CGP 54626 binding in GAERS and in non-epileptic rats

One of the interesting findings of this study is the observation that either saturation experiments with the $GABA_B$ antagonist [^{3}H]CGP 54626 or competition between this radioligand and the agonist R-(–)-baclofen uncovered several affinity states of $GABA_B$ receptors. The pharmacological and clinical significance of such multiple binding sites is still speculative (Wojcik & Holopainen, 1992) and the purpose of this study is not to analyse in detail the different binding parameters (Mathivet et al., to be published), but rather to use them as tools to investigate $GABA_B$-receptor-mediated transmission in GAERS and in controls. The second important finding is that all binding parameters of these different binding sites for the $GABA_B$ receptors investigated are similar in GAERS and in non- epileptic control rats.

Coupling to G proteins

$GABA_B$-receptor binding is inhibited by GTP through interaction with pertussis toxin-sensitive G proteins. Because G proteins appear to modulate many of the effects induced by activation of $GABA_B$ receptors (Dolphin, 1987), we investigated whether pertussis toxin could alter absence seizures. Intrathalamic injections of the toxin induced a time- and dose-dependent suppression of spike-and-wave discharges in GAERS (Mathivet et al., to be published). These results suggested that interaction between the $GABA_B$ receptor and its G protein is necessary for the generation of absence seizures. We examined the regulation of $GABA_B$ binding by Gpp(NH)p as an index of the interaction of $GABA_B$ receptors to G proteins. Hill et al. (1984) have shown that GTP decreased the affinity of the binding of agonists to the $GABA_B$ receptor, and did not affect the number of binding sites. The effect of Gpp(NH)p on [^{3}H] CGP 27492 binding and of the inhibition of CGP 54626 binding by R-(–)- baclofen revealed two different interactions between $GABA_B$ receptors and G proteins which were identical in GAERS and in congenic rats. This suggests that the two interactions of the $GABA_B$-binding site with the G-protein are similar in both strains.

Relevance to other models and to humans

The results of this investigation do not suggest that the physiological mediator of the genetic predisposition to absence seizures in GAERS is due to an alteration in GABA-ergic neurotransmission which is caused either by a change in the density of $GABA_B$ receptors, or by an alteration in the affinity for the agonist R-(–)-baclofen or by changes in the population of the different affinity states of $GABA_B$ receptors or a difference in interaction to the G protein.

These results are in line with clinical observations that baclofen can exacerbate absence seizures in patients with absence epilepsy but is unable to induce absence seizures in non-epileptic patients and that it does not induce spike-and-wave discharges in control animals.

In the lethargic (lh/lh) mice, Lin et al. (1993) observed an increased number of $GABA_B$ receptors as compared to wild (+/+) age-matched congenic mice. The different animal models of absence epilepsy and binding techniques used may explain the discrepancy between their observations and those of this study. On the other hand, the differences between the lethargic mice and GAERS may reflect clinical differences in absence epilepsy suggesting that $GABA_B$-receptor antagonists may be effective in different types of absence epilepsy.

Conclusion

On the basis of our results, the hypothesis that a dysfunction in $GABA_B$ receptors or an alteration in the interaction of these receptors to G proteins could account for the generation of spike-and-wave discharges in thalamo-cortical neurones of GAERS seems unlikely. However, there are some limitations to the interpretation of the results of this study. A small population of $GABA_B$ receptors with distinct pharmacological properties may be involved in the pathogenesis of absence seizures and could still be undetected by the $GABA_B$-receptor assays used in this study. The techniques of molecular biology have not yet led to the cloning of the $GABA_B$ receptor, and therefore the structural peculiarities of the putative subtypes of $GABA_B$ receptor are as yet unknown. The only possibility available at present to detect and characterize $GABA_B$-receptor subtypes is to use a combination of binding and pharmacological techniques.

Other alterations of $GABA_B$-mediated inhibitory transmission could be responsible for the pathological oscillatory properties observed in absence epilepsy. Alternatively, the dysfunction could be located at the level of neurotransmitter transport mechanisms or at the effector level.

In the last few years most research in epilepsy has focused on the *in vitro* analyses of neurotransmitter levels and enzyme activities, together with receptor affinities and densities in brain tissue. Comparatively few studies have examined signal transduction pathways beyond receptor levels in epilepsy. Investigation of the functional integrity of receptor mediated signal transduction is, therefore, essential for evaluating whether inhibitory neurotransmission mediated by $GABA_B$ receptors is altered in absence epilepsy.

References

Bittiger, H., Reymann, N., Hall, R. & Kane, P. (1988): CGP 27492, a new potent and selective radioligand for $GABA_B$ receptors. Proceeding of the 11th Meeting of the ENA, Zürich. **Abstr. 16.10,** Suppl. to *Eur. J. Neurosci.*

Bittiger, H., Froestl, W., Hall, R., Karlsson, G., Klebs, K., Olpe, H.-R., Pozza, M., Steinmann, M. & Van Riezen H. (1990): Biochemistry, electrophysiology and pharmacology of a new $GABA_B$ antagonist: CGP 35348. In: *$GABA_B$ receptors in mammalian function*, eds. N.G. Bowery, H. Bittiger & H.-R. Olpe, pp. 47–60. Chichester: John Wiley.

Bittiger, H., Reymann, N., Froestl, W. & Mickel, S.J. (1992): ^{3}H-CGP 54626: a potent antagonist radioligand for $GABA_B$ receptors. *Pharmacol. Commun.* **2,** 23.

Dolphin, A.C. (1987): Nucleotide binding proteins in signal transduction and disease. *Trends Neurosci.* **10,** 53–57.

Dolphin, A.C. & Scott, R.H. (1987): Calcium channel currents and their inhibition by (–)-baclofen in rat sensory neurones: modulation by guanine nucleotides. *J. Physiol.* **386,** 1–17.

Gloor, P. & Fariello, R.G. (1988): Generalized epilepsy: some of its cellular mechanisms differ from those of focal epilepsy. *Trends Neurosci.* **11,** 63–68.

Hill, D. R., Bowery, N.G. & Hudson, A.L. (1984): Inhibition of $GABA_B$ receptor binding by guanyl nucleotides. *J. Neurochem.* **42,** 652–657.

Hosford, D.A., Clark, S., Cao, Z., Wilson, W.A., Lin, F-H., Morrisett, R.A. & Huin, A. (1992a): The role of $GABA_B$ receptor activation in absence seizures of lethargic (*lh/lh*) mice. *Science* **257,** 398–401.

Hosford, D.A., Clark, S., Cao, Z., Wilson, W.A., Lin, F-H., Morrisett, R.A. & Huin, A. (1992b): Evidence for $GABA_B$ receptor activation in the lethagic (*lh/lh*) mouse model of absence seizures. *Pharmacol. Commun.* **2,** 123–124.

King, G.A. (1979): Effects of systemically applied GABA agonists and antagonists on wave-spike ECoG activity in rat. *Neuropharmacology* **18,** 47–55.

Knight, A.R. & Bowery, N.G. (1992): GABA receptors in rats with spontaneous generalized nonconvulsive epilepsy. *J. Neural Transm.* **[Suppl] 35,** 189–196.

Lin, F-H., Cao, Z. & Hosford, D.A. (1993): Selective increase in $GABA_B$ receptor number in lethargic (*lh/lh*) mouse model of absence seizures. *Brain Res.* **608,** 101–106.

Lowry, O.H., Rosebrough, N.J., Farr, A.L. & Randall, R.J. (1951): Protein measurement with the Folin phenol reagent. *J. Biol. Chem.* **193,** 265–275.

Marescaux, C., Vergnes, M. & Bernasconi, R. (1992a): GABA$_B$ receptor antagonists: potential new anti-absence drugs. *J. Neural Transm.* **[Suppl] 35,** 179–188.

Marescaux, C., Liu, Z., Bernasconi, R. & Vergnes, M. (1992b): GABA$_B$ receptors are involved in the occurrence of absence seizures in rats. *Pharmacol. Commun.* **2,** 57–62.

Marescaux, C., Vergnes, M. & Depaulis, A. (1992c): Genetic absence epilepsy in rats from Strasbourg – a review. *J. Neural Transm.* **[Suppl.] 35,** 37–69.

Munson, P.J. & Rodbard, D. (1980): LIGAND, a versatile computerized approach for characterization of ligand-binding systems. *Anal. Biochem.* **107,** 220–239.

Snead, O.C., Depaulis, A., Banerjee, P.K., Hechler, V. & Vergnes, M. (1992): The GABA$_A$ receptor complex in experimental absence seizures in rat: an autoradiography study. *Neurosci. Lett.* **140,** 9–12.

Wojcik, W.J. & Holopainen, I. (1992): Role of central GABA$_B$ receptors in physiology and pathology. *Neuropsychopharmacology* **6,** 201–214.

Vergnes, M. & Marescaux, C. (1994): Pathophysiological mechanisms underlying genetic absence epilepsy in rats. In: *Idiopathic generalized epilepsies: clinical, experimental and genetic aspects*, eds. A. Malafosse, P. Genton, E. Hirsch, C. Marescaux. D. Broglin & R. Bernasconi, pp. 151-168. London: John Libbey.

Chapter 18

The role of $GABA_B$-receptor activation in the lethargic (*lh/lh*) mouse model of primary generalized absence seizures

David A. Hosford, Fu-hsiung Lin, Zhen Cao, Diana L. Kraemer, Alex Huin, Eric Akawie, Yin Yin and John T. Wilson

Epilepsy Research Laboratory, Departments of Medicine (Neurology) and Neurobiology, Duke University and Durham Veterans Administration Medical Centers, Building 16, Room 20, 508 Fulton Street, Durham, North Carolina 27705, USA

Introduction

The need for animal models to study mechanisms and neural networks

The majority of patients with primary generalized absence (PGA) seizures are successfully treated with currently available antiabsence drugs (Berkovic, 1993). However, the development of newer anti-absence drugs would benefit both patients who are refractory to current anti-absence treatments, and those with unpleasant side effects of these treatments. The development of new anti-absence therapy will be facilitated by understanding the mechanisms and neural networks underlying PGA seizures. Animal models permit the elucidation of these mechanisms and networks, as well as the testing of potential new anti-absence drugs.

The rationale for studying *lh/lh* mice

Our goal at the outset of these studies was to seek an animal model with seizures that: (a) bore behavioural and pharmacological similarity to a specific type of human seizures; (b) were spontaneous, eliminating the possibility that the methods used to induce seizures might alter the mechanisms that were to be studied; and (c) would eventually allow us to exploit molecular biological techniques to determine the genetic regulation of the mechanism(s) underlying its seizures. Earlier descriptions of the lethargic (*lh/lh*) mutant mouse (Sidman *et al.*, 1965; Noebels, 1986) suggested that it would meet these criteria.

The *lh/lh* strain arose as a spontaneous mutation in a BALB/cGn strain at Jackson Labs. The strain has a single-locus mutation on chromosome 2 (Sidman *et al.*, 1965; Green, 1989), and expresses a phenotype of spontaneous seizures (Noebels, 1986), ataxia (Sidman *et al.*, 1965), and a defect in cell-mediated immunity (Dung, 1977). The phenotype currently resides in a B6C3HF1 background (the F_1 from C57Bl/6JEi × C3H/HESnJ males). Early studies conducted by Noebels *et al.* (1986) suggested that *lh/lh* mice had spontaneous spike-and-wave discharges similar to those observed in the tottering (*tg/tg*) model of seizures. In this study (first goal: see *Goals of this Study* below), we extended their observations by showing that seizures in *lh/lh* mice had behavioural, electrographic and pharmacological profiles similar to those of PGA seizures in humans.

The rationale for studying thalamocortical GABA$_B$ receptors

Ablation studies in humans with absence seizures (Jasper & Droogleever-Fortuyn, 1946) and in animal models (Pellegrini & Gloor, 1979) suggested that multiple thalamic nuclei could elicit epileptiform activity through widespread, diffuse pathways to the neocortex. More recently, studies using the penicillin model (Avoli, 1987) and *in vitro* systems (Steriade & Llinás, 1988) suggested that thalamic and neocortical neurons were equally important in generating volleys of oscillatory burst-firing. Steriade & Llinás (1988) implicated a thalamocortical circuit comprising reticular thalamic nucleus (NRT), thalamic relay neurons, and neocortical pyramidal cells.

Based on these findings, the search for mechanisms underlying absence seizures focused on mechanisms capable of triggering oscillatory burst-firing of thalamic neurons. Recent findings implicated low-threshold calcium (LTC) spikes elicited by activation of the T-type calcium channel (Coulter *et al.*, 1989a). Once activated, T-channels become inactivated and require a long-lasting hyperpolarization to reverse their inactivation (Coulter *et al.*, 1989b). The long-lasting IPSPs produced by activation of GABA$_B$ receptors are theoretically capable of reversing the inactivation of T-channels. Supporting this idea, GABA$_B$-receptor-mediated IPSPs in thalamic slices triggered LTC spikes that caused burst-firing of thalamic neurons (Crunelli *et al.*, 1989). Together, these data suggested the hypothesis that GABA$_B$ receptors in thalamic neurons could trigger absence seizures (Crunelli & Leresche, 1991).

Goals of this study

In this study we accomplished two goals. First, we validated an animal model of PGA seizures, the lethargic (*lh/lh*) mutant mouse. Our second goal was to use the *lh/lh* model of PGA seizures to: (i) test the role of GABA$_B$-receptor-mediated mechanisms in PGA seizures; (ii) study mechanisms underlying the role of GABA$_B$ receptors in these seizures; and (iii) begin to identify the neural network of structures in which GABA$_B$ receptors regulate the generation of PGA seizures. Identification of this neural network will facilitate further biochemical and electrophysiological studies of the mechanisms underlying the role of GABA$_B$ receptors in PGA seizures.

Methods

Colonization of lethargic (*lh/lh*) and wild mice

All of our colonies were initiated with stocks obtained from Jackson Labs. We maintain a colony of wild mice (+/+) that is coisogenic to *lh/lh*. The +/+ strain comprises all F_1 progeny of C57Bl/6JEi females × C3H/HeSnJ males; the colony yields about 30 +/+ newborn males per average month. We also maintain a colony of *lh/lh* mice. Male lh/+ (heterozygote) mice are bred with female lh/+ mice to produce 25 per cent *lh/lh* (about 30 male *lh/lh* per month) in the F_2 generation. By 3 weeks of age, *lh/lh* mice are easily distinguished from their phenotypically normal lh/+ and +/+ littermates by the presence of an ataxic gait. Because *lh/lh* mice are immunodeficient, both colonies are kept in an immunoprotected environment in the Duke University Vivarium.

Implantation of neocortical electrodes and subcortical cannulae

Male 8-week-old *lh/lh* mice were weighed, anaesthetized with sodium pentobarbital (50 mg/kg intraperitoneally (i.p.)), and placed into a stereotaxic holder fitted with a mouse incisor bar (David Kopf Instruments). Burr holes were drilled unilaterally (for studies including microinjections) or bilaterally (for studies without microinjections) over the frontal neocortex (1.5 mm lateral to the midsagittal suture and 1.5 mm anterior to bregma), and bilaterally over ventroanterolateral (VAL) thalamic relay nucleus (1.3 mm posterior to bregma; 1.6 mm lateral; all coordinates from Slotnick & Leonard (1975). Bipolar Teflon-coated microelectrodes (constructed from monopolar electrodes with a 0.011 inch outer diameter; A-M Products, Inc.) were lowered into the frontal neocortex (0.8 mm below dura). Subcortical guide cannulae (22-gauge; Plastic Products) were implanted bilaterally through their burr holes to a depth 0.5 mm dorsal to their intended target (final depth for VAL 3.6 mm below dura). Four screws, placed at the periphery of the skull, served as grounds for the electrodes and helped anchor a dental acrylic cap. After all surgical procedures, mice were allowed to recover for at least 7 days before experiments. After experiments animals were killed (100 mg/kg sodium pentobarbital i.p.). Cannula placements were verified histologically by a blinded observer who examined serial brain sections (stained with cresyl violet) for the most ventral position of the cannula tracks.

Analysis of absence seizure frequency in the presence of test drugs

At least 1 week after implantation, each group of mice (n = eight male 8-week-old *lh/lh* mice) underwent a series of six daily 3 h EEG recording sessions. Thirty min after each session began they were administered either vehicle (days 1, 3, and 5) or one of three doses of test drug (days 2, 4, and 6) via injection cannulae. Bilateral injection cannulae were lowered to their final targets under gentle hand-held restraint, and drug or vehicle was administered bilaterally at a rate of 0.25 µl/min to a total volume of 0.25 µl/site (Harvard infusion pump with Hamilton syringes). Cannulae were left in place an additional 2 min before they were withdrawn.

The following drugs were administered in testing antiepileptic drug efficacy: ethosuximide (100, 200 and 400 mg per kg i.p. in 0.9 per cent NaCl); trimethadione (100, 300 and 500 mg/kg i.p. in 0.9 per cent NaCl); clonazepam (3, 10 and 30 µg per kg i.p. in 40 per cent polyethylene glycol 400 mixed with 0.9 per cent NaCl); phenytoin (10, 20 and 40 mg/kg i.p. in 0.9 per cent NaCl); and carbamazepine (5, 10 and 20 mg/kg i.p. in 12.5 per cent propylene glycol). The following drugs were administered to test the role of $GABA_B$ receptors: (–)-Baclofen (0.5, 2.0 and 10 mg/kg i.p. in 40 per cent propylene glycol); CGP 35348 (25, 50 and 100 mg/kg i.p. in 0.9 per cent NaCl); and 2-hydroxysaclofen [2HS] (total dose 0.5, 2.5, or 10 µg in 0.9 per cent NaCl intraventricularly via cannulae implanted into both lateral ventricles 7 days previously by techniques similar to those used to implant microinjection cannulae).

During the 3 h EEG recording sessions, recording montages for each animal consisted of two monopolar derivations (each pole of the bipolar electrode to ground) and one bipolar derivation (one pole of the electrode to the other pole) for each electrode. Low- and high-frequency filters were set at 0.3 and 35 Hz, respectively; typical sensitivities ranged from 30–50 µV/mm. During these sessions the animals were observed for signs of sedation, increased ataxia, behavioural arrest, piloerection, and any stereotypic or clonic activity. This helped ensure that sedative effects of test drugs did not bias the actual seizure frequency. Animals were kept awake during these sessions by random, frequent hand-clapping by the technician.

EEGs were divided into 12 15-min epochs and the seizure frequency was counted by an observer blind to the drug treatment. Epileptiform bursts were counted as seizures only if they met all of four criteria: (1) bursts had a duration > 0.6 s; (2) bursts were comprised of truly epileptiform spikes (i.e. < 70 ms per spike); (3) bursts had a frequency 'typical' for that animal (5–6 Hz in all cases); (4) bursts were recorded in at least two channels simultaneously. Use of these criteria helped to exclude recording artifacts, and interobserver reliability was 90 per cent. To determine effects produced by a test compound, the seizure frequency of an animal during each of these 12 15-min epochs was divided by the seizure frequency in the corresponding epoch after vehicle administration. This normalized the effect in each animal against its own baseline seizure frequency, reducing interanimal variability. The mean change in seizure frequency during the epochs was then calculated for all the animals in the group.

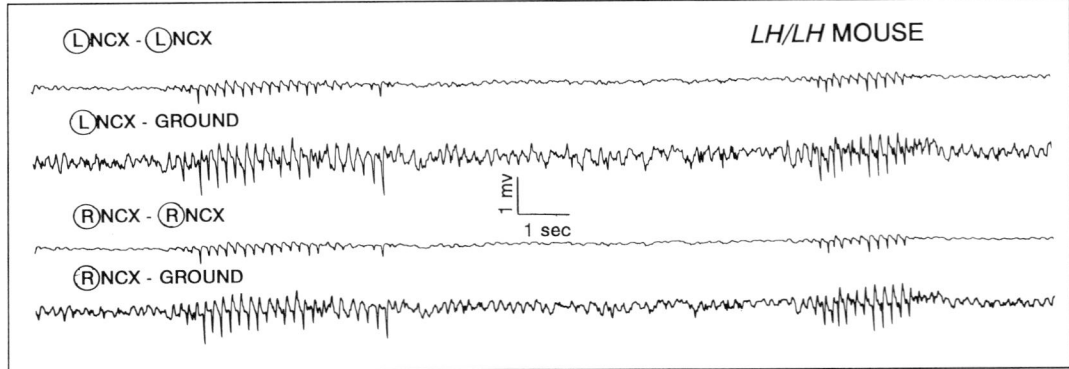

Fig. 1. EEG recording from frontal neocortex (NCX) of spontaneous seizures in an awake, freely moving lh/lh mouse. Electrographic bursts (seizures) arose from and returned to a normal waking background. EEG montages: bilateral bipolar recordings in frontal NCX; bilateral monopolar recordings, derived from one pole of each NCX electrode and a skull-screw reference (low- and high-frequency filters, 1 and 30 Hz).

Following the series of recordings, animals were killed (sodium pentobarbital, 100 mg/kg i.p.). Cannula placements were verified. Data were subjected to further analysis only if injection sites were present within the targeted structures.

Preparation of membranes and measurement of [^{3}H]baclofen binding

Male lh/lh and +/+ mice were anaesthetized with chloroform and decapitated. Brains were quickly removed, and the appropriate tissues were dissected over ice for further preparation. Neocortical tissue was homogenized and prepared using a series of cycles of resuspension, incubation, and centrifugation (Robinson et al., 1989)(buffer: 50 mM Tris HCl and 2.5 mM $CaCl_2$, pH 7.4 at 25 °C). The protein concentration of the final resuspension was 500–1500 µg/ml, measured by the method of Lowry (1951). $GABA_B$-receptor binding assays (adapted from Bowery et al. (1984)) were conducted as follows, using freshly prepared membranes. A quantity of membranes sufficient to contain 100 µg protein was added to incubation buffer (as above) containing [^{3}H]-baclofen (2–500 nM for Scatchard analyses; 10 nM for other experiments) and test drugs, either in the presence (nonspecific binding) or absence (total binding) of 500 µM GABA. The final incubation volume was 400 µl. Incubation was performed for 20 min at 25 °C. Incubation was terminated by centrifugation (15000 g for 10 min at 4 °C). The pellet was quickly washed three times, solubilized, and then counted with liquid scintillation spectrometry.

Preparation and analysis of baclofen-displaceable [^{3}H]GABA autoradiograms

The following procedure was modified from that of Bowery et al. (1987). lh/lh and +/+ mice were anaesthetized and decapitated; brains were quickly removed and frozen. Sections (16 µm) were cut at −18 °C and thaw-mounted onto acid-washed, gel-coated slides (Hosford et al., 1990). These slides were kept at −70 °C until the day of each experiment. Fingernail polish was used to paint wells around the sections on each slide, which were kept horizontal for the experiment. During preincubation, each section was covered with 200 µl of buffer (50 mM Tris-HCl with 2.5 mM $CaCl_2$, pH 7.4 at 25 °C) for 45 min at 25 °C. After the sections dried (20 min), sections were incubated for 45 min at 4 °C by applying 200 µl incubation buffer (buffer as above, with 20 nM [^{3}H]GABA (50 Ci/mmol; Dupont-NEN) and 10 µM isoguvacine (a $GABA_A$ agonist), either in the presence (nonspecific binding) or absence (total binding) of 100 µM baclofen). Each slide was then rapidly dipped into 2.5 per cent glutaraldehyde in acetone, and then twice into distilled water. Slides were dried under a stream of cool, filtered air (requires 30 s). They were apposed with tritium standards against [^{3}H]Ultrofilm (Amersham) at 4 °C for an exposure time of 3–4 weeks. Autoradio-

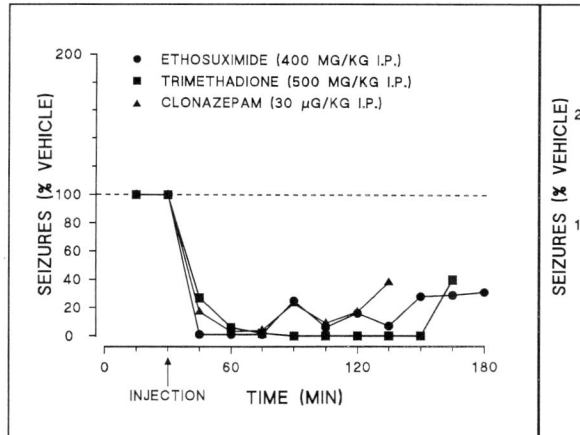 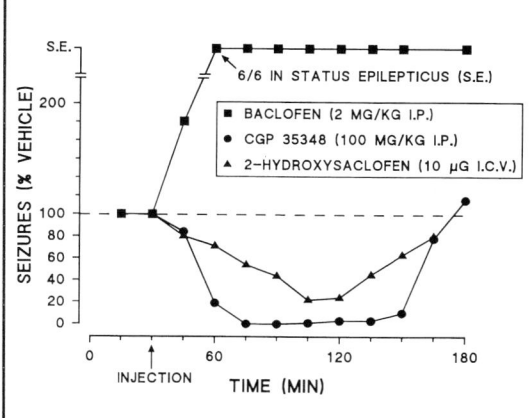

Fig. 2. Effects of antiepileptic drugs on seizure frequency in lh/lh mice. Graph depicts seizure frequency during each 15 min epoch after administration of ethosuximide (ETX), trimethadione (TMD), or clonazepam (CLO) as a percent of seizure frequency following administration of vehicle (VEH) (dotted line).

Fig. 3. Effects of GABA$_B$ receptor ligands ((−)baclofen, CGP 35348 and 2-HS) on seizure frequency in lh/lh mice, compared to effect produced by vehicle (dotted line). The seizure frequency during status epilepticus was arbitrarily assigned a score of 10 (a frequency 10 times that after vehicle); often the actual score was higher than 10.

grams were digitized and analysed using a computer-assisted image-analysis system (RAS/R1000; Loats, Inc.). Optical density (OD) measurements of the tritium standards allowed conversion of OD measurements into units of fmole/mg protein.

Results

Behavioural, electrographic and pharmacological features of seizures in *lh/lh* mice

We characterized seizures in *lh/lh* mice using behavioural, electroencephalographic (EEG), and pharmacological criteria. Ninety-four per cent (n = 96) of *lh/lh* (all ages observed, 5 weeks to 5 months) but no *lh/+* or *+/+* mice exhibited bilaterally synchronous electrographic bursts (seizures) of 5–6 Hz spike-wave complexes (Fig. 1). The mean seizure duration was 1.5 s (range, 0.6 to 5.0 s), and the mean seizure frequency was 127/h (range, 42 to 239/h). The seizures were accompanied by immobility and reduced responsiveness to external stimuli lasting the precise duration of the electrographic burst; no clonic activity was observed. These electrographic and behavioural characteristics of seizures in *lh/lh* mice are similar to those of PGA seizures in humans (Hosford et al., 1992).

To test the hypothesis that seizures in *lh/lh* mice were absence-like, we tested a series of anticonvulsants that were effective against either PGA or partial seizures. Compared to vehicle, anticonvulsants effective against PGA seizures in humans produced a dose-dependent reduction in seizure frequency (ethosuximide (ETX); trimethadione (TMD); clonazepam (CLO); only highest doses shown) (Fig. 2). In contrast, phenytoin and carbamazepine (anticonvulsants ineffective against PGA seizures but effective against partial seizures in humans) did not reduce seizure frequency. The inability of phenytoin to reduce seizure frequency was not caused by inadequate central nervous system concentrations, because the same doses of phenytoin significantly reduced ($P < 0.05$) tonic hindlimb extension during maximal electroshock seizures in *lh/lh* mice.

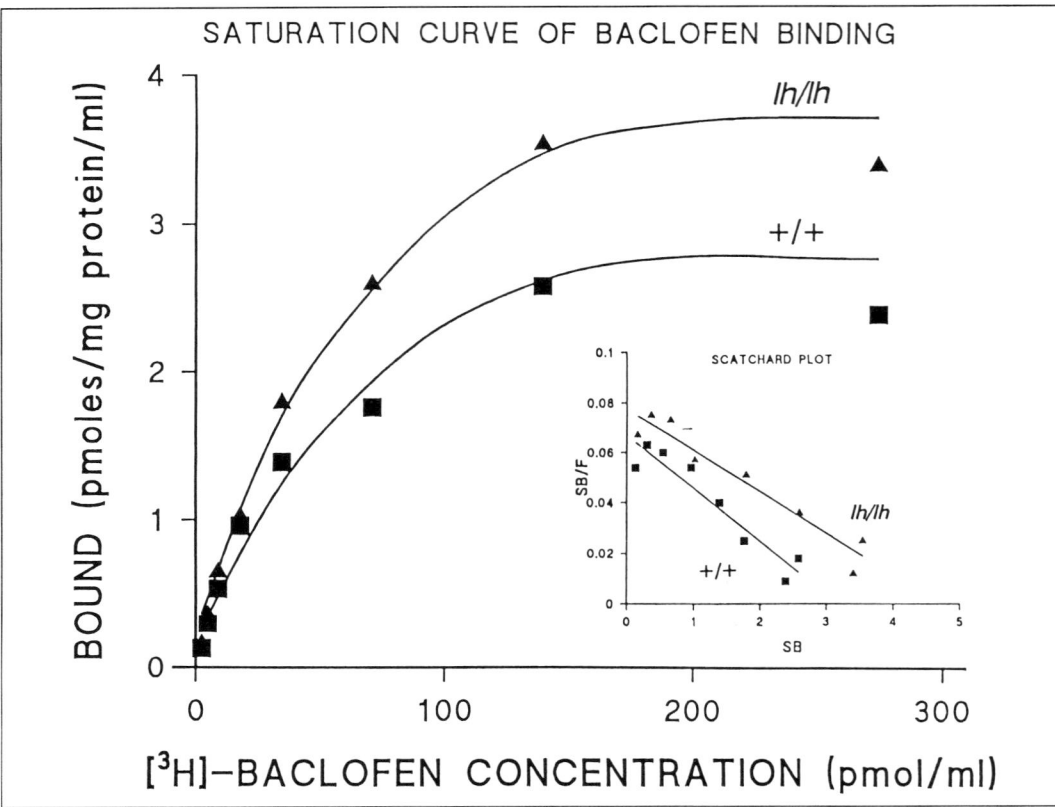

Fig. 4. GABA$_B$-binding isotherms and Scatchard analyses in neocortical membranes from matched lh/lh (solid triangles) and +/+ (solid squares) mice. When the increased binding in lh/lh mice (large figure) was analysed by the method of Scatchard (inset), there was a significant ($P < 0.02$) increase in maximum number of binding sites in lh/lh mice, but no change in the equilibrium dissociation constant.

Effects of compounds acting at GABA$_B$ receptors on seizures in *lh/lh* mice

To test the hypothesis that GABA$_B$-receptor activation was required for PGA seizures, we examined the effect of GABA$_B$-receptor agonists and antagonists on seizure frequency in *lh/lh* mice. Administration of the GABA$_B$ agonist (−)baclofen produced a significant dose-dependent increase in seizure frequency in *lh/lh* mice (Fig. 3). The same doses of baclofen produced sedation but no seizures in matched, nonepileptic +/+ mice, providing evidence against a nonspecific proconvulsant effect. Administration of the systemically active GABA$_B$-receptor antagonist CGP 35348 produced a dose-dependent abolition of seizures in *lh/lh* mice (Fig. 3). Moreover, administration of the structurally unrelated GABA$_B$-receptor antagonist 2HS (not systemically active; given i.c.v.) produced a dose-dependent suppression of seizure frequency (Fig. 3).

Kinetics of GABA$_B$-binding sites and coupling to G proteins

To test the hypothesis that an alteration in either binding affinity or number (B_{max}) of GABA$_B$ receptors underlies its enhanced activation in *lh/lh* mice, we measured GABA-displaceable [^{3}H]baclofen binding in neocortical membranes from *lh/lh* and +/+ mice. Scatchard analyses revealed a small (26 per cent) but significant increase in the number of GABA$_B$-binding sites from *lh/lh* mice compared to age-matched +/+ mice (Fig. 4); there was no significant difference in the equilibrium

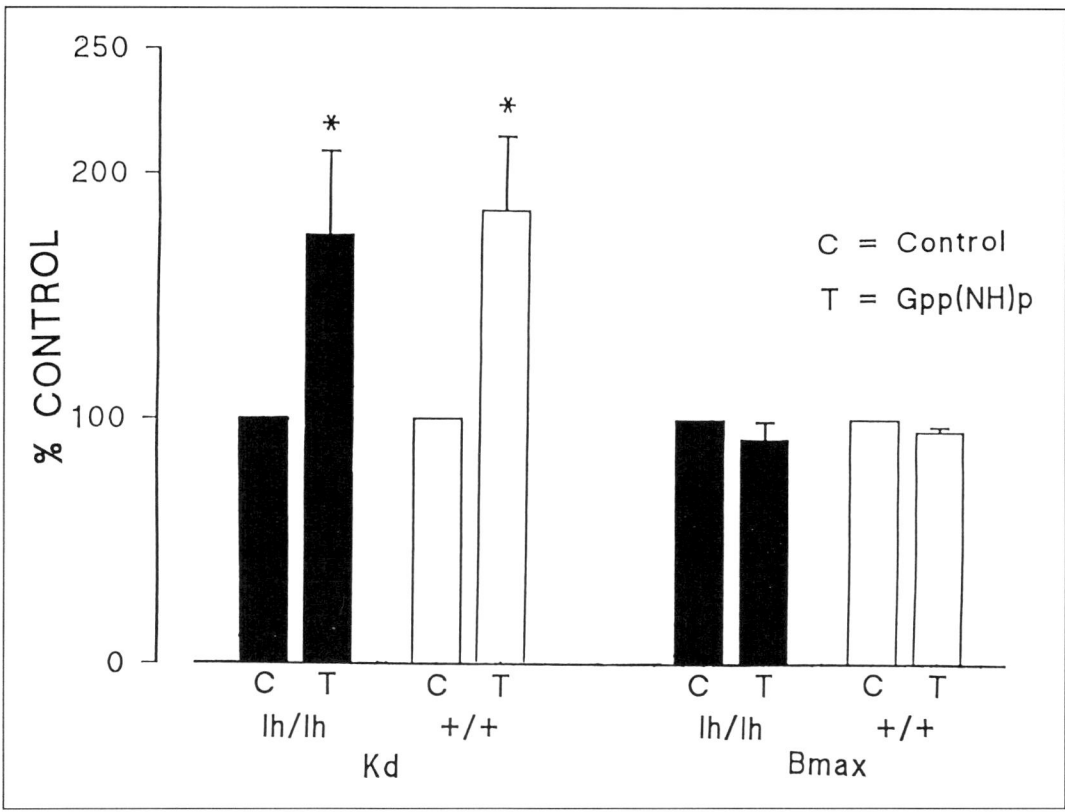

Fig. 5. Indirect measure of coupling of $GABA_B$-binding site to G proteins in membranes from matched lh/lh and +/+ mice. The irreversible GTP analogue Gpp(NH)pp ('T' condition) significantly ($P < 0.01$) increased the K_d of [^{3}H]baclofen binding compared to control binding ('C' condition) in membranes from both lh/lh and matched +/+ mice. There was no difference in the extent to which K_d was increased in the two strains of mice. There was no effect of Gpp(NH)p on the maximal number of sites in either strain of mice.

dissociation constant (K_d) of $GABA_B$ receptors. Interestingly, the B_{max} of $GABA_B$ receptors was positively correlated with seizure frequency in *lh/lh* mice. This increased number of $GABA_B$ receptors was selective, because Scatchard analyses of NMDA and $GABA_A$ receptor binding revealed no differences in the binding characteristics of these receptors in *lh/lh* and +/+ mice.

To test an alternative possibility that the enhanced effect of $GABA_B$-receptor activation stems from increased coupling of the receptor to G-proteins, we examined the ability of GTP analogues to inhibit $GABA_B$-receptor binding in membranes from *lh/lh* and +/+ mice. There was no difference in the ability of a GTP analogue to reduce the binding affinity of the $GABA_B$-binding site for [^{3}H]baclofen in membranes from *lh/lh* mice and matched controls (Fig. 5)(Lin et al., 1993).

$GABA_B$ autoradiograms, subcortical EEG recordings, and microinjection studies in *lh/lh* mice

To further characterize the regulatory role of $GABA_B$ receptors in PGA seizures, future studies will focus upon the neural network that generates these seizures, and in which $GABA_B$ receptors exert their pro-absence effect. To begin to identify the neuronal structures comprising this network, we accepted candidate neuronal structures if they passed three screening criteria: (i) those with an enriched density of $GABA_B$-binding sites; (ii) those passing the previous screen and able to gener-

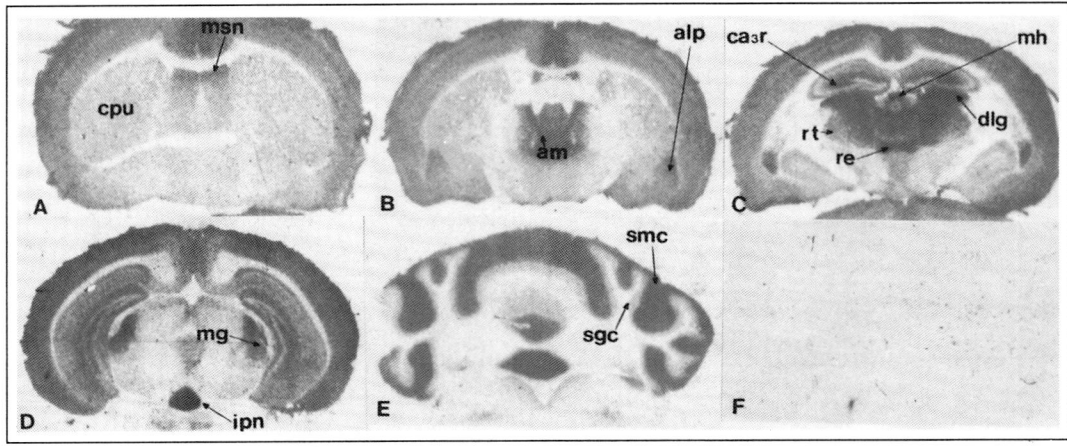

Fig. 6. Baclofen-displaceable [³H]GABA autoradiograms in slide-mounted coronal sections from 8-week-old male lh/lh mice. Structures labelled include alp (posterolateral amygdaloid nuc.), am (anteromedial thalamic nuc.), ca3r (stratum radiatum of hippocampal area CA3), cpu (caudate-putamen), dlg (dorsolateral geniculate nuc.), ipn (interpeduncular nuc.), mg (medial geniculate nuc.), mh (medial habenular nuc.), msn (medial septal nuc.), re (nuc. reuniens), rt (nuc. reticularis thalami), sgc (stratum granulosum of cerebellum), and smc (stratum moleculare of cerebellum). Panels A–E show total binding at five levels of brain; panel F is a representative figure of nonspecific binding.

ate PGA seizures synchronously with neocortex; (iii) those passing both screens and in which microinjections of baclofen or CGP 35348 enhanced or suppressed PGA seizures, respectively.

In the first screen, we used autoradiographic techniques to examine the anatomical distribution of baclofen-displaceable [³H]GABA binding in slide-mounted sections of *lh/lh* mouse brain (Fig. 6) (methods similar to Bowery et al., 1987). Quantitation of the autoradiograms showed that the density of GABA$_B$-binding sites was highly enriched in neocortical layers, stratum radiatum of

Table 1. Baclofen-displaceable [³H]GABA binding in lh/lh mouse brain

Region	Protein (fmol/mg)	Region	Protein (fmol/mg)
Telencephalon		**Diencephalon**	
Frontal neocortex		Thalamic nuclei	
Layers 1–3	209 ± 27	Lateral	220 ± 76
Layers 4–6	181 ± 22	Anterodorsal	173 ± 16
Septum		Anteromedial	234 ± 23
Lateral	147 ± 23	Anteroventral	191 ± 13
Medial	114 ± 20	Ventroanterolateral	197 ± 18
Neostriatum	93 ± 13	Ventromedial	300 ± 13
Hippocampus		Reticularis	132 ± 13
Dentate gyrus		Reuniens	278 ± 33
Str. gran.	118 ± 9	Dorsolat. genic.	259 ± 14
Str. molec.	192 ± 8	Medial genic.	307 ± 46
Area CA3		Medial habenula	242 ± 29
Str. pyram.	129 ± 10		
Str. rad.	223 ± 16	**Brainstem**	
Str. oriens	113 ± 14	Superior colliculus (superfic. grey)	237 ± 40
Area CA1		Substantia nigra	85 ± 17
Str. pyram.	109 ± 8	Interpedunc. nuc.	443 ± 86
S tr. rad.	126 ± 6		
Str. oriens	113 ± 13	**Cerebellum**	
Amygdaloid nuclei		Str. granulosum	123 ± 28
Posterolat.	163 ± 19	Str. moleculare	293 ± 56
Medial	114 ± 20		

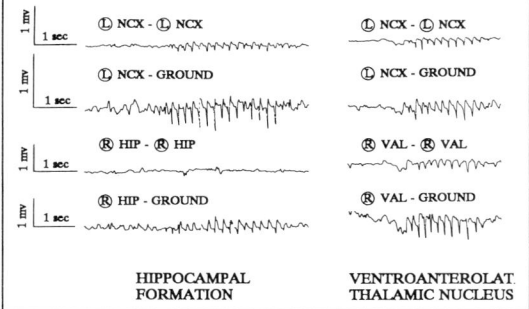

Fig. 7. EEG recordings from neocortex (NCX), hippocampal formation (HIP) and VAL thalamic nucleus. Settings are similar to those of Fig. 1. Note that seizures were recorded synchronously in bipolar derivations from neocortex and VAL, but not from hippocampal formation.

hippocampal area CA3, numerous thalamic subnuclei (particularly VAL and dorsolateral geniculate nuclei, and nucleus reuniens), posterolateral amygdaloid nucleus, interpeduncular nucleus, and stratum moleculare of cerebellum (Table 1)(Kraemer et al., 1992).

For the second screen we identified which of these neuronal structures generated PGA seizures, by recording from bipolar EEG electrodes implanted into each candidate neuronal structure. EEG recordings of seizures in 8-week-old lh/lh mice showed synchronous spike-and-wave discharges in neocortex and in VAL thalamic nucleus (n = 6 of 6; Fig. 7), but not in hippocampal formation (n = 0 of 6) or lateral amygdaloid nucleus (n = 0 of 6).

For the third screen we began to identify which of these structures had $GABA_B$ receptors that regulated PGA seizures, by microinjecting baclofen or its vehicle bilaterally into these structures and recording the effects on PGA seizures. When we microinjected baclofen (3–300 ng/side in 0.25 µl) into VAL thalamic nucleus of 8-week-old male lh/lh mice, baclofen produced a dose-dependent increase in seizure frequency (Fig. 8). Studies are still underway in other sites.

Discussion

Principal findings

This study resulted in four principal findings. First, lh/lh mice are a valid model of PGA seizures in humans. Second, there is an apparent requirement for $GABA_B$ receptors in the expression of PGA seizures in lh/lh mice. Third, one mechanism underlying this striking role of $GABA_B$ receptors may be the increased density of $GABA_B$-binding sites that we measured in lh/lh mice compared to matched controls. Fourth, the VAL thalamic relay nucleus is one of the structures within the neural network which generates PGA seizures, and in which $GABA_B$ receptors regulate those seizures.

Validation of lh/lh mice as a model of primary generalized absence seizures

Taken together, the similarity of the behavioural, electrographic, and pharmacological features of seizures in lh/lh mice to these seizures in humans validated lh/lh mice as a model of PGA seizures (Hosford et al., 1992). There are several other well-studied models of PGA seizures. The Genetic Absence Epilepsy-prone Rat of Strasbourg (GAERS) has spontaneous absence seizures and an antiepileptic drug sen-

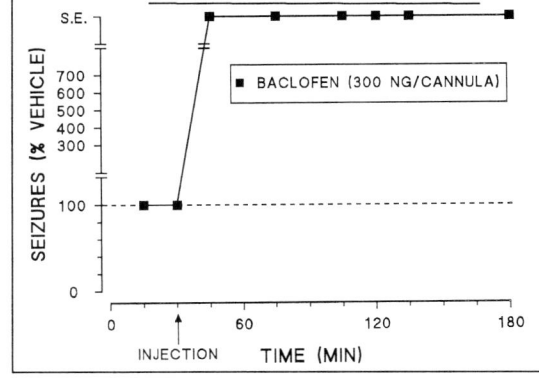

Fig. 8. Effect of microinjecting (–)baclofen bilaterally into the VAL thalamic nucleus on seizure frequency in lh/lh mice. Compared to vehicle (dotted line) microinjection of baclofen (300 ng/cannula) significantly ($P < 0.05$) suppressed PGA seizure frequency in 8-week-old male lh/lh mice (n = 6). Effects were dose-dependent; only highest doses are shown. Only mice with cannula sites in VAL are included.

sitivity similar to that of *lh/lh* mice (Vergnes et al., 1982; Marescaux et al., 1992b). However, the behavioural and electrographic features of these two models are somewhat different. First, the behavioural features of PGA seizures in GAERS include a lowering of the head and a myoclonic twitching of the vibrissae (Marescaux et al., 1992b); these features are reminiscent of human PGA seizures with a myoclonic component (Panayiotopoulos et al., 1989; Berkovic et al., 1993). In contrast, the PGA seizures in *lh/lh* mice are accompanied by immobility, without twitching of any kind (Hosford et al., 1992); these features are more reminiscent of childhood absence seizures in humans (Panayiotopoulos et al., 1989; Berkovic et al., 1993). Second, the spike-and-wave discharges of GAERS have a frequency of 7–11 Hz (Vergnes et al., 1982), whereas those of *lh/lh* mice have a frequency of 5–6 Hz (Hosford et al., 1992). The mechanisms underlying these differences appear to reside in the biophysical properties of ion channels in thalamic relay neurons. These ion channels, which generate the oscillatory burst-firing of spike-and-wave discharges, are critically dependent upon membrane potential (Steriade et al., 1993). GABAergic interneurons provide one of the main determinants of membrane potential, and hence powerfully regulate both the propensity and the frequency of thalamocortical burst-firing. The density of these thalamic interneurons varies widely across species (Steriade et al., 1990), providing a plausible reason that the frequency of burst-firing should also vary widely across species.

The tottering (*tg/tg*) mouse also has spontaneous PGA seizures that are well-characterized (Noebels et al., 1986). The behavioural and electrographic profiles and antiepileptic drug sensitivity of *tg/tg* mice are quite similar to those of *lh/lh* mice. However, *tg/tg* mice also exhibit a second seizure type with a clonic component (Sidman et al., 1965; Noebels et al., 1986).

None of these different features that distinguish the several models of PGA seizures invalidate them as models of human PGA seizures. Instead, the diversity of animal models with their unique genetic bases and mechanisms underlying PGA seizures needs to be studied, in the hope that some of these mechanisms may be applicable to a subpopulation of the heterogenous group of humans with PGA seizures.

Requirement for GABA$_B$ receptors in absence seizures of *lh/lh* mice

At least one of the mechanisms that can generate PGA seizures appears to require GABA$_B$ receptors, because of our finding that administration of GABA$_B$ antagonists abolished seizures in *lh/lh* mice. Interestingly, administration of baclofen to *lh/lh* mice produced PGA status epilepticus at doses which did not affect matched +/+ mice. This finding may indicate that GABA$_B$ receptors in *lh/lh* mice are qualitatively different than those in their nonepileptic littermates.

Similar findings were obtained independently when GABA$_B$ antagonists were administered in two pharmacological models of PGA seizures (Snead, 1992) and in the GAERS model (Marescaux et al., 1992a). Together, these findings offer the hope that GABA$_B$-receptor antagonists may represent a new class of anti-absence drugs in human patients.

Increased number of GABA$_B$ receptors in *lh/lh* mice

Our finding of increased numbers of GABA$_B$-binding sites in neocortical membranes of *lh/lh* mice is significant for several reasons. First, it offers a possible mechanism that might underlie the generation of these seizures. If GABA$_B$-receptor-mediated IPSPs are required for the deinactivation of T-channels, thereby increasing the likelihood that thalamic neurons will participate in oscillatory burst-firing, then increased numbers of these receptors in the appropriate synapses could powerfully increase the chances of generating PGA seizures. Second, the quantitative increase in the numbers of these binding sites in *lh/lh* mice parallels the qualitative difference implied by the profound effect of baclofen administration in this strain. Thus, GABA$_B$ receptors in *lh/lh* mice may be both qualitatively and quantitatively different than those in their nonepileptic littermates. No change in GABA$_B$-receptor binding was found in studies of pharmacological models or in GAERS. The lack of increased GABA$_B$-binding density in these models underscores the differences between these models and *lh/lh* mice, further indicating the need to study all of these models.

When we indirectly measured and compared the coupling of GABA$_B$ receptors to G-proteins in *lh/lh* and +/+ mice, we found no evidence to support a change in coupling between the strains. Thus, there was no evidence of a further 'amplification' of GABA$_B$-receptor-mediated effects in *lh/lh* mice, beyond that conferred by the increased numbers of binding sites (Lin et al., 1993).

Neural network underlying absence seizures in *lh/lh* mice

To further characterize the regulatory role of GABA$_B$ receptors in the neural network that generates PGA seizures, we screened candidate neuronal structures for those that: (i) had enriched GABA$_B$-binding sites; (ii) generated PGA seizures; and (iii) had GABA$_B$ receptors that regulated the seizures. These studies are still ongoing, but our preliminary finding is that VAL thalamic nucleus is one of the structures in this neural network in *lh/lh* mice. Similar experiments are underway in other candidate thalamic nuclei (e.g. nucleus reuniens and NRT), based on the results of our GABA$_B$ autoradiograms and subcortical EEG recordings.

Interestingly, studies conducted in the GAERS model also suggested that lateral thalamic nuclei such as VAL are important to the generation of PGA seizures in that model (Vergnes et al., 1990; Liu et al., 1991; Vergnes & Marescaux, 1992). It will be important to continue to use these and other models to compare the neural networks which generate PGA seizures and in which GABA$_B$ receptors regulate these seizures. The mechanisms underlying the behavioural and electrographic differences of these models must be explained in order to begin to understand possible mechanisms underlying similar features of PGA seizures in human patients.

In conclusion, in these studies we obtained four principal findings. First, we characterized the behavioural and electrographic features, and antiepileptic drug sensitivity of spontaneous seizures expressed in lethargic (*lh/lh*) mutant mice. These features validated *lh/lh* mice as a model of primary generalized absence (PGA) seizures in humans. Second, we found that GABA$_B$ antagonists abolished PGA seizures in *lh/lh* mice, suggesting that GABA$_B$ receptors are required for their expression, and offering therapeutic promise in the treatment of humans with these seizures. Third, we found increased numbers of GABA$_B$-binding sites in neocortical membranes of *lh/lh* compared to matched control mice. The increased density of GABA$_B$-binding sites may underlie the requirement for these receptors in PGA seizures of *lh/lh* mice. Fourth, we began to determine the structures that comprise the neural network that generates PGA seizures, and in which GABA$_B$ receptors regulate these seizures. VAL thalamic nucleus is one of the structures of this network. Together, these findings show that *lh/lh* mice are a model in which to study the mechanisms underlying PGA seizures, and in which to test potential new anti-absence drugs.

Acknowledgement

We thank Drs Nevin Lambert, Darryl V. Lewis, James O. McNamara, David Mott, H. Scott Swartzwelder, and Wilkie A. Wilson, Jr. for helpful discussions of these experiments. We also thank Ms Betty Worrell and Ms Sarah Sneed for administrative assistance. These studies were funded by grants to DAH from the Epilepsy Foundation of America, NIH (NINDS), and Veterans Administration; and by a grant to F-HL from NINDS.

References

Avoli, M. (1987): Mechanisms of generalized epilepsy with spike-and-wave discharge. *EEG* (Suppl. **39**), 184–190.

Berkovic, S.F. (1993): Childhood absence epilepsy and juvenile absence epilepsy. In: *The treatment of epilepsy: principles and practice*, ed. E. Wyllie, pp. 547–551. Philadelphia: Lea & Febiger.

Bowery, N.G., Hill, D.R., Hudson, A.L., Price, G.W., Turnbull, M.J. & Wilkin, G.P. (1984): Heterogeneity of mammalian GABA receptors. In: *Actions and interactions of GABA and benzodiazepines*, ed. N.G. Bowery, pp. 81–108. Raven Press: New York.

Bowery, N.G., Hudson, A.L. & Price, G.W. (1987): GABA$_A$ and GABA$_B$ receptor site distribution in the rat central nervous system. *Neuroscience* **20**, 365–383.

Coulter, D.A., Huguenard, J.R. & Prince, D.A. (1989a): Characterization of ethosuximide reduction of low-threshold calcium current in thalamic neurons. *Ann. Neurol.* **25**, 582–593.

Coulter, D.A., Huguenard, J.R. & Prince, D.A. (1989b): Calcium currents in rat thalamocortical relay neurones: kinetic properties of the transient, low-threshold current. *J. Physiol.* **414**, 587–604.

Crunelli, V. & Leresche, N. (1991): A role for GABA$_B$ receptors in excitation and inhibition of thalamocortical cells. *Trends Neurol. Sci.* **14**, 16–21.

Crunelli, V., Lightowler, S. & Pollard, S.E. (1989): A T-type Ca^{2+} current underlies low-threshold Ca^{2+} potentials in cells of the cat and rat lateral geniculate nucleus. *J. Physiol.* **413**, 543–561.

Dung, H.C. (1977): Deficiency in the thymus-dependent immunity in 'lethargic' mutant mice. *Transplantation* **23**, 39–43.

Green, M.C. (1989): Catalog of mutant genes and polymorphic loci. In: *Genetic variants and strains of the laboratory mouse*, 2nd ed, eds. M.F. Lyon & A.G. Searle, pp. 12–403. Oxford: Oxford University Press.

Hosford, D.A., Bonhaus, D.W. & McNamara, J.O. (1990): A radiohistochemical measure of [^{3}H]-TCP binding to the activated NMDA-receptor-gated ion channel in rat brain. *Brain Res.* **516**, 192–200.

Hosford, D.A., Clark, S., Cao, Z., Wilson, W.A., Lin, F-H., Morrisett, R.A. & Huin, A. (1992): The role of GABA$_B$ receptor activation in absence seizures of lethargic (*lh/lh*) mice. *Science* **257**, 398–401.

Jasper, H.H. & Droogleever-Fortuyn, J. (1946): Experimental studies on the functional anatomy of petit mal epilepsy. *Res. Publ. Assoc. Res. Nerv. Ment. Dis.* **26**, 272–298.

Kraemer, D.L., Lin, F-H., Cao, Z. & Hosford, D.A. (1992): Anatomic distribution of GABA$_B$ receptors in the lethargic (*lh/lh*) mouse model of epilepsy. *Epilepsia* **33**, (Suppl. 3), 32.

Lin, F-H., Cao, Z. & Hosford, D.A. (1993): Selective increase in GABA$_B$ receptor number in lethargic (*lh/lh*) mouse model of absence seizures. *Brain Res.* **608**, 101–106.

Liu, Z., Vergnes, M., Depaulis, A. & Marescaux, C. (1991): Evidence for a critical role of GABAergic transmission within the thalamus in the genesis and control of absence seizures in the rat. *Brain Res.* **545**, 1–7.

Lowry, O.H., Rosebrough, N.J., Farr, A.L. & Randall, R.J. (1951): Protein measurement with the Folin phenol reagent. *J. Biol. Chem.* **193**, 265–275.

Marescaux, C., Vergnes, M. & Bernasconi, R. (1992a): GABA$_B$ receptor antagonists: potential new anti-absence drugs. *J. Neural Transm.* [Suppl.] **35**, 179–188.

Marescaux, C., Vergnes, M. & Depaulis, A. (1992b): Genetic absence epilepsy in rats from Strasbourg – a review. *J. Neural Transm.* [Suppl.] **35**, 37–69.

Noebels, J.L. (1986): Mutational analysis of inherited epilepsies. In: *Basic mechanisms of the epilepsies*, eds. A.V. Delgado-Escueta *et al. Adv. Neurol.* **44**, 97–113.

Panayiotopoulos, C.P., Obeid, T. & Waheed, G. (1989): Differentiation of typical absences in epileptic syndromes: a video EEG study of 224 seizures in 20 patients. *Brain* **112**, 1039–1056.

Pellegrini, A. and Gloor, P. (1979): Effects of bilateral partial diencephalic lesions on cortical epileptic activity in generalized penicillin epilepsy in the cat. *Exp. Neurol.* **66**, 285–308.

Robinson, T.N., Cross, A.J., Green, A.R., Toczek, J.M. & Boar, B.R. (1989): Effects of the putative antagonists phaclofen and δaminovaleric acid on GABA$_B$ receptor biochemistry. *Br. J. Pharmacol.* **98**, 833–840.

Sidman, R.L., Green, M.C. & Appel, S.H. (1965): *Catalog of the neurological mutants of the mouse*. Cambridge, MA: Harvard University Press.

Slotnick, B. & Leonard, C.M. (1975): *A stereotaxic atlas of the albino mouse forebrain*. Rockville, MD, ADAMHA Press.

Snead, O.C. (1992): Evidence for GABA$_B$-mediated mechanisms in experimental generalized absence seizures. *Eur. J. Pharmacol.* **213**, 343–349.

Steriade, M., Jones, E.G. & Llinás (1990): Intrinsic circuitry in the thalamus and cortex. In: *Thalamic oscillations and signaling*, eds. M. Steriade, E.G. Jones & R.R. Llinás, pp. 69–112. New York: John Wiley & Sons.

Steriade, M., McCormick, D.A. & Sejnowski, T. (1993): Thalamocortical oscillations in the sleeping and aroused brain. *Science* **262**, 679–685.

Steriade, M. & Llinás, R.F. (1988): The functional states of the thalamus and the associated neuronal interplay. *Physiol. Rev.* **68**, 649–742.

Vergnes, M. & Marescaux, C. (1992): Cortical and thalamic lesions in rats with genetic absence epilepsy. *J. Neural Trans.* (Suppl.) **35**, 71–83.

Vergnes, M., Marescaux, C. & Depaulis, A. (1990): Mapping of spontaneous spike-and-wave discharges in Wistar rats with genetic generalized non-convulsive epilepsy. *Brain Res.* **523**, 87–91.

Vergnes, M., Marescaux, C., Micheletti, G., Reis, J., Depaulis, A., Rumbach, L. & Warter, J.M. (1982): Spontaneous paroxysmal electro-clinical patterns in rat: a model of generalized non-convulsive epilepsy. *Neurosci. Lett.* **33**, 97–101.

Chapter 19

Potential role of intrinsic and GABA$_B$ IPSP-mediated oscillations of thalamic neurons in absence epilepsy

Vincenzo Crunelli[*], Jonathan P. Turner[*], Stephen R. Williams[*], Alice Guyon[†] and Nathalie Leresche[†]

[*]*Department of Physiology, University of Wales, College of Cardiff, Cardiff, UK* and [†]*Département de Neurobiologie Cellulaire, Institut des Neurosciences, Université P. & M. Curie, Paris, France*

Introduction

The functional integrity of cortical and thalamic structures as well as of the corticothalamic loop play a key role in the expression and spread of spike-and-wave discharges (SWDs), the bilaterally synchronous, high-voltage, low-frequency (2–4 Hz) activity that is the main EEG feature of patients suffering from absence epilepsy (Avoli *et al.*, 1990). In particular, unilateral lesions of the lateral thalamic nuclei have been found to abolish both spontaneous and drug-induced spike-and-wave discharges in the ipsilateral cortex of animals that had their corpus callosum transected (Vergnes & Marescaux, 1992), and both in humans and in epileptic-prone animals spike-and-wave discharges appear in the thalamus before than the cortex (Williams, 1953; Vergnes & Marescaux, 1992). In an attempt to elucidate the processes responsible for spike-and-wave discharges in the thalamus and the mechanism of action of anti-absence drugs, such as ethosuximide (ETX) and valproate, we have studied the cellular mechanisms underlying the rhythmic electrical activity of thalamocortical (TC) neurons both in normal animals, and, recently, in a genetic model of absence epilepsy, the Genetic Absence Epilepsy Rats from Strasbourg (GAERS) (Marescaux *et al.*, 1992b).

Thalamic oscillations

The firing of thalamocortical neurons changes according to the behavioural state, both in experimental animals and in man (Lamarre *et al.*, 1971; Fourment *et al.*, 1985; Steriade *et al.*, 1990). While tonic single-action potential firing is observed during wakefulness, high-frequency (100–450 Hz) bursts of action potentials occurring at low-frequency (0.5–4 Hz) are mainly observed during the deep stage of slow wave sleep (δ sleep). However, such high-frequency bursts occurring rhythmically at a low-frequency are also present during wakefulness in thalamic cells of patients

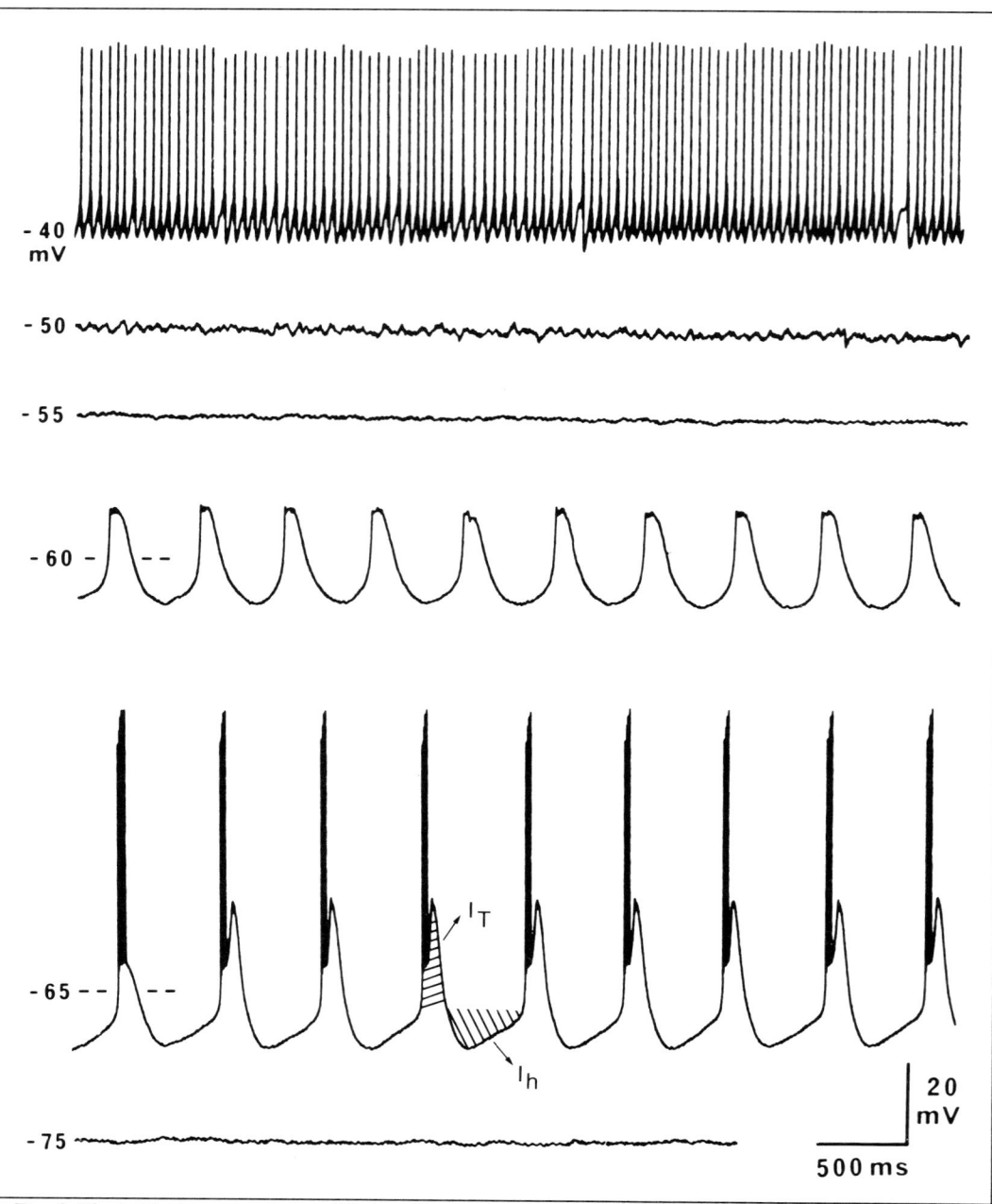

Fig. 1. The intrinsic pacemaker oscillation. The trace marked −65 mV show the pacemaker oscillation recorded in a thalamocortical neuron of the cat dorsal lateral geniculate nucleus. The contribution of the two currents I_T and I_h to the generation of the pacemaker oscillation is highlighted by the shaded areas. In the trace marked −60 mV, the pacemaker oscillation is seen without action potentials since the amplitude of the low-threshold Ca^{2+} potential does not reach threshold for firing. At −55 and at −75 mV no intrinsic activity is present, while above −50 mV single action potential firing is observed. Each trace was obtained using different steady current injection that depolarized or hyperpolarized the cell from −40 to −75 mV.

suffering from (and in animal models of) different neurological diseases, e.g. Parkinson's disease (Buzsaki et al., 1990), and chronic central pain (Lenz et al., 1988). Indeed, in different experimental models of absence epilepsy, the spike-and-wave discharges observed in the EEG and thalamus coincides with high-frequency burst firing occurring at low-frequencies in thalamocortical neurons (Avoli et al., 1990; Vergnes & Marescaux, 1992).

Experimental evidence accumulated in the last 10 years has now demonstrated that the high-frequency bursts of action potentials present in thalamocortical neurons are generated by a low threshold Ca^{2+} potential, i.e. the large amplitude depolarization that is evoked only after a period of membrane hyperpolarization to potentials more negative than −65mV (Jahnsen & Llinas, 1984a,b; Deschênes et al., 1984; Crunelli et al., 1987). In the past, the process responsible for the low-frequency, rhythmic appearance of high-frequency burst firing (i.e of low-threshold Ca^{2+} potentials) was thought to require synaptic drive involving EPSPs and $GABA_A$-receptor-mediated IPSPs originating from the rhythmic recruitment of GABA-containing thalamic neurons (Andersen & Anderson, 1968; Steriade et al., 1990). Indeed, this series of synaptic events has been demonstrated to underlie the generation of the sleep spindles, where each low-threshold Ca^{2+} potential is generated after a few $GABA_A$ IPSPs (Steriade et al., 1985). In addition, at least two other mechanisms have now been shown to be able to produce a rhythmic, low-frequency oscillation of the membrane potential that leads to the generation of high-frequency burst firing in TC neurons. The first is an intrinsic mechanism (i.e. without any synaptic activation) where the interplay of voltage-dependent currents is responsible for the generation of rhythmic low-threshold Ca^{2+} potentials (Leresche et al., 1990; McCormick & Pape, 1990; Soltesz et al., 1991); the second is a synaptic mechanism that involves the periodic occurrence of $GABA_B$-receptor-mediated IPSPs and low-threshold Ca^{2+} potentials (Crunelli & Leresche, 1991).

Intrinsic oscillations

The intrinsic oscillation evoked by thalamocortical neurons that is of particular interest for the present discussion is the pacemaker oscillation (Fig. 1) (Leresche et al., 1990). It consists of the rhythmic generation of low-threshold Ca^{2+} potentials occurring at a frequency of 0.5–4 Hz (mean: 1.8 Hz) that are often crowned by single, or a burst of 2–7, action potentials (intraburst frequency: 100–450 Hz) (Leresche et al., 1991). Apart from the Na^+ and the K^+ currents responsible for the action potentials, two other voltage-dependent currents are essential for the pacemaker oscillation to occur: the low-threshold Ca^{2+} current, I_T (responsible for the low-threshold Ca^{2+} potential) (Crunelli et al., 1989), and the Na^+/K^+ inward rectifying current, I_h (responsible for the slow depolarization and the after-hyperpolarization that precedes and follows a low-threshold Ca^{2+} potential, respectively) (Fig. 1) (McCormick & Pape, 1990; Soltesz et al., 1991). Starting from the most hyperpolarized level of an oscillation cycle, activation of I_h produces a slow pacemaker depolarization until the threshold voltage of activation of I_T is reached. Since the hyperpolarization has provided the requirements in terms of time and voltage to de-inactivate I_T, a low threshold Ca^{2+} potential is generated, which, in turn, evokes a single or a high-frequency burst of action potentials. The transient nature of I_T, together with the leakage current, then terminates the depolarization and hyperpolarizes the cell (McCormick & Pape, 1990; Soltesz et al., 1991). Since during the depolarization associated with a low-threshold Ca^{2+} potential I_h partly de-activates, at the end of a low threshold Ca^{2+} potential there will be less I_h activated (i.e. less inward current) than at its beginning, and, as a consequence, the neurone hyperpolarizes to a potential more negative than the threshold voltage of I_T. The membrane potential will thus reach the peak of the hyperpolarization, and, since the preceding depolarization has provided the time and voltage requirements necessary for partial de-activation of the I_h channels, I_h could be re-activated and the cycle restarts again (for a detailed explanation of this mechanism see Soltesz et al. (1991)). The ability of I_T and I_h to generate the pacemaker oscillation with little or no contribution from a Ca^{2+}-activated K^+ conductance is sup-

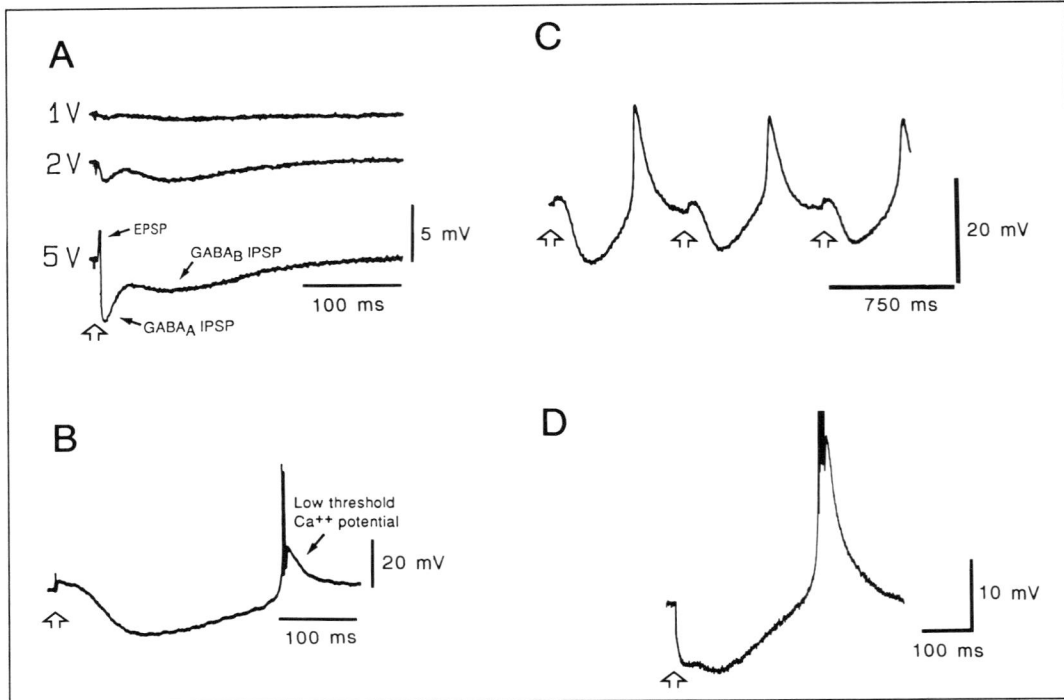

Fig. 2. The $GABA_B$ IPSP-mediated oscillation. (a) Intracellular voltage records from a thalamocortical neuron of the rat dorsal lateral geniculate nucleus show the EPSP, $GABA_A$ and $GABA_B$ sequence obtained by increasing electrical stimulation of the optic tract (open arrow) in a slice preparation. (b) In this thalamocortical neuron, electrical stimulation of the optic tract produced a large $GABA_B$ IPSP that was capable of evoking a low-threshold Ca^{2+} potential and associated burst of action potentials. No $GABA_A$ IPSP is present in this record since the experiment was performed in the presence of the $GABA_A$ receptor antagonist, bicuculline (50 μM). (c) Repetitive stimulation of the optic tract (open arrows) mimicking the $GABA_B$ IPSP-mediated oscillation in a thalamocortical neuron of the cat dorsal lateral geniculate nucleus. In both A, B and C, the $GABA_B$ IPSP is generated by the interneurons present in the dorsal lateral geniculate nucleus since the other intrathalamic source of GABA (i.e. the neurons of the nucleus reticularis thalami) was not present in these slices. (d) The intracellular voltage record shows a $GABA_A$ and $GABA_B$ IPSP sequence evoked by electrical stimulation of the GABA-containing cells of the nucleus reticularis thalami in a neuron of the rat ventrobasal complex. The hyperpolarization associated with these synaptic potentials then evokes a low-threshold Ca^{2+} potential and associated burst of action potentials. 2-Amino-5-phosphonovaleric acid (100 μM) and 6-cyano-7-nitroquinoxaline-2,3-dione (20 μM) were present during this experiments to abolish the EPSP evoked by the concomitant activation of the corticothalamic afferent passing through the nucleus reticularis thalami.

ported by the results of computer simulations of the activity of thalamocortical neurons obtained using different biophysical models (Tóth & Crunelli, 1992; McCormick & Huguenard, 1992).

From a functional point of view, two of the most important consequences of this intrinsic mechanism are that: (i) this low-frequency oscillation of thalamocortical neurons can be simply achieved by changing the level of tonic depolarization imposed onto these neurons (i.e. without the involvement of rhythmic, low-frequency synaptic inputs) (Fig. 1); (ii) the upper limit of the frequency range of the pacemaker oscillation is set by the biophysical properties of I_T and I_h and may not exceed 4–6 Hz in rats and cats.

There are differences between thalamic nuclei in their ability of producing the pacemaker oscillation *in vitro*. Thus, in a standard perfusion medium containing 2 mM Ca^{2+} and 1 mM Mg^{2+}, very few thalamocortical neurons (1–4 per cent) in the rat and cat dorsal lateral geniculate nucleus generate the pacemaker oscillation, while 50–100 per cent of thalamocortical neurons in the rat and cat ventrobasal complex have been found to produce this type of oscillation. Note, however, that an increase in the extracellular $[Ca^{2+}]/[Mg^{2+}]$ ratio from 2 to 7 results in a larger number (50 per cent in the rat, 58 per cent in the cat) of thalamocortical neurons in the dorsal lateral geniculate nucleus showing the pacemaker oscillation. Similar results have also been reported *in vivo*, where thalamocortical neurons in the lateral and ventrolateral nuclei have been shown to produce intrinsic oscillation more consistently than those in the dorsal lateral geniculate nucleus (Nuñez et al., 1992). It thus appears that the thalamic nuclei that are more prone to produce the pacemaker oscillation are those thalamic nuclei (i) from which the more robust and consistent thalamic spike-and-wave discharges can be recorded (Marescaux et al., 1992b), and (ii) whose lesions leads to the abolishment of spike-and-wave discharges in the EEG (Pellegrini & Gloor, 1979; Vergnes & Marescaux, 1992).

It is also worth stressing that the pacemaker oscillation does not always occur continuously but it can also appear every 5–25 s for periods lasting from 1.5 to 28 s (Leresche et al., 1990, 1991). We have shown that changes in the properties of I_h can reversibly transform the continuous pacemaker oscillation into this intermittent oscillation. Indeed, the pacemaker oscillation can even be abolished (or made to appear) by controlling the size of I_h via selective changes in the level of β-adrenoreceptor activation (Soltesz et al., 1991). Thus, a particular type of intrinsic oscillation is not peculiar to a group of thalamocortical neurons but is part of a continuum of intrinsic activities that depend not only on the level of membrane polarization but also on the fine tuning between the relative proportion/kinetics of I_T and I_h, and their modulation by neurotransmitters.

$GABA_B$-receptor-mediated oscillation

Synaptic activation of post-synaptic $GABA_B$ receptors evokes in thalamocortical neurons a late, long-lasting, K^+ dependent IPSP, which generally follows the classical EPSP–$GABA_A$ IPSP sequence (Fig. 2a) (Crunelli et al., 1988; Soltesz et al., 1988, 1989; Crunelli & Leresche, 1991). For the present discussion, it is important to highlight the following features of the thalamic $GABA_B$ IPSP mediated by the thalamic interneurons:

(i) its latency of onset (20–50 ms) and its duration (100–300 ms) are longer than the $GABA_A$ IPSP;

(ii) its amplitude shows a frequency-dependent decrease that, unlike thalamic $GABA_A$ IPSPs, is never greater than 30 per cent, even at those frequencies (4–10Hz) of activation characteristic of certain types of thalamic rhythmic activity *in vivo*;

(iii) its amplitude is not linearly related to the membrane potential: it has a maximum in the voltage region of –55 to –65mV and it decreases both at more hyperpolarized and depolarized potentials (Fig. 3);

(iv) blockade of $GABA_A$ IPSPs by bicuculline, picrotoxin or penicillin markedly increases the amplitude of the $GABA_B$ IPSP (Fig. 2b) (for an explanation of this effect see Crunelli et al., 1988; Soltesz et al. (1989)).

On the basis of these properties of the thalamic $GABA_B$ IPSP, we have suggested that these potentials are well suited for the high-frequency burst-firing excitation of thalamocortical neurons that requires the activation of a low-threshold Ca^{2+} potential, i.e. that $GABA_B$ IPSPs have a 'priming role' for burst-firing excitation (Fig. 3) (Crunelli & Leresche, 1991). Thus, the relatively long latency to onset, time to peak and duration as well as the voltage region of maximal amplitude of a $GABA_B$ IPSP give rise to a hyperpolarization with voltage- and time-dependent features ideal to provide the necessary removal of inactivation of I_T (Crunelli et al., 1989), so that, on repolarization of the membrane, a low-threshold Ca^{2+} potential with associated burst firing is generated (Fig. 2b,c, Fig. 3).

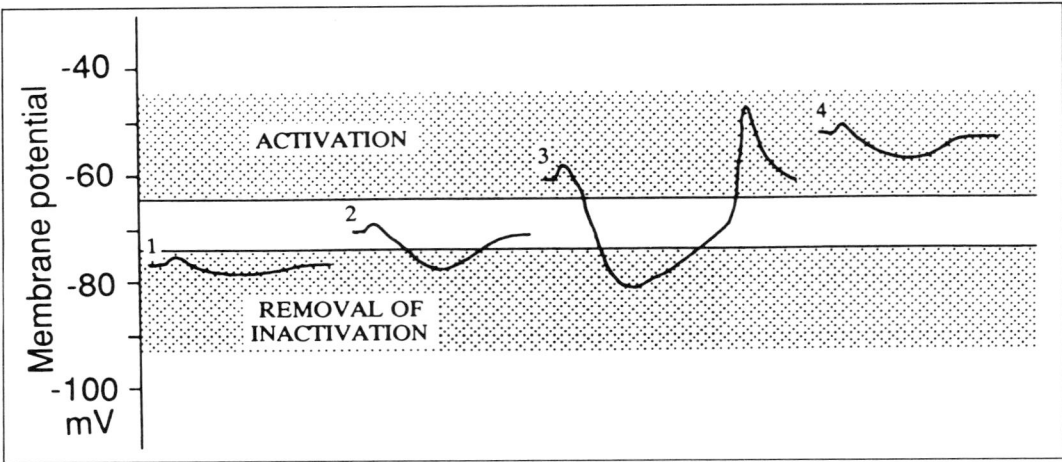

Fig. 3. Schematic diagram showing the relationship between the amplitude of $GABA_B$ IPSPs and the activation/inactivation properties of I_T. The shaded area above $-65mV$ indicates the voltage region where I_T can be activated (activation) while the shaded area below $-70mV$ (removal of inactivation) indicates the voltage region where the removal of inactivation of I_T occurs. The four schematic traces show typical examples of EPSP and $GABA_B$ IPSP evoked by stimulation of the optic tract (the $GABA_A$ IPSP has been omitted for clarity). In trace 1 and 2, the $GABA_B$ IPSP does not reach the activation region of I_T and does not evoke a low-threshold Ca^{2+} potential. In trace 3, the $GABA_B$ IPSP is large enough to reach the voltage region where inactivation of I_T is removed and, on repolarization of the membrane to its original level, the voltage activation range of I_T, thus evoking a low-threshold Ca^{2+} potential. In trace 4, the $GABA_B$ IPSP is in the voltage activation region, but because of its smaller amplitude, it does not reach the voltage region where inactivation of I_T can be removed and thus it does not cause a low-threshold Ca^{2+} potential.

Thus, a rhythmic sequence of $GABA_B$ IPSPs and low-threshold Ca^{2+} potentials represents an alternative mechanism to the intrinsic pacemaker oscillation by which low-frequency oscillation of the membrane potential and associated burst-firing can be produced by thalamocortical neurons (Fig. 2c). The absence of a large $GABA_B$ IPSPs at all levels of membrane potentials will also ensure that this mechanism of low-frequency burst-firing will only be operational in a relatively small region of membrane potentials (Fig. 3). Finally, as it is the case for the intrinsic pacemaker oscillation, the upper frequency limit of the $GABA_B$ IPSP-mediated oscillations will be dictated by the biophysical properties of the low-threshold Ca^{2+} potential and its underlying current, I_T, and hence will not exceed 4–6 Hz in rat and cat.

Since our original observations on the $GABA_B$ IPSPs generated by the GABA-containing interneurons of the dorsal lateral geniculate nucleus, evidence has also been accumulating on the similarity of the properties of these $GABA_B$ IPSPs and those evoked by the GABA-containing cells of the nucleus reticularis thalami. For instance, the nucleus reticularis-mediated $GABA_B$ IPSP is able to generate, alone or in combination with a $GABA_A$ IPSP, a low-threshold Ca^{2+} potential and associated burst-firing in thalamocortical neurons of the rat ventrobasal complex (Fig. 2d) (Turner & Crunelli, 1992). Recent results from thalamic slices of the ferret *in vitro* have also shown that in the presence of bicuculline thalamocortical neurons of the dorsal lateral geniculate nucleus functionally connected to neurons of the perigeniculate nucleus (i.e. the visual portion of the nucleus reticularis thalami) generate a sequence of $GABA_B$ IPSPs and low-threshold Ca^{2+} potentials (Von Krosigk et al., 1993). Extracellular multi-unit recordings, performed simultaneously in the same area as the intracellular recordings, have shown a pattern of activity reminiscent of a thalamic spike-and-wave discharge. Clearly, this findings support our hypothesis that the $GABA_B$ IPSP-mediated oscillation might be the mechanism underlying the thalamic spike-and-wave discharges (Crunelli & Leresche, 1991), at least as far as the penicillin model of absence epilepsy is concerned.

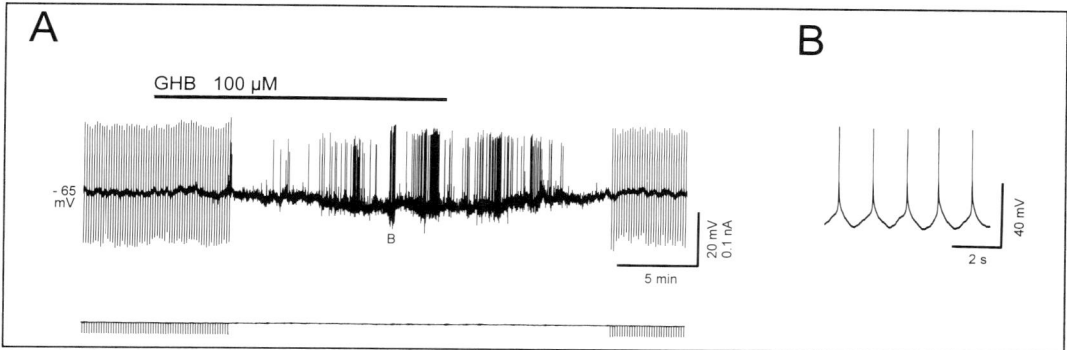

Fig. 4. The intrinsic pacemaker oscillation evoked by γ-hydroxybutyric acid (GHB) in a TC neurone of the rat dorsal lateral geniculate nucleus. A. The top trace is a chart record showing that application of γ-hydroxybutyric acid produces a small and slow hyperpolarization that brings the cell into the membrane potential region where the intrinsic pacemaker oscillation is evoked. Downward deflections at the beginning and at the end of the trace represent the response of the neurone to a current pulse (bottom trace). B. Enlargement of part of the trace in A shows the pacemaker oscillation at a fast time base.

Pharmacological manipulation of GABA$_B$ receptors in absence epilepsy

Systemic as well as intrathalamic injection of GABA$_B$ receptor agonists and antagonists potentiate and block, respectively, the spike-and-wave discharges in different genetic and pharmacological models of absence epilepsy (Marescaux et al., 1992a; Hosford et al., 1992; Snead, 1992), except in the stargazer mouse (Qiao & Noebels, 1992). This finding is corroborated by the data showing that baclofen, the selective GABA$_B$ agonist, and progabide, a pro-GABA drug, aggravate absence epilepsy in humans (Gloor & Fariello, 1988; Bowery et al., 1990). In addition, in the lethargic mouse (but not in GAERS) the number of GABA$_B$ binding sites in some cortical and thalamic nuclei is higher than in their matched, non-epileptic controls (Hosford et al., 1992, 1993). All these results have been interpreted in support of our hypothesis that the GABA$_B$ IPSP-mediated oscillation underlies spike-and-wave discharges, i.e. by blocking the GABA$_B$ receptors the antagonists would abolish the GABA$_B$ IPSPs, and thus eliminate the hyperpolarization necessary for the activation of I_T and the generation of low-threshold Ca^{2+} potentials and burst firing. Indeed, such possibility is supported by the results obtained in the ferret *in vitro* where the GABA$_B$-mediated oscillation recorded during perfusion with bicuculline could be abolished by the selective GABA$_B$ antagonist 2-OH-saclofen (Von Krosigk et al., 1993).

Except for the latter results, however, all the data obtained with GABA$_B$ agonists and antagonists are also compatible with an intrinsic mechanism (i.e. the pacemaker oscillation) underlying the electrical activity of thalamocortical neurons during the spike-and-wave discharges of absence epilepsy. For instance, tonic activation of GABA$_B$ receptors could hyperpolarize a thalamocortical cell to the membrane potential region where the intrinsic pacemaker oscillation occur (see Fig. 1). This possibility is supported by the results of recent experiments using γ-hydroxybutyrate (GHB), an endogenous substance (Roth & Giarman, 1970; Gold & Roth, 1977) whose systemic injection in animals is known to produce a pattern of spike-and-wave discharges similar to the human absence epilepsy (Godshalk et al., 1976; Snead, 1978a, b). When tested on thalamic cells *in vitro*, small concentrations of γ-hydroxybutyrate hyperpolarize thalamocortical neurons into a membrane potential region where they evoke the pacemaker oscillation (Fig. 4) (Williams et al., 1993). The action of γ-hydroxybutyrate is blocked by CGP 35348, a selective GABA$_B$ antagonist (Crunelli et al., 1992), but not by tetrodotoxin, demonstrating that the effects of γ-hydroxybutyrate are mediated by a direct action on the post-synaptic GABA$_B$ receptors present on the thalamocortical neurons. This result supports previous biochemical and electrophysiological evidence indicating that γ-hydroxybutyrate interacts with $GABA_B$ receptors in the hippocampus and cortex (Bernasconi et al., 1992; Xie & Smart, 1992). More importantly, the ability of γ-hydroxybutyrate to induce the pacemaker oscillation suggests that this type of intrinsic activity might be the electrical activity of TC neurons underlying thalamic spike-and-wave discharges in the γ-hydroxybutyrate model of absence epilepsy.

Another potential mechanism by which $GABA_B$ receptors might affect spike-and-wave discharges is via a direct modulation of I_T, since it has been shown that small concentrations of baclofen decrease the low-threshold Ca^{2+} current of rat sensory neurons (Scott et al., 1990). Using patch electrode recordings, however, baclofen (2 and 50 μM) has been found to have no effect on I_T, excluding therefore the possibility that the aggravation and blocking of spike-and-wave discharges by $GABA_B$ agonists and antagonists, respectively, takes place via a $GABA_B$ receptor-mediated modulation of I_T.

The site and mechanism of action of ethosuximide: I_T or not I_T?

As mentioned in the previous sections, the low-threshold Ca^{2+} potential and its underlying current, I_T, are essential for the burst firing of thalamocortical neurons, and thus for the spike-and-wave discharges, independent of whether they are generated by the intrinsic mechanism (i.e. the pacemaker oscillation) or the synaptic mechanism (i.e. the $GABA_B$ IPSP-mediated oscillation). Indeed, drugs used in the treatment of human absence epilepsy and effective against the experimental models of this disease, i.e. ethosuximide (ETX) and dimethadione, were shown to decrease I_T in thalamocortical neurons of the rat ventrobasal complex (VB) (Coulter et al., 1989a,b, 1990), and, more recently, in neurons of the nucleus reticularis thalami (Huguenard & Prince, 1992). In particular, therapeutic concentrations of ethosuximide were shown to produce a voltage-dependent, maximum decrease of 40 per cent in the peak amplitude of I_T. The effects of ethosuximide on the low-threshold Ca^{2+} potential itself were less impressive (Coulter et al., 1990): this finding, however, could be explained by the fact that, because of the regenerative properties and the steep activation curve of I_T, it would be rather difficult in current-clamp experiments to detect differences in the waveform of the low-threshold Ca^{2+} potential that are due to a 40 per cent maximum decrease of the underlying current. Since that original series of publications, however, numerous reports from different groups have now shown a lack of action of ethosuximide on the low-threshold Ca^{2+} current present in freshly isolated or cultured neurons including both thalamocortical and cortical neurons (Pfrieger et al., 1992; Sayer et al., 1993; Thompson & Wong, 1991).

We thus decided to re-investigate the effect of ethosuximide on I_T in rat thalamic neurons using patch-electrode recordings in brain slices. In 10 and five thalamocortical neurons of the rat dorsal lateral geniculate nucleus and the ventrobasal complex, respectively, as well as in three neurons of the nucleus reticularis thalami, we have so far been unable to detect any effect of ethosuximide (0.5–1 mM) on the peak amplitude, the activation/inactivation properties and the kinetics of I_T in normal Wistar rats as well as in GAERS. Preliminary experiments using intrathalamic application of therapeutic concentrations of ethosuximide have also shown no effect on the number and severity of spike-and-wave discharges in GAERS (M. Vergnes & C. Marescaux, unpublished observations). Since it is well established that the ability of TC cells to generate burst firing during spike-and-wave discharges (as well as in other pathological conditions or physiological functions) depends on the presence of a low-threshold Ca^{2+} potential, these results question the validity of the initial observation regarding the effect of ethosuximide on I_T, and re-open the question of the mechanism(s) and site(s) of action of this anti-absence medicine.

Electrophysiological analysis of TC cells in the GAERS

Recently, we have also started to look at the electrical properties of thalamocortical neurons in GAERS using patch-electrode recordings in a slice preparation (Guyon et al., 1993). In particular,

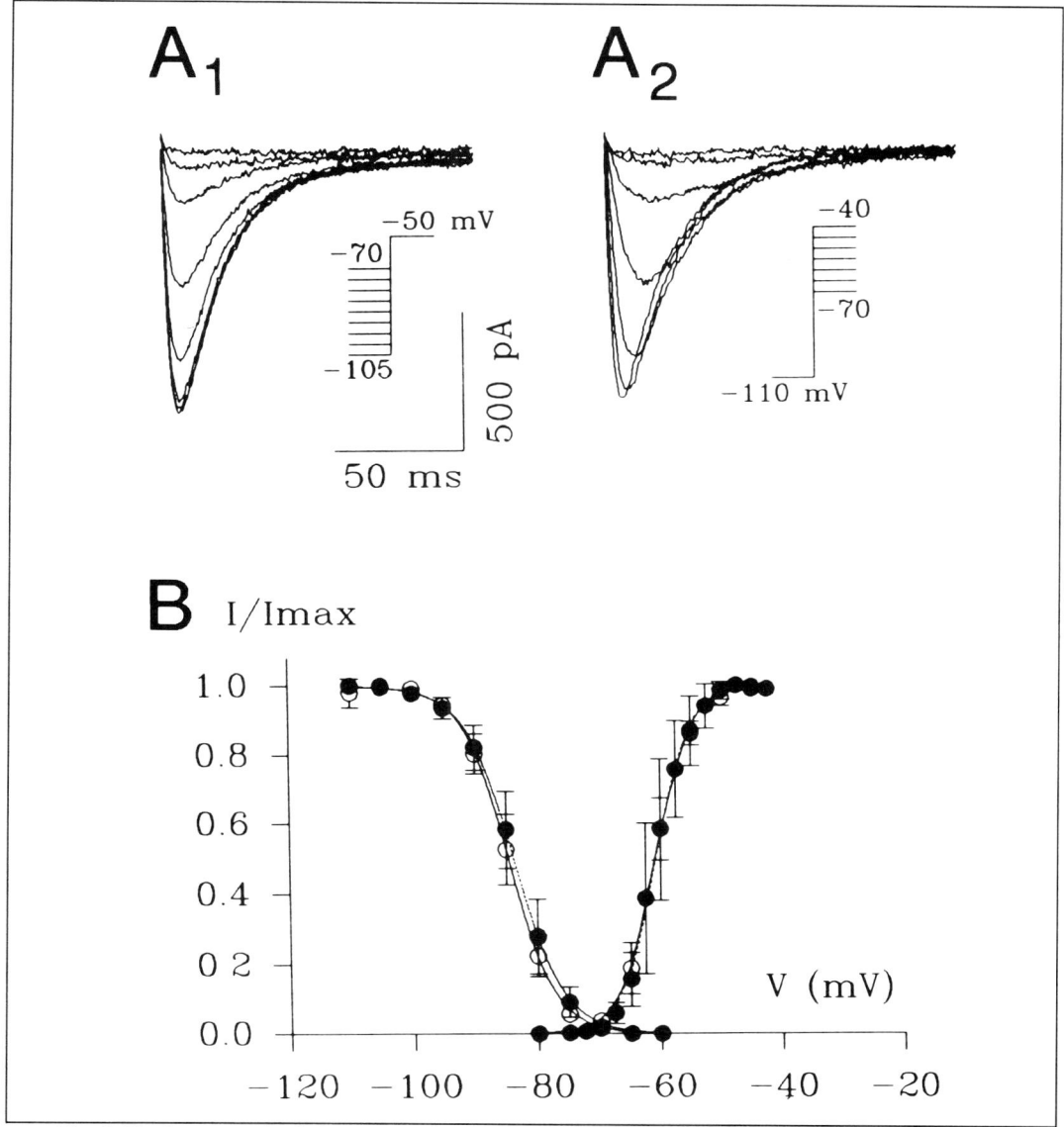

Fig. 5. The I_T current in thalamocortical neurone of Genetic Absence Epilepsy Rats from Strasbourg (GAERS) and their matched, non-epileptic controls. (a) Examples of the I_T current evoked in GAERS by the voltage protocols illustrated and used to construct the activation (A_1) and inactivation (A_2) curves depicted in B. (b) Steady-state activation and inactivation curves of the I_T current recorded in GAERS (white circles, solid line) and their non-epileptic controls (black circles, broken line) (bars indicate standard error of the mean, n = 5 for each group) show no difference between these two group of animals. Curves were fitted to the experimental points using the equation $I/I_{max} = 1/1 + exp((V-V_0)/K$.

we have investigated the possibility that differences in I_T might be responsible for the occurrence of spike-and-wave discharges in these epileptic animals. For instance, a larger maximal conductance and/or a more hyperpolarized half-activation value of I_T might allow smaller depolarizations to trigger low-threshold Ca^{2+} potentials in these animals. However, we have found no difference in the peak amplitude of I_T, nor in its activation/inactivation properties or its kinetics between thalamocortical neurons of GAERS and their non-epileptic, matched controls (Fig. 5) (Guyon et al., 1993). Since for technical reasons these experiments have been conducted in 12–28-day-old GAERS, the possibility that an abnormality of I_T might occur later in development cannot be totally excluded at the present time. Nevertheless, the similarity in the characteristics of I_T between GAERS and non-epileptic controls at 2–4 weeks of age clearly indicates that at this stage of development a dysfunction of I_T is not involved in the series of events leading to the development of spike-and-wave discharges later in life.

Conclusions and outlook

At present the available evidence does not indicate conclusively whether an intrinsic oscillation or a $GABA_B$ IPSP-mediated oscillation is the thalamic mechanism underlying the spike-and-wave discharges of human absence epilepsy. It is likely that in the penicillin model the $GABA_B$-mediated oscillation is responsible for the thalamic spike-and-wave discharges, while in the γ-hydroxybutyrate model the pacemaker oscillation might underlie the thalamic spike-and-wave discharges. What is ever more apparent, therefore, is the problem of the similarities/differences of the cellular mechanism generating the thalamic spike-and-wave discharges in the different models of absence epilepsy, and not only between the genetic and pharmacological models, but also within each of these two groups. The fact that all models are sensitive to the same anti-absence medicine or $GABA_B$ antagonist does not imply that the mechanisms underlying the spike-and-wave discharge are similar. Indeed, our present knowledge of the cellular and molecular processes underlying burst discharge in the thalamus clearly suggests that different mechanisms could generate the same output (i.e. high-frequency burst firing occurring at low frequencies) in thalamocortical neurons. On the other hand, the understanding of the mechanism by which this similar burst firing output of thalamocortical neurons could give rise to different EEG activities according to the physiological or pathological condition (e.g. slow wave sleep, Parkinson's disease, absence epilepsy, etc.) is still an intriguing problem to solve.

After the explosion of new information generated in the last 4 years by the *in vitro* work focussing on the type and properties of the voltage-dependent and transmitter-gated currents with which the thalamocortical neurons are endowed, it will perhaps be useful to assess the *in vivo* situation in different species and in the different experimental models of absence epilepsy. Another problem that remains unresolved is the different frequency of the cortical and thalamic spike-and-wave discharges observed between different species/models. It will also be useful to reconsider the mechanism of action of ethosuximide and the other, chemically different, medicines that are effective against human absence epilepsy. The role of the thalamocortical loop, as well as of the cortex itself, has also been neglected in recent years both by the *in vivo* and *in vitro* experiments. Whatever the approach, it is evident that the next few years are going to generate interesting new information in this field, hopefully leading to the development of new types of anti-absence medicines.

Acknowledgment

We thank Mr R.M. Jones and Mr T.M. Gould for their skilful technical assistance. The work described in this chapter was supported by the Wellcome Trust (grants 015032, 019135 and 037089) and the CNRS.

References

Andersen, P. & Andersson, S.A. (1968): *Physiological basis of alpha rhythm*, New York: Appleton-Century-Crofts.

Avoli, M., Gloor, P., Kostopoulos, G. & Naquet, R. (1990): *Generalized epilepsy: neurobiological approaches*. Boston: Birkhauser.

Bernasconi, R., Lauber, J., Marescaux, C., Vergnes, N., Martin, P., Rubio, V., Leonhardt, T., Reyman, N. & Bittiger, H. (1992): Experimental absence seizures: potential role or γ-hydroxybutyric acid and GABA$_B$ receptors. *J. Neural. Transm. (Suppl)* **35**, 155–177.

Bowery, N.G., Bittiger, H. & Olpe, H.R. (1990): *GABA$_B$ receptor in mammalian function*, Chichester: J. Wiley & Sons.

Buzsaki, G., Smith, A., Berger, S., Fisher, L.J. & Gage, F.H. (1990): Petit mal epilepsy and parkinsonian tremor: hypothesis of a common pacemaker. *Neuroscience* **36**, 1–14.

Coulter, D.A., Huguenard, J.R. & Prince, D.A. (1989a): Specific petit mal anticonvulsants reduce calcium currents in thalamic neurons. *Neurosci. Lett.* **98**, 74–78.

Coulter, D.A., Huguenard, J.R. & Prince, D.A. (1989b): Characterization of ethosuximide reduction of low-threshold calcium current in thalamic neurons. *Ann. Neurol.* **25**, 582–593.

Coulter, D.A., Huguenard, J.R. & Prince, D.A. (1990): Cellular action of petit mal anticonvulsants: implication of thalamic low-threshold calcium current in generation of spike-wave discharge. In: *Generalized epilepsy: neurobiological approaches*, eds. M. Avoli, P. Gloor, G. Kostopoulos & R. Naquet, pp. 425–435. Boston: Birkhauser.

Crunelli, V., Kelly, J. S., Leresche, N. & Pirchio, M. (1987): The ventral and dorsal lateral geniculate nucleus of the rat: intracellular recordings *in vitro*. *J. Physiol.* **384**, 587–601.

Crunelli, V., Haby, M., Jassik-Gerschenfeld, D., Leresche, N. & Pirchio, M. (1988): Cl$^-$ and K$^+$ dependent inhibitory postsynaptic potentials evoked by interneurones of the rat lateral geniculate nucleus. *J. Physiol.* **399**, 153–176.

Crunelli, V., Lightowler, S. & Pollard, C.E. (1989): A T-type Ca^{2+} current underlies low-threshold Ca^{2+} potentials in cells of the cat and rat lateral geniculate nucleus. *J. Physiol.* **413**, 543–561.

Crunelli, V. & Leresche, N. (1991): A role for GABA$_B$ receptors in excitation and inhibition of thalamocortical cells. *Trends Neurosci.* **14**, 16–21.

Crunelli, V., Emri, Z., Leresche, N., Kekesi, K.A., Soltesz, I., Toth, K., Turner, J. P. & Juhasz, G. (1992): GABA$_B$ receptors in the thalamus assessed by *in vivo* and *in vitro* experiments. *Pharmacol. Comm.* **2**, 113–116.

Deschenes, M., Paradis, M., Roy, J.P. & Steriade, M. (1984): Electrophysiology of neurones of lateral thalamic nuclei in cat: resting properties and burst discharges. *J. Neurophysiol.* **51**, 1196–1219.

Fourment, A., Hirsch, J.C. & Marc, M.E. (1985): Oscillations of the spontaneous slow-wave sleep rhythm in the lateral geniculate nucleus relay neurons of behaving cats. *Neuroscience* **14**, 1061–1075.

Gloor, P. & Fariello, R.G. (1988): Generalized epilepsy: some of its cellular mechanisms differ from those of focal epilepsy. *Trends Neurosci.* **11**, 63–68.

Godshalk, M., Dzljic, M.R. & Bonta, I.L. (1976): Antagonism of gamma hydroxybutyrate-induced hypersynchronization in the ECoG by anti-petit mal drugs. *Neurosci. Lett.* **3**, 1173–1178.

Gold, B.I. & Roth, R.H. (1977): Kinetics of the *in vivo* conversion of γ-[^{3}H]-aminobutyric acid to γ-[^{3}H]-hydroxybutyric acid by rat brain. *J. Neurochem.* **29**, 1069–1073.

Guyon, A., Vergnes, M. & Leresche, N. (1993): Thalamic low threshold calcium current in a genetic model of absence epilepsy. *NeuroReport* **4**, 1231–1234.

Hosford, D.A., Clark, S., Cao, Z., Wilson, W.A. Jr., Lin, F-H., Morrisett, R.A. & Huin, A. (1992): The role of GABA$_B$ receptor activation in absence seizures of lethargic (*lh/lh*) mice. *Science* **257**, 398–401.

Hosford, D.A., Lin, F-H., Cao, Z., Kraemer, D. & Huin, A. (1993): Neural network of absence seizures in lethargic (*lh/lh*) mice: use of GABA$_B$ autoradiograms, EEG recordings and microinjections. *Soc. Neurosci. Abstr.* **19**, 598.5.

Huguenard, J.R. & Prince, D.A. (1992): A novel T-type current underlies prolonged Ca^{2+}-dependent burst firing in GABAergic neurons of rat thalamic reticular nucleus. *J. Neurosci.* **12**, 3804–3817.

Jahnsen, H. & Llinas, R.R. (1984a): Electrophysiological properties of guinea-pig thalamic neurones: an *in vitro* study. *J. Physiol.* **349**, 205–226.

Jahnsen, H. & Llinas, R.R. (1984b): Ionic basis for the electroresponsiveness and oscillatory properties of guinea-pig thalamic neurones *in vitro*. *J. Physiol.* **349**, 227–247.

Lamarre, Y., Filion, M. & Cordeau, J.P. (1971): Neuronal discharges of the ventrolateral nucleus of the thalamus during sleep and wakefulness in the cat. I. Spontaneous activity. *Expl. Brain Res.* **12**, 480–498.

Lenz, F.A., Tasker, R.R., Kwan, H.C., Dostrovsky, J.O. & Murphy, J.T. (1988): Single unit analysis of the human thalamic ventral nuclear group: correlation of thalamic 'tremor cells' with the 3–6Hz component of parkinsonian tremor. *J. Neurosci.* **8**, 754–764.

Leresche, N., Jassik-Gerschenfeld, D., Haby, M., Soltesz, I. & Crunelli, V. (1990): Pacemaker-like and other types of spontaneous membrane potential oscillations of thalamocortical cells. *Neurosci. Lett.* **113**, 72–77.

Leresche, N., Lightowler, S., Soltesz, I., Jassik-Gerschenfeld, D. & Crunelli, V. (1991): Low frequency oscillatory activities intrinsic to rat and cat thalamocortical cells. *J. Physiol.* **441**, 155–174.

McCormick, D.A. & Huguenard, J.R. (1992): A model of the electrophysiological properties of thalamocortical relay neurons. *J. Neurophysiol.* **68**, 1384–1400.

McCormick, D.A. & Pape, H.C. (1990): Noradrenergic and serotoninergic modulation of a hyperpolarization-activated cation current in thalamic relay neurones. *J. Physiol.* **431**, 319–342.

Marescaux, C., Vergnes, M. & Bernasconi, R. (1992a): $GABA_B$ receptor antagonists: potential new-antiabsence drugs. *J. Neural. Transm. (Suppl.)* **35**, 179–188.

Marescaux, C., Vergnes, M. & Depaulis, A. (1992b): Genetic absence epilepsy in rats from Strasbourg – a review. *J. Neural. Transm. (Suppl)* **35**, 37–69.

Nuñez, A., Amzica, F. & Steriade, M. (1992): Intrinsic and synaptically generated delta (1–4 Hz) rhythms in dorsal lateral geniculate neurons and their modulation by light-induced fast (30–70 Hz) events. *Neuroscience* **51**, 269–284.

Pellegrini, A. & Gloor, P. (1979): Effects of bilateral partial diencephalic lesions on cortical epileptic activity in generalized penicillin epilepsy in the cat. *Exp. Neurol.* **66**, 285–308.

Pfrieger, F.W., Veselovsky, N.S., Gottman, K. & Lux, H.D. (1992): Pharmacological characterization of calcium currents and synaptic transmission between thalamic neurons in vitro. *J. Neurosci.* **12**, 4347–4357.

Qiao, X. & Noebels, J.L. (1992): $GABA_B$ receptor-independent spike-wave epilepsy in the mutant mouse stargazer. *Pharmacol. Comm.* **2**, 125.

Roth, R.H. & Giarman, N.J. (1970): Natural occurrence of γ-hydroxybutyrate in mammalian brain. *Biochem. Pharmacol.* **19**, 1087–1093.

Sayer, R.J., Brown, A.M., Schwindt, P.C. & Crill, W.E. (1993): Calcium currents in acutely isolated human neocortical neurons. *J. Neurophysiol.* **69**, 1596–1606.

Scott, R.H., Wootton, J.F. & Dolphin, A.C. (1990): Modulation of neuronal T-type calcium channel currents by photoactivation of intracellular guanine 5'-o-(3-thio)triphosphate. *Neuroscience* **38**, 285–294.

Snead, O.C. (1978a): Gamma hydroxybutyrate in the monkey I. Electroencephalographic, behavioral and pharmacokinetic studies. *Neurology* **28**, 636–642.

Snead, O.C. (1978b): Gamma hydroxybutyrate in the monkey II. Effect of chronic oral anticonvulsant drugs. *Neurology* **28**, 643–648.

Snead, O.C. (1992): Evidence for $GABA_B$-mediated mechanisms in experimental generalized absence seizures. *Eur. J. Pharm.* **213**, 343–349.

Soltesz, I., Haby, M., Leresche, N. & Crunelli, V. (1988): The $GABA_B$ antagonist phaclofen inhibits the late K^+-dependent IPSP in cat and rat thalamic and hippocampal neurones. *Brain Res.* **448**, 351–354.

Soltesz, I., Lightowler, S., Leresche, N. & Crunelli, V. (1989): On the properties and origin of $GABA_B$ IPSPs recorded from morphologically identified projection cells of the cat lateral geniculate nucleus. *Neuroscience* **33**, 23–33.

Soltesz, I., Lightowler, S., Leresche, N., Jassik-Gerschenfeld, D., Pollard, C.E. & Crunelli, V. (1991): Two inward currents and the transformation of low frequency oscillations of rat and cat thalamocortical cells. *J. Physiol.* **441**, 175–197.

Steriade, M., Deschênes, M., Domich, L. & Mulle, C. (1985): Abolition of spindle oscillations in thalamic neurons disconnected from the reticularis thalami. *J. Neurophysiol.* **54**, 1473–1497.

Steriade, M., Jones, E.G. & Llinas, R.R. (1990): *Thalamic oscillations and signaling*, pp. 431. New York: J.Wiley & Sons.

Thompson, S.M. & Wong, R.S. (1991): Development of calcium current subtypes in isolated rat hippocampal pyramidal cells. *J. Physiol.* **439**, 671–689.

Tóth, T. & Crunelli, V. (1992): Computer simulation of pacemaker oscillations of thalamocortical cells. *NeuroReport* **3**, 65–68.

Turner, J.P. & Crunelli V. (1992): The characterization of the input from the nucleus reticularis thalami to the ventro-basal thalamus of the rat. *Soc. Neurosci. Abstr.* **18,** 427.15.

Vergnes, M. & Marescaux, C. (1992): Cortical and thalamic lesions in rats with genetic absence epilepsy. *J. Neural. Transm. (Suppl)* **35,** 71–83.

Von Krosigk, M., Bal, T. & McCormick, D.A. (1993): Cellular mechanisms of a synchronized oscillation in the thalamus. *Science* **261,** 361–364.

Williams, D. (1953): A study of thalamic and cortical rhythms in petit mal. *Brain* **76,** 50–69.

Williams, S.R., Turner, J.P. & Crunelli, V. (1993): γ-Hydroxybutyrate hyperpolarizes rat thalamocortical cells by a direct action on GABA$_B$ receptors. *Soc. Neurosci. Abstr.* **19,** 219.10.

Xie, X.M. & Smart. T.G. (1992): γ-Hydroxybutyrate hyperpolarizes hippocampal neurones by activating GABA$_B$ receptors. *Eur. J. Pharmacol.* **212,** 291–294.

Chapter 20

Genetic and phenotypic heterogeneity of inherited spike-and-wave epilepsies

Jeffrey L. Noebels

Associate Professor of Neurology, Neuroscience, and Molecular Genetics, Developmental Neurogenetics Laboratory, Department of Neurology, Section of Neurophysiology, Baylor College of Medicine, Houston, Texas, USA

Introduction

Genetic models of absence epilepsy provide a unique resource for experimental investigations into the natural causes, intervening mechanisms, and secondary neuropathological effects of inherited spike-wave synchronization. Single locus gene mutations that have been mapped on chromosomes of the mouse are of particular value (Noebels, 1979), since they permit the neuronal circuits altered by individual epilepsy genes to be analysed reproducibly before and after seizures begin in the developing brain. The isolation of multiple mutants all sharing a specific epileptic phenotype creates a *model system* that adds further analytic power, since comparisons of the patterns of primary and secondary excitability defects can help to define necessary and sufficient elements of the disorder. These elements can ultimately be correlated with homologous genetic absence syndromes in man.

The search for relevant genes and molecular mechanisms in animals and man is beginning to accelerate despite the drawback that the generalized cortical spike-and-wave discharges accompanying the behavioural absence episodes represent the only specific phenotypic marker for this major category of childhood-onset epilepsy. Early *in vivo* animal experiments first pinpointed a candidate pacemaker mechanism for 3 s cortical oscillations following stimulation of intralaminar thalamic nuclei (Jasper & Droogleever-Fortuyn, 1947), and subsequent depth recordings in patients confirmed that the thalamus was a constant participant in spontaneous cortical 3/s spike-and-wave seizures (Williams, 1953). Intracellular and patch clamp recordings in isolated thalamic neurons are now beginning to provide the crucial molecular and synaptic details required to model their rhythmic firing properties (Steriade *et al.* 1990; Crunelli & Leresche 1991; Huguenard & Prince 1992; Lytton & Sejnowski, 1992; von Krosigk *et al.*, 1993), and there is strong evidence that the excitability of reticular (Avanzini *et al.*, 1993) and cortical (Fisher & Prince, 1977; Gloor *et al.*, 1990) neurons are also critical to the generation of the synchronous network discharge.

These studies of normal and model networks all portray epileptiform spike-and-wave seizures as a unitary excitability disturbance arising within the 'centrencephalic' (Penfield & Jasper, 1947;

Penfield, 1952) or more specifically defined 'cortico-reticular' (Gloor, 1968) systems of the brain, but the pattern has never been accepted as a marker of a single neurological disease, and the actual causes for instability within the proposed circuit are unknown. In studies of both affected human pedigrees and genetic animal models of absence epilepsy, a variety of distinct clinical syndromes have been identified that all share the generalized spike-and-wave discharge in the neocortex as a common electrophysiological trait. One of the most intriguing questions still facing both groups of investigators is whether the basic mechanisms underlying the generation of this discharge pattern in different pedigrees and experimental models are truly identical, and if not, whether there is overlap at some level of nervous system organization where the syndromes share a genetic, molecular, or cellular mechanism in common. Since the human seizure disorders appear at differing ages while the brain is still immature, seizure-induced plasticity may contribute to secondary phenotypic divergence in these brains. It is therefore also of specific interest to determine how the primary molecular errors, and the age-dependent synchronous discharges they generate, interact with normal programs of synaptogenesis and development within the affected neural circuits.

We have used a strategy comprising mutational and cellular analysis of the electrocortical spike-and-wave pattern to explore some of these issues. In so doing, we have found that in mice, a generalized spike-and-wave seizure pattern can be inherited as a result of a defect at a single genetic locus, and that many such loci exist. We have determined that this genetic heterogeneity is accompanied at the neurobiological level by some general similarities, as well as some clear phenotypic differences (Table 1), in the nature of the intervening defects expressed within the epileptic neuronal networks. Finally, we have uncovered evidence that a sustained history of spike-and-wave seizures can lead to varying degrees of abnormal synaptic reorganization in the developing brain. This chapter summarizes examples of distinguishing features between experimental genetic epilepsy models within ten principal categories.

Table 1. Genetic and phenotypic diversity of inherited spike-and-wave epilepsies

1. Locus heterogeneity
2. Allelic heterogeneity
3. Gene dose
4. Variability in developmental onset
5. Morphology of spike-wave discharge
6. Regional cerebral synchronization patterns
7. Selective neurotransmitter imbalances
8. Distinct *in vitro* network excitability defects
9. Pharmacogenetic variation
10. Variable patterns of seizure induced gene expression

Locus heterogeneity

Using a simple search strategy to identify genes linked to spike-and-wave epilepsy phenotypes, we have been systematically screening for mapped single locus murine mutants with cortical excitability defects (Noebels, 1979, 1984b, 1986). Over 110 mapped mutations have been studied to date. This survey has so far revealed five autosomal recessive gene loci (*lethargic*, chr 2; *tottering*, chr 8; *ducky*, chr 9; *mocha*, chr 10; *stargazer*, chr 15) in the mouse associated with the spontaneous appearance of generalized, paroxysmal spike-and-wave discharges in the cortical EEG (Fig. 1). Each discharge arises out of a normal pattern of background EEG rhythms, and is associated with a stereotyped clinical seizure, consisting of sudden arrest of movement and an occasional myoclonic jerk of the neck or jaw, with immediate resumption of normal behaviour at the end of the cortical discharge. The seizures begin in the young mouse, persist throughout adulthood, and are rapidly suppressed by ethosuximide.

Although the clinical features of the seizure phenotype in the five mutants are essentially identical,

Chapter 20 Genetic and phenotypic heterogeneity of inherited spike-and-wave epilepsies

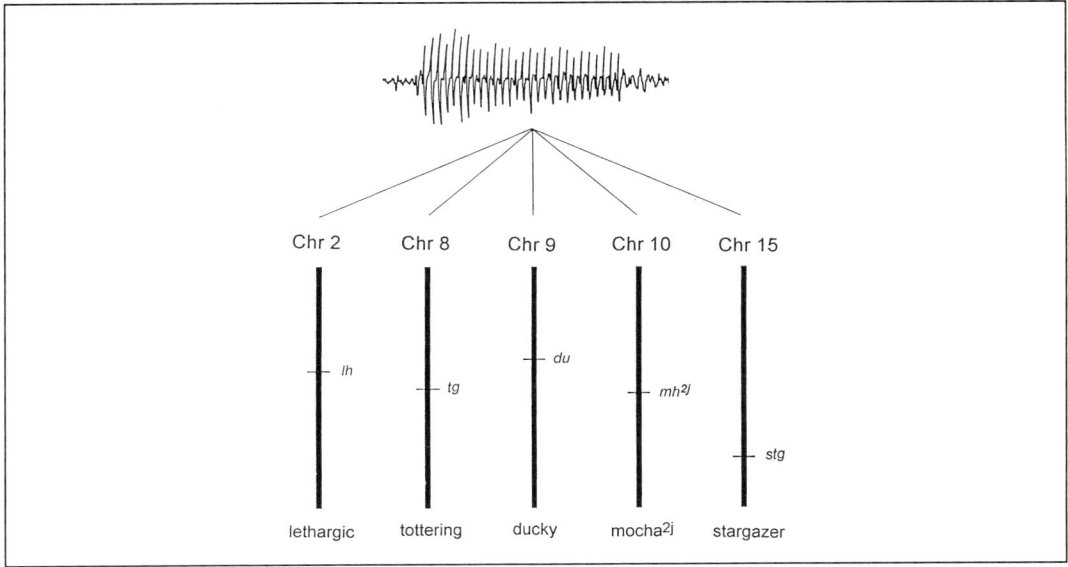

Fig. 1. Chromosomal positions of five independent recessive mutations in the mouse expressing generalized spike-and-wave discharges.

large differences in seizure frequency and in the remainder of the accompanying neurological disorder in each mutant are immediately apparent, and can be readily distinguished by characteristic clinical signs and deficits. For example, *tg, du, lh*, and *stg* mutants all show a prominent gait ataxia with varying degrees of severity specific for each gene locus. Homozygous *tg, du* and *lh* mutants also show intermittent (1–2 day) episodes of focal myoclonus linked to activation of specific brain-stem reticular nuclei but with no correlated EEG discharge (Sidman *et al.*, 1965; Noebels & Sidman, 1979). *Stargazer* mutants have impaired vestibular function with frequent head tossing movements and inability to swim (Noebels *et al.*, 1990). Mocha^{2J} homozygotes show no ataxia, and in this mutant model the seizures appear in isolation from other evident neurological abnormality.

Allelic heterogeneity

Different genetic alleles at a specific chromosomal locus may represent functionally independent point mutations, diverse rearrangements, or even variable length deletions of one or more contiguous genes. Allelic heterogeneity can produce epileptic mutants mapping to the same locus that differ phenotypically either in degree, temporal onset, or in the spectrum of accompanying clinical abnormalities. The *tottering* mutant and its two alleles, *leaner* (tg^{la}) and *roller* (tg^{rol}) provide instructive examples, although their significance will not be entirely appreciated until the genes have been cloned. Similar spike-and-wave discharges have been recorded in *tg*, tg^{la}, and tg/tg^{la} (Fig. 2), and all three alleles show gene-linked noradrenergic hyperinnervation (Levitt & Noebels, 1981; Muramoto *et al.*, 1982). Ataxia becomes noticeable at two weeks postnatal in *roller* and *leaner* mutants, but not earlier than 4 weeks of age in *tottering* mice. Routine histopathological survey of the *tottering* brain reveals no gross cytopathological features, however *leaner* and *roller* both show severely hypoplastic cerebella with striking granule cell loss in the anterior lobe. While the *tottering* homozygote is least severely affected and *leaner* the most; the tg/tg^{la} double heterozygote is closer to the *leaner* phenotype, and like its tg^{la}/tg^{la} counterpart, can be recognized 2 weeks earlier in development. There have been several known remutations to the *tg* and *stg* locus, but these mice have not yet been carefully examined.

IDIOPATHIC GENERALIZED EPILEPSIES

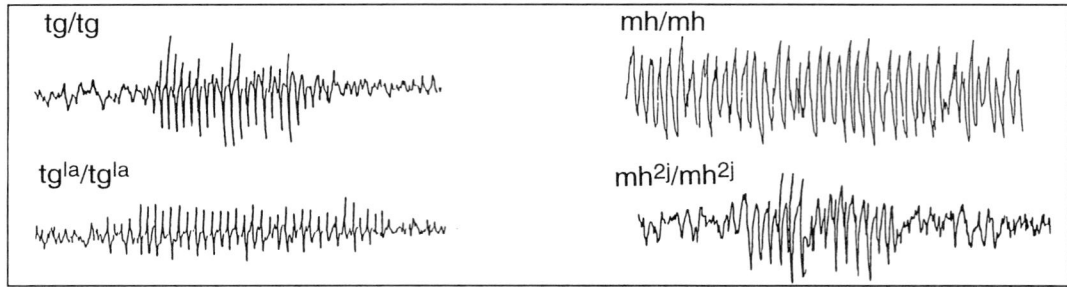

Fig. 2. Similarities and differences in EEG phenotypes expressed in different alleles at the same locus. Left: Synchronous spike-and-wave discharges in tg/tg and tg^{la}/tg^{la} are morphologically similar, but more frequent in tg/tg^{la} and tg^{la}/tg^{la} mutants. Right: In contrast, mocha (mh/mh) mutants show constant 6 s rhythmic oscillations, while the allelic mh^{2j}/mh^{2j} homozygotes show infrequent 6 s spike-wave activity. (Noebels, 1984b; Noebels & Sidman, 1989).

The mutant mouse *mocha* and its paired allele *mocha*^{2J} provide a second example of allelic heterogeneity in the control of cortical excitability. In this allelic pair, the original coat colour mutant, *mocha*, shows a striking hypersynchronous pattern of constant, generalized cortical theta rhythms (Noebels & Sidman, 1989), while the remutation *mocha*^{2J} displays intermittent 6 s spike-and-wave seizure discharges arising on an unaltered electrocortical background (Fig. 2). The phenotypic differences in cortical rhythmic activity between these two alleles are striking, and raise interesting questions regarding the potential for common mechanisms modulating the generation of cortical spikes and persistent wave-like rhythms.

Gene dose

Extended EEG recordings from clinically unaffected heterozygous neurological mutants can, in certain cases, reveal evidence of trace levels of abnormal synchronous discharge activity. Thus adult *tg, stg, du* and *mh*^{2J} heterozygotes might show a single spike-and-wave discharge during an 8 h recording period (J.L. Noebels, unpublished), an event sufficiently rare to impede systematic study. In some mutants, the discharge may be of a somewhat different morphology (Fig. 3). In nearly all cases, the discharge is diminished in duration and amplitude; and in every case the spontaneous seizure frequency in the heterozygote is reduced by 50–100-fold relative to the homozygous mutant

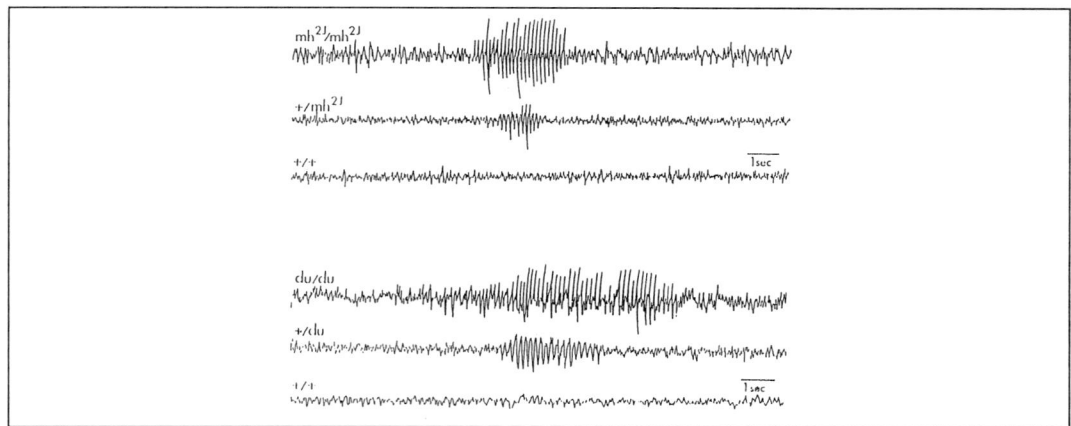

Fig. 3. Evidence for co-dominance of the spike-and-wave phenotype at selected loci. Rare discharges of a generally similar (+/mh2j) or different (+/du) morphology can be detected in prolonged recordings from heterozygotes (J.L. Noebels, unpublished data).

Chapter 20 Genetic and phenotypic heterogeneity of inherited spike-and-wave epilepsies

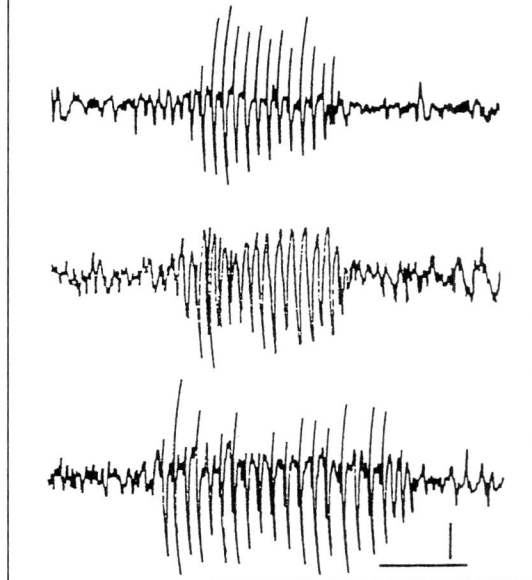

Fig. 4. Spike-and-wave discharge morphology in adult tottering *mutant. Individual components of the burst are variably present at different recording times in the same mutant. Upper primarily spike burst, middle: primarily wave burst, lower: spike-and-wave burst. Bar = 1 s, 100 µV (Noebels, 1986).*

littermate. It is not yet certain whether this 'leakage' or co-dominant effect of a single defective copy of the mutant allele is present at all of the recessive murine epileptic mutant loci. Very prolonged recordings from the +/+ homozygous mice on the parental background strains have never revealed any spontaneous discharge activity.

Variability in developmental onset

Age of onset is a major parameter distinguishing human generalized absence syndromes, and this variable may also prove informative in experimental genetic models (Noebels & Tharp, 1995). In two mutations, *tg* and *stg*, the time of onset is roughly identical in each mutant, with brief episodes of EEG discharges appearing in the third postnatal week (postnatal days 16–19). Within 1 week, the spontaneous discharge rate rises to the respective adult level (Noebels, 1984a; Qiao & Noebels, 1993). Two genetic models developed in inbred rat strains (Vergnes et al., 1986; Coenen & Van Luitjelaar, 1987) never show cortical seizures prior to 1 month of age, but begin to progressively display seizures after that time at considerably later, postpubertal, ages. These differing ontogenetic profiles may signal either the action of distinct epileptogenic mechanisms at the molecular level, or a multigenic threshold effect controlled by the selective maturation of other central neuromodulatory systems in the different background strains.

Seizure severity, assessed by the mean frequency and duration of individual cortical discharges, is apparently also gene-linked in epileptic mutant mice, although different multigenic strain effects could contribute to the differences observed. In our studies, spontaneous seizure rates in the five mutants on their respective inbred backgrounds are in the order, $stg>>tg>>lh>mh^{2J}>du$ (Qiao & Hoebels, 1991; J.L. Noebels, unpublished data), however definitive comparisons require the transfer of each mutation onto the same inbred genetic background.

Morphology of spike-and-wave discharge

The morphology of the cortical discharge is remarkably uniform across the five mutants studied, although minor variations have been noted. In *tottering* mice, prolonged recordings from over 80 homozygotes revealed that the amplitude of the spike or wave within a discharge is subject to variation. The changes can occur reversibly in the same mouse during a single recording session, suggesting that alterations in the degree of cerebral synchronization, and not the recording electrodes, are the source of variability (Fig. 4). No significant changes are seen in spike frequency during the discharge, however in *stg* mice a relatively unusual pattern of complex prolonged discharge has been noted (Noebels *et al.*, 1990). In these mice, the baseline 6/s spike-and-wave discharge may accelerate roughly twofold; alternatively the discharge will begin with fast spiking and decelerate to the baseline rate. It was repeatedly observed that during periods of faster spiking, the mouse could initiate locomotor activity, in sharp contrast with the behavioural arrest seen during the typical 6/s discharge. It is worth noting that inbred rat strains with spike-and-wave/behavioural arrest seizures typically show higher baseline discharge rates (range 7–11 spikes/s, Vergnes *et al.* (1990)) than the mouse mutants.

Regional cerebral synchronization patterns

Cortical mapping studies of the EEG spike-and-wave discharge in man, rat and mouse demonstrate a steady decrease in spike amplitude along an anterior–posterior gradient. In the *stargazer* mutant, EEG recordings with monopolar electrodes referred to an indifferent reference electrode, reveal that discharges are strongly predominant over frontal cortical areas, smoothly diminishing in amplitude more posteriorly (Qiao, 1992). High-amplitude discharges are also seen in the olfactory bulbs, as they are in humans (Angeleri *et al.*, 1964), and using bipolar depth electrodes, discharges are present in basal ganglia, lateral thalamus and hippocampus. Hippocampal involvement is also seen in *tottering* mice (Noebels, 1984a), but not in *lethargic* (Hosford *et al.*, 1992) or in the inbred GAERS rat model (Vergnes *et al.*, 1990). In the mouse, hippocampal discharges are likely to be mediated through synchronizing input from ventral midline thalamic nuclei (in particular, the rhomboid and reuniens nuclear groups) along with perforant path activity from the adjacent entorhinal cortex (Wouterlood *et al.*, 1990). There is no recent electroanatomy of human generalized absence seizures, however several published depth electrode studies reveal that limbic system pathways, including hippocampus, amygdalar nuclei and olfactory cortex, participate with the thalamus and neocortex in the spike-and-wave synchronization of typical generalized absence epilepsy, as well as secondary bilateral synchrony (Angeleri *et al.*, 1964; Rossi *et al.*, 1968; Niedermeyer *et al.*, 1969). Cerebral metabolic mapping studies reveal diffuse increases during clinical (Engel *et al.*, 1985) and experimental (Nehlig *et al.*, 1991) spike-wave seizures, but have not disclosed any specific regional activation abnormalities. Mapping neural circuits by their expression of the immediate early gene proteins c-Fos and c-Jun has also not contributed any detailed information on selective pathway activation in inbred rat (Willoughby *et al.*, 1993) or mutant models (Nahm & Noebels, 1993) of generalized absence seizures.

Selective neurotransmitter imbalances

Detailed comparisons of central noradrenergic pathways in two epileptic mutants, *tottering* and *stargazer*, demonstrate how a major brain neuromodulatory pathway can contribute differently to their respective neuronal excitability phenotypes. The *tottering* mutant develops a paroxysmal spike-and-wave seizure disorder controlled by a gene-linked proliferation of noradrenergic locus coeruleus axon terminals in target regions of the *tg* brain (Levitt & Noebels, 1981). Neonatal correction of the inherited hyperinnervation with a selective neurotoxin (6-OHDA) prevents the expression of epilepsy (Noebels, 1984a), demonstrating that the excess noradrenergic innervation is likely to represent the primary gene-linked epileptogenic lesion. Intracellular microelectrode studies in *in vitro* brain slices reveal that *tg* mutant neurons show a latent hyperexcitability defect revealed during network burst-firing (Helekar & Noebels, 1991) that includes a reduction in the Ca^{2+}-mediated potassium after hyperpolarization mediated by β-adrenoreceptor activation. Increased NE release could also promote synchronous network hyperexcitability by other mechanisms, including disinhibition, as it has been shown to do in cortical (Waterhouse *et al.*, 1980), hippocampal (Doze *et al.*, 1991), and thalamic relays (Rogawski & Agajhanian, 1980). While excess activation of the β-adrenoreceptor facilitates neuronal bursting *in vitro* (Noebels & Rutecki, 1990), other excitability defects have also been identified (Kostopoulos & Psarropoulou, 1990; Helekar & Noebels, 1992, 1994).

The *stargazer* mutant shows a more severe spike-and-wave seizure disorder than the *tottering* mouse. Unlike the latter, no proliferative noradrenergic abnormalities are identifiable in *stg* brain, and neonatal depletion of noradrenaline has no effect on subsequent seizure expression (Qiao &

Chapter 20 Genetic and phenotypic heterogeneity of inherited spike-and-wave epilepsies

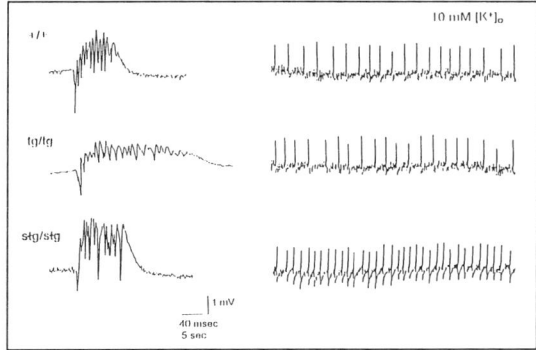

Fig. 5. Distinct repolarization defects in isolated neuronal networks revealed by convulsant-induced bursting in tottering (prolonged burst duration, left) and stargazer (accelerated discharge rate, right) mutants. (Noebels & Rutecki, 1991; Namgung & Noebels, 1992).

Noebels, 1991). The persistence of seizures following neonatal 6-OHDA treatment in the *stg* mice also confirms that their failure to appear in *tg* mutants following treatment is not due to a non-specific antiepileptic effect of the toxin on the developing brain (neonatal 6-OHDA treatment lowers the *convulsant* threshold for seizures in normal brain (Chauvel & Trottier, 1986), but rather to a selective correction of the epileptogenic effects of the *tg* inborn error. These data indicate that the two mutant genes express spike-and-wave seizures modulated by different intervening neurotransmitter pathways in the developing brain.

Distinct *in vitro* network excitability defects

Inherited synchronization defects in epileptic mutant brains have been shown to persist in isolated CNS networks maintained *in vitro* (Noebels & Rutecki, 1990), and can be specifically uncovered during convulsant-induced bursting. While the passive neuronal membrane properties of mutant neurons may be unaffected (Helekar & Noebels, 1991), comparisons of network firing behaviour under activating conditions demonstrate that abnormalities in synaptic excitability differ markedly between mutants sharing the spike-and-wave seizure phenotype.

Extracellular microelectrode studies in *tg* neurons reveal that synchronous bursting in the CA3 region of hippocampus induced by elevated extracellular potassium is characterized by a striking prolongation of the network burst duration compared to that of the wild type. The baseline frequency (i.e. the repetition rate) of the bursting remains unaltered by the *tg* mutation. In contrast, synchronous firing in *stg* neurons under identical conditions shows the exact opposite pattern (Fig. 5). Hippocampal networks in *stg* slices bathed in elevated extracellular potassium show a burst response similar in duration to the wild type, but a significant acceleration of the baseline 'interictal' bursting frequency (Namgung & Noebels, 1991). These data provide evidence for distinct repolarization defects associated with the expression of the two genetically heterogeneous spike-and-wave seizure disorders.

Pharmacogenetic variation

Although not all patients with generalized spike-and-wave epilepsies are seizure-free with ethosuximide treatment (Browne et al., 1975), the drug has proven effective in suppressing cortical spike-and-wave discharges in virtually every genetic model where it has been assessed, and anticonvulsants that are typically ineffective as anti-absence therapy in humans are generally ineffective in these experimental models as well (Heller et al., 1983; Vergnes et al., 1990; Hosford et al., 1992). The recent development of a potent selective $GABA_B$ receptor antagonist has contributed a new molecular target for the pharmacological treatment of absence epilepsy (Vergnes & Marescaux, Ch. 15) as well as an additional phenotype for characterizing its various syndromes. The $GABA_B$ antagonist CGP 35348 effectively blocks spontaneous spike-and-wave seizures in the *lethargic* mutant mouse (Hosford et al., 1992) as well as the GAERS inbred rat strain (Liu et al., 1992). In contrast, although ethosuximide (50–150 mg/kg i.p.) produces an immediate and complete cessation of spike-and-wave discharge activity in *stg* mice for a period of several hours (with a gradual return of seizure activity as the serum level declined), CGP 35348 at doses of 50–500 mg/kg

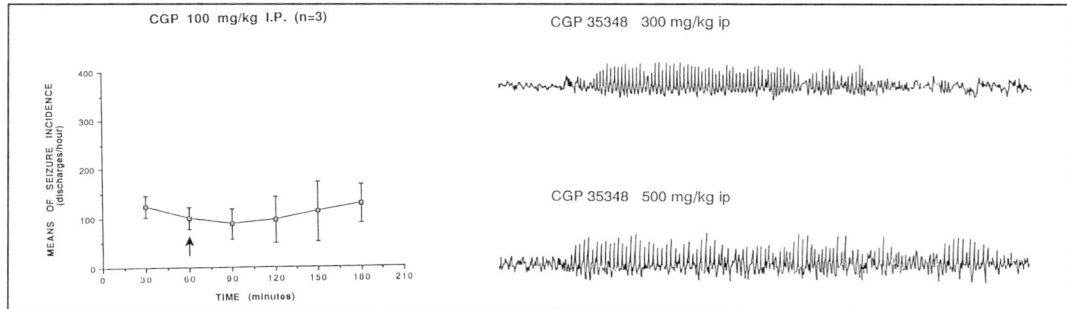

Fig. 6. Pharmacogenetic diversity in experimental spike-and-wave epilepsy models demonstrated by lack of sensitivity to the $GABA_B$ antagonist CGP 35348 at doses well in excess of those reported to block absence in other genetic models (Qiao & Noebels, 1992).

i.p. does not alter seizure morphology (Fig. 6) or frequency over a similar time period (Noebels & Qiao, 1992). Higher doses depressed the amplitude and slowed the frequency of background EEG rhythms. These data suggest that central $GABA_B$-receptor activity is not a critical mechanism underlying the spike-and-wave pattern of epileptogenesis in the *stargazer* mutant, and therefore does not constitute a final common pathway mediating the generation of murine 6–7 s spike-and-wave bursting.

Variable patterns of seizure-induced gene expression

Since seizures induce the expression of nervous system genes (Gall *et al.*, 1991), it can be anticipated that a prolonged history of epilepsy might steadily deregulate levels of neural gene expression within bursting neural circuits, modify their patterns of excitability and connectivity, and create secondary cerebral pleiomorphisms that vary between experimental models. Several parameters that could contribute to distinctive patterns of change in the mutants include: the anatomy of the discharging circuits; the age of onset of ictal activity; and the severity of the seizures.

One clear example of this multifactorial plasticity is illustrated by the phenomenon of aberrant mossy fibre sprouting in the inner molecular layer of the dentate gyrus, a process that has been described in human hippocampal epilepsy (Sutula *et al.*, 1989; Houser *et al.*, 1990; Babb *et al.*, 1991) and that has recently been found in striking excess in adult *stg* mutants. The aberrant mossy fibre reorganization is not observed at the time of *stg* seizure onset, but increases steadily with age, consistent with secondary seizure-induced fibre outgrowth induced by the prolonged history of spike-and-wave epileptogenesis (Qiao & Noebels, 1993). A similar pattern of mossy fibre sprouting in adult *tg* mice can be detected, but only to a minimal degree (Stanfield, 1989; Qiao & Noebels, 1993). Although the temporal onset of the seizure disorder and the general spike-and-wave morphology of hippocampal spike-and-wave discharges are essentially identical in both mutants, the mean frequency and duration of the spike-and-wave discharges are markedly elevated in *stg* mice, resulting in a seizure index approximately double that of *tg* mutants. These data suggest that secondary patterns of brain plasticity may distinguish the different models of spike-and-wave epileptogenesis.

Conclusion

In conclusion, defined single-locus mutations in the mouse provide a model system for the genetic analysis of spike-and-wave epilepsies that is beginning to reveal the extent of genotypic and phenotypic diversity that is likely to be associated with this important category of childhood epilepsy. Comparative developmental studies reveal at least four fundamental properties underlying the heredity of this specific cortical synchronization trait. First, a defect at a single gene locus is sufficient to produce a spontaneous, generalized spike-and-wave seizure disorder. Second, the EEG trait itself is genetically heterogeneous, and can arise from recessive mutations at more than one chromosomal locus. Third, the intervening cellular excitability mechanisms underlying the generation of spike-and-wave cortical discharges by mutations at these loci are not necessarily identical. Fourth, each of the mutant genes gives rise to distinct syndromes, each with a characteristic seizure frequency, sensitivity to antiepileptic drugs, and severity of the associated neurological phenotype. These epilepsy syndromes may differ because of the nature of the primary mutant molecular errors, the time of onset in the developing brain, and the degree of secondary seizure-dependent plasticity in the affected neural circuits.

Acknowledgements

Supported by NIH NS 29709, 11535 and the Blue Bird Circle Foundation for Pediatric Neurology. The author thanks S. Helekar, X. Qiao, and W. Nahm for their contribution to this research.

References

Angeleri, F., Ferro-Milone, F. & Parigi, S. (1964): Electrical activity and reactivity of the rhinencephalic, pararhinencephalic and thalamic structures: prolonged implantation of electrodes in man. *Electroencephalogr. Clin. Neurophysiol.* **16**, 100–129.

Avanzini, G., Vergnes, M., Spreafico, R. & Marescaux, C. (1993): Calcium-dependent regulation of genetically determined spike-and-waves by the reticular thalamic nucleus of rats. *Epilepsia* **34**, 1–7.

Babb, T.L., Kupfer, W.R., Pretorius, J,K,, Crandall, P.H. & Levesque, M.F. (1991): Synaptic reorganization by mossy fibers in human epileptic fascia dentata. *Neuroscience* **42**, 351–363.

Browne, T.R., Dreifuss, F.E., Dyken, P.R., Goode, D.J., Penry, J.K., Porter, R.J., White, B.G. & White, P.T. (1975): Ethosuximide in the treatment of absence (petit mal) seizures. *Neurology* **25**, 515–524.

Chauvel, P. & Trottier, S. (1986): Role of noradrenergic ascending system in extinction of epileptic phenomena. *Adv. Neurol.* **44**, 475–487.

Coenen, A.M.L. & Van Luitjelaar, E.L.J.M. (1987): The WAG/Rij rat model for absence epilepsy: age and sex factors. *Epi. Res.* **1**, 297–301.

Crunelli, V. & Leresche, N. (1991): A role for $GABA_B$ receptors in excitation and inhibition of thalamocortical cells. *TINS* **14**, 16–21.

Doze, V.A., Cohen, G.A. & Madison, D.V. (1991): Synaptic localization of adrenergic disinhibition in the rat hippocampus. *Neuron* **6**, 889–890..

Engel, J. Jr, Kuhl, D.E. & Phelps, M.E. (1985): Local cerebral metabolic rate for glucose during petit mal absences. *Ann. Neurol.* **17**, 121–128.

Fisher, R.S. & Prince, D.A. (1977): Spike-wave rhythms in cat cortex induced by parental penicillin. I. Electroencephalographic features. *Electroencephalogr. Clin. Neurophysiol.* **42**, 608–624.

Gall, C.M., Lauterborn, J., Bundman, M., Murray, K. & Isackson, P. (1991): Seizures and the regulation of neurotrophic factor and neuropeptide gene expression in brain. In: *Genetic strategies in epilepsy research*, eds. E. Anderson, I. Leppik & J. Noebels, pp. 225–246. Amsterdam: Elsevier.

Gloor, P. (1968): Generalized cortico-reticular epilepsies. Some considerations on the pathophysiology of generalized bilaterally synchronous spike-and-wave discharge. *Epilepsia* **9**, 249–263.

Gloor, P., Avoli, M. & Kostopoulos, G. (1990): Thalamocortical relationships in generalized epilepsy with bilaterally synchronous spike-and-wave discharge. In: *Generalized epilepsy: neurobiological approaches*, eds. M. Avoli, P. Gloor, G. Kostopoulos & R. Naquet, pp. 190–212. Boston: Birkhauser.

Helekar, S.A. & Noebels, J.L. (1991): Synchronous hippocampal bursting unmasks latent network excitability alterations in an epileptic gene mutation. *Proc. Natl. Acad. Sci. (USA)* **88**, 4736–4740.

Helekar, S.A. & Noebels, J.L. (1992): A burst dependent excitability defect elicited by potassium at the developmental onset of spike-wave seizures in the tottering mutant. *Dev. Brain Res.* **65**, 205–210.

Helekar, S.A. & Noebels, J.L. (1994): Analysis of voltage-gated and synaptic conductances contributing to a gene-linked prolongation of depolarizing shifts in the epileptic mutant mouse tottering. *J. Neurophysiol.* **71**, 1–10.

Heller, A.H., Dichter, M.A. & Sidman, R.L. (1983): Anticonvulsant sensitivity of absence seizures in the tottering mutant mouse. *Epilepsia* **25**, 25–34.

Hosford, D.A., Clark, S., Cao, Z., Wilson, W., Lin, F-H., Morisett, R.A. & Huin, A. (1992): The role of GABA$_B$ receptor activation in absence seizures of lethargic (lh/lh) mice. *Science* **257**, 398–401.

Houser, C.R., Miyashiro, J.E., Swartz, B.E., Walsh, G.O., Rich, J.R. & Delgado-Escueta, A.V. (1990): Altered patterns of dynorphin immunoreactivity suggest mossy fiber reorganization in human hippocampal epilepsy. *J. Neurosci.* **10**, 267–282.

Huguenard, J.R. & Prince, D.A. (1992): A novel T-type current underlies prolonged Ca^{2+}-dependent burst firing in GABAergic neurons of the rat thalamic reticular nucleus. *J. Neurosci.* **12**, 3804–3817.

Jasper, H.H. & Droogleever-Fortuyn, J. (1947): Experimental studies of the functional anatomy of petit mal epilepsy. *Assoc. Res. Nerv. Ment. Dis. Proc.* **26**, 272–298.

Kostopoulos, G. & Psarropoulou, K. (1990): *In vitro* electrophysiology of a genetic model of generalized epilepsy. In: *Generalized epilepsy: neurobiological approaches,* eds. M. Avoli, P. Gloor, G. Kostopoulos & R. Naquet, pp. 137–160. Boston: Birkhauser.

Levitt, P. & Noebels, J.L. (1981): Mutant mouse tottering: selective increase of locus coeruleus axons in a defined single locus mutation. *Proc. Natl. Acad. Sci. (USA)* **78**, 4630–4634.

Liu, Z., Vergnes, M., Depaulis, A. & Marescaux, C. (1992): Involvement of intrathalamic GABAb neurotransmission in the control of absence seizures in the rat. *Neuroscience* **48**, 87–93.

Lytton, W.W. & Sejnowski, T.J. (1992): Computer model of ethosuximide's effect on a thalamic neuron. *Ann. Neurol.* **32**, 131–139.

Muramoto, O., Ando, K. & Kanazawa, I. (1982): Central noradrenaline metabolism in cerebellar ataxic mice. *Brain Res.* **237**, 387–395.

Nahm, W.K. & Noebels, J.L. (1993): Immediate-early gene protein expression in a mutant mouse model of spike-wave epilepsy, stargazer. *Neurosci. Abstr.* **19**, 1030.

Namgung, U. & Noebels, J.L. (1991): Hippocampal CA3 pyramidal cells of the epileptic mutant mouse stargazer display a distinctive gene-linked hyperexcitability. *Neurosci. Abstr.* **17**, 170.

Nehlig, A., Vergnes, M., Marescaux, C. Boyer, S. & Lannes, B. (1991): Local cerebral glucose utilization in rats with petit mal-like seizures. *Ann. Neurol.* **29**, 72–77.

Niedermeyer, E., Laws, E.R. & Walker, A.E. (1969): Depth EEG findings in epileptics with generalized spike-wave complexes. *Arch. Neurol.* **21**, 51–58.

Noebels, J.L. (1979): Analysis of inherited epilepsy using single locus mutations in mice. *Fed. Proc.* **38**, 2405–2410.

Noebels, J.L. (1984a): A single gene error in noradrenergic axon growth synchronizes central neurons. *Nature* **310**, 409–411.

Noebels, J.L. (1984b): Isolating single genes of the inherited epilepsies. *Ann. Neurol.* **16**, S18–21.

Noebels, J.L. (1986): Mutational analysis of the inherited epilepsies. In: *Basic mechanisms of the epilepsies: molecular and cellular approaches,* eds. A.V. Delgado-Escueta, A.A. Ward & D.M. Woodbury, pp. 97–114. New York: Raven Press.

Noebels, J.L. & Sidman, R.L. (1979): Inherited epilepsy: spike-wave and focal motor seizures in the mutant mouse tottering. *Science* **204**, 1334–1336.

Noebels, J.L. & Sidman, R.L. (1989): Persistent hypersynchronization of neocortical neurons in the Mocha mutant mouse. *J. Neurogen.* **6**, 53–56.

Noebels, J.L. & Rutecki, P.A. (1990): Altered hippocampal network. Excitability in the hypernoradrenergic mutant mouse tottering. *Brain Res.* **524**, 225–230.

Noebels, J.L., Qiao X., Bronson, R.T., Spencer, C. & Davisson, M.T. (1990): Stargazer: a new neurological mutant in the mouse on chromosome 15 with prolonged cortical seizures. *Epi. Res.* **7**, 129–135.

Noebels, J.L. & Tharp, B. (1995): Absence seizures in developing brain. In: *Brain development and epilepsy,* eds. S. Moshe, J.L. Noebels, P. Schwartzkroin & J. Swann. New York: Oxford University Press (in press).

Penfield, W.G. & Jasper, H.H. (1947): Highest level seizures. *Assoc. Nerv. Ment. Dis. Proc.* **26**, 252–271.

Penfield, W.G. (1952): Epileptic automatism and the centrencephalic integrating system. *Assoc. Nerv. Ment. Dis. Proc.* **30**, 513–528.

Qiao, X. (1992): Developmental analysis of excitability and plasticity in an epileptic mutant mouse, stargazer. PhD Dissertation, Baylor College of Medicine.

Qiao, X. & Noebels, J.L. (1991): Genetic heterogeneity of inherited spike-wave epilepsy: two mutant gene loci with independent cerebral excitability defects. *Brain Res.* **555**, 43–50.

Qiao, X. & Noebels, J.L. (1992): GABA-$_B$ receptor independent spike-wave epilepsy in the mutant mouse stargazer. *Pharmacol. Abstr.* **18**, 553.

Qiao, X. & Noebels, J.L. (1993): Developmental analysis of hippocampal mossy fiber outgrowth in a mutant mouse with inherited spike-wave seizures. *J. Neurosci.* **13**, 4622–4635.

Rogawski, M.A. & Agajhanian, G.K. (1980): Activation of lateral geniculate neurons by norepinephrine: mediation by an α-adrenergic receptor. *Brain Res.* **182**, 345–359.

Rossi, G.F., Walter, R.D. & Crandall, P.H. (1968): Generalized spike-and-wave discharges and nonspecific thalamic nuclei. *Arch. Neurol.* **19**, 174–183.

Sidman, R.L., Green, M.C. & Appel, S.H. (1965): *Catalog of the neurological mutants of the mouse.* Cambridge, MA: Harvard University Press.

Stanfield, B.B. (1989): Excessive intra- and supragranular mossy fibers in the dentate gyrus of tottering (tg/tg) mice. *Brain Res.* **480**, 294–299.

Steriade, M., Jones, E.G. & Llinas, R.R. (1990): *Thalamic oscillations and signaling.* New York: John Wiley and Sons.

Sutula, T., Cascino, G., Cavazos, J., Parada, I. & Ramirez, L. (1989): Mossy fiber synaptic reorganization in the epileptic human temporal lobe. *Ann. Neurol.* **26**, 321–330.

Vergnes, M., Marescaux, C., Depaulis, A., Micheletti, G. & Warter, J.M. (1986): Ontogeny of spontaneous petit mal like seizures in Wistar rats. *Dev. Brain Res.* **30**, 85–87.

Vergnes, M., Marescaux, C., Depaulis, A., Micheletti, G. & Warter, J.M. (1990): Spontaneous spike-wave discharges in Wistar rats: a model of genetic generalized non-convulsive epilepsy. In: *Generalized epilepsy: neurobiological approaches*, eds. M. Avoli, P. Gloor, G. Kostopoulos & R. Naquet. pp. 238–253. Boston: Birkhauser.

von Krosigk, M., Bal, T. & McCormick, D.A. (1993): Cellular mechanisms of a synchronized oscillation in the thalamus. *Science* **261**, 361–364.

Waterhouse, B., Moises, H.C. & Woodward, D. (1980): Noradrenergic modulation of somatosensory cortical neuronal responses to iontophoretically applied putative neurotransmitters. *Exp. Neurol.* **69**, 30–49.

Williams, D. (1953): A study of thalamic and cortical rhythms in 'petit mal'. *Brain* **76**, 50–69.

Willoughby, J.O., Mackenzie L., Hiscock, J.J. & Sagar, S. (1993): Non-convulsive spike-wave discharges do not induce Fos in cerebro-cortical neurons. *Molec. Brain Res.* **18**, 178–180.

Wouterlood, F.G., Saldana, E. & Witter, M.P. (1990): Projection from the nucleus reuniens thalami to the hippocampal region: light and electron microscopic tracing study in the rat with the anterograde tracer *Phaseolus vulgaris*-leucoagglutinin. *J. Comp. Neurol.* **296**, 179–203.

Part IV
Juvenile myoclonic epilepsy and related syndromes

Chapter 21

Impulsive petit mal

D. Janz and W. Christian[1]

Aus der Nervenabteilung der Ludolf-Krehl-Klinik der Universität Heidelberg, Germany
(Director: Prof. Dr P. Vogel)

Impulsions, secousses, commotions épileptiques (Herpin, 1867), petit mal moteur (Delasiauve, 1854; Féré, 1890), myoclonies épileptiques (Rabot, 1899), intermittierende Myoklonusepilepsie (Lundborg, 1903), regionäre Zuckungen (Muskens, 1926), myoclonic epilepsy (Lennox, 1945), épilepsie myoclonique bénigne ou fonctionnelle (Sole-Sagarra, 1952), myoclonic petit mal (Penfield, 1954).

There are epileptic equivalents that look like a sudden contraction caused by intense fright. Patients report that – mostly after getting up in the morning – during their morning wash or breakfast, they experience unprovoked jerks, causing them to drop their razor, their coffee cup or whatever they are holding. This can happen once or several times in succession, or even escalate into a succession of jerks. The jerks can be mild enough to escape the attention of onlookers, but they can also be strong enough to make the patients fall, although they will immediately stand up again. As long as these jerks are the only symptoms, no doctor will be called, because they are infrequent, are the subject of shame or are not perceived as abnormal. And if the doctor is asked about these phenomena, he will most often state that they are caused by 'nervousness'. Having said this, abstinence from alcohol and regular, sufficient sleep will be recommended, as the medical interview will have shown that these are likely precipitating factors; at this stage of the disease, such recommendations may, even in the absence of accurate diagnosis, lead to cure. Most often, however, the significance of these symptoms will only become apparent following the first generalized grand mal seizure, which is characterized by a particularly intense tonic phase, a long apnoea and a cyanosis that will appear to be life-threatening. Following this, the jerks that had preceded the dramatic seizure by months or years will be diagnosed, in retrospect, as a petit mal forerunner. A detailed description of this type of petit mal is missing in the epilepsy literature and would be justified due to its practical significance only. Furthermore, our investigations led us to find that this condition has such a typical clinical presentation that no diagnosis other than Unverricht–Lundborg disease comes to

---

1 *Translation by Pierre Genton MD from the original paper 'Impulsiv-Petit mal' (Janz, D. & Christian, W. (1957): Impulsiv-Petit mal. J. Neurol. (Zeitschrift f Nervenheilkunde)* **176**, *346–386). The translator thanks Professor D. Janz for his very kind help.*

mind, a much less common but better known disorder with which it has occasionally been mistaken in spite of important differences. This mistake rests less on factual than on terminological grounds.

Herpin (1867) was the first to name and precisely describe these previously known clinical phenomena (Delasiauve, 1854; Reynolds, 1865): 'The model of this variety of seizure precursors is a jerk ('secousse') that rattles the whole body like an electric shock'. He described the 14-year-old son of a doctor who suffered such seizures from age 13; they were first limited to the upper part of the body, then generalized. 'Whenever he stands or walks, he may fall . . . He gets up again immediately. He drops or throws whatever he is holding in his hands'. Full-blown seizures appeared later, that were triggered by 'sudden and forced awakening'. Delasiauve (1854), Féré (1890), Binswanger (1899) and Gowers (1901) mention in their monographs such 'sudden jerks' as the expression of prodromes, auras or aborted seizures (motor petit mal), without trying to differentiate the phenomenological and disease-specific aspects.

In 1881, Friedreich coined the term 'paramyoclonus multiplex' to describe the hitherto unclear observation of a 50-year-old man with 'clonic cramps of a number of symmetrical muscles of the upper and lower extremities, that were triggered by great fear, remitted remarkably rapidly after a duration of several years, disappeared during sleep and voluntary motion and did not hinder in the least the muscular strength and coordination'. His description opened the floodgates for reports of cases featuring involuntary jerks, although the underlying conditions were as unrelated as hysteria, tics, chorea, encephalitis, Parkinsonism and systematic diseases affecting the spinal cord. From the 'chaos of motor neuroses' and from the opaque background of the numerous publications, Unverricht (1895) then crystallized a specific condition, which he described in five siblings in 1891 and in three siblings from another family in 1895. The disease began between the ages of 7 and 15 and was characterized by the combination of nightly epileptic seizures of a particular type and of specific, '*blitz*-like, arrhythmic, isolated jerks involving single, functionally unconnected muscles of either side; these jerks could be partially controlled by will, were increased by psychological excitement and disappeared completely during sleep'. Hence the terminology he chose, 'Myoklonie', to which he later added 'familial': the familial occurrence was the proof that this condition was not hysteria, a criticism that had been voiced against the cases reported by Friedreich and others. He considered the epileptic seizures to be complications. In his detailed discussion of the differential diagnosis of this condition, he did not mention the preparoxysmal jerks of epileptics (known in these days as 'secousses'), although a clinician like him, with a large experience in epilepsy, must have known about them. It can be concluded from this that the condition he described as 'Myoklonie' and the 'secousses' described by Herpin were, in his mind, different phenomena that could not be mistaken for each other.

This clarity was short-lived. In 1899, Dide (cited in Lundborg, 1903) and Rabot quite simultaneously introduced the concept of 'myoclonia' into the vocabulary of epilepsy. Dide, from a semiological point of view (*La myoclonie dans l'épilepsie*), compared the 'clonic jerks, that sometimes are limited to a sudden shrug, and sometimes entail a sudden movement of the limbs' (one recognizes here Herpin's 'secousses') with the 'rhythmic contractions, vibrations and choreiform movements', the latter looking more like Unverricht's Myoklonie. Rabot, on the other hand, was more concerned with the nosological aspects (*De la myoclonie épileptique*), and with the meaning of the manifestations he considered to be 'secousses myocloniques' as epileptic equivalents; he described these as 'petit mal moteur', in contrast to the much more frequent 'petit mal intellectuel'. However, his clinical histories contain what had been described by Herpin and what we intend to study in more detail. This is one of his clinical reports:

> 'At age 15, a now 24-year-old baker's apprentice experienced his first epileptic seizure at work. He remained seizure-free on bromide for 2 years, then again had seizures that were generally announced by myoclonic jerks. These jerks usually began in the morning, after he woke up. They lasted until a seizure occurred, i.e. generally 1–2 h, but could last 24 h or more. The jerks were not affected by walking or lying down. They stopped when the seizure

occurred. He compared them to an electric shock that took him by surprise. The jerks caused all the muscles of the body to contract quickly and violently. If he happened to be seated, he would jump in his chair. If he was standing, he was suddenly overwhelmed and fell to his knees. His consciousness was completely unimpaired, but every act of will was impeded. The sentence he was speaking was interrupted by the seizure. Before he was treated, he was seized almost every day between 6 and 7 a.m. by almost continuous myoclonic jerks'.

A few years later, in 1902, Clark & Prout suggested the term 'myoclonus epilepsy' for their cases of Unverricht's Myoklonie, which Clark had reported in 1900 as 'paramyoclonus multiplex with epilepsy'. Thus Lundborg found that two different entities had been described under the same name, when he had to choose the right name for a disease he described and thoroughly studied throughout its evolution in 18 members of a peasant family. He chose to give more importance to criteria drawn from the long-term evolution, over those drawn from the symptomatology. He consequently decided to describe 'progressive, familial myoclonus epilepsy' as identical with Unverricht's 'Myoklonie' and closer to 'essential epilepsy' than to the 'sporadic, intermittent myoclonic epilepsy of the Rabot type'. Brissaud (1903) found no support for his opinion: according to him, the term 'myoclonia' was ill-chosen to describe the 'large jerks of the limbs' in the Herpin–Rabot type, because it was meant to describe an 'isolated contraction of a muscle or a muscular group', and not the global jerking of limbs. Muskens (1926) went so far as to call any type of jerking myoclonic, which was but a short step away from his statement that the enlarged concept of 'myoclonic epilepsy' represented the 'core and type of true epilepsy'. This would be of no consequence, except for the classification of petit mal forms by Lennox (1945) still widely accepted until now. Lennox upheld the concept of 'myoclonic epilepsy' for 'falls and jerks that cause isolated contractions of axial muscles and usually one or both arms, even the trunk', even though he warned against the confusion of this form with the 'extremely uncommon' myoclonus epilepsy. This most confusing common denomination of basically different clinical entities was recently settled by the proposal of Sole-Sagarra (1952), who called both forms myoclonic epilepsy and only distinguished between a 'benign or functional' and a 'malign or degenerative' form.

Personal patients

Our study is based on the examination of 47 patients. This group includes all the cases with the type of jerks described above, seen among 1712 patients with epilepsy who were systematically evaluated over the past 10 years; of these, 1252 had no identifiable cause for epilepsy while 460 had a known aetiology (Table 1). The duration of the disease was 1.5–33 years (mean 10.3 years), the age at the last evaluation was between 14 and 55 (mean 26); 23 were males, 24 females.

Table 1. Distribution and aetiology of the different forms of minor seizures

Type of seizure	Idiopathic	Symptomatic	Total
Propulsive petit mal	52 = 4.2%	24 = 5.2%	76 = 4.4%
Pyknoleptic petit mal (54% = retropulsive petit mal)	110 = 8.1%	11 = 2.4%	121 = 7.1%
Impulsive petit mal	47 = 3.75%	0	47 = 2.7%
Oral petit mal (including dreamy state)	265 = 21.2%	65 = 14.1%	330 = 19.2%
Adversive petit mal	30 = 2.4%	7 = 1.5%	37 = 2.2%
Crepuscular attacks (without oral or adversive petit mal)	8 = 0.6%	1 = 0.2%	9 = 0.5%
Indifferent absences	18 = 1.4%	3 = 0.7%	21 = 1.2%
Jacksonian and adversive seizures	45 = 3.6%	123 = 26.7%	168 = 9.8%
Unclassifiable equivalents	69 = 5.5%	22 = 4.8%	91 = 5.3%
Pure grand mal epilepsies	608 = 47.9%	204 = 44.2%	812 = 47.4%
Total	1525	460	1712

Characteristics of the minor seizures

In their reports, the patients always mention three significant moments: the sudden occurrence, 'like an electric shock', the brief duration, 'like a flash of lightning', and the lack of direction of the movements, 'like a startle provoked by fright'. The intensity can vary objectively and subjectively: from a inner shrug, that can hardly be witnessed by others, to a sudden thrust, to a massive jerk. It always includes, at first, the shoulders and arms, mostly in a symmetrical fashion, less commonly the legs or the head, but never without the arms. The jerks always affect the limbs or segments of limbs, never isolated muscles or muscular groups, which is why the denomination of 'myoclonia' is wrong. The phenomenon is often described as a blow that goes through all limbs, and only closer questioning or examination will show that first and foremost the arms jerk from the shoulders, either inwards or outwards, which causes objects that the patient is holding or that are close to fly away or to be thrown away. At times, the patient will experience a blow in his neck or a shock in his head. If the impulse is stronger, the knees will collapse. This can cause merely kneeling or cause the patient to fall 'as if struck by lightning', but he will rise again immediately to his feet. The diaphragm and/or the belly muscles will often be involved, which explains why an inspiratory noise occurs, that may sound like a hiccup or like a yell, mimicking, like the other motor phenomena, a natural reaction of fright.

The patients experience the jerks mostly in full consciousness. During violent jerks, however, they will be 'slightly benumbed', 'momentarily away' or 'shortly absent'. When they fall to the ground, they may remain lying there for a short while 'stunned' and without contact. But the rule is that consciousness is never altered before the jerks, only during the moment of the shock, and that it returns not longer than 1–2 s later.

The possibility of a loss of consciousness depends on the intensity of the jerks, not on their duration. Consciousness and motor phenomena behave, in this type of petit mal, in a manner exactly opposite to pyknoleptic petit mal, in which the 'absence' is in the foreground, while the (retropulsive) movements are very mild. The fact that a clouding of consciousness may occur during the violent jerks does not allow us to describe these as 'motor petit mal'. As they do not represent myoclonias (as already mentioned), but movements of the trunk and limbs, they should not be called 'myoclonic petit mal' either, the latter is all the more inadequate, as it has previously been used to describe such different ictal symptoms as the lightning-like attacks of propulsive petit mal (Janz & Matthes, 1955), the nystactic twitchings found in pyknoleptic absences that happen mainly in retropulsive petit mal (Janz, 1955), or as the true myoclonias in myoclonus epilepsy.

We propose to describe this type of minor seizures as 'impulsive petit mal' (impulsio = shock), mainly because there is nothing in the foreground that masks the characteristic symptom of the shock-like jerks, and because this description is linguistically linked to the descriptions of the two forms of petit mal that precede this one in their age-dependency, i.e. propulsive petit mal and retropulsive petit mal; these three forms are pathogenetically linked within a petit mal triad (Lennox, 1945; Janz, 1955).

Rhythmicity

Even though the frequency of jerks may vary greatly between cases and also during the course of the disease in a given case, the manner in which they recur merits further precision, especially in comparison with the other forms of petit mal. The jerks seldom remain isolated, they often occur in series of two, three or four in a short, but irregular sequence. In cases of rapid evolution, or after a long course, a particular sequence of jerks can occur as a 'salvo', to use the patients' own term. To illustrate the pattern of their recurrence, one can compare the short, but irregular and unpredictable intervals between jerks with those found between flashes of lightning when several storms collide. At times, the jerks follow each other so closely that for minutes, or even, with some breaks,

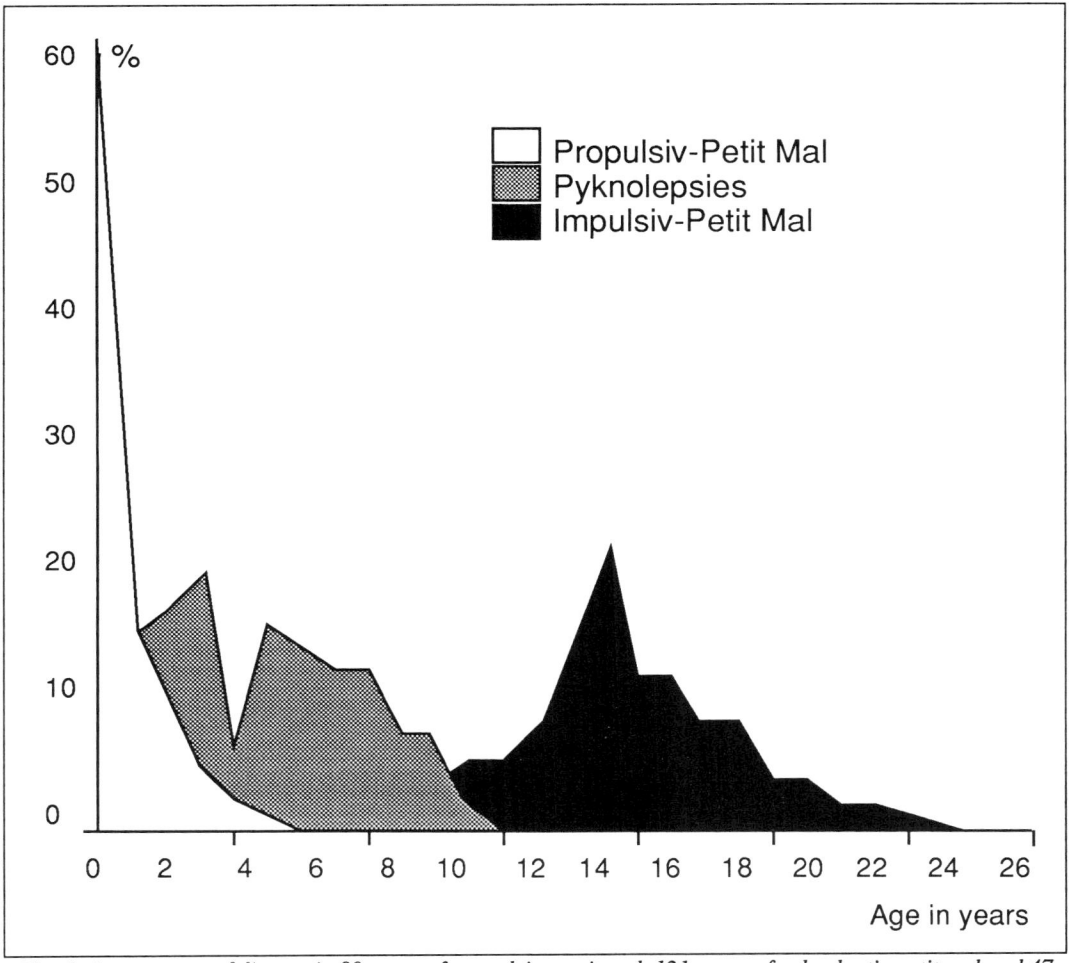

Fig. 1. Age at onset of disease in 89 cases of propulsive petit mal, 121 cases of pyknoleptic petit mal and 47 cases of impulsive petit mal.

for hours, one can speak of a petit mal status during which, in contrast to grand mal status, the consciousness is only minimally clouded.

Even petit mal can lead to status-like events, and each type of petit mal has its own type of increased occurrence of seizures, series of attacks or status. A status of propulsive petit mal is characterized by intervals between attacks that become progressively shorter, then progressively longer; retropulsive petit mal (as usually in pyknoleptic petit mal) is characterized by the linking of individual seizures to one another after identically short intervals, and this form is commonly referred to as petit mal status; impulsive petit mal, on the contrary, is characterized by a chaos of more or less rapid jerks, sometimes in volleys, sometimes as consecutive isolated events, sometimes melting into a tonic rigidity.

While isolated jerks are mostly associated with aimless but coordinated symmetrical motor impulses, impulsive petit mal status is strikingly characterized by uncoordinated jerking that at times predominantly affects the shoulders and arms, at other times the trunk or the legs, and includes the diaphragm. There are no autonomic symptoms in impulsive petit mal. When the jerks become frequent and tend to produce a status, the patients experience palpitation and sweating. When one witnesses such a status, one will never be able to see the involuntary play of isolated muscles or groups of muscles, but one may think of a chorea or of a hysterical display, seeing these sudden, violent, ample, balancing moves, until – because it is most often the case – a major epileptic seizure ends the performance.

Age of onset

Impulsive petit mal begins at a precise age, between age 10 at the earliest and age 23 at the latest. In two-thirds of cases, the age of onset falls between the narrower range of 14 to 18 years. Propulsive petit mal begins within the first year of life, in the latest cases until age 5. Retropulsive petit mal and the other forms of pyknoleptic petit mal begin between age 4 and age 12, most often between the ages of 6 and 8 (Fig. 1).

The existence of a close relationship between age and type of seizure indicates the influence that the biological background has on the clinical manifestations and on the evolution of the disease.

The myoclonus epilepsy of Unverricht–Lundborg begins at an age that is intermediary between that of pyknolepsy and that of impulsive petit mal, i.e. mostly between 9 and 11, never before the ages of 6, and never after 15: this fact alone may determine the differential diagnosis between myoclonus epilepsy and impulsive petit mal.

Prevalence

Among 1712 epilepsy cases personally evaluated in the past 10 years, we found 47 patients with the epileptic equivalents described above (i.e. 2.7 per cent of the total or 3.75 per cent of all idiopathic cases). Epilepsies with impulsive petit mal are thus comparatively rare, but nevertheless much more common than the Unverricht–Lundborg type of myoclonus epilepsy, of which we have observed only four cases over the same period (Table 1).

There are no comparable data from other sources. Gibbs & Gibbs (1952) found 133 epilepsies with so-called myoclonic fits among 11600 electrocencephalographically evaluated cases of epilepsy. But their clinical definition is much too wide and cannot be compared to ours. Among the six cases they cite as examples, they mention two for which the diagnosis of propulsive petit mal can be suggested and the diagnosis of impulsive petit mal firmly rejected.

Aetiology

From Table 1, it appears that no brain damage was found as the causal factor. Epilepsies with impulsive petit mal thus represent the only type of epilepsy in which the symptoms alone exclude the presence of a symptomatic epilepsy.

Six patients had reported head trauma as a possible cause, with onset of the seizures 12 years (one case), 2 months (4 cases) or immediately after the accident. In all cases, this had been but a slight commotio cerebri that had not been accompanied by neurological signs or symptoms, either at the time of the trauma or at the time of our evaluation.

Heredity

Eight patients had a family history of epilepsy (Table 2). In two, it was their father, in two an uncle, in one each the brother, the mother, and the great-grandmother, and in the last case the daughter, the mother, the grandfather and the great-uncle on the mother's side. The diagnosis of epilepsy in these family members was fairly secure, but the exact type of epilepsy in the families was not investigated. However, it is certain that there are identical types of epilepsy among siblings, as in propulsive petit mal (Zellweger & Hess, 1950; Janz & Matthes, 1955) and in pyknolepsies (Hansen,

1939 cited in Rhode, 1939; Lennox & Davies, 1950). Ballet & Bloch (1903), Dawidenkov (1926) and Filimonoff (1927) have each reported on siblings with epilepsies that can be diagnosed, from their descriptions, as impulsive petit mal. The sibling pairs reported by Sepilli (1896, cited in Bresler, 1986) and Austregesilio & Ayres (1914) probably belong to this entity and not to the Unverricht–Lundborg type of myoclonus epilepsy, which, with respect to its familial character, is consequently also not a significant differential diagnostic characteristic.

Table 2. Epilepsies in the families

Type of seizure	Idiopathic	Symptomatic	Total
Propulsive petit mal	7 = 13.5%	1 = 4%	8 = 10.5%
Pyknolepsies	20 = 18%	1 = 9%	21 = 17%
Impulsive petit mal	8 = 17%	–	8 = 17%
Oral petit mal (including dreamy state)	40 =15%	1 = 2%	41 = 12%

Course

In most cases (43 per cent) there are only petit mal seizures over months and years, before the onset of the first major seizure (after a mean of 3.3 years). Often (32 per cent), the disease begins almost simultaneously with petit mal and grand mal. Sometimes (25 per cent) grand mal is the first seizure type, the minor seizures occurring soon after, although a latency of 2, 3, 5 and 8 years was found, respectively, in four patients. We have seen only two cases in which the petit mal seizures were the only seizure type encountered, after a course of 2 and 15 years, respectively. The first case is a female medical student, whose twitchings became conspicuous during an undergraduate lesson, the other is a housekeeping employee in our hospital, who experienced, at 2–7 week intervals, jerks during the morning that bothered her very little, although she usually dropped her cleaning tools or her cup of coffee, until we personally became aware of her and confirmed the diagnosis with an electroencephalogram. The fact that these two patients did not come to us spontaneously leads us to think that, as in the first years of the course in pyknolepsies, the purely petit mal course is probably much more common, but usually escapes attention or remains undiagnosed. The jerks are mostly isolated, as equivalents. They can also initiate the major seizures as prodromes, in which cases the patients may sometimes conclude, from the violence of the jerks, that a major seizure is likely to happen. On the whole, one can find a certain antagonism, according to the following rule: the more frequent the minor seizures, the rarer the major seizures, and vice versa. In cases where major seizures are frequent, the minor attacks will only appear as introduction to the grand mal. Infrequently, minor attacks will completely subside in favour of the major seizures during the course of the disease.

Other authors, especially Muskens (1926), have stressed as very characteristic the predominant occurrence of the jerks in most patients during the morning, soon after awakening (so called 'matutinal' jerks). The timing is not significant itself, but rather the fact of gaining full consciousness after awakening: this is proved by the fact that the patients also experience seizures when they awaken from sleep at another time of the day, e.g. after an afternoon nap. As the jerks may occur while the patient is still lying supine, it appears that the triggering moment is not getting up, i.e. moving from the supine to the upright position, but rather by awakening from sleep. Even patients who have made a habit of remaining some time in bed in the morning, do not fear the act of getting up, rather an abrupt awakening and an urge to wake up. Four patients had also experienced jerks in the afternoon or in the evening – when they were overtired, according to them. Jerks never occurred during sleep in this form of the disease, as they do in myoclonus epilepsy. The physiological jerks present in every normal person at the onset of sleep have nothing to do with impulsive petit mal. In these patients, they are neither more violent nor more frequent than in normals, and they are completely unrelated in their physiopathology. According to Gibbs & Gibbs (1952), such hypnagogic jerks are not associated with electroencephalographic changes. In their distribution over the day, the major seizures behave like the minor ones. They can thus be distinguished from the grand mal seizures occurring in the course of propulsive petit mal, that occur mostly (72 per cent) during sleep (Janz & Matthes, 1955), or in myoclonus epilepsy, where they always occur during sleep (Janz, 1953a), while grand mal seizures occurring in pyknolepsies occur in 90 per cent of the cases as awakening seizures (Janz, 1953b). In impulsive petit mal, grand mal seizures are always awakening seizures.

To be more precise: 20 patients experienced their major seizures exclusively after awakening (longest follow-up: 11 years); 15 other patients also had rare major seizures in the late afternoon, in two cases also during sleep. In seven patients, there was a balance between awakening and late afternoon seizures, that existed from the onset or had occurred during the course; in two of these, major seizures tended to be more frequent in the late afternoon than in the morning after some time. Three patients, who had begun with awakening epilepsy, later had seizures mostly during sleep (two cases) or without any particular pattern ('diffuse seizures').

'Impulsive grand mal'

The jerks can introduce a generalized tonic–clonic seizure suddenly or, when they repeatedly increase and decrease, at irregular intervals, more in a crescendo. After a major discharge, which is often perceived by the patient as a liberation or a release, even in the presence of headache and tiredness, the jerks may disappear for days or weeks. Lundborg (1903) saw this as a major criterion for a different diagnosis from 'progressive myoclonus epilepsy' and proposed to consider this type as 'intermittent'. In this condition, the major seizure has distinctive traits: lack of sensory aura, symmetry, remarkable violence and duration of the tonic seizure that often leads to opisthotonos, and consequently intense cyanosis plus frequent bilateral biting of the tongue. Loss of urine is very uncommon.

Most of the time, a major epileptic seizure has, in a given patient, a stable symptomatology, although it may show some typical differences between patients and between different types of epilepsies; such differences have not yet been studied extensively. Unverricht (1895) and Lundborg (1903) have described as 'tetaniform' the particular character of the major seizure in their myoclonus epilepsy: consciousness remains for a long time, fading only at the acme of the ever-increasing intensity of the seizure, at the stage of exhaustion. We had insisted on the sometime emprosthonic posture during grand mal in patients with propulsive petit mal (Janz & Matthes, 1955). To be more precise, the grand mal seizures found in patients with impulsive petit mal were as follows: six patients had noticed a feeling of uneasiness in their head between awakening and the onset of the major seizure. A sensory aura was never reported. In 18 patients, the seizure began with an initial cry, that was variously described as a grunt, a croak, a moan, either short or lasting. In 12 patients, we know the position during the seizure. In nine, it was clear opisthotonos, with upward rolling of the eyes and extended extremities. The contractions were always symmetrical and were introduced only in three cases by a lateralized deviation of the head, that occurred as the patient was no longer conscious. The intensity and duration of the tonic *vs.* clonic phase was noteworthy, as was the often menacing cyanosis, that was not limited, as in most other cases, to the lips. The sudden onset often leads to falls, with injuries, according to the direction of the fall, on the face or, more commonly, on the back of the head. Loss of urine never occurred in 25 cases, seldom in 13, and during each seizure in only one case. Drooling and foaming occurred in half of the cases, biting of the tongue or lips always or very frequently in 25 cases, rarely or never in 14. Following the seizure, and in spite of headache, cramps and fatigue, the patients often report a feeling of liberation, especially when the seizure followed a period of heaviness and numbness.

Triggering factors

Both the onset and course of this type of epilepsy seem particularly dependent on environmental factors. In more than half of our cases (28), we found that the first seizure had been preceded by unaccustomed lack of sleep and sudden, provoked awakening (23, including seven by nocturnal air-raid warning or air attacks) or by excessive intake of alcohol. Other precipitating factors are less convincing. In only three cases was a major physical effort made responsible; in one case the first seizure coincided with menarche. Even when the precipitating factor of the first seizure was no longer known, distinct causes for later seizures were found in every patient, the major role being played by lack of sleep (40), excessive intake of alcohol (19), or early awakening or getting out of bed unusually quickly (18). Among 19 women, eight suggested a certain relationship between seizures and the menses. Psychological stress or physical exhaustion were incriminated only five and three times, respectively. One of the patients had seizures provoked by intermittent light stimulation (driving along rows of trees or along fences in the sun).

These clinical data are useful for treatment, as some patients will experience seizures only if provoked in these ways; they have also led us to use sleep deprivation as a diagnostic tool for the precipitation of seizures. We advise the patients not to go to bed earlier than 1 a.m. for 1–2 nights and to drink strong coffee or a bottle of wine before that. Such provocation was tried in eight cases and resulted in the occurrence, the next or following morning, of jerks followed by a major seizure, even in patients with spontaneously rare events. Only once did we obtain only subclinical EEG changes. For the electroencephalographic proof of the specific EEG changes, a single night of provocation was always sufficient, the EEG being recorded on the following morning, if possible soon after awakening. Pregnancies regularly inhibit seizures. Among four women with five pregnancies, we found that none, even without medication, experienced minor or major attacks; however, these recurred immediately following delivery, mostly during the sleep- deprived period of breastfeeding.

Constitution of the patients

It is unfortunate that we can only reproduce impressions instead of the expected comparative data; we will nevertheless give an incomplete account of the psychological and bodily analogies found in this condition. We will summarise the physical constitution of 38 patients. We will first stress that nearly two-thirds of the patients (23) must be described as asthenic, only five as predominantly athletic and four as dysplastic. A pronounced pyknic habitus was never found, although six patients presented a stocky and heavy body type. Among the asthenics, 12 were markedly gracile and fine-limbed, the others markedly strong-boned with protruding skeletal profiles. Even those described as predominantly athletic or dysplastic had marked asthenic traits (flat thorax, long face). We were able to assess objectively the apparent anomalies of the skeletal build, at least in one detail: we have noted evident markers on the radiographs of the skull and compared these findings to those encountered in other types of genuine epilepsies and in normals (Table 3).

Table 3. Frequency of abnormalities of the skull

Abnormal findings in:	Sclerosis	Thick calotta	Internal hyperosteosis
33 patients with impulsive petit mal	25%	43%	11%
100 healthy subjects	8%	11%	2%
240 other types of idiopathic epilepsies	11%	9%	2%

In patients with impulsive petit mal, we found, with increased prevalence compared to normals and to other epileptics, a sclerosis of the crown (thickening of the lamina externa and of the lamina interna at the expense of the diploë), an overall thickening and an hyperostosis of the tabula interna. Sclerosis means that the diploë was thinner than the lamina externa and lamina interna, from a ratio of l. ext./diploë/l. int. of 3/2/3 to a complete disappearance of the diploë. A 'thick crown' was noted when the thickness of the os frontale and os parietale totalled more than 16 mm (measured at the metopion on the profile and at the middle between tuber parietale and longitudinal sinus on the frontal radiograph). Internal hyperostosis gathers findings of clear frontal nebula and internal frontal hyperostosis. Other markers such as a tendency to calcification of intracranial organs (epiphysis, plexus, falx) and changes of the sella such as sellar bridges, did not differ among patients with impulsive petit mal and patients with other types of epilepsies.

There is one point on which a similar finding will be made in all patients with impulsive petit mal, as long as one does not rely entirely on interviewing the patients, but also takes into account the clinical observation of in-patients and the interviews with their relatives: namely, their behaviour concerning sleep. They all awake with difficulty in the morning, take some time to become fully conscious and remain sleep-drugged for an even longer time. Every one of them will report that it is difficult to wake, that he/she would rather remain in bed for a while, that 'sleep sticks to their limbs', that they first 'act fully automatically', 'in a haze', 'with a flabby head'. Many of them have adapted to this, and remain for some time in bed and have their breakfast there. Others, who cannot afford to, stick their head into cold water or drink strong coffee. All stress that they require 'much sleep' and most of them that they sleep soundly. But in our experience, these patients forget they do not recognize that – as a rule – they go to sleep too late and therefore may reach deep sleep only late in the night. It appears that the characteristic change is represented not so much by the quantity of sleep as by the displacement of the sleep period within the 24 h the of day. This sleep profile of late sleep and late awakening, overrepresented among awakening epilepsies, is the rule in impulsive petit mal, a condition, given the timing of the grand mal seizures, that can also be ascribed to the awakening epilepsies. In our experience, as already hypothesized by Schulte (1955), this sleep profile is primary, i.e. founded in the constitution of the patients, and not secondary, i.e. a consequence of the epilepsy. The sleep typology is an indicator for the circadian performance, the change of capacity for activity and need for rest over the 24 h period. In patients with awakening epilepsy, especially in those with impulsive petit mal, the ability to perform is constantly in danger of being exceeded, as these patients find it difficult to adapt themselves to the daily rhythm of activities, because of the shift of their activity and passivity markers. Excessive demands, caused by even later bedtime, earlier rising in the morning, forced awakening, emotional or drug-induced stimulation, overuse of bodily or mental energy, will thus lead to new seizures. From this point of view, seizures may have an emergency function for a autonomic system that is beyond its performance ability, and the increased awareness caused by the jerks, or the sleepiness that follows a major seizure, may have a significant role in provoking some kind of relaxation. Consequences can be drawn from these findings, and a better observance of the daily rhythms will have therapeutic value – the patients being too rarely able to follow such guidelines on their own initiative.

As described by us earlier in patients with awakening epilepsy, and contrary to 'typical epileptic behaviour', their mental behaviour is very often characterized by unsteadiness, lack of discipline, hedonism and indifference towards their disease. As patients with impulsive petit mal behave in a similar manner psychologically, we feel that it is possible to describe a typology. Only one patient was mentally retarded. Most were of average intellectual ability, none was extraordinarily gifted. As they are all quick to learn and judge, are flexible and adaptable, they succeed in school and professional learning. But they promise more than they can deliver. Among 19 men with a professional career known to us, 10 were downgraded to unskilled work from prior positions as clerks, craftsmen, professional workers or students. Even if a responsibility can be ascribed to the psychic and social trauma associated with epilepsy, and if the onset of the disease occurred mostly during the delicate years of schooling, we nevertheless think that a pathological lack of ambition and endurance is responsible for this negative evolution. Their behaviour often has negative effects on their therapy. They will declare that they adhere to all prescriptions, but in fact often forget to attend control visits and to take their medication regularly. They often appear self-assured and bragging, the girls and women coquettish and seducing, but can also act decidedly mistrustfully and be timid, frightened and inhibited. Their labile feelings of self-worth leads them to be both eager to help, to invite, to give, on the one hand, and to be able to react in an exaggeratedly sensitive way on the other hand. Their mood changes rapidly and frequently. This makes their contact both charming and difficult. They are easy to encourage and to discourage, they are gullible and unreliable. Their suggestibility makes contacts easy but makes trust difficult. This personality profile plays along a scale, from likeable nonchalance or timidity, through a psychasthenic syndrome, to the extremes represented by sensitive or reckless psychopathy. In spite of this antisocial stigma, only two patients required institutional care. All the others found their place in society, the best adjustment being found by those who fulfilled their propensity for change as salesman, messenger, traveller, musician, circus hand, as soldier's girl, servant, saleswoman, secretary, or maid. It must be noted that none had a stable, independent profession, although all earned a living (except for four patients who had been institutionalized, one who had invalidity benefits and two younger patients still in the care of their parents).

Electroencephalographic (EEG) findings (without the figures)

The clinical individualization of the minor epileptic attacks described here as impulsive petit mal is confirmed by characteristic EEG findings. The seizure itself has a very particular, specific bioelectric correlate; moreover, typical changes can also be found in the interictal state. From an EEG point of view, this form of epilepsy can also be delimited from other epilepsies. In general, 3/s spike-and-waves (SW) are considered the specific epileptic potentials of pyknoleptic absences and of retropulsive petit mal, or of all types of minor epileptic seizures of childhood. Slow spike-and-waves are said to be characteristic of residual epilepsies. Our own opinion, which does not fully coincide with the currently expressed opinions, will not be expressed here, but will be the subject of another work. Let is be said that for impulsive petit mal, the multispike-wave (MSW) complex is pathognomic.

When we compared the EEG findings, we firstly proceeded from a purely clinical point of view and did not make any further selection. The starting point was the clinical picture. With time, we recognized that the clinical type of seizure was always associated with the same characteristic equivalent, so that later, even without knowledge of the clinical course, we were able to suspect impulsive petit mal from the EEG findings alone. We have evaluated a total of 38 patients with 63 EEG tracings. In these patients, the close relationship between the clinical manifestations and the time period following awakening or early morning hours, led us to perform the examinations preferably during this period of the day, as we expected to raise the chances of a positive EEG finding. Fourteen patients (39 per cent) experienced their petit mal attacks during the EEG recording. It must be noted that the attack was seldom isolated: as a rule, the attacks recurred at 2–3 min intervals, often during 1–2 h. Characteristic subclinical changes were found in 35 (93 per cent) of the patients.

No significant EEG changes were obtained in two patients only: one had already been seizure-free for 2 years and both were on antiepileptic treatment. The very high percentage of positive EEG findings must be noted: it is much higher than in any other form of epilepsy.

When we assess an EEG recording, we ask: what is the overall appearance of the curve? are there one or several, more or less evident, general changes? is there a dysrhythmia? are there focal changes? are there specific epileptic potentials that are characteristic for this form of epilepsy? If yes, how do they look? It must be noted that slight general changes of the background activity were found in only four patients (10 per cent), although with the exception of two patients) all had experienced major generalized epileptic attacks besides the minor ones; these major attacks occurred as awakening epilepsies, which, in our experience, are more commonly associated with general changes of the background activity than are the sleep epilepsies. We even found in most of our impulsive petit mal patients a remarkably regular EEG with a comparatively frequent (10–11 Hz) α-rhythm. It is known that the frequency of the background activity depends on the present age of the patient, until an age that differs between individuals. The good expression of the α-rhythm and the disappearance of the slow waves shows that impulsive petit mal is a form of epilepsy that manifests itself comparatively late, at least later than the age of pyknolepsy, at a time, thus, when the background α-rhythm is already firmly established. The clinical facts are thus confirmed by the EEG findings. In other forms of petit mal epilepsy, general changes of the background activity are both more frequent and more pronounced. We also must stress that no focal abnormality was found in any case. This also confirms the clinical data, according to which evidence for a symptomatic process was found in none of the cases.

The question pertaining to the form of the specific EEG changes in impulsive petit mal must start from the association between the clinical seizure and its bioelectric correlate. The seizure has a characteristic bioelectric equivalent on the EEG curves, which cannot be ignored. We nearly always found the paroxysmal occurrence, out of a normal background activity, of a herd of spikes of increasing amplitude, followed by slow waves of varying frequency and amplitude. This produces a pattern of spike-and-wave complexes with preceding, following or superimposed spikes. One can speak of a multiple-spike-wave complex, or of a polypointe-onde (Gastaut, 1950; Gastaut and Roger, 1951). The number of spikes is most variable and ranges between 5 and 20. According to our present experience, they are obviously correlated with the intensity, not with the duration, of the attack. Further justification of the term 'impulsive petit mal' can be found here as well, in contrast to the usual description of myoclonic jerks, for a single jerk in an isolated muscle has a different bioelectric correlate. Stronger motor manifestations are thus associated with frequent, sharp ictal spikes, and with flat, slow post-discharges. In milder manifestations, one will find a reduced amount of spikes, but larger slow waves. The amplitudes of the spikes reach 150–300 μV, their frequency varies between 12 and 15 Hz, and they are negatively oriented. The slow waves have a mean length of 200–250 ms, which corresponds to a frequency of 3–5 Hz. Their amplitude lies between 200–350 μV and but seldom surpasses 400 μV. The clinical dependency of the number of mostly initial spikes (series of spikes) described above certainly represents a statistical correlation. The statement that no clinically manifest impulsive petit mal occurs without multispikes should be impossible to refute. The total multispike-wave complex is also quite variable in its form and duration. The paroxysmal bioelectric phenomenon can span 2 s, or persist over 10 s, even if the clinical attack has lasted but 1–1.5 s. Using simultaneous recording of the electromyogram, we were able to demonstrate the multiple spikes that occur synchronously with the clinical phenomena are often preceded by groups of irregular, slow, 2–3 Hz sharp waves that are subclinical prodromic events. These slow waves can be interrupted by isolated or paired spikes. The same sequences of irregular slow waves also appear after the paroxysm, so that, from a bioelectric point of view, the clinical attack appears to be characterized by a crescendo–decrescendo course.

Besides their form, the localization of these specific ictal potentials is of interest. In agreement with the bilaterality of the jerks, bilateral, symmetrical discharges are found that predominate frontally and centrally. The EEG changes are less evident over the other brain areas, where they are of shorter duration, with a smaller number of spikes and with a lower amplitude. The initial point of emergence of the discharges is mostly the frontal or the central region. The propagate to the parietal, temporal or occipital areas with a marked time lag. A close synchrony, as known in pyknoleptic absences or in retropulsive petit mal, could not be observed in impulsive petit mal. One has the impression that the subcortical steering of impulsive petit mal is much less rigorous than in seizures associated with the 3-Hz spike-and-wave, but that the cortical activity plays a more important role, and that inhibitory mechanisms – if we consider the slow wave of the spike-and-wave complex as a inhibitory phenomenon, in the sense of Jung (1953) – have less meaning in impulsive petit mal. Phenomenologically, impulsive petit mal stands somewhere between the pure absence seizure, which is defined by a clear clouding of consciousness and a lack of motricity, and the full-blown generalized epileptic seizure, which is associated with its massive motor discharges. This alternative can be deciphered from the EEG findings, as both clinical and bioelectric components are represented in impulsive petit mal. Grinker *et al.* (1938) considered 'myoclonia and absence as opposed variants of grand mal'. In order to explain why seizures associated with regular 3-Hz spike-and-wave discharges last as a rule much longer than impulsive petit mal, energetic points of view could be called upon: following Jung again, the potential maximal activity may be diminished by exhaustion in the motor phenomenon in impulsive petit mal, compared with the pure alteration of consciousness in the absence type of seizure. The slow post-discharges that follow the multispike complexes are evidence for the existence of inhibitory phenomena that are capable of preventing a full-blown major seizure. A biological compensatory mechanism can be recognized here too. The relevance of these hypotheses cannot be confirmed by clinical and EEG observations alone. But we are convinced that energetic principles are involved, because we have seen on several occasions – especially following certain methods of provocation – that a series of impulsive petit mal with steadily shortening intervals between attacks and steadily decreasing amounts of slow (inhibitory) waves has led the way to a generalized major seizure.

The simultaneous recording of the electromyogram nearly always confirmed the correlation, in time, between the muscular and the cortical discharges. This seems important to us, because such close association is not found in myoclonus epilepsy, where major epileptic seizures coexist with purely muscular jerks.

Compared with other forms of petit mal, impulsive petit mal is singled out on the EEG by the irregularity of the whole complex, by its duration, by the number of spikes and by the lack of a close synchrony. Concerning the subclinical EEG changes, we noted that several spikes nearly always preceded a slow wave. Often, only a single complex will be seen, with a frequency between 3.5–4.5 Hz, in all cases nearly always greater than 3 Hz.

As the frequency of the epileptic potentials is dependent upon age, this finding must mean that the interictal EEG changes found in impulsive petit mal have also appeared after the age of pyknolepsy. They are bilaterally symmetrical, but are often found only over a limited brain area, mostly frontally or precentrally. A certain periodicity can be seen. Epileptic potentials with a single spike can also happen; the complex will nevertheless be faster than 3 Hz. We have never seen 2 Hz spike-and-wave discharges, or typical biphasic waves or sharp waves, as in the so-called psychomotor seizures or 'Dämmerattacken'. Conversely, we never found multispike-wave complexes in patients with 'temporal epilepsy'. In two of our patients, we also found, besides the characteristic multispike-waves, runs of regular, synchronous 3 Hz spike-and-wave discharges. In both patients, retropulsive petit mal occurred at times other than impulsive petit mal, and either ictal type could be differentiated by the ictal EEG recording (see 'Differential Diagnosis').

We found that, by and large, the EEG changes remained constant in a given individual. Practically no differences were found in the intensity and form of the EEG changes between the different EEG recordings performed in the same patient over time. However, our control EEGs were performed over periods that do not exceed several years.

A statistical overview of the EEG findings is as follows: in 38 patients with a clinically firm diagnosis of impulsive petit mal, we performed 63 EEGs. In six, standard EEGs allowed us to record clinical seizures, in nine other patients the seizures happened following certain methods of provocation. Twenty-two patients already exhibited on the standard EEG the specific multispikes and waves, in 30 patients (96 per cent) they could be observed after provocation (hyperventilation, sleep deprivation). In 96 per cent, the findings were positive, which allows us to establish a precise diagnosis based on the EEG. These numbers show that certain methods of provocation will markedly increase the percentage of positive EEG findings. During hyperventilation, a procedure that we systematically carry out in all patients, seizures occurred on three occasions; on eight occasions, characteristic EEG changes appeared that had not been present on the standard recording. An effect of hyperventilation is thus evident, although it is not as specific as in pyknolepsies associated with

3 Hz spike-and-wave discharges. During sleep EEG, which we performed on three occasions, we were unable to find specific EEG changes.

The specific provocative method for impulsive petit mal or subclinical bioelectric associated phenomena is sleep deprivation following absorption of significant amounts of coffee of alcohol. This was evident from our clinical observations; the precise procedure has been described in the clinical section. The triggering effect is self-evident and surpasses the effects of the other methods, even of the combination of light and cardiazol proposed by Gastaut (1950). His so-called myoclonic threshold is not a precisely defined value; it may vary significantly in normals. Anyhow, a lowering of the myoclonic threshold is not by itself pathognomonic for the myoclonic form of epilepsy.

The special standing of impulsive petit mal among minor epileptic seizures is thus also secured from the EEG point of view. The differential diagnosis must nevertheless discuss the delimitation from other conditions that are associated with jerks: first and foremost from myoclonus epilepsy, the startle reaction, and hypnagogic jerks, but also from the absences described as indifferent (Janz, 1955), which begin between the age of the pyknoleptic retropulsive petit mal and impulsive petit mal. Here too, the EEG contributes to the differential diagnosis.

Contrary to impulsive petit mal, the true hereditary myoclonus epilepsy is characterized by a clear, most often pronounced global alteration of the EEG; we have evaluated four cases of myoclonus epilepsy. The α-rhythm is replaced by slow theta and δ waves, that are interrupted by recurring groups of sharp δ waves and spikes (Delay et al., 1947), that may be associated with muscular discharges or not. In myoclonus epilepsy, the number of spike series within the spike-and-waves complex is smaller, and the strict correlation between the EEG and electromyographic discharges is missing. In one of our female patients, we noted that the epileptic EEG potentials either preceded or followed the muscular discharges, and were seldom time-locked to the latter – a finding also described by Jung. The EEG of myoclonus epilepsy is therefore strikingly different from the EEG of impulsive petit mal.

Hypnagogic jerks are not associated with EEG changes (Gibbs & Gibbs, 1952). The jerks described as pure 'startle syncinesias' (Alajouanine & Gastaut, 1955), that can be elicited by unexpected motor or sensory stimuli, can be associated with sharp waves, typical epileptic potentials of the spike-and-waves type or no change at all.

In this context, we find it worthy of interest – without dwelling too much on this subject – to raise the following question: do dissociated sleep components (according to the idea of Bonhoeffer (1928)) manifest themselves in impulsive petit mal, a condition characterized by awakening jerks? Their association with a belated and dissociated (in its sensorimotor aspects) awakening, their provocation by sleep deprivation and their purely motor, tonic character, which take the appearance of a short stretching movement upon awakening, seem to point in that direction.

The (sensorally and motorally) indifferent absences are not only clinically situated between retropulsive petit mal and impulsive petit mal; the EEG also shows that they belong to neither of these forms, as the epileptic potentials are less regular and more frequent in indifferent absences than in pyknoleptic petit mal; unlike impulsive petit mal, they fail to exhibit the multispike pattern.

In the symptomatic myoclonias of subacute leucoencephalitis, the EEG shows periodic, large slow waves or complexes with a large biphasic wave followed by slow components, the initial biphasic sharp wave being often associated with myoclonias (Cobb & Hill, 1950; Radermecker, 1950; Thiry et al., 1953; Dreyer, 1956).

Treatment (abridged)

This condition necessitates a particularly well-planned and rigorous therapeutic approach, in which three perspectives play an important part:

(1) the tendency of these patients to be reckless and indifferent towards any kind of rule must be kept in mind and must be taken into account;
(2) the external factors that regularly provoke the seizures must be avoided as far as possible;
(3) adequate medication at the effective dosage must be chosen and prescribed for as long as needed.

Point 1: our experience has shown that these patients, when left to themselves, follow the medical prescription for only a short period and then become careless; it is thus advisable to delegate the responsibility of the practical administration of treatment to a family member who has some authority over the patient. Because of this, the intervals between follow-up visits of the patient and his helper should not be too long, and one should not tire of repeating the rules of treatment, even when it has already be proved effective. Frequently, the disorder in the family circumstances makes the therapeutic approach so much more difficult in that a long stay in a hospital or institution should be organized at the beginning, during which social measures may be taken.

Point 2: the history will clearly show what is to be permitted, to be forbidden or to be regulated. Alcohol must be strictly forbidden in any form and quantity. There is no known deleterious effect of smoking, nor of the type and quantity of food: there is thus no need to impose any type of restriction in these fields. The most important point is the regulation of sleep, both its timing and duration. The patients should never sleep less than 8–9 h. Even more important is the instruction that they should go to bed around 9 p.m., always before 10 p.m., and that they should arise in the morning not too early, but also not too late, because this might reduce their need for sleep on the following evening. Stimulants like tea or coffee will not have to be completely forbidden, but it would be wise to allow them in the morning and to forbid them in the evening.

Point 3: if full remission of seizures is the therapeutic goal (which it is for us), medication will have to be used even in the mildest cases. In spite of this, one should never abstain from asking both patient and family whether they are ready to endure years of medication, to awaken their own sense of responsibility. The choice and the dosage of the medication will be determined by efficacy and tolerability.

We have performed over 50 treatments using the seven following medications:

- Anirrit* (methyldibromstyrylhydantoin 0.18 g + phenylethylbarbituric acid 0.02 g)
- Antisacer* (diphenylhydantoin 0.1 + phenylethylbarbituric acid 0.025 + K bromide 0.4 g + caffeine citric. 0.0125 g + atropine sulphate 0.00025 g)
- Comital-L* (phenylethylbarbituric acid 0.05 + methylphenylbarbit. 0.05 + diphenylhydantoin 0.05 g)
- Luminal* (phenylethylbarbituric acid 0.1 g)
- Mesantoin* (methylethylphenylhydantoin 0.1 g)
- Zentropil* (diphenylhydantoin 0.1 g)
- Zentronal* (same + phenylethylbarbituric acid 0.015 g).

(* denotes trade name)

No medication was absolutely efficacious, none was absolutely without effect. When the composition of the different preparations is considered, it appears that Luminal* and the predominantly barbituric Comital-L* are more efficient than the preparations containing exclusively hydantoins. The differences between preparations predominantly based on barbiturates and those predominantly based on hydantoins are not major, but still relevant; this type of epilepsy responds better to barbiturates than to hydantoins (Table 4). It seems thus justified to initiate the treatment with Luminal*, preferably with increasing daily dosage to obtain habituation to the initially sedative effect: 0.15 to 0.2 g Luminal* in the evening and three or four tablets of Coffeminal* (each containing 0.05 g Luminal* + 0.025 g caffeine) in the morning. In our experience, these patients tolerate Luminal* better than patients with other forms of epilepsy, which may be due to their particular constitution. If the necessary dosage provokes sleepiness and if no habituation occurs after several weeks, then one can go over to Comital-L*, with an average of four tablets per day. Whether hydantoins can succeed in isolated cases after the failure of barbiturates remains to be investigated.

Table 4. Summary of therapeutic effects of medications. The various preparations have been categorized according to their predominant content (barbiturates or hydantoins)

		I + II	III + IV	Total
Predominantly barbiturates		PM 21 = 91%	2 = 9%	23
		GM 15 = 79%	4 = 21%	19
Predominantly hydantoins		PM 15 = 71%	6 = 29%	21
		GM 12 = 63%	7 = 37%	19

Class I + II = satisfactory (class I: seizure-free, class II = seizure frequency diminished > 75 per cent); Class III + IV = unsatisfactory (Class III: diminished > 50 per cent; Class IV: no effect or worse). PM = petit mal; GM = grand mal.

Prognosis

In one case, a spontaneous cure occurred 4 years after the onset of the disease, without any treatment, and no relapse occurred in the eight following years. In six patients, the course could be described as mild, with either only minor seizures (two cases) or major seizures at intervals of several years. Four patients had to be institutionalized. One of these was in a mental hospital when he came to our attention. In two cases, domestic difficulties were the main motive for the referral to the mental hospital. Both had been clinically treated on several occasions and had been seizure-free for a long time. At home, they regularly relapsed. The fourth case was a vagrant, who was again lost to our follow-up after he had passed through several mental institutions. A female patient died from an intercurrent disease. In all other cases who had a moderately severe course before therapy, the intensive treatment resulted in their personal further development or employment, or, as in 12 patients, who had been unable to work for months or years, in their resuming a previous job.

Differential diagnosis

Impulsive petit mal can be easily distinguished from startle ('syncinesie-sursaut' according to Alajouanine & Gastaut (1955)) or from hypnagogic myoclonias: both these are not systematically localized, both concern mostly and alternatively one side of the body and can involve only the lower limbs, while impulsive petit mal is dependent on the time of the day and is not provoked by stimulation. It is more difficult to convince the patients themselves and their family that impulsive petit mal is not 'only nervous', but rather of an epileptic nature, and that it requires treatment.

The differentiation from Unverricht–Lundborg's myoclonus epilepsy is not as difficult as the melding of both conditions under the category of 'myoclonus epilepsy' seemingly implies. One has to keep in mind its most important features: onset between the ages of 6 and 15 (in most cases, between 9 and 11), the occurrence of major seizures mostly during sleep and the clinical characteristics of these seizures: the patient awakens, experiences a cluster of clonic jerks while he is still fully conscious and overwhelmed by fear, at the acme of which he becomes progressively hypertonic, the loss of consciousness occurring only as the convulsive manifestations resolve. In this myoclonus epilepsy, the jerks are mostly asynchronous and asymmetrical, do not occur at any preferential time of the day, are enhanced by intention-directed movement, by sensory stimulation and by psychological stress and concern either muscular groups, isolated muscles or muscular fibres without major displacement; they can also extend to the muscles of the face, tongue and throat.

However, it remains an open question whether symptoms from both conditions may occur in some patients, or whether either form may evolve into the other, as Lundborg (1903) thought. We have indeed recently seen a 35-year-old patient who experienced, with increasing frequency, typical impulsive petit mal and grand mal attacks after awakening, and in whom, during a status of impulsive jerks that evolved into a grand mal seizure, we also noted isolated, asymmetrical and asynchronous jerking of the face, neck, eyelids and mouth, that recurred on occasions 2 days later, independent of the jerks of the arms and shoulders.

Other forms of minor epilepsy that comprise jerks can also be delineated from impulsive petit mal: propulsive petit mal (Blitz-, Nick-, Salaam-attacks) because of the particular, propulsive-emprosthonic form of the movement, while these Blitz- or Nick-attacks occur in series and not in salvoes and begin at another age (1–5 years, mostly between 6–10 months).

In some cases, impulsive petit mal can be distinguished from retropulsive petit mal only with difficulty, especially in cases when the latter also comprises 'jerking' movements of the arms from the shoulder downwards, or when both forms of petit mal are associated, as we observed in four patients. This association points to a close nosological and pathophysiological relationship, that is also expressed electroencephalographically.

As retropulsive petit mal, we describe a form of minor seizures that occur only in a pyknoleptic fashion (i.e. several times per day) and that is the most frequent (54 per cent) among all forms of pyknoleptic petit mal (i.e. those with propulsive, adversive, indifferent or oral symptomatology). Its symptomatology is characterized by a nystagmic upward deviation of the eyes and by a more or less pronounced clonic backward movement of the head. In more intense forms, it may lead to jerk-like elevations and flexion of the arms and to a backward bending of the trunk, which leads the patients to make a few steps backwards, as if to maintain their balance, and sometimes to fall back. Even if the vertical upward gaze represents the leading symptoms in most cases, there are also less common cases in which – especially when the age of onset is at the end of the age span of the onset of pyknolepsy (4–12 years) – the eyes and head remain quiet and straight while only the flexed arms jerk. Here the pyknoleptic jerks differ from the impulsive jerks only because they are milder, rhythmic-saccadic and accompanied by an absence.

We also know of two cases that have begun more in the form of pyknoleptic retropulsive petit mal with involvement of the eyes and head, but whose symptomatology evolved over the years to more impulsive jerks, involving the shoulders and arms more. This change of symptomatology, which may be considered insignificant, but which is very meaningful from the pathophysiological point of view, has since then been observed in the comparison of the ictal symptomatology between patients and within the clinical evolutions of the same patients, although it never came to a radical change of the ictal type, including the four patients who presented both forms successively. Impulsive petit mal was never related to other classical forms such as adversive petit mal, oral petit mal (Hallen, 1954), or psychomotor seizures: this underlines the significance of the relationship between impulsive petit mal and retropulsive petit mal.

Pathophysiology and nosology

This clinico-phenomenological relationship seems to furnish the most natural starting point for a pathophysiological approach to impulsive petit mal. From our experience, we can confirm the opinion of Lennox (1945) according to whom the petit mal triad, which is defined electrophysiologically by variants of the spike-and-wave complex, is represented clinically by the Blitz-Nick-Salaam seizures, the pyknoleptic attacks and the so-called myoclonic fits. But beyond this, the symptomatology of the forms of paroxysms is characterized by a certain pattern of movement, that leads to an propulsive-emprosthonic position in the Blitz-Nick-Salaam seizures and to a retroflexion in the majority of pyknoleptic attacks. In consequence, the movement pattern characteristic of impulsive petit mal would be a stretching movement evolving out of the trunk and shoulders.

The symptomatology of these three types of seizures is thus comparable, in so far as the eyes, head, trunk and extremities show a pattern of movement that occur in a sagittal plane. Related to the functional level, this means that the seizures involve the statics of the body, each in its particular way: propulsive petit mal provokes a forward and inward bending, retropulsive petit mal an upward and backward bending and impulsive petit mal an extension. From this, one can conclude that the underlying central nervous system mechanisms originate from a single functional structure, i.e. that the midbrain circuits that control the statics of the body are responsible for the symptomatology of the so-called static petit mal triad.

To support this theory, one can point to the fact that the clinical picture of these fits does not include cortical symptoms (distal, lateralized, sensitive and sensory) or diencephalic (autonomic, vasomotor, oral motor or sensory, emotional) ones. There is however no proof from autopsy findings, no histological data are available for propulsive petit mal, no anatomical data for retropulsive petit mal – or for pyknolepsies in general – and the pathological–anatomical data published for possible cases of impulsive petit mal that were reported as myoclonus epilepsies cannot be identified with certainty, due to the lack of precise clinical data.

Startle reaction provoked by acoustic stimulation, which so much resemble impulsive petit mal, can occur in 'midbrain creatures' (Edinger & Fischer (1913); Gamper (1926); Strauss, 1929), and this proves that the implied reflex arch cannot run anteriorly of the midbrain structures. Strauss thinks that this type of startle is based on a sudden stimulation of the red nucleus.

The experimental neurophysiology was yet unable to clearly establish which brain structure is responsible for the production of myoclonic jerks. The corresponding electrophysiological phenomena speak for an increased activity of the subcortical zones. The dentate, the olives and the central lemniscal pathways were repeatedly implied in the genesis of myoclonias. Electrical stimulation of the central lemniscal pathway during animal experimentation leads to jerks of the face and eyes. Stimulation of the *Bindearme* provokes ispilateral, arrhythmic movements. Myorhythmias of the velum have been observed in lesions of the olives. Anatomical observations in myoclonus epilepsy find the most constant lesions in the cerebellum. It has been hypothesized that an inhibition, or a modulation, which is produced there between the afferent and efferent pathways, is suppressed. Myoclonias can also be provoked by an irritation of the pyramidal system (Van Bogaert *et al.*, 1950). On the basis of electrophysiological analyses, it was thought that the centre for myoclonias was located in the substantia reticularis – an extensive formation in the pons and tegmentum. The modified impulses (Radermecker, 1950) could thus reach the spinal cord via the reticulospinal tract and possibly trigger there automatisms of the motor neurons (Hassler, 1953).

The experimental data do not yet allow us to locate the anatomical centre of myoclonias clearly. The ictal symptomatology of impulsive petit mal can, however, give some clues as to the origin of this type of jerks: in our opinion, a model is given by the features of the decerebrate rigidity known in clinical practice and in animal experiments. This is constituted by a complex of symptoms that is based on a mixture of pyramidal and extrapyramidal changes of the muscular tone and that appears clinically as a spastic tetraplegia with retraction of the head. If one compares the symptomatology of impulsive petit mal with the picture of decerebrate rigidity, the similarity between these states leads one to consider impulsive petit mal as a paroxysmally occurring rudiment of decerebrate rigidity, or, in the same sense, as abortive cerebellar fits (Jackson, 1906). In this context, one must also note that impulsive grand mal develops very symmetrically, at times as the consequence of an increasing occurrence of impulsive petit mal, at times as a locked-in syndrome, with an extreme tonic rigidity and an enormous livid coloration of the face, which is seldom seen, with such intensity, in other forms of grand mal.

The problems that are touched upon here concern the basis of the muscular tone and the centres of motor coordination. The symmetry of the clinical manifestations points to a central organ, and firstly to the midbrain, as this is the place were the positional tone will be modified. One should thus make a centrally located, unique structure responsible for the occurrence of impulsive petit mal, a structure that normally guarantees the positional tone, that is subjected to a particular demand at the age of onset of impulsive petit mal, and that is also concerned in other clinically analogous phenomena, e.g. in decerebrate rigidity and in the cerebellar fit.

All the data that can participate in a better comprehension of impulsive petit mal epilepsy, from the neurophysiological and from the neuropathological point of view, justify the theory according to which the symptomatology of this form of epilepsy depends on midbrain structures.

The seizures of this petit mal triad are thus apparently caused by the impairment of a common function and by the manifestations of a common structure. This automatically raises the following question: why does the respectively propulsive, retropulsive or impulsive variant express itself exclusively, according to each clinical variant, within this common theme? One should further ask: in individual cases, why does their respective variant express itself only fragmentarily, i.e. only in the head or arms, or only in the head, or in the arms, or in the eyes ?

When many attacks are observed in the same patient, one must recognize that the possible nuances are due, not to a random mix of different symptoms, but rather to a varying intensity of similar symptoms. For the physiology of the seizures, the comparison of symptoms shows that the clinical picture of the seizures is determined, not by the random addition of equivalent and isolated elementary functions, e.g. for the head, eyes, arms, but rather by a stronger or weaker action of a single functional system that links head, eyes and arms. One can recognize here that the symptomatology of the minor attacks is due to a physiological performance, confirming what had already been proven by Hallen (1952; 1954, 1955) for the jacksonian seizure and for oral petit mal, and already formulated in the following way by Jackson (1888) for epileptic seizures in general: 'the epileptic process is but an exaggeration – although a large one – of normal nervous discharges, of normal physiological processes'. However, we see the concept of discharge as inappropriate for the minor seizures, as it evokes an explosion that might nonetheless account for the process of the major seizure. Minor seizures appear more as the weakened and crippled rendering of physiological processes. As they are but a fragment of the whole involved performance, they may be understood as evocation of the more significant, as signs of the comprehensive, as parts of the whole. From the permanent comparison between symptoms, one can learn to read them as syllables of the language of an organ – not unlike the meaning of foreign characters. Then, even if the experimental basis is still missing, one will admit that the performance of the maintenance of body position represents the physiological basis that is affected, in different pathologic ways, in the seizures of the petit mal triad. The pathological character of the seizures is neither their apparently random symptomatology, which indeed responds to a physiological order, nor the motor discharge, the excessive character of a completed movement, because other natural phenomena as surprise, fear, anger are also accompanied by expansive motricity, nor is it the fragmentary character, since we often enough limit ourselves to bare hints of expressive movement. It is rather the interruption of a seemingly natural ongoing process by a basically physiological, but untimely and senseless performance.

Selbach (1953) has tried to explain the chronological conditions required for the seizure to appear as the necessary consequence of an ongoing evolution. According to his concepts, which are derived from the model of a time-base oscillation (*Kippschwingung*), the seizure represents the solution of an unbearable conflict between the rival autonomic partners, its goal being relaxation. The dynamic conditions that are required for a major or only a minor seizure to happen is the proper domain of the EEG. The EEG shows the rhythmic regulatory–stimulatory processes to be the concurrence of facilitation and inhibition, of activation and braking, of collectivization and individualization. It follows that the seizure represents the complete or incomplete collapse of proper brain activity following a decreased capacity of inhibition.

We have endeavoured to account for the conditions that determine the symptomatology of the seizures:

In order to answer the question why only the propulsive, retropulsive or impulsive variant appears, one must consider the significance of the close relationship between the given seizure type and the age of onset. The specificity for age, already noted by Jung for the corresponding variants of the spike-and-wave complex, justify an explanation based on biology. The hypothesis according to which the seizures are based on disturbed development or maturation of the brain will be more closely analysed from the standpoint of the ictal symptomatology; a disturbed relationship between midbrain and whole brain may be the main factor involved here.

In future research on these patients, it will be necessary to pay special attention to the existence of signs of abnormal relationship between midbrain and static development on the one hand, and between the whole brain and general development on the other hand. The fact that the age of occurrence of the three static seizure forms coincides with the three stages when the acquisition of the upright stance and growth are particularly rapid and accentuated is sufficiently conspicuous to make us suspect that an acquired or inherited dysfunction, that is clinically largely compensated for, might, in these periods of particular stress, lead to paroxysmal derailments.

We have already shown that such associations can be even more apparent, as in propulsive petit mal (Janz & Matthes, 1955): the main age at clinical manifestation (4–10 months) coincides exactly with the period where three important stages of static development occur, i.e. holding of the head (fourth month), sitting up (sixth month) and standing up (ninth–10th month) (Pfaundler, 1946). The total age of manifestation, that reaches until the fifth year, encompasses the period during which further static differentiation occurs, until the final form of the symmetrical act of getting up from the supine position, which is specific to humans (Peiper, 1949; Schaltenbrand & Lust, 1926). When one considers these performances, the seizures appear as countersensical misperformances. The propulsive movement is exactly opposite to the movement of getting up. Both the pathological process of the seizure and the biological performance act on the same neurophysiological level: this also emerges from the observation that static development will especially suffer when seizures are frequent, first by stagnation, then by loss of already acquired capacities, while the other motricity and the trophicity remain unaffected. The specific paroxysmal, and later even interictals after-effects of propulsive petit mal (Jackson, 1876) affect the static function. If, with Jackson, we try to describe the physiological meaning of the ictal misperformance, we must admit that the seizure depicts a certain position, 'as if the body was trying to regain the intrauterine position' (Lederer, 1926). In propulsive petit mal, a posture is thus paroxysmally reinstated which was the dominant one during the foetal period. The observation according to which the seizure also presents a falling back to a position that is ontogenetically anterior remained inexplicable, until comparative developmental physiology proved the infant to still be a foetal being from the biological point of view. Following Portmann (1956), human development is specifically singled out among higher mammals by the fact that man comes into the world physiologically premature and completes his foetal development only at the end of the first year of life, the so-called extrauterine early year. Thus propulsive petit mal not only represents a countersensical misperformance of static function, but also an actualization of a fact that can only be understood biologically.

We have repeated these relationships following the model provided by the propulsive variant, because it can be an example of how to study the pathophysiological and biological significance of the retropulsive and impulsive variants. In the pattern of retropulsion, one would rather see an 'exaggeration of a physiological process', in the sense of Jackson, if one interprets the upward and backward movements as an excessive prolongation of the process of striving to be upright. This misperformance is again countersensical, from the biological point of view, if one keeps in mind that, at the age of predilection of retropulsive petit mal (6–8 years), the process of getting up has just reached its completion and that intensive growth is taking place. At that age, a development occurs, that has been described as the first change of the 'Gestalt' (Hetzer, 1936; Zeller, 1952). If we nevertheless ask ourselves about the previous ontogenetic motor motive that may be reactualized, however fragmentarily, in retropulsive petit mal, one must evoke the transition from crawling to standing up. Then it again appears to be significant, as the same motor pattern that predominates in retropulsive petit mal is evident here: upward gaze, retroflexion of the head and elevation of the flexed arms.

We know least about the developmental significance of impulsive petit mal. Its age of predilection, at 10–20, mostly between 14–17, years encompasses the phase of sexual development, but also the time of the second change of the 'Gestalt', that is marked by a particularly intensive lengthwise growth, that ends in our climate at around the age of 19. The sexual evolution may not be of particular significance for the onset of the disease, as only one case experienced the first symptoms at menarche. The fact that the disease occurs on the average 1 year earlier in girls (15.42 years) than in boys (16.61) is more in favour of the significance of the growth pulse, which begins later and lasts longer in boys. However, our (non-systematic) enquiries about the age of accelerated growth and the age of the first seizure did not show any clear relationship. In spite of that, a relationship can be suspected between the marked acceleration of growth, that is part of the global development, and the specific ictal pattern, which we analysed as a stretching movement. If, again, the stretching during a seizure is an unnatural exaggeration of the physiological age-related performance, the interpretation of impulsive petit mal as a regression to a prior ontogenetic pattern is not possible without arbitrariness, unless one remembers that the increased growth of the first change of the 'Gestalt' is allegedly a stretching of the upper half of the body, which indeed constitutes the symptomatology of impulsive petit mal.

References

Austregesilio, A. & Ayres, O. (1914): Myoclonie et Epilepsie (Syndrome de Unverricht). *Rev. Neurol.* **27**, 746.

Alajouanine, Th. & Gastaut, H. (1955): La syncinésie-sursaut et l'épilepsie-sursaut à déclenchement sensoriel ou sensitif inopiné. I. Les faits anatomo-cliniques (15 observations). *Rev. Neurol.* **93**, 29.

Ballet, G. & Bloch, P. (1903): Les secousses musculaires, manifestation larvée de l'épilepsie. *Rev. Neurol.* 735.

Binswanger, O. (1899): *Die Epilepsie.* Vienna: Alfred Hölder.

Van Bogaert, L., Radermecker, J. & Titeca, J. (1950): Les syndromes myocloniques. *Folia. psychiatr. néerl.* **53**, 650.

Bonhoeffer, K. (1928): Über Dissoziation von Schlafkomponenten bei Postencephalitikern. *Wien. Klin. Wochenschr.*, 979.

Bresler (1896): Über Spinalepilepsie. *Zentralbl. Neurochir.* **15**, 1015.

Brissaud, M. (1903): Diskussionsbemerkung zum Vortrag von Ballet & Bloch (s.d.)

Clark, L. (1900): Paramyoclonus multiplex associated with epilepsy. *Arch. Neurol. Psychopath.* **2**, 473.

Clark, L. & Prout, T.P. (1902): The nature and pathology of myoclonus epilepsy. *Am. J. Insanity* **59**, 185.

Cobb, W. & Hill, D. (1950): Electroencephalogram in subacute progressive encephalitis. *Brain* **73**, 392.

Dawidenkov, S. (1926): Über eine ticähnliche Myoclonie bei 2 Brüdern. *Z. Neur.* **103**, 403.

Delasiauve, L.J.F. (1854): *Traité de l'épilepsie.* Paris: Masson.

Delay, J., Fischgold, H., Pichot, P. & Verdeaux, G. (1947): L'épilepsie myoclonique de type Unverricht. Etude génétique. Constatations électro-encéphalographiques. *Rev. Neurol.* **79**, 430.

Dide (1899): *La myoclonie dans l'épilepsie.* Cited in Lundborg.

Dreyer, R. (1956): Hirnelektrischer Befund bei einem anatomisch gesicherten Fall von Leukoencephalitis van Bogaert. *Nervenarzt* **27**, 227.

Edinger, L. & Fischer, B. (1913): Ein Mensch ohne Grosshirn. *Pflügers Arch. ges. Physiol.* **152**, 535.

Féré, Ch. (1890): *Die Epilepsie.* übers. von Ebers. Leipzig.

Féré, Ch. (1900): *Les Epilepsies et les Epileptianes.* Paris: Alcan.

Filimonoff, J.N. (1927): Ein cigenartiger, der Unverricht–Lundborgschen Krankheit nahestchender Fall von familiärer Erkrankung. *Zges. Neurol. Psychiat.* **108**, 86.

Friedreich, N. (1881): Neuropathologische Beobachtungen: Paramyoclonus multiplex. *Virchows Arch. Path. Anat.* **86**, 421.

Gamper, E. (1926): Bau und Verrichtungen eines menschlichen Mittelhirn. *Wesens. Z. ges Neurol. Psychiat.* **102, 154,** 104–149.

Gastaut, H. (1950): Die kombinierte Aktivierung des EEG mit Cardiazol und intermittierendem Licht. *Verh. dtsch Ges. inn. Med.* **56,** 82.

Gastaut, H. & Roger, A. (1951): Les formes expérimentales de l'épilepsie: III: provocation chez l'homme non épileptique des éléments cliniques et électrographiques du petit mal: myoclonies et absences polypointes et pointeondes. *Rev. Neurol.* **84,** 1.

Gastaut, H. & Remond, A. (1952): Etude électrencéphalographique des myoclonies. *Rev. Neurol.* **86,** 596.

Gibbs, E.L. & Gibbs, F.A. (1952): *Atlas of Electroencephalography*, Vol. 2: *Epilepsy*. pp. 100–108. Cambridge, MA: Addison–Wesley.

Gowers, W.R. (1901): *Epilepsy and other chronic convulsive diseases*. London: Churchill.

Grinker, R.R., Serota, H. & Stein, S.J. (1938): Myoclonic epilepsy. *Arch. Neurol.* **40,** 968.

Hallen, O. (1952): Über Jackson-Anfälle. *Dtsch. Z. Nervenheilk.* **167,** 143.

Hallen, O. (1954): Das Oral-Petit mal. *Dtsch. Z. Nervenheilk.* **171,** 236.

Hallen, O. (1955): Zur Frage des Oral-Petit mal. (Entgegnung auf die Bemerkungen von E. Niedermeyer). *Dtsch. Z. Nervenheilk.* **172,** 535.

Hansen: Cited in Rohde.

Hassler, R. (1953): Erkrankungen des kleinhirns. In: *Handbuch der inneren Medizin*, eds. G. Von Bergmann, W. Frey & H. Schweigk, 5. Band: Neurologie, 3. Teil, pp. 782–783. Berlin: Springer.

Herpin, Th. (1867): *Des accès de l'épilepsie*. Paris: J. Ballière et Fils.

Hetzer, H. (1936): *Die seelischen Veränderungen des Kindes bei dem 1. Gestaltwandel*. Leipzig: Hirzel.

Jackson, H. (1876): On epilepsies and the after effects of epileptic discharges. *W. Riding Lunatic Asylum Reports* **105** (5).

Jackson, H. (1888): On a particular variety of epilepsy (intellectual aura), one case with symptoms of organic brain disease. *Brain* **11,** 179 Footnote 3.

Jackson, H. (1906): Case of tumour of middle lobe of cerebellum-cerebellar paralysis with rigidity-cerebellar attitude-occasional tetanus-like seizures. *Brain* **29,** 425.

Janz, D. & Matthes, A. (1955): *Die Propulsiv-Petit-mal-Epilepsie*. Basel, New York: S. Karger.

Janz, D. (1953a): 'Nacht'-oder 'Schlaf'-Epilepsien als Ausdruck einer Verlaufsform epileptischer Erkrankungen. *Nervenarzt* **24,** 361.

Janz, D. (1953b): 'Aufwach'-Epilepsien. (Als Ausdruck einer den 'Nacht'- oder 'Schlaf'-Epilepsien gegenüberzustellenden Verlaufsform epileptischer Erkrankungen). *Arch. Psychiatr. Z. Neur.* **191,** 73.

Janz, D. (1955): Die klinische Stellung der Pyknolepsie. *Dtsch. med. Wochenschr.* **1955,** 1392.

Jung, R. (1953): Augemaine Neurophysiologie. In: *Handbuch der inneren Medizin*, eds. G. Von Bergmann, W. Frey & H. Schweigk, 5. Band: Neurologie, 1. Teil, pp. 139–144. Berlin: Springer.

Lederer, M. (1926): Beitrag zur Kenntnis der Nickkrämpfe. *Jb. Kinderheilk.* **113,** 275.

Lennox, W.G. (1945): The petit mal-epilepsies. *J.A.M.A.* **129,** 1069.

Lennox, W.G. & Davies, J.P. (1950): Clinical correlates of the fast and slow spike-wave electrencephalogram. *Am. J. Pediatr.* **5,** 626.

Lundborg, H. (1903): *Die progressive Myoclonusepilepsie (Unverrichts Myoclonie)*. Upsala: Almquist u. Wiksell.

Muskens, J.J. (1926): *Epilepsie*. Berlin: Springer.

Peiper, A. (1949): *Die Eigenart der kindlichen Hirntätigkeit*. Leipzig: Thieme.

Penfield, W. & Jasper, H. (1954): *Epilepsy and the functional anatomy of the human brain*. Boston: Little, Brown & Co.

Pfaundler, M.F. Lust (1946): *Krankheiten des Kindesalters*. 3. Aufl.: München: Urban u. Schwarzenberg.

Portmann, A. (1956): *Zoologie und das neue Bild des Menschen*. Hamburg: Rowohlt.

Rabot (1899): *De la myoclonie épileptique*. Thèse de Paris. Cited in Lundborg.

Radermecker, J. (1950): Considérations sur la physiopathologie des myoclonies et d'autres phénomènes dites d'excitation Fol. *Psychiatr. néerl.* **53,** 691.

Reynolds, J.R. (1861): *Epilepsy: its symptoms, treatment and relation to other chronic convulsive diseases.* London: Churchill.

Rhode, M. (1939): Beitrag zur Kenntnis der Pyknolepsie. *Z. ges Neurol. Psychiat.* **164,** 516.

Schaltenbrand, G. (1926): Über die Entwicklung des Menschlichen Aufstehens und dessen Störung bei verschiedenen Nervenkrankheiten. *Dtsch. Z. Nervenheilk.* **89,** 82.

Schulte, W. (1955): Der Schlaf der Epileptiker, Schizophrenen und Manisch-Depressiven. *Dtsch. med. Wochenschr.* **80,** 1872.

Selbach, H. (1953): Die cerebralen Anfallsleiden. In: *Handuch der innere Medizin,* 5. Band: Neurologie, 3. Teil, eds. G. Von Bergmann, W. Frey & H. Schweigk, pp. 1082–1227. Berlin: Springer

Seppilli, G. (1895): *Un caso di mioclonia Familiare associata all'epilepsia. Riv. Sper. Freniat.* **21,** 326.

Sole-Sagarra, J. (1952): Epilepsie myoclonique maligne familiale. *Schweiz. Arch. Neurol.* **79,** 259.

Strauss, H. (1929): Das Zusammenschrecken. Experimentell-kinematographische Studie zur Physiologie und Pathophysiologie der Reaktiv bewegungen. *J. Psychol. Neur.* **39,** 111.

Thiry, S., Tinant, M., Massaut, C. & Remack, L. (1953): Etude électroclinique d'un nouveau cas de leucoencéphalite sclérosante subaiguë. *Acta Neurol. Psychiatr. Belg.* **53,** 746.

Unverricht, H. (1891): Die Myoclonie. Leipzig,Vienna: Franz Deuticke.

Unverricht, H. (1895): Über familiäre Myoclonie. *Dtsch. Z. Nervenheilk* **7,** 32.

Zeller, W. (1952): *Konstitution und Entwicklung.* Göttingen: Psychologische Rundschau.

Zellweger, H. & Hess, U.R. (1950): Familiäre Blitz, Nick – und Salamkrämpfe. *Helvet. Paediatr. Acta* **5,** 85.

Chapter 22

Juvenile myoclonic epilepsy and related syndromes: clinical and neurophysiological aspects

Pierre Genton*, Xavier Salas Puig†, Antonio Tunon†, Carlos Lahoz†
and Maria Del Socorro Gonzalez Sanchez*

Centre Saint Paul, 13258 Marseille 09, France; †Department of Neurology, Hospital General de Asturias, 33006 Oviedo, Spain

Introduction

The clinical picture that is nowadays considered typical of juvenile myoclonic epilepsy (JME) was described a long time ago; it was the merit of Janz & Christian (1957) to pinpoint 'impulsive petit mal' as a comparatively frequent, characteristic and often misdiagnosed form of epilepsy. A translation into English of their original article is included in this volume (Ch. 21); it gives all the references that were published prior to their landmark paper. It was the merit of Delgado-Escueta and his group (Delgado-Escueta & Enrile-Bacsal, 1984; Greenberg et al., 1988) to make the international community aware of this syndrome, that had already been recognized by European epileptologists, and to initiate the molecular genetic research.

Juvenile myoclonic epilepsy is one of the most common types of epilepsies, and certainly a very common form of idiopathic generalized epilepsy (IGE): in the recent experience of our centre, it represents 23.3 per cent of all IGEs, 4 per cent of all epilepsy cases and 4.4 per cent of all classifiable epilepsies (Roger et al., Chapter 2). Given the biased referral basis of our centre, that selects severe epilepsies, these numbers are probably underestimating the actual prevalence of juvenile myoclonic epilepsy; similar biases are found in other reports. Among hospitalized patients with epilepsy, Simonsen et al. (1976) found 3.4 per cent with juvenile myoclonic epilepsy, Janz (1969) found 4.3 per cent in his specialized clinic, and Tsuboi (1977) found 5.4 per cent among patients followed in a German University Department. The prevalence of juvenile myoclonic epilepsy may in fact be twice as high, as reported in probably less selected epilepsy populations by Gooses (1984) (11.9 per cent), Wolf & Gooses (1986) (11.4 per cent), and Obeid & Panayiotopoulos (1988) (10.7 per cent). Underlining the effect of patient selection, Loiseau et al. (1991) reported a different prevalence of 4.8 per cent of juvenile myoclonic epilepsy among outpatients with epilepsy seen in a private practice, *vs.* 3.5 per cent among hospitalized in-patients. Although frequent, it is often misdiagnosed, or diagnosed retrospectively after a long evolution (Panayiotopoulos et al., 1991; Grünewald et al., 1992).

Many reviews on the clinical and neurophysiological features of juvenile myoclonic epilepsy have been published in recent years (Delgado-Escueta & Enrile-Bacsal, 1984; Asconapé & Penry, 1984; Wolf, 1985; Dinner et al., 1987; Salas-Puig et al., 1990; Janz, 1991; Wolf, 1992a; Serratosa & Delgado-Escueta, 1993; Grünewald & Panayiotopoulos, 1993). In the past few years, considerable efforts have been concentrated on the search for the location of the gene(s) involved in the transmission of the trait that results, in some patients, in the clinical syndrome of juvenile myoclonic epilepsy. Both clinicians and geneticians have underlined the heterogeneity of clinical phenotypes involved in families with probands. There is still an obvious need for a clear definition of this syndrome and of its limits with other types of epilepsies: we shall thus try to focus on the clinical and neurophysiological certainties and uncertainties, in order to try and help those involved in the screening of patients and their families.

Our recent experience is based on 82 cases of juvenile myoclonic epilepsy diagnosed between 1986 and 1994 at the Centre Saint Paul, Marseille; the main demographic and clinical characteristics of the patients have been reported on Table 1. We also studied the electroencephalographic data collected in a distinct group of 85 cases evaluated in the Department of Neurology of Oviedo.

Table 1. Clinical data of 82 patients

Sex ratio	34M/48F
Age at onset of seizures	
Mean age ± SD	14.5 ± 4.3
Range	7–33
Boys	15.6 ± 4.5
Girls	14.2 ± 3.2
First seizure:	
GTCS	n = 29
Mean age ± SD	15.1 ± 4.6
Range	7–33
Sex ratio	19M/10F
Myoclonic jerks	n = 44
Mean age ± SD	15.3 ± 2.6
Range	10–20
Sex ratio	12M/32F
Absences	n = 9
Mean age ± SD	11.7 ± 3.2
Range	7–16
Sex ratio	3M/6F
Association of seizure types	
Myoclonic jerks only	9
Jerks + absences	2
Jerks + GTCS	51
Jerks + GTCS + absences	20

GTCS = Generalized tonic–clonic seizures.

Juvenile myoclonic epilepsy: the clinical syndrome

Family history and genetics

The genetic aspects of juvenile myoclonic epilepsy will be dealt with elsewhere in this volume (see Delgado-Escueta et al., Ch. 24 and Janz et al., Ch. 25). From a purely clinical point of view, however, it must be stressed that a family history of epilepsy should be looked for as a diagnostic feature, but that a majority of patients will appear as isolated cases; in our patients, we found only

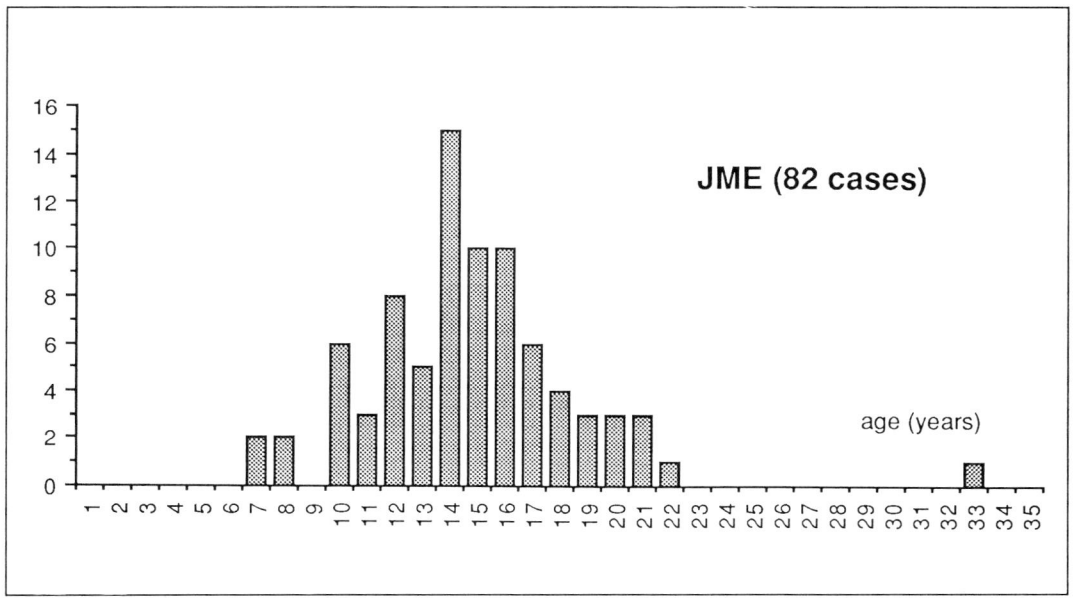

Fig. 1. Age at onset of juvenile myoclonic epilepsy in a cohort of 82 consecutive patients diagnosed at the Centre Saint Paul between 1986 and 1994.

25/82 (30 per cent) patients with a history of epilepsy, including 13 cases with first-degree relatives (16 per cent); a firm diagnosis of juvenile myoclonic epilepsy was made in first-degree relatives of only four families of our probands, the most frequent seizure history found in relatives being one of infrequent generalized tonic–clonic seizures (GTCS) (eight cases, 32 per cent).

Personal history

A typical juvenile myoclonic epilepsy patient will have no significant personal history prior to the onset of epilepsy. Febrile seizures during early childhood are found in a small minority of cases (8/82, 10 per cent in our experience, vs. only 4.4 per cent for Janz (1991)). Significant mental or psychiatric problems were present in six cases (7.3 per cent). A personal medical history, including potential factors of cerebral damage, is not considered significant for the diagnosis (Wolf, 1992a).

Sex distribution and age-dependence

We found a female predominance (58.5 per cent) among our patients, as did other authors (Mai et al., 1990: 66 per cent), but others found a male predominance (33 vs. 20 females: Delgado-Escueta & Enrile-Bacsal, 1984). Most authors have stressed an equal sex distribution (Janz, 1969; Tsuboi, 1977).

Juvenile myoclonic epilepsy is clearly an age-related epileptic syndrome; the age at onset of the first seizure in our patients is shown in Fig. 1. The incidence is practically limited to the second decade of life, with a peak around the age of puberty (14–15); the age of onset is slightly less in female patients (Table 1), which probably reflects the earlier onset of puberty in girls.

Clinical symptoms of epilepsy

As initially described by Janz & Christian (1957), two main seizure types are found, i. e. jerks and generalized tonic–clonic seizures (GTCS). The major, diagnostic feature is represented by massive myoclonic jerks, occurring preferentially after awakening. These jerks remain the only seizure type in only a few patients (4/82, 5 per cent in our experience), and are the first seizure type encountered in a majority of the cases (44/82, 54 per cent). The jerks are of varying intensity, are often reported as tremor, but can lead to falls. They are usually not accompanied by loss of consciousness. Myoclonic status, or prolonged episodes of jerks, may occur in some patients (7.3 per cent in the series of Salas-Puig et al. (1990).

Generalized tonic–clonic seizures are found in a majority of cases (71/82 cases, 87 per cent); our data are in accordance with data from the larger series quoted above (Janz, 1969; Tsuboi, 1977; Obeid & Panayiotopoulos, 1988) (80–95 per cent). Generalized tonic–clonic seizures are often preceded by massive myoclonic jerks – thus being in fact clonic–tonic–clonic seizures (Delgado-Escueta & Enrile-Bacsal, 1984) – and share the same circadian distribution as the jerks. They are often the motivation for the first medical consultation, even though they may only occur several years after the first jerks. They are the first seizure type in a significant proportion of patients (29/82, 35 per cent in our series), apparently more often in males.

Absences were not considered a major feature in the original description of juvenile myoclonic epilepsy; they occur less commonly (22/82 cases, 27 per cent in our series), but may be underestimated as they may escape the attention of the patient's entourage; their occurrence in juvenile myoclonic epilepsy patients is usually found to be low (10 per cent for Janz (1969); 14 per cent for Tsuboi (1977); 18 per cent for Obeid & Panayiotopoulos (1988)). They are infrequent, occurring typically less than several times per week. They are apparently associated with an earlier onset of juvenile myoclonic epilepsy (Table 1), and their clinical incidence thus appears to be age-related. A more systematic approach and a closer description of the features of absences may be found in as many as 38 per cent of patients when systematic, long-term video-EEG monitoring is used. This method probably yields a more exact evaluation of the occurrence of absences in juvenile myoclonic epilepsy.

Some patients may experience clinical photosensitivity (i. e. myoclonic jerks triggered by visual stimulation, especially television and videogames, in association with the spontaneously occurring attacks). We found four patients (5 per cent) (one male, three female) with clinically obvious photosensitivity; this feature was not specifically studied in the literature, since most data on photosensitivity are restricted to findings during EEG evaluation using stroboscopic light stimulation; such data show that the prevalence of photoparoxysmal responses is much higher (see below).

No other types of seizures were found in our patients. A majority of patients will experience a combination of seizures, with relatively frequent jerks and infrequent generalized tonic–clonic seizures being the most common combination (51/82, 62 per cent in our series). However, a proportion of juvenile myoclonic epilepsy cases (including family members of patients we evaluated) may experience only infrequent jerks and may totally escape medical attention and diagnosis. Systematic studies of large pedigrees, with clinical and EEG assessment of relatives of probands, have provided some interesting data in this respect (see Delgado-Escueta et al., Ch. 24).

The circadian distribution of the seizures is one of the major clinical characteristics of juvenile myoclonic epilepsy, which was already clear to Janz & Christian (1957). Touchon et al. (1982) have stressed, in their systematic survey, the existence of a peak of occurrence of seizures at awakening, in the morning in most cases, during intermediate nocturnal awakening in others, with a lesser peak during the evening.

Another important characteristic is the existence of clear precipitating factors, with lack of sleep being the major cause of increased morning jerks and occurrence of generalized tonic–clonic seizures. A typical history will be that of an adolescent boy or girl who has been experiencing 'tremor' and clumsiness during breakfast or in the bathroom after awakening for several months or even years, and who is brought by his/her parents to the doctor's attention after the first generalized tonic–clonic seizures, which occurred on 1 January, after a night of revelling (and drinking) and a very short period of sleep. In most Western and developed nations, acute excessive intake of alcohol is often associated with sleep deprivation, but the precise role of alcohol *per se* has not been evaluated in juvenile myoclonic epilepsy. Other precipitating factors have been quoted, including illicit drugs and psychotropic medications like amitriptyline (Resor & Resor, 1990); however, such triggers for seizures are present in only a minority of patients.

Associated disorders

In contrast to the group of myoclonic epilepsies considered to be 'progressive' (review in Genton & Roger, 1993), juvenile myoclonic epilepsy is a stable condition and is not associated with progressive deterioration, either mental or neurological. According to the original description by Janz & Christian (1957), patients often have an unstable personality, which may lead to social maladjustment (and to lack of compliance with treatment); their findings have been corroborated by later publications in the German literature, but not by other authors. It must however be stressed that juvenile myoclonic epilepsy (as other types of epilepsy, and of IGE) may be fortuitously associated with severe psychiatric conditions and/or with mental retardation (7.3 per cent of the patients in our series). The use of illicit drugs may increase the occurrence of jerks and seizures, as may alcohol (implicated by Janz & Christian (1957) in 40 per cent of their patients, vs. 30 per cent according to Penry et al. (1989)). Hyperthyroidism has also been considered an aggravating factor (Su et al., 1993). However, no particular medical or psychiatric condition can be considered as significantly associated.

Neurological examination and neuroimaging

Juvenile myoclonic epilepsy is not associated with any neurological abnormality; in spite of the abnormal (or 'borderline') skull radiographs initially reported by Janz & Christian, modern neuroimaging techniques have consistently failed to show any abnormal findings. In our recent series of 82 cases, 42 patients had had at least one CT scan, and three had abnormal findings (two due to perinatal damage, one to traumatic lesions); seven patients with normal CT scans had also had at least one MRI, one with multifocal white matter anomalies also ascribed to sequelæ of perinatal brain damage. Serratosa & Delgado-Escueta (1993) report that MRI imaging and PET studies were consistently normal in their patients.

Evolution and prognosis

Juvenile myoclonic epilepsy is not a severe condition, and was described as 'benign juvenile myoclonic epilepsy' (Wolf, 1985) before the present denomination was universally adopted. It does indeed not qualify as a 'benign' condition, as another major feature of this condition is represented by its pharmacodependency: even in easily totally controlled cases, the discontinuation of drug therapy after several years of remission leads to a very high rate of relapse, probably close to 90 per cent (Janz et al., 1983; Delgado-Escueta & Enrile-Bacsal, 1984; Baruzzi et al., 1988; Mai et al., 1990). The present data suggest that juvenile myoclonic epilepsy is a lifelong condition, although some patients may experience long remissions or a certain abatement of ictal phenomena with increasing age.

The symptoms may be exacerbated in the menstrual period in some women, and jerks may diminish during pregnancy (Janz & Christian, 1957; Asconapé & Penry, 1984), but these phenomena have not been systematically studied; after delivery, there is often an increased risk for seizures, due to the usual lack of sleep associated with the first weeks of breastfeeding.

Treatment

Valproate is now considered the drug of choice for the treatment of juvenile myoclonic epilepsy, replacing phenobarbital and primidone, that were considered efficient (in contrast to phenytoin) in the earlier reports (Janz, 1969). Valproate used alone (monotherapy) leads to total control of seizures in about 80 per cent of the patients (Janz, 1991). In patients with some degree of resistance, clonazepam may be used in cotherapy (Obeid & Panayiotopoulos, 1989); this drug seems particularly effective for myoclonic jerks, less against generalized tonic–clonic seizures. Adjunctive treatment (using intermittent clonazepam, clobazam or acetazolamide) may be useful in women with a clear catamenial exacerbation of ictal manifestations (Genton & Ganeva, 1993).

Carbamazepine has been considered to have a deleterious effect in juvenile myoclonic epilepsy, increasing the occurrence of jerks and of subclinical interictal changes. The efficacy of newer anticonvulsant drugs, such as vigabatrin, lamotrigine, felbamate or gabapentin, has not been specifically assessed in juvenile myoclonic epilepsy.

As the occurrence of jerks and of generalized tonic–clonic seizures is closely related, in most cases, to precipitating factors like sleep deprivation, most patients should be advised to keep to reasonable sleep schedules; others should be given adequate counselling when most of the ictal phenomena are due to photic stimulation (see Takahashi, Ch. 27). As some forms of juvenile myoclonic epilepsy indeed seem less severe than others, some patients may choose to forsake the regular intake of medication; this attitude may be justified in particular in patients who experience only isolated, infrequent jerks, and who tolerate valproate and/or alternative medications poorly.

Juvenile myoclonic epilepsy: electroencephalographic aspects

Very characteristic interictal and ictal EEG findings were reported in the original description of 'impulsive petit mal' (Janz & Christian, 1957). Their findings were confirmed by all later studies, and we will try here to underline the most important EEG changes found in juvenile myoclonic epilepsy.

The EEG data were gathered from a cohort of 85 patients with juvenile myoclonic epilepsy evaluated in Oviedo, Spain. The patients (44 were male, 41 female) were aged 13 to 63 (mean: 27.9 years) and followed over 0.5–24 years (mean: 4.8 years).

Fully normal standard EEG recordings were found, at one point, in 88 per cent of the patients, although characteristic changes were present at other times. Janz & Christian (1957) found normal EEG in 12 per cent of their patients, Tsuboi (1977) in 7 per cent only, and many authors have stressed the possibility of normal EEG in juvenile myoclonic epilepsy patients (up to 26 per cent for Obeid & Panayiotopoulos (1988). Considering only the first standard EEG performed in newly referred patients, we found fully normal tracings in only 27 per cent (Gonzalez Sanchez *et al.*, 1994). Hyperventilation may strongly activate the interictal changes (Tsuboi, 1977).

The background activity was normal in all, except seven (8 per cent) who showed some amount of theta slowing; such changes were only present in periods of poor seizure control and/or of polytherapy; in all these patients, the background activity returned to normal when a better control of seizures was achieved. Slowing of background activity was also reported in some patients by Janz & Christian (1957).

The interictal EEG showed generalized SW discharges of varying periodicity (Fig. 2): 3 Hz SW were found in 16 per cent of the patients, 4–5 Hz SW in 82 per cent, and poly-SW discharges in 45 per cent; a single patient could exhibit various types of SW discharges over the years. The slower, 3 Hz variety, may be found predominantly in patients who have absence seizures (Panayiotopoulos *et al.*, 1989).

A photoparoxysmal response was obtained in 28 patients (33 per cent) (Fig. 3), 70 per cent of them were females. Juvenile myoclonic epilepsy is the IGE syndrome with the highest rate of photoparoxysmal responses (Wolf, 1992), a trait that is present in 27–42 per cent of the patients, more frequently in females. Eye closure facilitated the paroxysmal discharges during intermittent photic stimulation in 19 (22 per cent) of our patients, a prevalence that is in accordance with previous data (Guirao *et al.*, 1987; Salas-Puig *et al.*, 1990; Gigli *et al.*, 1991). However, a smaller number of patients have clinical photosensitivity.

Myoclonic status, with numerous jerks in succession over a prolonged period of time, may occur in certain circumstances (Fig. 4), including drug withdrawal.

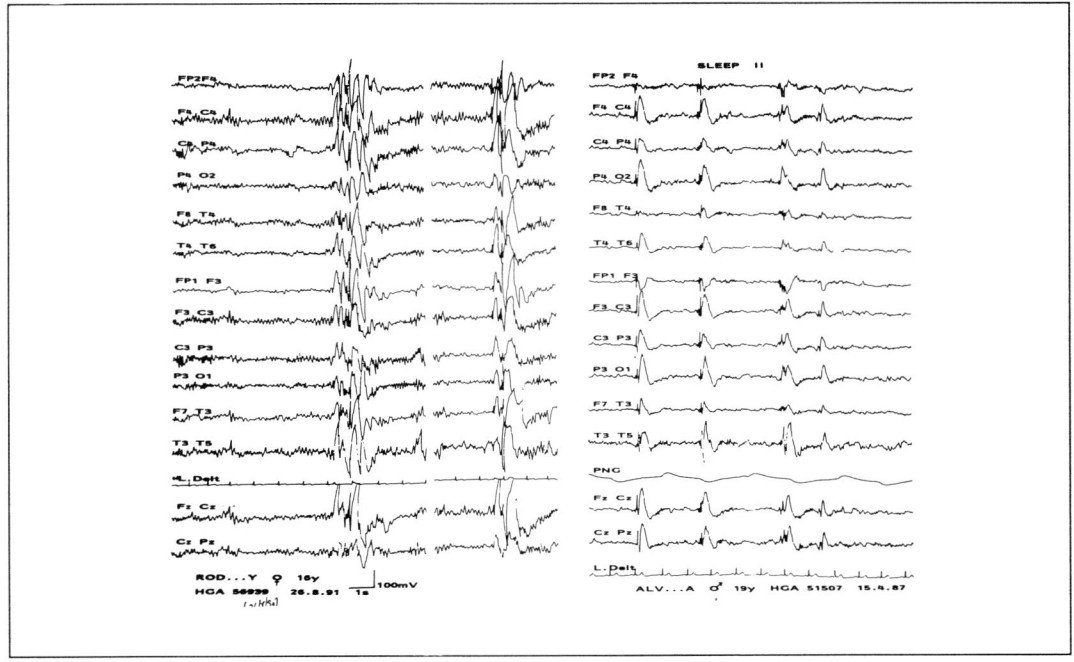

Fig. 2. Female patient aged 16 years. Since the age of 13, she has had daily myoclonic jerks on awakening. Two generalized tonic–clonic seizures occurred following sleep deprivation. The EEG shows a typical pattern of juvenile myoclonic epilepsy with normal background activity and generalized spike-, polyspike-and-wave discharges. Right: male patient aged 19 suffering from recent onset of myoclonic jerks on awakening. Typical EEG pattern during light non-REM sleep, with successive, subclinical poly-pike-and-wave discharges.

Sleep EEG were obtained during 4 h naps after partial sleep deprivation in 68 patients (80%); non-REM sleep periods were recorded; 3 Hz SW were found in 9 per cent of the patients, 4–5 Hz SW in 88 per cent, and poly-SW discharges in 57 per cent; all patients recorded during sleep had abnormal EEGs, including 3 with previously normal waking EEGs. The activation of generalized SW and polySW is considered to predominate during nREM sleep, being highest during stages 3–4, while REM sleep is associated with abolition of the SW discharges (Gigli et al., 1991). The discharge rate is particularly high during intermediate awakenings, the most important activation occurring after the final morning awakening, especially when the night period has been shortened by a provoked arousal (Touchon et al., 1982; Touchon, 1982). This activation profile (Fig. 5) closely parallels the timing of seizures in juvenile myoclonic epilepsy, and sleep deprivation, which is the major triggering factor of seizures in juvenile myoclonic epilepsy, was already advocated as an efficient activation method by Janz & Christian (1957).

Focal EEG abnormalities were present in 13 patients (15 per cent): these were mostly asymmetrical paroxysmal discharges that could change from one hemisphere to the other during the same recording, or between successive recordings. In no patient, however, were these focal changes the only finding, and generalized paroxysms were found either in the same recording or in successive ones. Focal changes may indeed be frequent in the EEGs of juvenile myoclonic epilepsy patients: a prospective study found such changes in up to 55 per cent of the patients (Aliberti et al., 1993), and focal and/or asymmetrical abnormalities may be found in 29 per cent of the patients on the first standard EEG performed (Gonzalez-Sanchez et al., 1994).

Spontaneous jerks were recorded in six patients and were always associated with generalized

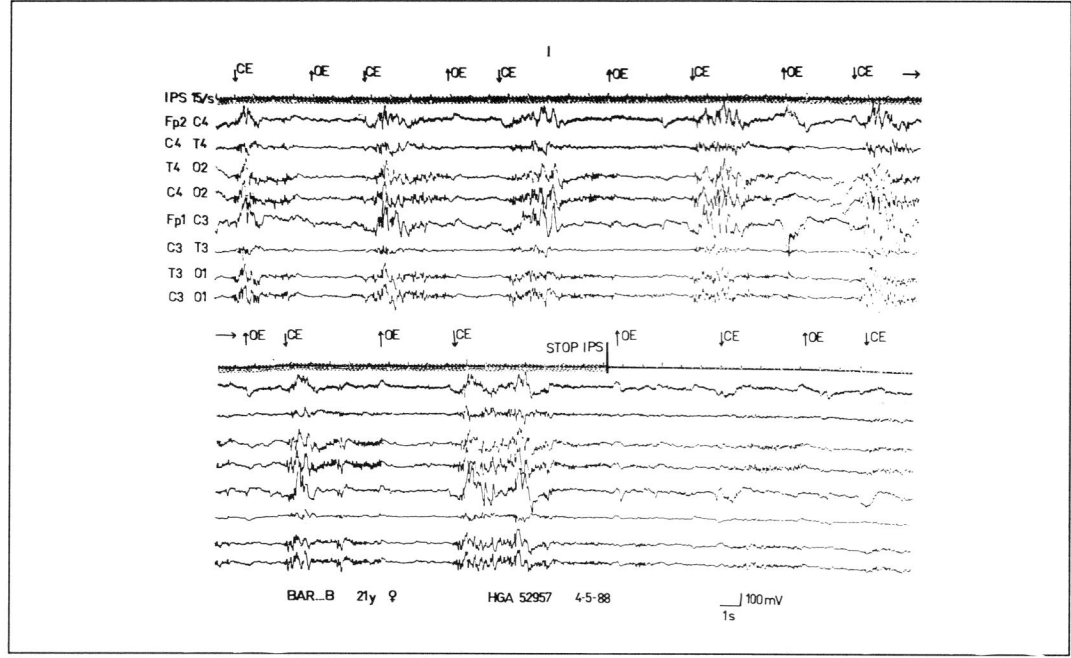

Fig. 3. Female patient aged 23 years. Since the age of 16 she has had myoclonic seizures on awakening, only one generalized tonic–clonic seizure and no clinical photosensitivity. The EEG recording shows spike and poly-spike wave discharges during photic stimulation, enhanced by eye closure. There is no effect of eye closure outside the intermittent photic stimulation.

poly-SW discharges. Absences were recorded in nine patients (four of whom had never been aware of absences); a generalized tonic–clonic seizure was recorded in three patients, and a myoclonic status epilepticus in one. Ictal manifestations, and their recording on the polygraphic EEG, can be facilitated by sleep deprivation and by awakening (Touchon, 1982).

The EEG evaluation of juvenile myoclonic epilepsy patients is thus both easy and difficult:

– when the clinical diagnosis has not been made, there are numerous pitfalls, including the possibility of normal EEG tracings and the high prevalence of focal or atypical changes, and this may delay the diagnosis (Grünewald *et al.*, 1992);

– when the diagnosis of juvenile myoclonic epilepsy is suspected clinically, on the contrary, it seems quite easy to confirm it by obtaining the typical interictal and ictal changes using sleep and sleep deprivation EEG.

Prolonged EEG, polygraphic and video monitoring, associated with sleep and sleep deprivation, is the most useful neurophysiological method of diagnosis in juvenile myoclonic epilepsy; it will allow the clinician to record the characteristic interictal and ictal changes, and should be performed whenever the diagnosis is suspected.

Related types of IGEs

The discussion concerning the existence of either a continuum or a series of discrete, distinct epileptic entities within the category of IGE has been resolved (see Roger *et al.*, Ch. 2). The typical clinical picture of childhood absence epilepsy (CAE), in particular, can be easily separated from juvenile myoclonic epilepsy, on clinical and on genetic grounds, in spite of reports of cases evolving

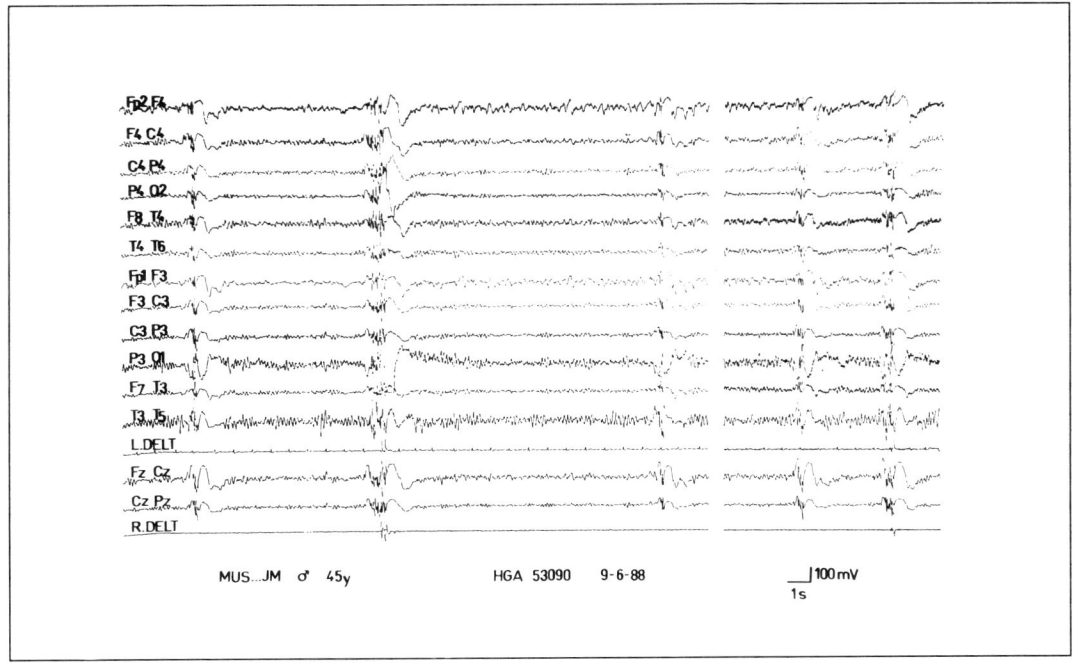

Fig. 4. Male patient aged 45 years. Since the age of 12 he has had frequent myoclonic seizures on awakening and generalized tonic–clonic seizures. He has suffered several myoclonic status epilepticus related to sodium valproate withdrawal. On the EEG recording, myoclonic status epilepticus is shown on awakening. Generalized polyspike-and-wave discharges related with myoclonus are recorded with deltoid muscle polygraphy (L. Delt, R. Delt).

from childhood absence epilepsy to juvenile myoclonic epilepsy (Rabe, 1961). Janz (1969) reported that 4.6 per cent of all childhood absence epilepsy patients evolved into juvenile myoclonic epilepsy, but this report predates the present nosological revision of absence epilepsies. The distinction between benign myoclonic epilepsy of infancy, other forms of IGEs with myoclonic attacks, and juvenile myoclonic epilepsy, will be discussed by Guerrini *et al.*, in Chapter 23. We shall thus discuss mainly the different syndromes of IGE that are most often associated with an onset in adolescence or adulthood.

Juvenile absence epilepsy (JAE)

Juvenile absence epilepsy (Janz, 1969; Wolf, 1992b) was separated from childhood absence epilepsy on the basis of later onset of absences, equal sex distribution (contrary to female predominance in childhood absence epilepsy), and non-pycnoleptic absences. Juvenile absence epilepsy appears, in the words of Wolf (1992), as an 'intermediate syndrome' between childhood absence epilepsy and juvenile myoclonic epilepsy: both the clinical ictal and the EEG interictal and ictal patterns are intermediary. The differences with childhood absence epilepsy are represented (in addition to those quoted above) by a lesser sensitivity to hyperventilation, by a lower proportion of patients with photosensitivity than in juvenile myoclonic epilepsy, by the very high proportion of patients who will experience generalized tonic–clonic seizures, often occurring at awakening (83 per cent according to Janz (1969)), and by the association in 8–16 per cent of myoclonic jerks. Although some of the patients categorized as having juvenile absence epilepsy might indeed be considered to have a condition that is very similar to juvenile myoclonic epilepsy, no definite

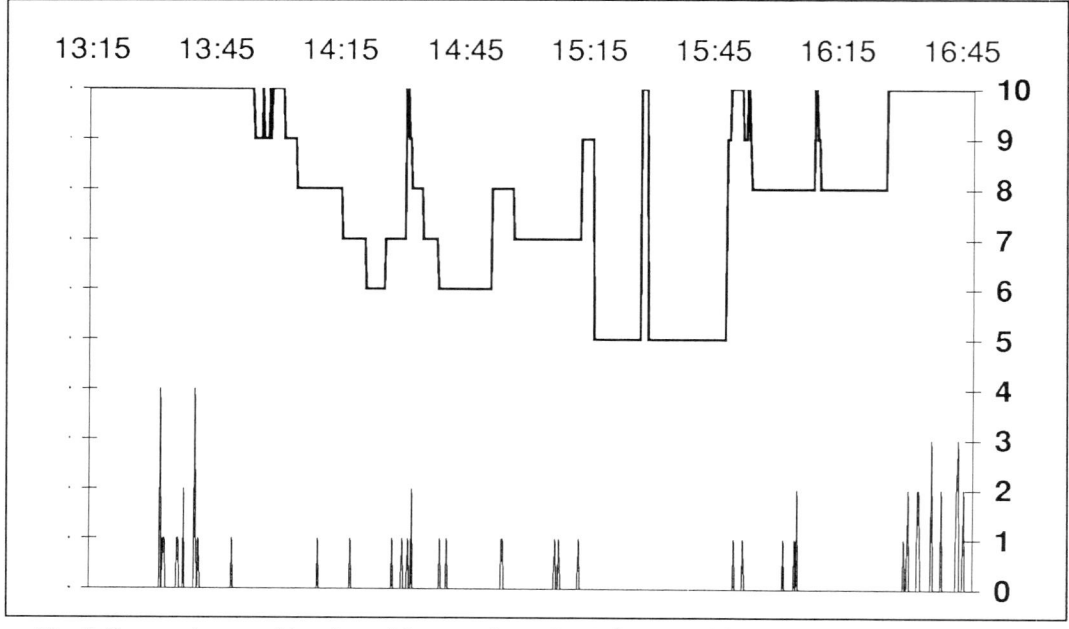

Fig. 5. Twenty-six year old patient with onset of morning jerks at age 14 and of generalized tonic–clonic seizures, often preceded by jerks, at age 16. Diagnosis of grand mal epilepsy, treated by phenobarbital with persisting morning jerks. Quantification of the number of spike-and-wave discharges per 20 s epoch during an afternoon nap following partial sleep deprivation (4 h of sleep during the preceding night); sleep stages: from top to bottom, awake, stages 1–4 of nREM sleep, REM sleep. Presence of spontaneous poly-spike-and-wave discharges during waking, no important activation during sleep, absence of abnormalities during a long REM period, but recurrence during intermediate awakenings and clear activation after the final awakening.

statement can be made at this stage; ongoing large scale studies on the genetic family background of juvenile absence epilepsy and juvenile myoclonic epilepsy patients will probably provide an answer.

Epilepsy with generalized tonic–clonic seizures on awakening

Epilepsy with generalized tonic–clonic seizures on awakening (Janz, 1969; Wolf, 1992c) shares many of the features considered characteristic for juvenile myoclonic epilepsy. The major problem encountered when dealing with this syndrome is that most cases with infrequent generalized tonic–clonic seizures will be ascribed to this category, whether or not the seizures show a clear circadian dependency. This syndrome is characterized by a slight male preponderance, a broad range of the age of onset (66 per cent of the cases commencing their epilepsy between the ages of 9 and 24 (Janz, 1969)) and the possible occurrence, besides infrequent generalized tonic–clonic seizures, of minor seizures in the form of absences (46–63 per cent of the cases) or myoclonic jerks as in juvenile myoclonic epilepsy (6–27 per cent). The precipitating factors of seizures are identical with those described in juvenile myoclonic epilepsy, and the EEG is often of the juvenile myoclonic epilepsy type, showing interictal irregular polyspike-wave discharges. This syndrome must clearly be differentiated from focal epilepsies with rare generalized tonic–clonic seizures seizures, in which the EEG is often normal, and the existence of typical generalized EEG changes is of paramount importance for the diagnosis. Given the frequent occurrence of this syndrome in families of patients with a juvenile myoclonic epilepsy proband, this condition appears to be closely related to juvenile myoclonic epilepsy and might represent a minor form of the latter.

Other epilepsies with infrequent generalized tonic–clonic seizures that are not specifically linked to the sleep–wake cycle are quite common (see Roger et al., Ch. 2); they are often found in families of juvenile myoclonic epilepsy probands; the seizure frequency is low in many cases, and some patients may experience only a single generalized tonic–clonic seizure in their lifetime; in many cases, triggering factors such as fatigue, sleep deprivation, drug withdrawal and/or acute excess of alcohol may be found. Whenever a generalized interictal EEG pattern is found, these cases will be considered as 'awakening grand mal' or as a non-classified form of IGE with generalized tonic–clonic seizures. As for the former syndrome, they may also represent a minor expression of juvenile myoclonic epilepsy.

Finally, the occurrence of myoclonic jerks in association with a generalized EEG interictal and ictal pattern may be found in elderly patients (Gram et al., 1988). Different clinical situations may indeed occur: some patients will be diagnosed in old age only, but have had a lifelong history of jerks and generalized tonic–clonic seizures, with onset in adolescence, as in most cases with juvenile myoclonic epilepsy; others will have an apparently very late onset of a seemingly typical generalized and idiopathic epilepsy with jerks as the presenting symptoms. The latter may in some cases be categorized as juvenile myoclonic epilepsy, in others, to the contrary, to late-onset myoclonic epilepsy with a very different prognosis; a clinical picture that much resembles that of juvenile myoclonic epilepsy has recently be reported as 'senile myoclonic epilepsy' in elderly Down syndrome patients (Genton & Paglia, 1994), and may also occur in Alzheimer patients, but such cases are rarely well documented.

Conclusion

Juvenile myoclonic epilepsy is both a frequent and a very characteristic epileptic syndrome, that will probably be diagnosed more frequently and more rapidly in the future because of the increasing awareness of this syndrome.

Among the various types of IGEs with onset from late childhood to early adulthood, the typical, full-blown clinical and electrophysiological picture of juvenile myoclonic epilepsy probably represents a 'hard core' at the fringe of which some phenotypic variants occur. Typical cases of epilepsy with generalized tonic–clonic seizures on awakening, and other forms of IGE with infrequent generalized tonic–clonic seizures may share the EEG markers of juvenile myoclonic epilepsy and are often found in families with juvenile myoclonic epilepsy probands: in the present state of our knowledge, we may be tempted to consider these syndromes as minor forms of juvenile myoclonic epilepsy. This may also be the case for some of the 'photogenic' epilepsies, when the clinical and the EEG expression are compatible with the markers characteristic for juvenile myoclonic epilepsy, and for some forms of juvenile absence epilepsy, with the same reservations. In the two latter syndromes, it may be postulated that factors other than those implicated in typical juvenile myoclonic epilepsy, either inherited or acquired, play a role.

Most of the recent data point to a lack of relationship between childhood absence epilepsy and juvenile myoclonic epilepsy; some observations reporting a transition from childhood absence epilepsy to juvenile myoclonic epilepsy around the time of puberty are troubling, but such reports have not been too well documented. Childhood absence epilepsy is probably a very heterogeneous group, and the most typical, 'pure', cases can already be easily separated from the juvenile myoclonic epilepsy group of conditions, on both clinical and genetic grounds (Bianchi et al., 1994).

In clinical practice, juvenile myoclonic epilepsy can be easily and firmly diagnosed by careful interviews with the patient and witnesses of the attacks, and by EEG, with the help, if necessary, of long-term EEG-video monitoring using sleep and/or sleep deprivation recordings. An accurate diagnosis of juvenile myoclonic epilepsy is important, as it carries a very precise prognosis and leads to effective therapy.

For research purposes, a well-documented family history is important. Given the comparative unreliability of EEG data, it may seem difficult – or costly – to screen out subjects considered as 'carriers', i. e. presenting with subclinical EEG changes and no ictal symptoms. From a clinical point of view, it appears that two strategies are justified in the search for the genetic mechanism of juvenile myoclonic epilepsy and related syndromes: either the study of isolated individuals with a very firm diagnosis of juvenile myoclonic epilepsy (of which large numbers can be collected), or the study of adequately assessed large families with several juvenile myoclonic epilepsy probands; studies concentrating of the smaller, nuclear families found in most industrialized societies may be less fruitful.

References

Aliberti, V., Grünewald, R.A. & Panayiotopoulos, C.P. (1994): Focal electroencephalographic abnormalities in juvenile myoclonic epilepsy. *Epilepsia* 35, 297–301.

Asconapé, J. & Penry, J.K. (1984): Some clinical and EEG aspects of benign juvenile myoclonic epilepsy. *Epilepsia* 25, 108–114.

Baruzzi, A., Procaccianti, G., Tinuper, P. & Lugaresi, E. (1988): Antiepileptic drug withdrawal in childhood epilepsies: preliminary results of a prospective study. In: *Diagnostic and therapeutic problems in pediatric epileptology*, eds. C. Faienza & G.L. Prati, pp. 117–123. Amsterdam: Elsevier.

Bianchi, A., Tiezzi, A., Buzzi, G., Severi, S. & Zolo, P. (1994): Childhood absence epilepsy: an analysis of the 'pure' syndromic subform. *Epilepsia* 35 (Suppl. 7), 9.

Delgado-Escueta, A.V. & Enrile-Bacsal, F. (1984): Juvenile myoclonic epilepsy of Janz. *Neurology* 34, 285–294.

Dinner, D.S., Lüders, H., Morris, H.H. & Lesser, R.P. (1987): Juvenile myoclonic epilepsy. In: *Epilepsy: electroclinical syndromes*, eds H. Lüders & R. P. Lesser, pp 131–149. Berlin: Springer Verlag.

Genton, P. & Ganeva, G. (1993): Epilepsie cataméniale: mythe et réalité. *Epilepsies* 5, 147–154.

Genton, P. & Roger, J. (1993): Progressive myoclonus epilepsies. In: *The treatment of epilepsy. Principles and practice*, ed. E. Wyllie, pp. 571–583. Philadelphia, London: Lea and Febiger.

Genton, P. & Paglia, G. (1994): Epilepsie myoclonique sénile? Myoclonies épileptiques d'appartion tardive dans le syndrome de Down. *Epilepsies* 6, 5–11.

Gigli, G.L., Calia, E., Luciani, L., Diomedi, M., De La Pierre, L., Marciani, M.G. & Sasanelli, F. (1991): Eye closure sensitivity in juvenile myoclonic epilepsy: polysomnographic study of electrocencephalographic epileptiform discharge rates. *Epilepsia* 32, 677–683.

Gonzales Sanchez, M.S., Genton, P., Bureau, M., Dravet, C. & Saltarelli, A. (1994): Misleading aspects of the first standard EEG in juvenile myoclonic epilepsy. *Epilepsia* 35, (suppl. 7), 10.

Gooses, R. (1984): *Die Beziehung der Fotosensibilität zu den verschiedenen epileptischen Syndromen*. Thesis, Berlin.

Gram, L., Alving, J., Sagild J.C. & Dam, M. (1988): Juvenile myoclonic epilepsy in unexpected age groups. *Epil. Res.* 2, 137–140.

Greenberg, D.A., Delgado-Escueta, A.V., Widelitz, H., Sparkes, R.S., Treiman, L., Maldonado, H.M., Park, M.S. & Terasaki, P.I. (1988): Juvenile myoclonic epilepsy (JME) may be linked to the BF and HLA loci on human chromosome 6. *Am. J. Med. Genet.* 31, 185–192.

Grünewald, R.A., Chroni, E. & Panayiotopoulos, C.P. (1992): Delayed diagnosis of juvenile myoclonic epilepsy. *J. Neurol. Neurosurg. Psychiatry* 55, 497–499.

Grünewald, R.A. & Panayiotopoulos, C.P. (1993): Juvenile myoclonic epilepsy: a review. *Arch. Neurol.* 50, 594–598.

Guirao, I.P., Behe, I. & Wolf, P. (1987): Epileptic discharges after eye closure: relation to epileptic syndromes. In: *Advances in epileptology*, vol. 16, eds P. Wolf, M. Dam, D. Janz & F. E. Dreifuss, pp. 255–258. New York: Raven Press.

Janz, D. & Christian, W. (1957): Impulsiv petit-mal. *Dtsch Z. Nervenheilk.* 176, 346–386.

Janz, D. (1969): *Die Epilepsien*. Stuttgart: Thieme Verlag.

Janz, D (1991): Juvenile myoclonic epilepsy. In: *Comprehensive epileptology*, eds. M. Dam & L. Gram, pp. 171–185. New York: Raven Press.

Janz, D., Kern, A., Mössinger, H.J. & Puhlmann, H.U. (1983): Rückfallprognose nach Reduktion der Medikamente bei Epilepsiebehandlung. *Nervenarzt.* **54**, 525–529.

Loiseau, P., Duché, B. & Loiseau, J. (1991): Classification of epilepsies and epileptic syndromes in two different samples of patients. *Epilepsia* **32**. 303–309.

Mai, R., Canevini, M.P., Pontrelli, V., Tassi, L., Bertin, C., Di Marco, C. & Canger, R. (1990): L'epilessia mioclonica giovanile di Janz: analisi prospettiva di un campione di 57 pazienti. *Boll. Lega. Ital. Epil.* **70/71**, 307-309.

Obeid, T. & Panayiotopoulos, C.P. (1988): Juvenile myoclonic epilepsy: a study in Saudi Arabia. *Epilepsia* **29**, 280–282.

Obeid, T. & Panayiotopoulos, C.P. (1989): Clonazepam in juvenile myoclonic epilepsy. *Epilepsia* **30**, 2603–2606.

Panayiotopoulos, C.P., Obeid, T. & Waheed, G. (1989): Absences in juvenile myoclonic epilepsy: a clinical video-EEG study. *Ann. Neurol.* **25**, 391–397.

Panayiotopoulos, C.P., Tahan, R. & Obeid, T. (1991): Juvenile myoclonic epilepsy: factors of errors involved in the diagnosis and treatment. *Epilepsia* **32**, 672–676.

Penry, J.K., Dean, J.C. & Riela, A.R. (1989): Juvenile myoclonic epilepsy: long-term response to therapy. *Epilepsia* **30** Suppl. 4, 19–23.

Rabe, F. (1961): Zum Wechsel des anfallscharaktars epileptischer Anfälle. *Dtsch Z. Nervenheilk.* **182**, 201–230.

Resor, S.R. & Resor, L.D. (1990): The neuropharmacology of juvenile myoclonic epilepsy. *Clin. Neuropharmacol.* **13**, 465–491.

Salas-Puig, X., Camara da Silva, A.M., Dravet, C. & Roger, J. (1990): L'épilepsie myoclonique juvénile dans la population du Centre Saint Paul. *Epilepsies* **2**, 108–113.

Serratosa, J.M. & Delgado-Escueta, A.V. (1993): Juvenile myoclonic epilepsy. In: *The treatment of epilepsy. Principles and practice*, ed. E. Wyllie, pp. 552–570. Philadelphia: Lea and Febiger.

Simonsen, N., Mollgaard, V. & Lund, M. (1976): A controlled clinical and electroencephalographic study of myoclonic epilepsy (impulsiv-petit mal). In: *Epileptology*, ed. D. Janz, pp. 41–48. Stuttgart: Thieme Verlag.

Su, Y.H., Izumi, T., Kitsu, M. & Fukuyama, Y. (1993): Seizure threshold in juvenile myoclonic epilepsy with Graves' disease. *Epilepsia* **34**, 488–492.

Touchon, J. (1982): Effect of awakening on epileptic activity in primary generalized myoclonic epilepsy. In: *Sleep and epilepsy*, eds. M.B. Sterman, M.N. Shouse & P. Passouant, pp. 239–248. New York: Academic Press.

Touchon, J., Besset, A., Billiard, M. & Baldy-Moulinier, M. (1982): Effects of spontaneous and provoked awakening on the frequency of polyspike and wave discharges in 'bilateral massive epileptic myoclonus'. In: *Advances in epileptology*, Vol. 13, eds. H. Akimoto, M. Kazamatsuri, M. Seino & M. Ward, pp. 269–272. New York: Raven Press.

Tsuboi, T. (1977): *Primary generalized epilepsy with sporadic myoclonias of myoclonic petit mal type*. Stuttgart: Thieme Verlag.

Wolf, P. (1985): Benign juvenile myoclonic epilepsy. In: *Epileptic syndromes in infancy, childhood and adolescence*, eds. J. Roger, Ch. Dravet, M. Bureau, F.E. Dreifuss & P. Wolf, pp. 242–246. London: John Libbey.

Wolf, P. (1992a): Juvenile myoclonic epilepsy. In: *Epileptic syndromes in infancy, childhood and adolescence*, 2nd edn, eds. J. Roger, M. Bureau, Ch. Dravet, F.E. Dreifuss A. Perret & P. Wolf, pp. 313–327. London: John Libbey.

Wolf, P. (1992b): Juvenile absence epilepsy. In: *Epileptic syndromes in infancy, childhood and adolescence*, 2nd edn, eds. J. Roger, M. Bureau, Ch. Dravet, F.E. Dreifuss, A. Perret & P. Wolf, pp. 307–312. London: John Libbey.

Wolf, P. (1992c): Epilepsy with grand mal on awakening. In: *Epileptic syndromes in infancy, childhood and adolescence*, 2nd edn, eds. J. Roger, M. Bureau, Ch. Dravet, F.E. Dreifuss, A. Perret & P. Wolf, pp. 329–341. London: John Libbey.

Wolf, P. & Gooses, R. (1986): Relation of photosensitivity to epileptic syndromes. *J. Neurol. Neurosurg. Psychiatry* **49**, 1386–1391.

Chapter 23

Idiopathic generalized epilepsies with myoclonus in infancy and childhood

Renzo Guerrini[*], Charlotte Dravet[†], Giuseppe Gobbi[‡], Stefano Ricci[§] and Olivier Dulac[¶]

[*]*Istituto di Neuropsichiatria e Psicopedagogia dell' Età Evolutiva dell' Università di Pisa-Istituto Scientifico 'Fondazione Stella Maris', Pisa, Italy;* [†]*Centre Saint Paul, Marseille, France;* [‡]*Servizio di Neuropsichiatria Infantile, Ospedale di Reggio Emilia, Italy;* [§]*Servizio di Neurofisiologia, Istituto Scientifico Ospedale Pediatrico Bambino Gesù, Rome, Italy and* [¶]*Hôpital Saint Vincent de Paul, Paris, France*

Introduction

According to the classification of epilepsies and epileptic syndromes (Commission, 1989) benign myoclonic epilepsy in infancy (BME) (Dravet & Bureau, 1981) is the only form of idiopathic generalized epilepsy (IGE) with onset before adolescence that is characterized predominantly by myoclonus. Juvenile myoclonic epilepsy (JME) is another better known IGE with prominent myoclonus, but which typically begins during adolescence. Another generalized epilepsy with myoclonus was defined by Doose et al. (1970) as myoclonic–astatic epilepsy, but whether it is idiopathic or cryptogenic is still open to debate. Myoclonus is frequent in IGEs and may be prominent in some affected children. Despite the phenotype of IGE, myoclonic epilepsies of childhood cannot be considered as a separate syndrome, and their classification and prognosis have been unclear.

Non-myoclonic forms of epilepsy are classified by aetiology, general clinical context, and the clinical and EEG pattern. However the semiological approach, and mere occurrence of myoclonus with epilepsy, has constituted the only inclusion criterion in many studies of epilepsies with myoclonus (Loiseau et al., 1974; Doose, 1985). More recently, attempts have been made to define syndromes in which myoclonus can be the sole and defining symptom (Aicardi, 1980; Dravet et al., 1982; Sheffner, 1982; Dravet et al., 1985; Dalla Bernardina et al., 1987, 1992; Chiron et al., 1988; Aicardi & Levy-Gomes, 1989; Lombroso, 1990). Certain syndromes have been included in the international classification (Commission, 1989). Despite these attempts, there is still a great deal of confusion and in clinical practice, many cases are difficult to classify. For example, although all the patients reported by Doose (1992) as myoclonic–astatic epilepsy have myoclonus, it is only a minor symptom in some of them who have daily convulsive seizures, prolonged absence, or myoclonic status; whereas it is the principal feature in some children with prominent and disabling myoclonic–astatic seizures leading to injury. In addition, some of the patients reported by Doose are neurologically and cognitively normal and their epilepsy is idiopathic, while others are mentally retarded and have a non-idiopathic epilepsy. Because of these different clinical manifestations and the variable course and outcome, myoclonic–astatic epilepsy is classified as a large syndrome group among age-related cryptogenic or symptomatic generalized epilepsies (Commission, 1989). Dulac et al. (1990) described a childhood-onset benign myoclonic epilepsy as a clearly defined form of IGE. This demonstrates that idiopathic cases do exist in this age group and, if separated from the heterogeneous group of myoclonic–astatic epilepsy, would fill a large part of the syndromic void existing in the classification of idiopathic epilepsies with myoclonus starting from the age range of benign myoclonic epilepsy in infancy to that of juvenile myoclonic epilepsy.

In this chapter we will attempt to summarize the current knowledge of idiopathic generalized epilepsies predominantly characterized or accompanied by myoclonus, starting in infancy or childhood, before the age of onset of juvenile myoclonic epilepsy.

Benign myoclonic epilepsy of infancy

Dravet and Bureau defined this syndrome in 1981, after which only isolated cases or small groups of patients were reported from Europe (Dalla Bernardina et al., 1983; Colamaria et al., 1987; Salas-Puig et al., 1990; Todt & Muller, 1992; Dravet et al., 1992a, b), for a total of 38 cases. This syndrome is, however, probably more frequent than commonly recognized, with many cases likely unreported. As it has been recently described, is relatively straightforward, and responds well to antiepileptic drugs (AEDs), potential authors may believe that further reports would contribute little. Furthermore, benign myoclonic epilepsy in infancy could go unrecognized in centres where polygraphic EEG is not carried out routinely. Reports from the USA, where polygraphic studies are much less common than in Europe, have been scanty (Lombroso, 1990).

The incidence of benign myoclonic epilepsy in infancy is not known. Among patients with seizure onset in the first 3 years, benign myoclonic epilepsy represented 0.46 per cent of new admissions among 1987 and 1989 at the Centre Saint-Paul (Dravet et al., 1992a), 0.5 per cent of those referred to the Institute of Developmental Neuropsychiatry of the University of Pisa between 1990–1992, and 2 per cent of 504 consecutive patients reported by Dalla Bernardina et al. (1983).

The age at onset of benign myoclonic epilepsy in infancy ranges from 4 months to 3 years. Rare cases with identical clinical and EEG characteristics have been reported with seizure onset up to 5 years (Jeavons, 1977; Delgado-Escueta et al., 1990). There has been a 2:1 preponderance of males. Approximately one third of the patients have family histories of epilepsy or febrile convulsions. Other conditions have occasionally coexisted without being responsible for the syndrome: single cases have been reported with diabetes (Colamaria et al., 1987), Down's syndrome (Guerrini et al., 1990a), and haemophilia (see below – case report no. 2).

Some of the patients reported by Dravet & Bureau (1981) were mentally retarded when evaluated at ages between 10 and 15 years (Dravet et al., 1990, 1992a,b). Such retardation was correlated mainly with delay in beginning anti-epileptic drugs and repetition of myoclonic seizures, although other factors were likely to have contributed (Dravet et al., 1992b). However, particular caution is necessary in evaluating the origin of cognitive deficit in patients with generalized epileptic myoclonus. Mild to moderate mental retardation as the only neurological deficit is difficult to identify in the first year of life, before the onset of myoclonus, and can be associated with static encephalopathies on a genetic basis (see below).

The seizures of benign myoclonic epilepsy in infancy consist of brief generalized myoclonic jerks, either singly or repeated in groups of two or three. Intensity and frequency vary from patient to patient and in the same patient but seizures typically occur many times a day. In the mildest form, jerks are only identified polygraphically, without any obvious clinical manifestations. Jerks during sleep are often mistaken for nonepileptic sleep myoclonus. If the child is standing or sitting, the jerks often cause nodding with upward gaze deviation and eyelid myoclonus, accompanied by slight abduction of the arms or bending of the elbows. The child may stagger if standing, especially up to

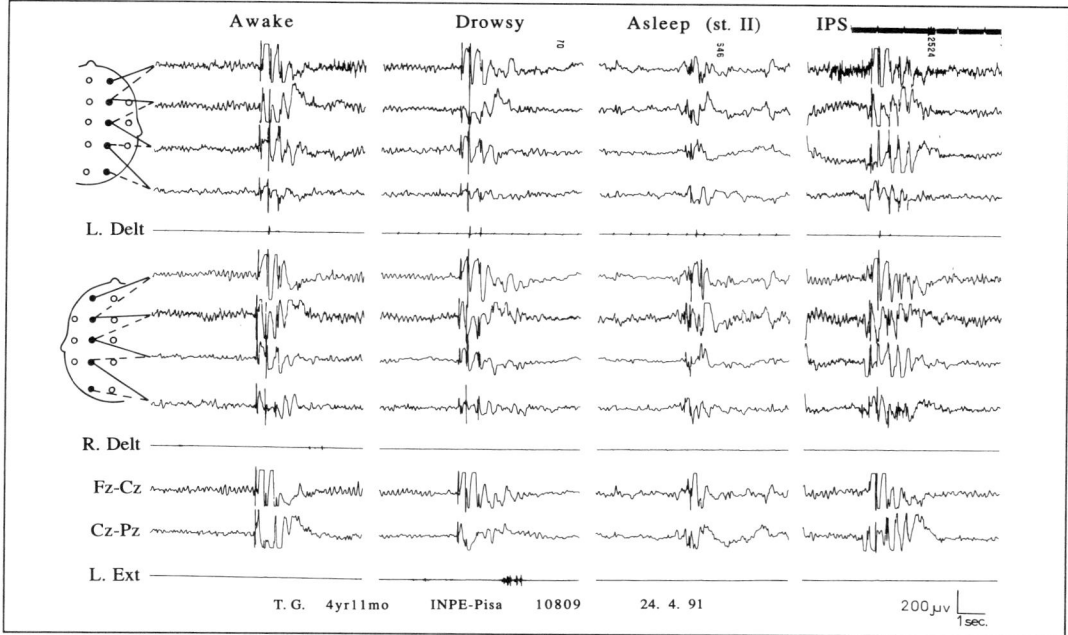

Fig. 1. Case 1: benign myoclonic epilepsy in infancy. Child with mild myoclonic jerks since the age of 1 year. Spontaneous discharges while awake and asleep and photic-induced discharges are very similar, as are the EMG correlates.

the second year of life when walking is still unstable. Though falls are unusual, when they occur the child falls onto the buttocks and gets up immediately to continue activity.

The myoclonic jerks are never accompanied by other seizures, even if not treated early. Absences have never been observed. Two patients from the series of Dravet et al. (1992b) had generalized tonic–clonic seizures in adolescence after withdrawal of anti-epileptic drugs. However, this happens too rarely to have any bearing on the usual duration of drug treatment, which should be stopped before school age.

Reflex form of benign myoclonic epilepsy in infancy

Most cases of benign myoclonic epilepsy in infancy have no triggering factors. However, 10 per cent have photic-induced jerks (Dravet et al, 1992b) clinically indistinguishable from spontaneous jerks (Fig. 1), and some children have reflex myoclonus triggered by tactile (Fig. 2) or sudden acoustic stimuli, with or without spontaneous jerking (Revol et al., 1989; Deonna & Despland, 1989; Ricci et al., 1993a, b). These may thus be either forms of benign myoclonic epilepsy in infancy with reflex seizures or true reflex epilepsies. Ricci et al., (1993b) found that four of 17 children with benign myoclonic epilepsy in infancy had reflex myoclonus, two of whom had a pure reflex form. Onset ranged from 4 to 11 months. Jerks could be provoked during sleep or while awake and acoustic stimuli were the most effective. In two children who were not treated, the jerks disappeared 4 months after onset. In the two treated children, valproate (VPA) stopped myoclonic jerks within 2 months. Ictal and interictal EEGs were identical to those of other patients with benign myoclonic epilepsy in infancy.

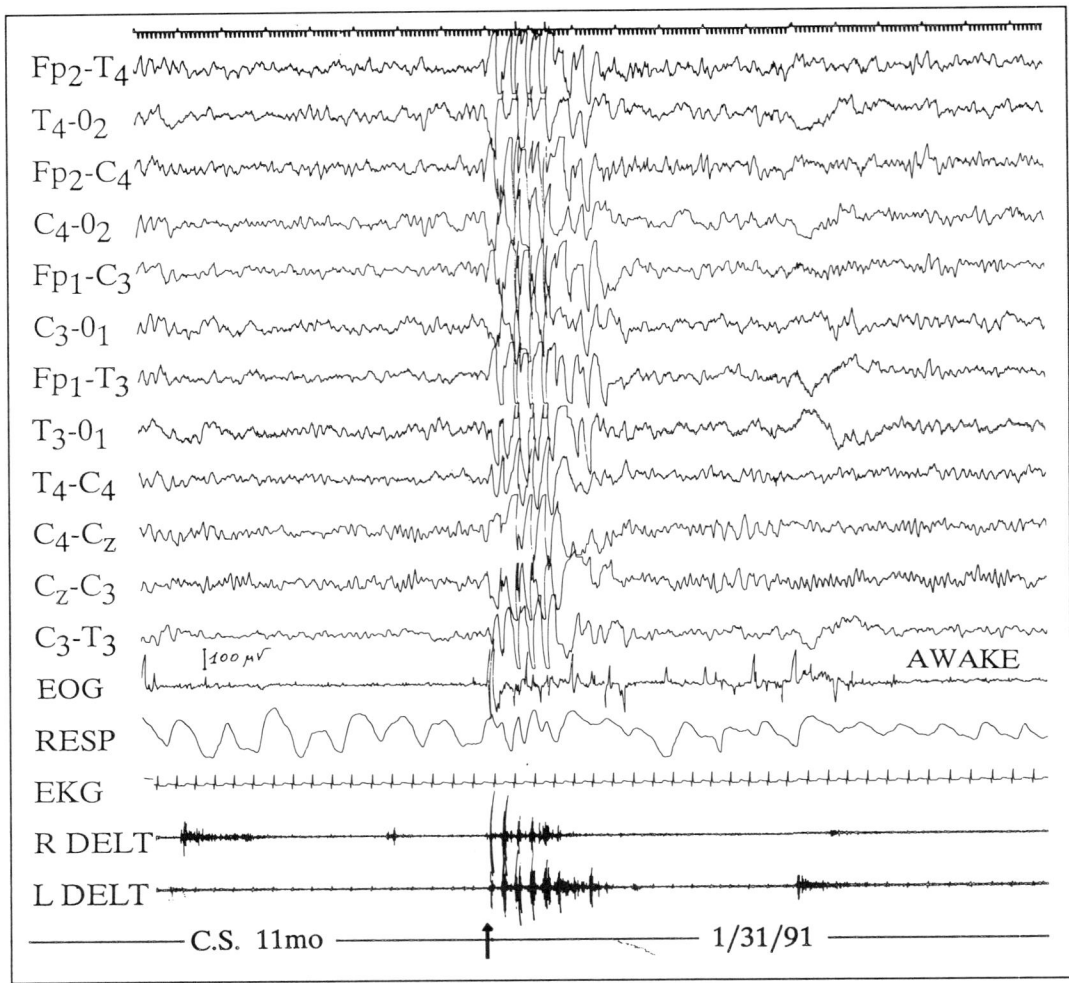

Fig. 2. Case 3: pure reflex form of benign myoclonic epilepsy in infancy. A bout of rhythmic jerks is recorded in response to sudden touch. A brief burst of diffuse polyspike and wave complexes accompanies the jerks.

Childhood-onset myoclonic epilepsy similar to benign myoclonic epilepsy in infancy

We observed six patients with idiopathic generalized epileptic myoclonus beginning between 2.5 and 5 years with jerks, either isolated or in short series, predominating in axial muscles and not causing falls (Fig. 3). Age at onset of myoclonus was determined retrospectively by questioning the parents. Four patients had a family history of epilepsy or febrile seizures. No other types of spontaneous seizures occurred. However, one child had had a febrile convulsion and another had absence seizures with irregular jerks during hyperventilation. In two, intermittent photic stimulation caused myoclonic jerks that were identical to spontaneous ones. All these children had generalized spike and wave or polyspike and wave EEG complexes during myoclonus. The background EEG activity was normal and interictal abnormalities were extremely rare. Myoclonus was more frequent during drowsiness, but was so mild that it could have been missed without a polygraphic recording. In all children the jerks disappeared completely with valproate. They are now aged 5–9 years and their development is normal. Magnetic resonance imaging (MRI) performed in two was normal.

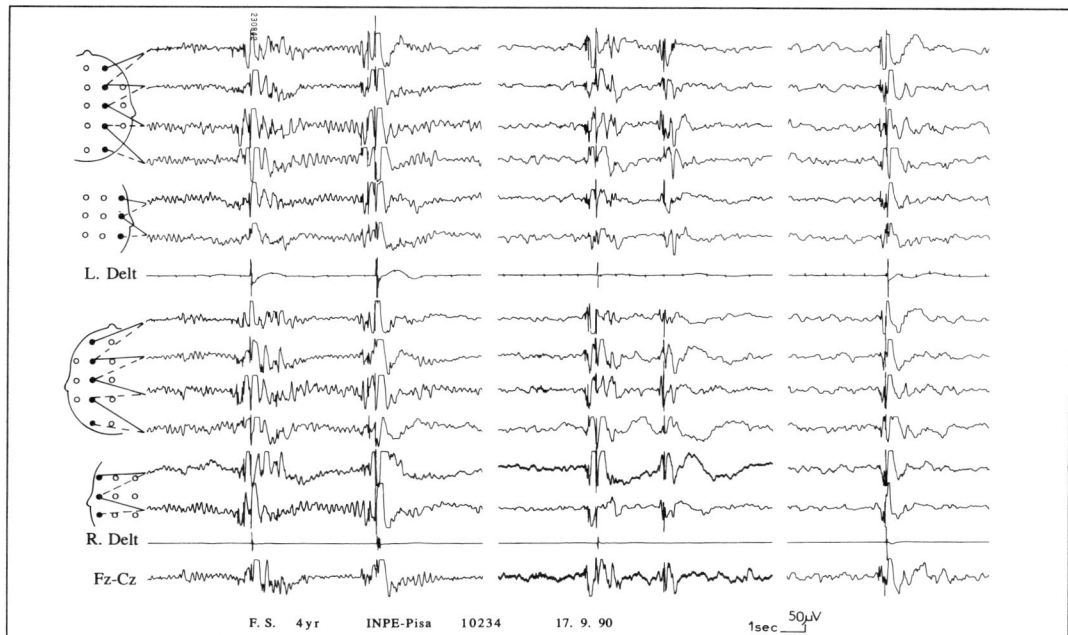

Fig. 3. Case 4: childhood-onset benign myoclonic epilepsy. Isolated jerks of epileptic myoclonus are recorded while the patient is drowsy (left) and asleep (middle and right). The jerks are clinically indistinguishable from sleep myoclonus.

These patients have an IGE with clinical and EEG features very similar to those of benign myoclonic epilepsy in infancy, but with a slightly later onset. Similar cases have been reported by Jeavons (1977). Maton et al. (1990) reported seven patients with myoclonic–astatic seizures with onset in infancy and childhood, numerous generalized EEG discharges, and slowing of background EEG activity associated with a favourable outcome and normal cognitive development. Four of their patients had no other types of seizure. Although rare, such cases suggest that there is a continuum of clinical expression of 'fragments' of idiopathic generalized epilepsy with myoclonus throughout childhood.

Eyelid myoclonus with absences

This form of epilepsy is discussed in the chapter on absence epilepsies. After the first description by Jeavons (1977), few authors have dealt with this form of epilepsy (Dalla Bernardina et al., 1989; Appleton et al., 1993), which is not yet included in the international syndrome classification. Its definition as a separate epileptic syndrome would be difficult in patients with onset in late childhood or adolescence because their electroclinical manifestations overlap those of juvenile myoclonic epilepsy.

Generalized myoclonus in children with static encephalopathies

Generalized myoclonus as the only manifestation of epilepsy in an otherwise healthy child is usually carefully studied to identify the characteristics that will guide both treatment and prognosis. Occasional myoclonic jerks occurring in a child with a static encephalopathy will probably be considered an infrequent and unimportant symptom, especially if it is not disabling. However, when systematically searched for in the mentally retarded population, generalized epileptic myoclonus appears to be rather common. At the Institute for Developmental Neuropsychiatry of the University of Pisa and at the Infancy and Childhood Neuropsychiatry Service of Reggio Emilia, where polygraphic video-EEG recordings are performed routinely in wakefulness and sleep in patients with static encephalopathies with or without epilepsy, we found 11 patients with previously overlooked generalized myoclonus whose clinical and ictal EEG manifestations were indistinguishable from those of benign myoclonic epilepsy in infancy (Fig. 4). The fixed neurological signs were either of genetic (chromosomal abnormalities or multiple congenital anomalies/mental retardation syndromes) or perinatal origin. We believe that this condition is a mild manifestation of a symptomatic epilepsy, rather than a chance or causal association of idiopathic generalized epilepsy traits and a fixed encephalopathy (Guerrini et al., 1990b). There is no clear aetiological link between any specific genetic abnormality and myoclonus, with the possible exception of Angelman yndrome that could represent a genetic model of cortical myoclonus (Guerrini et al., 1994).

Severe generalized myoclonus may also occur as a form of status epilepticus in patients with fixed encephalopathies (Chiron et al., 1988; Dalla Bernardina et al., 1992).

True myoclonic–astatic epilepsy

Epilepsy with myoclonic–astatic (MA) seizures is included in the classification of epilepsies and syndromes as a generalized cryptogenic or symptomatic form with onset between ages 7 months and 6 years. Since the classification was published (Commission, 1989), and since the concepts that inspired it were discussed in print (Roger et al., 1985; Henriksen, 1985), there has been growing evidence that the patients classified by Doose as having myoclonic–astatic epilepsy contain a large subgroup with idiopathic epilepsy or 'primarily generalized seizures' (Doose et al., 1970; Doose, 1985, 1992). Myoclonic–astatic epilepsy is distinct from Lennox–Gastaut syndrome (LGS) (Beaumanoir & Dravet, 1992; Dulac & N'Guyen, 1993), but different syndromes characterized by myoclonus appear to be present in patients considered to have myoclonic–astatic epilepsy. Children with massive myoclonus as the only clinical feature and a favourable outcome are likely to have benign myoclonic epilepsy or a similar form with later onset. Those with frequent and prolonged unilateral alternating febrile and afebrile clonic seizures from the first year of life and myoclonic attacks after some years probably have severe myoclonic epilepsy in infancy (Dravet et al., 1992c).

However, a rather large subset of patients with what we call 'true myoclonic–astatic epilepsy' shares some distinct electroclinical features but has a variable outcome (Dulac et al., 1990; Dulac, 1993). Dulac et al. (1990, 1993) studied 28 patients referred over 12 years with a follow-up of at least 3 years, with non-progressive myoclonic epilepsy beginning between ages 1 and 10 years, normal development and neuroimaging, and no evidence of metabolic disease. Patients with benign myoclonic epilepsy in infancy, absence epilepsy with eyelid myoclonus, juvenile myoclonic epilepsy, or Lennox–Gastaut syndrome were excluded. There was a strong male predominance (five girls, 23 boys) and 11/28 had a family history of epilepsy or febrile seizures. Seizures began between 18 months and 4 years with generalized clonic or tonic–clonic seizures, or drop attacks due to massive myoclonus (Fig. 5). Each type of seizure tended to be isolated or occur in clusters. Within a few months the children began to have several types of seizures, including atypical absences, generalized clonic or tonic–clonic seizures, massive myoclonus, and episodes of status epilepticus.

These authors recognized two distinct prognostic groups: in 17 patients, epilepsy lasted less than 3 years; the other 11 had an unfavourable prognosis.

In the group with favourable prognosis, the status epilepticus consisted of episodes of stupor with repeated massive myoclonus, tonic–clonic, and atonic absence seizures lasting for about 4–5 days. After these episodes, the seizures soon became considerably less frequent and, following a few convulsive seizures the epilepsy resolved. Although children continued to be hyperactive for some months, recovery was rapid and treatment could be suspended despite the transient period of severe

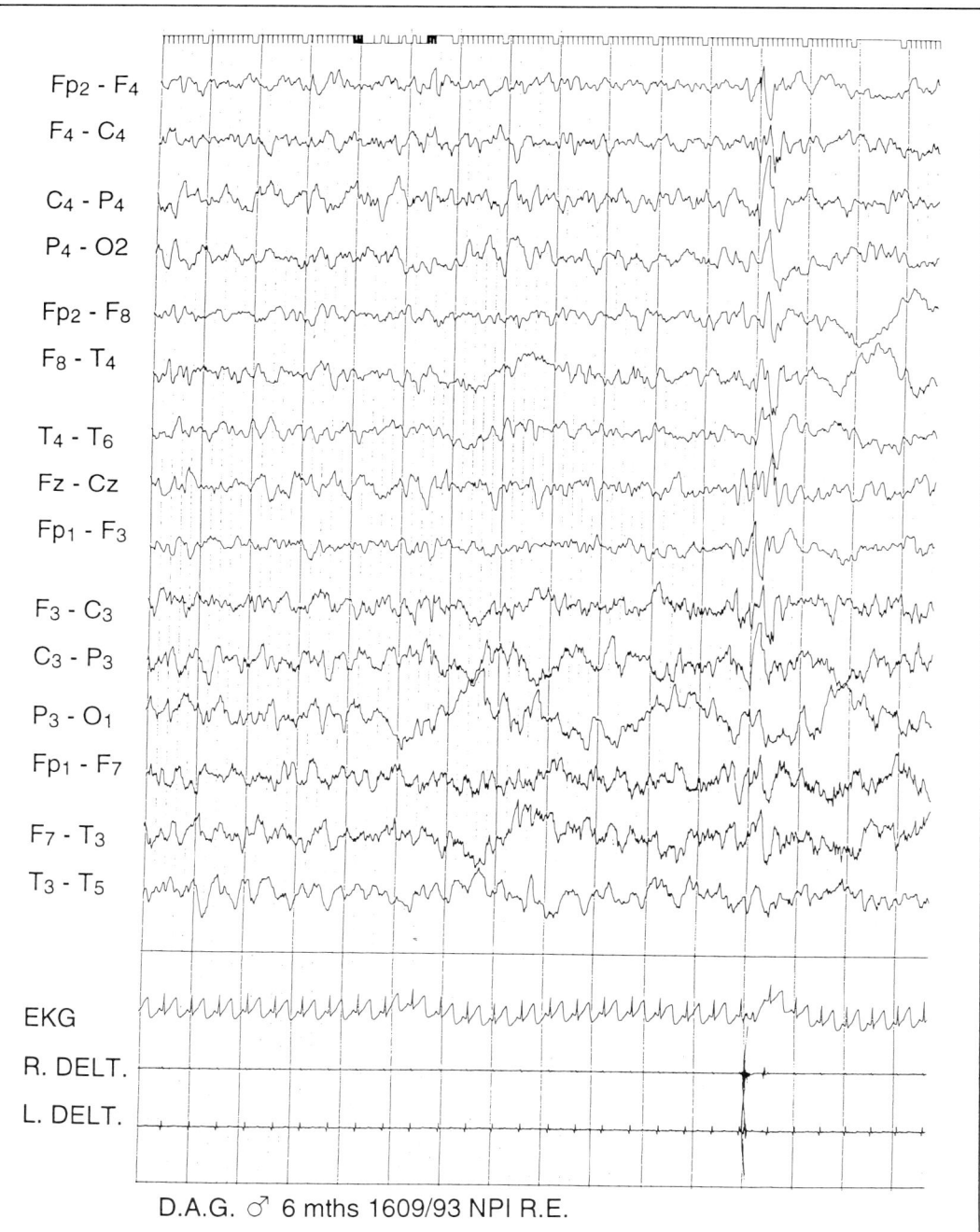

Fig. 4. Six-month-old child with history of intrapartum hypoxia and neonatal seizures treated with phenobarbital. Spastic quadriparesis and mild diffuse cortical and subcortical atrophy at MRI. From the age of 10 weeks, onset of jerks of all four limbs, isolated or in short clusters. The EEG showed the myoclonic jerks to be related to the spike of a generalized spike and wave complex, more evident over the central regions. Valproate and ethosuximide controlled myoclonus. No relapse occurred after 1 year of follow-up.

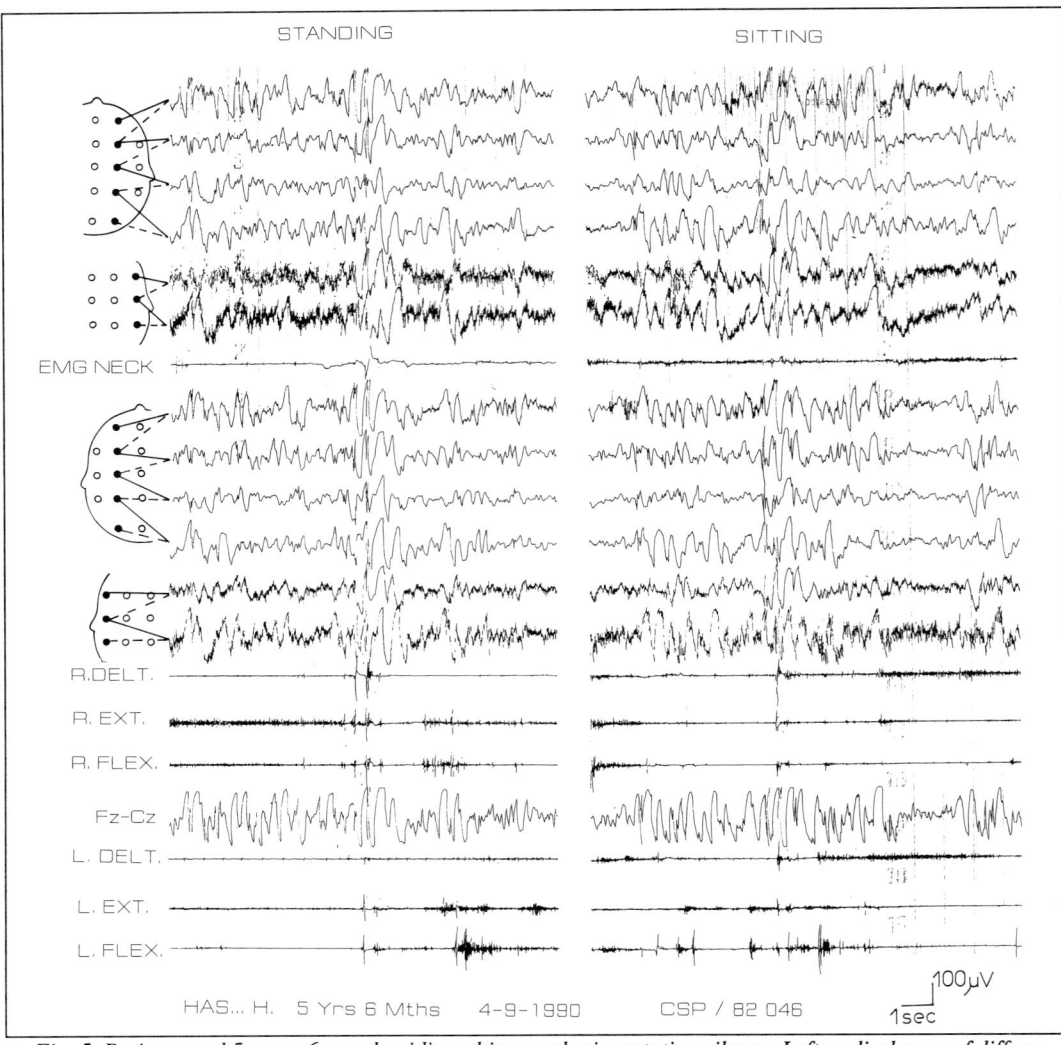

Fig. 5. Patient aged 5 years 6 months; idiopathic myoclonic–astatic epilepsy. Left: a discharge of diffuse spikes and polyspikes is accompanied by two myoclonic potentials, each followed by a post-myoclonic EMG silence. Clinically, the patient falls abruptly due to positive and negative motor phenomena. Right: a mild myoclonic contraction while he is seated causes a jerk without a fall.

seizures. Mean duration of the active epilepsy was 14 months and all patients were seizure-free after 3 years. In the group with unfavourable prognosis, the episodes of status epilepticus consisted of confusion, hypotonia with stupor, drooling and erratic distal or facial myoclonus, combined with tonic seizures, all lasting up to one month. Numerous episodes of status could occur before the seizures became less frequent. The patients continued to have brief tonic seizures during sleep for years, especially between 4:00 and 6:00 a.m. (Fig. 6).

In the early stages of the disease, the myoclonus is mainly massive in cases with favourable outcome and erratic in those with unfavourable outcome. There are, however, cases with favourable outcome in which erratic myoclonus coexists with generalized jerks (Case 5, Fig. 7). The appear-

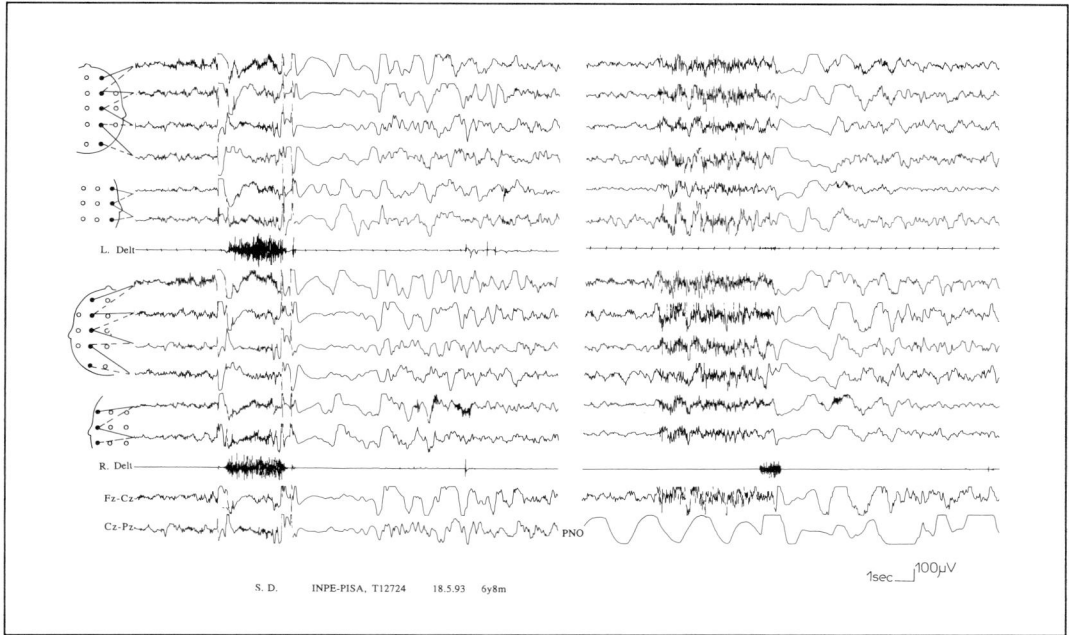

Fig. 6. Patient aged 6 years 8 months; idiopathic myoclonic-astatic epilepsy. Brief tonic seizures appearing near the end of the night. Left: a brief tonic seizure accompanied by diffuse low-voltage theta activity, preceded and followed by generalized spike and wave complexes corresponding to myoclonic potentials on the EMG. Right: low-voltage fast activity is superimposed on delta and theta sleep activity. A very short tonic contraction appears at the end of the discharge. These tonic seizures were found by video-EEG monitoring but were so mild as to have been unrecognized by the parents.

ance of tonic seizures in the second stage of the disease seems to be correlated with a worse prognosis.

Some features suggest that the aetiology and pathophysiology of myoclonic–astatic epilepsy and those of Lennox–Gastaut syndrome are different. Lennox–Gastaut syndrome is often symptomatic, while myoclonic–astatic epilepsy is by definition idiopathic. Tonic seizures which are a diagnostic feature of Lennox–Gastaut syndrome, are observed only in cases of myoclonic–astatic epilepsy with poor prognosis. Even in such patients the EEG recruiting rhythms of Lennox–Gastaut syndrome are not clearly recognizable, and the rhythmic slow spike and wave complexes typical of Lennox–Gastaut syndrome do not occur. Response to treatment is also different. Lamotrigine and steroids that are often useful in Lennox–Gastaut syndrome (Aicardi & Chevrie, 1986; Schlumberger *et al.*, 1994) do not affect myoclonic epilepsy. However such differences may not be always clear-cut and some of us wonder whether some of these patients really have Lennox–Gastaut syndrome with some unusual tonic seizures, which in these patients are infrequent, brief, and occur near the end of nocturnal sleep. Beaumanoir & Dravet (1992) pointed out that tonic seizures are not present at the onset of Lennox–Gastaut syndrome, which tends to begin with falls and atypical absences. Further studies of larger series with video EEG-polygraphic monitoring will probably clarify any early differences between myoclonic–astatic epilepsy with unfavourable outcome and cryptogenic Lennox–Gastaut syndrome.

Conclusions

Some idiopathic generalized epilepsies of which myoclonus is the only symptom begin in infancy

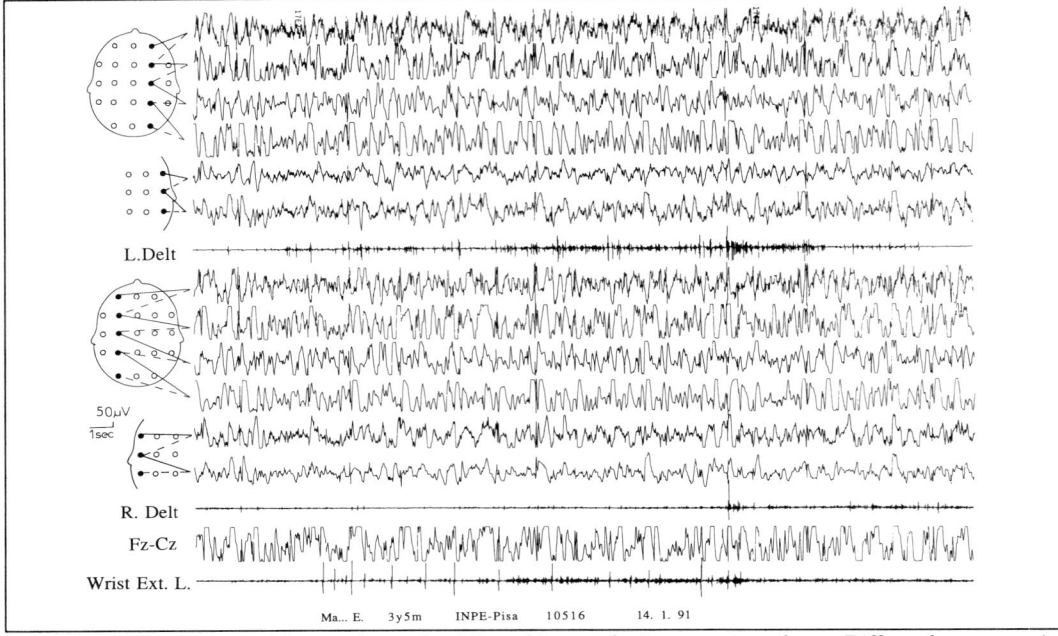

Fig. 7. Case 5: patient aged 3 years 5 months; idiopathic myoclonic–aastatic epilepsy. Diffuse slow waves, interspersed with high voltage, diffuse, irregular slow spike and wave complexes. The EMG channels show arrhythmic, focal and generalized myoclonic potentials on a background of mild tonic contraction. Clinically, the child is unresponsive and staring, with irregular distal jerks and arrhythmic nodding or whole body jerks leading to falls.

or childhood. Seizure onset is typically around 3 years, but may occur up to age 5. These forms appear to be quite homogeneous, are easily controlled by therapy, and tend to last only a few years.

Others, beginning in childhood and described in the past as myoclonic–astatic epilepsies, are characterized by the occurrence of myoclonus, absences, and convulsive seizures. In these children, one seizure type is more common from time to time than another. Usually patients with more than one seizure type are more resistant to anti-epileptic drugs.

The idiopathic generalized epilepsies with onset between 5 and 10 years of age are almost exclusively absence epilepsies (Fig. 8), and those with onset after age 10 are juvenile myoclonic epilepsy. There does not seem to be any age-related transition from one form of myoclonic epilepsy to another in the same patient.

When considering epilepsies with generalized myoclonus, we emphasize that the syndromes are defined by clinical and EEG criteria and that there is no reason to exclude cases that appear to be transiently intractable from the idiopathic group. Myoclonic–astatic epilepsy, as defined here, should therefore be included among the idiopathic generalized epilepsies.

Appendix

Several case reports illustrate the different types of epilepsy considered in this chapter.

Benign myoclonic epilepsy in infancy

Case 1. This boy was born at term after a normal pregnancy as the only child of healthy parents. Early development was normal. At 9 months haemophilia was diagnosed. From age 1, the child had

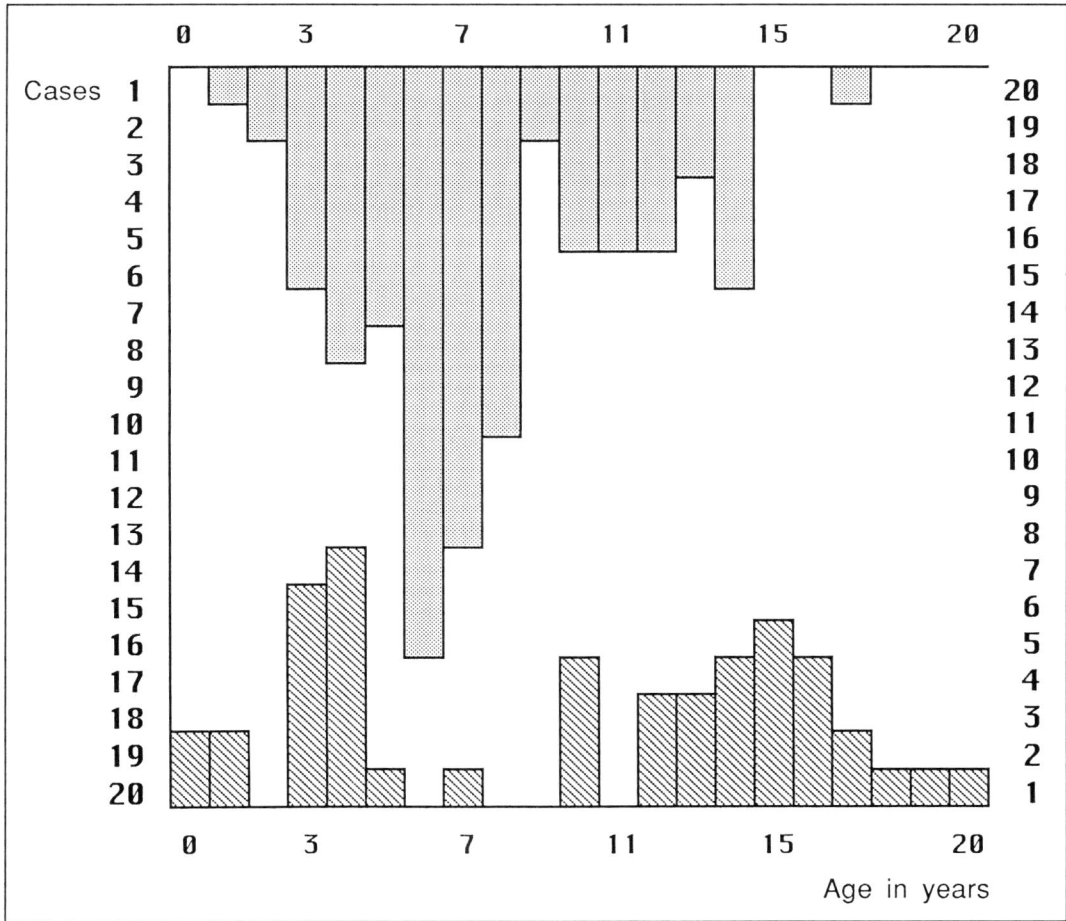

Fig. 8. Age of onset and number of cases of idiopathic absence epilepsies (above) and of idiopathic myoclonic epilepsies (below) on a population of 137 consecutive patients showing these types of epilepsy, seen between 1988 and 1993 at Institute of Developmental Neuropsychiatry at University of Pisa and Centre Saint Paul at Marseilles. Note that of 50 patients, in whom onset occurred between ages 5 and 9 years, only two had myoclonic epilepsies.

episodes of eye fluttering and head shaking, sometimes with jerking of the whole body without falling, most frequently while watching television. These could occur many times a day, but some days they were not noticed at all. The jerks were not disabling and the parents thought that they were tics. At 5 years the family doctor suggested an EEG which showed spontaneous and photic-induced generalized polyspike and wave activity associated with massive myoclonic jerks (Fig. 1). Clobazam 5 mg twice daily controlled the myoclonus. When last seen at age 8, no relapses had occurred, and the child had a normal cognitive level but was hyperactive.

Case 2. This patient had a negative family history. Pregnancy and delivery were normal. At 20 months he had a febrile convulsion. Between 20 months and 2 years he began to have nodding with leg jerks many times a day. Interictal EEG was normal but generalized spike and wave and polyspike and wave activity occurred during the jerks. Diazepam, phenobarbital, and ethosuximide were ineffective. Valproate was begun at 2 years 7 months. The jerks disappeared completely and the EEG became normal. Valproate was withdrawn at 8 years. He remained seizure-free at age 16, with a normal EEG. Cognitive development was normal, but schooling was difficult because of hyperactivity.

Reflex form of benign myoclonic epilepsy in infancy

Case 3. This 4-year-old boy was born after a normal pregnancy and delivery. His mother had had absences from age 8 to 15 years. From 10 months he had massive jerks triggered by acoustic stimuli, 10–20 times a day. Effective triggers were unexpected and loud noises (doors slamming, hands clapping, or objects falling to the ground), particularly in a quiet environment. Sometimes unexpected touch was also effective. Jerks were bilateral and symmetrical, involved the limbs, were accompanied by head nodding and upward gaze deviation, and were isolated or in brief bouts of three to eight, lasting up to 3–4 s. Consciousness was impaired during the longer series. Video-EEG-polygraphy showed the jerks to be accompanied by diffuse spikes or polyspike and wave activity, with the myoclonic potentials coinciding with the polyspikes (Fig. 2). Interictal EEGs were normal. The child was not treated and the seizures disappeared 4 months after onset. A single brief febrile convulsion occurred at 18 months of age. Cognitive and motor development were normal.

Childhood-onset benign myoclonic epilepsy

Case 4. This girl was born after a normal pregnancy and delivery. Her elder sister had symptomatic temporal lobe epilepsy. Initial development was normal. At age 4, her parents noted many episodes per day of axial jerking, occurring either singly or in clusters of 3–4. Video-EEG recording showed generalized polyspike and wave complexes with massive symmetrical jerks in wakefulness and the first stages of slow-wave sleep (Fig. 3). Seizures stopped with administration of valproate. At age 8, she is still being treated and has not had any further seizures. Schooling is normal.

Idiopathic myoclonic–astatic epilepsy

Case 5. This boy was born after a normal pregnancy and delivery. A paternal uncle had idiopathic generalized epilepsy. After normal development, the child had a generalized tonic–clonic seizure during sleep at 2 years 7 months. EEG background activity was normal; rhythmic 4 Hz activity was recorded over both centroparietal regions. Generalized polyspike and wave activity was recorded interictally and with major jerks. Phenobarbital was prescribed. He then had many nocturnal and infrequent diurnal generalized tonic–clonic seizures and frequent myoclonic–astatic seizures with falls. Episodes of status epilepticus occurred, lasting days, characterized by stupor with loss of contact, staring, mild tonic arm abduction, irregular muscular jerks and massive myoclonus (Fig. 7). Ethosuximide added to phenobarbital had no effect: carbamazepine worsened the myoclonus. When clonazepam was added at 3 years 8 months, myoclonic–astatic seizures and episodes of status ceased. He had several more generalized seizures during sleep but has been seizure-free on phenobarbital and clonazepam from age 4. Schooling was normal. At age 7 the EEG showed only occasional spike and wave activity during sleep.

References

Aicardi, J. (1980): Course and prognosis of certain childhood epilepsies with predominantly myoclonic seizures. In: *Advances in epileptology: The Xth Epilepsy International Symposium*, eds. J.A. Wada & J.K. Penry, pp. 159–163. New York: Raven Press.

Aicardi, J. & Chevrie J.J. (1986): Lennox–Gastaut syndrome and myoclonic epilepsies in infancy and early childhood. In: *Intractable epilepsy: clinical and experimental aspects*, eds. P.L. Morselli & P. Schmidt, pp. 157–166. New York: Raven Press.

Aicardi, J. & Levy-Gomes, A. (1989): The myoclonic epilepsies of childhood. *Cleveland Clin. J. Med.* **56 (Suppl. 1)**, S34–S39.

Appleton, R.E., Panayiotopoulos, C.P., Acomb, B.A. & Beirne, M. (1993): Eyelid myoclonia with typical absences: an epilepsy syndrome. *J. Neurol. Neurosurg. Psychiatry* **56,** 1312–1316.

Beaumanoir, A. & Dravet, C. (1992): The Lennox–Gastaut syndrome. In: *Epileptic syndromes in infancy, childhood and adolescence*, 2nd edn, eds. J. Roger, M. Bureau, C. Dravet, F.E. Dreifuss, A. Perret & P. Wolf, pp. 115–132. London, Paris: John Libbey Eurotext Ltd.

Chiron, C., Plouin, P., Dulac, O., Mayer, M. & Ponsot, G. (1988): Epilepsies myocloniques des encephalopathies non progressives avec états de mal myocloniques. *Neurophysiol. Clin.* **18,** 513–524.

Colamaria, V., Andrighetto, G., Pinelli, L., Olivieri, A., Alfieri, P. & Dalla Bernadina, B. (1987): Iperinsulinismo, ipoglicemia ed epilessia mioclonica benigna del lattante. *Boll. Lega It. Epil.* **58/59,** 231–233.

Commission on Classification and Terminology of the International League Against Epilepsy. (1989): Proposal for revised classification of epilepsies and epileptic syndromes. *Epilepsia* **30,** 389–399.

Dalla Bernardina, B., Colamaria V., Capovilla, G. & Bondavalli, S. (1983): Nosological classification of epilepsies in the first three years of life. In: *Epilepsy an update on research and therapy*, eds. G. Nisticò, R. Di Perri & H. Meinardi, pp. 165–183. New York: Alan Liss.

Dalla Bernardina, B., Capovilla, G., Chiamenti, C., Trevisan, E., Colamaria V. & Fontana, E. (1987): Cryptogenetic myoclonic epilepsies of infancy and early childhood: nosological and prognostic approach. In: *Advances in epileptology*, Vol. 16, eds. P. Wolf, M. Dam, D. Janz, & F.E. Dreifuss, pp. 175–179. New York: Raven Press.

Dalla Bernardina, B., Sgrò, V., Fontana, E., Cellino, M.R., Moser, C., Zullini, E., Grimau-Merino, R. & Blasi-Esposito, S. (1989): Eyelid myoclonias with absences. In: *Reflex seizures and reflex epilepsies*, eds. A. Beaumanoir, R. Naquet & H. Gastaut, pp. 193–200. Genève: Médecine et Hygiène.

Dalla Bernardina, B., Fontana, E., Sgrò, V., Colamaria, V. & Elia, M. (1992): Myoclonic epilepsy ('myoclonic status') in non-progressive encephalopathies. In: *Epileptic syndromes in infancy, childhood and adolescence,* 2nd edn, eds. J. Roger, M. Bureau, C. Dravet, F.E. Dreifuss, A. Perret, & P. Wolf, pp. 89–96. London, Paris: John Libbey Eurotext Ltd.

Delgado-Escueta, A.V., Greenberg, D., Weissbecker, K., Liu, A., Treiman, L., Sparkes, R., Parlk Min, S., Barbetti, A. & Terasaki P. (1990): Gene mapping in the idiopathic generalized epilepsies: juvenile myoclonic epilepsy, childhood absence epilepsy, epilepsy with grand mal seizures, and early childhood myoclonic epilepsy. *Epilepsia* **31 (Suppl. 3),** S19–S29.

Deonna, T. & Despland, P.A. (1989): Sensory-evoked (touch) idiopathic myoclonic epilepsy of infancy. In: *Reflex seizures and reflex epilepsies*, eds. A. Beaumanoir, R. Naquet & H. Gastaut, pp. 99–102. Genève: Médecine et Hygiène.

Doose, H., Gerken, H., Leonhardt, R., Voelzke, E. & Voelz, Ch. (1970): Centrencephalic myoclonic–astatic petit mal. Clinical and genetic investigations. *Neuropaediatrie* **2,** 59–78.

Doose, H. (1985): Myoclonic astatic epilepsy of early childhood. In: *Epileptic syndromes in infancy, childhood and adolescence*, eds. J. Roger, C. Dravet, M. Bureau, F.E. Dreifuss & P. Wolf, pp. 78–88. London, Paris: John Libbey Eurotext Ltd.

Doose, H. (1992): Myoclonic astatic epilepsy of early childhood. In: *Epileptic syndromes in infancy, childhood and adolescence,* 2nd edn, eds. J. Roger, M. Bureau, C. Dravet, F.E. Dreifuss, A. Perret & P. Wolf, pp. 103–114. London and Paris: John Libbey Eurotext Ltd.

Dravet, C. & Bureau, M. (1981): L'épilepsie myoclonique bénigne du nourrisson. *Rev. Electroencephalog. Neurophysiol. Clin.* **11,** 438–444.

Dravet, C., Roger, J., Bureau, M. & Dalla Bernardina, B. (1982): Myoclonic epilepsies in childhood. In: *Advances in epileptology: XIIIth Epilepsy International Symposium,* eds. H. Akimoto, H. Kazamatsu, M. Seino & A. Ward, pp. 125–127. New York: Raven Press.

Dravet, C., Boniver, C., Santanelli, P., Bureau, M. & Roger, J. (1985): Myoclonic epilepsies in the first three years of life. *XVIth Epilepsy International Congress,* (Abstract). Hamburg.

Dravet C. (1990): Les épilepsies myocloniques bénignes du nourrisson. *Epilepsies* **2,** 95–101.

Dravet, C., Bureau, M. & Roger, J. (1992a): Benign myoclonic epilepsy in infants. In: *Epileptic syndromes in infancy, childhood and adolescence* 2nd edn, eds. J. Roger, M. Bureau, C. Dravet, F.E. Dreifuss, A. Perret & P. Wolf, pp. 67–74. London and Paris: John Libbey Eurotext Ltd.

Dravet, C., Bureau, M. & Genton, P. (1992b): Benign myoclonic epilepsy of infancy: electroclinical symptomatology and differential diagnosis from the other types of generalized epilepsy in infancy. In: *The benign localized epilepsies in early childhood*, Epilepsy Res. Suppl. 6, eds. R. Degen & F. Dreifuss, pp. 131–135. Amsterdam: Elsevier.

Dravet, C., Bureau, M., Guerrini, R., Giraud, N. & Roger, J. (1992c): Severe myoclonic epilepsy in infants. In: *Epileptic syndromes in infancy, childhood and adolescence*, 2nd edn, eds, J. Roger, M. Bureau, C. Dravet, F.E. Dreifuss, A. Perret, & P. Wolf, pp. 75–88. London, Paris: John Libbey Eurotext Ltd.

Dulac, O., Plouin, P., Chiron, C. (1990): Forme 'bénigne' d' épilepsie myoclonique chez l'enfant. *Neurophysiol. Clin.* **20**, 115–129.

Dulac, O. (1993): Idiopathic myoclonic epilepsy in childhood. In: *Idiopathic generalized epilepsies: clinical, experimental and genetic aspects*. International Workshop, April 1993 (Abstracts).

Dulac, O. & N' Guyen, T. (1993): The Lennox–Gastaut syndrome. *Epilepsia* **34 (Suppl. 7)**, S7–S17.

Guerrini, R., Genton, P., Bureau, M., Dravet, C. & Roger, J. (1990a): Reflex seizures are frequent in patients with Down syndrome and epilepsy. *Epilepsia* **31**, 406–417.

Guerrini, R., Bureau, M., Mattei, M.G., Battaglia, A., Galland, M.C. & Roger, J. (1990b): Trisomy 12p: a chromosomal disorder associated with generalized 3 Hz spike and wave discharges. *Epilepsia* **31**, 557–566.

Guerrini, R., Bonnani, P., Thomas, P. & Suisse, G. (1994): Status myoclonicus and cortical tremor in Angelman Syndrome. *Epilepsia* **35 (Suppl. 7)**, 88.

Henriksen, O. (1985): Discussion on myoclonic epilepsies and Lennox–Gastaut syndrome. In: *Epileptic syndromes in infancy, childhood and adolescence*, eds. J. Roger, C. Dravet, M. Bureau, F.E. Dreifuss & P. Wolf, pp. 101–105. London and Paris: John Libbey Eurotext Ltd.

Jeavons, P.M. (1977): Nosological problems of myoclonic epilepsies in childhood and adolescence. *Dev. Med. Child Neurol.* **19**, 3–8.

Loiseau, P., Legroux, M., Grimond, P., du Pasquier, P. & Henry, P. (1974): Taxonometric classification of myoclonic epilepsies. *Epilepsia* **15**, 1–11.

Lombroso, C.T. (1990): Early myoclonic encephalopathy, early infantile epileptic encephalopathy and benign and severe infantile myoclonic epilepsies: a critical review and personal contributions. *J. Clin. Neurophysiol.* **7**, 380–408.

Maton, B., Hirsch, E., Finck, S., Boulay C., Kurtz, D. & Marescaux C. (1990): Benign form of childhood epilepsy with astatomyoclonic seizures. *Epilepsia* **31 (Suppl. 5)**, 607, (Abstract).

Revol, M., Isnard, H., Beaumanoir, A. & Ducommun, Y. (1989): Touch evoked myoclonic seizures in infancy. In: *Reflex seizures and reflex epilepsies*, eds. A. Beaumanoir, R. Naquet & H. Gastaut, pp. 103–105. Genève: Médecine et Hygiène.

Ricci, S., Cusmai, R., Fusco, L., Cilio, R. & Vigevano, F. (1993a): Reflex myoclonic epilepsy of the first year of life. *Epilepsia* **34 (Suppl. 6)**, 47, (Abstract).

Ricci, S., Cusmai, R., Fusco, L., Claps, D. & Vigevano, F. (1993b): Studio video-EEG di bambini con mioclono riflesso da stimolo acustico e tattile. *Boll. Lega It. Epil.* 84.

Roger, J., Dravet, Ch., Bureau, M., Dreifuss, F.E. & Wolf, P. (1985): *Epileptic syndromes in infancy, childhood and adolescence*. London, Paris: John Libbey Eurotext Ltd.

Salas-Puig, J., Ramos Polo, E., Macarron Vincente, J. & Hernandez Lanoz, C. (1990): Benign myoclonic epilepsy of infancy. Case report. *Acta Pediatr. Scand.* **79**, 1128–1130.

chlumberger, E., Chavez, F., Palacios, L., Rey, E., Pajot, N. & Dulac, O. (1994): Lamotrigine in treatment of 120 children with epilepsy. *Epilepsia* **35**, 359–367.

Sheffner, D. (1982): Myoclonic seizures: etiology and differential diagnosis. In: *Advances in epileptology: XIIIth Epilepsy International Symposium*, eds. H. Akimoto, H. Kazamatsu, M. Seino & A. Ward, pp. 125–127. New York: Raven Press.

Todt, H. & Müller, D. (1992): The therapy of benign myoclonic epilepsy in infants. In: *The benign localized and generalized epilepsies in early childhood*, Epilepsy Res. Suppl. 6, eds. R. Degen & F. Dreifuss, pp. 131–139. Amsterdam: Elsevier.

Chapter 24

Juvenile myoclonic epilepsy: is there heterogeneity?

A.V. Delgado-Escueta[*†‡], A. Liu[*†‡], J. Serratosa[*†‡], K. Weissbecker[§], M.T. Medina[*‡¶], M. Gee[*†], L.J. Theiman[*†‡] and R.S. Sparkes[*¥]

[*]*California Comprehensive Epilepsy Program and* [†]*Neurological and Research Service, Suite 3405, West Los Angeles VA Medical Center (W127B), Wilshire and Sawtelle Boulevards, West Los Angeles, California 90073, USA;* [‡]*Department of Neurology, UCLA School of Medicine;* [§]*Biometry and Genetics, Louisiana State University;* [¶]*National Autonomous University of Honduras, Tegucigalpa, Honduras*

Introduction

Juvenile myoclonic epilepsy or JME (Herpin–Janz Syndrome) is a specific and common form of adolescent onset non-progressive idiopathic generalized epilepsy characterized by myoclonias, tonic–clonic or clonic–tonic convulsions and absences. Ictal EEGs show high amplitude multispikes followed by slow waves during myoclonias, and interictal EEGs manifest 3.5-6 Hz diffuse multispike–wave complexes. Although considered a single distinct clinical syndrome, three lines of evidence suggest genotypic heterogeneity: (1) clinical and EEG affectedness in pedigrees of juvenile myoclonic epilepsy, (2) segregation analysis, and (3) genetic linkage mapping.

Clinical and EEG affectedness in 115 pedigrees of juvenile myoclonic epilepsy favours heterogeneity

We observed 8 possible subphenotypes of juvenile myoclonic epilepsy based on the affectedness of the proband and family members (See Table 1). Clinical features of patients were the first signs of possible heterogeneity. All patients have myoclonias; 5 per cent have myoclonias only, 95 per cent have grand mal convulsions. One-third of patients also manifest absences of childhood, early childhood or juvenile onset. In addition to these common features of juvenile myoclonic epilepsy, we observed sudden drops in six patients and only rare myoclonias in another eight patients. When the clinical phenotypes of affected non-proband family members are examined, further subgroups can be recognized. Most commonly, juvenile myoclonic epilepsy is present in affected non-proband family members (47 of 115 pedigrees). In 25 families, non-proband family members have only have grand mal. In another 21 families, absences of juvenile of childhood or early childhood onset affected nonproband family members with or without grand mal. EEGs identified asymptomatic siblings with 3.5–6 Hz spike wave complexes in six pedigrees and nonspecific epileptiform patterns in non-proband members of another eight families. Based on the combinations of affectedness in members, we subdivided families into eight subgroups (see Table 1).

Table 1. Subgroups of 115 JME families*: based on affectedness of proband and affected family members

	Description of subphenotypes	No. of enrolled families (typed)
I	Proband and affected family members have JME: MS + TC ± absences, adolescent onset in all affected family members	47
IIa	Proband has JME and asymptomatic sibling has EEG 3.5–6 Hz multispike wave complexes	6
IIb	Proband has JME and asymptomatic sibling(s) has EEG non-specific epileptiform patterns	2
III	Proband has JME but affected family members have GMTC convulsions	25
IV	Proband has JME but affected family members have CA (6) or ECAE (1) of juvenile absence (15) with or without GMTC	21
V	Proband has GMTC, MS and drop attacks, adolescent onset	6
VI	Proband has GMTC and rare MS, adolescent onset	3
VII	Proband has CA and GMTC, during adolescence rare MS appear. CA or GMTC is present in affected family members	3
VIII	Proband has juvenile absence, GMTC, and rare MS; all start at adolescence	2
	Total	115

MS: myoclonic seizures; JME: juveile myoclonic epilepsy; CA: childhood absence; ECAE: early childhood absence epilepsy; GMTC: grand mal tonic clonic seizures. Nonspecific EEG patterns are irregular 3 and 4–7 Hz spike and slow wave formations, 4–7 Hz sharp and slow wave formations and rhythmic 6–12 Hz paroparoxysms mixed with spikes. *Only 55 families, so far, have had EEGs in all nuclear members.

Segregation analysis : heterogeneity vs. autosomal dominant transmission with incomplete penetrance with sporadic cases

We validated the clinical and EEG trait of 249 family members of 55 families collected from our epilepsy clinics. Families were ascertained through a patient (proband or index case) with juvenile myoclonic epilepsy. These juvenile myoclonic epilepsy patients were originally referred for diagnosis and treatment. Table 2 summarizes the data base and basis for classifying affectedness in these 55 families during segregation analysis.

Since every sibship had been ascertained by only one proband, the proportion of affected siblings or the segregation ratio was estimated for each mating group by using the proband method described by Weinberg in 1912 and provided with an error formula by Fisher in 1934 to correct for ascertainment bias. The ascertainment method was unambiguously single selection.

We examined which mode of transmission could best explain most, if not all, information we obtained from the nuclear families of our 55 sibships (Table 3). Every sibship was ascertained by only one proband and the progeny of all mating types were analysed statistically. Initial estimation of all pedigrees across all mating types fits the expectation of recessive inheritance ($P = 0.2518$; SE = 0.03681), but the segregation ratio dropped considerably ($P = 0.1511$) when we excluded all paroxysmal forms of EEGs, specific and non-specific. This ratio is similar to that obtained by Panayiotopoulos and Obieb in Saudi Arabian families who did not have their EEGs examined. Matings between unaffecteds (both simplex and multiples pedigrees) also yielded a significantly lower estimate of the segregation ratio ($P = 0.1782$) than the expected 0.25 in recessive inheritance. Because two possible reasons for an underestimated P are mixtures of sporadic cases amongst the simplex families and exclusion of the EEG juvenile myoclonic epilepsy trait in asymptomatics, we restricted statistical analyses to sibships with more than one clinically affected sib. Estimates ($P = 0.2647$) fit the expectation of fully penetrant autosomal recessive inheritance, regardless of mating type. Interestingly, matings between affecteds and unaffecteds provided further proof of an autosomal recessive inheritance ($P = 0.40625-0.4492$) whether we analysed clinical affectedness on non-specific EEG paroxysms separately or together. When we separated clinical from EEG affectedness by restricting statistical analyses to six sibships whose asymptomatic siblings exhibited

Table 2. Data base and basis for classifying affectedness during seregation analysis

(a) 40 normal by normal matings

No. of families	Clinically affected	EEG affectedness	Family classification
24	Proband only	Normal EEGs on all members except patient or proband	Simplex by clinical and EEG
8	Proband and sibling	Proband and one sibling by 3.5–6 Hz multispike wave complexes	Multiplex clinically and by specific EEG pattern
6	Proband only	Proband and one sibling by 3.5–6 Hz multispike wave complexes	Multiplex by specific EEG paroxysms only
2[1$^\Delta$]	Proband only	Proband and one sibling have non-specific epileptiform EEG paroxysms	Multiplex by non-specific EEG paroxysms only

(b) 15 normal by affected matings

No. of families	Clinically affected	EEG affectedness	Family classification
4	Proband and one parent		
9	Proband, one parent & sibling		
1*	Proband only		
2[1*†]	Proband only		
[3]‡	Proband and sibling		

Total: 55 families

* These families would be classified as simplex and normal by normal matings when non-specific epileptiform EEG paroxysms are excluded. † One of these two pedigrees are represented under both mating types (they are the same pedigree).
‡ These three families would be classified as multiplex clinically under normal by normal mating when nonspecific epileptiform EEG paroxysms in parents are excluded and were originally counted under the eight pedigrees multiplex by clinical and specific EEG paroxysms.

the 3.5–6 Hz multispike wave trait, the segregation ratio fitted best the criteria of dominant inheritance.

Our present segregation analyses suggests two possibilities. The first possibility is that genetic heterogeneity exists within our population. A majority of families with autosomal recessive mode of inheritance and a minority of families with autosomal dominant mode of inheritance could be admixed with sporadic cases (non-hereditary or dominant new mutations) in our population. Recent genetic linkage mapping performed on our families have indicated genetic heterogeneity, (see below), one group genetically linked to chromosome 6p markers in the Bf-HLA region and another group which showed no such linkage. The second possibility is that an incompletely penetrating autosomal dominant gene is responsible for the clinical juvenile myoclonic epilepsy phenotype while same dominant gene is fully penetrant for the EEG 3.5–6 Hz multispike wave phenotype. In families who show linkage to chromosome 6p, the best lod scores reported by Greenberg et al. (1988) during linkage mapping have been obtained with the autosomal dominant model.

Genetic linkage mapping: is there an epilepsy locus in chromosome 6p? Is there genotypic heterogeneity?

At the *Human Gene Mapping 9 Workshop* in 1987 we reported that juvenile myoclonic epilepsy may be linked to the Bf-HLA loci in chromosome 6p (Greenberg et al., 1988). Using clinical and EEG characteristics in the identification of affected family members, we reported a maximum lod score of 3.05 at a recombination fraction of 0.10 under a recessive model of inheritance assuming a penetration of 0.6 using HLA and Bf (properdin factor) as markers. We obtained these results from 22 nuclear families, of which 11 were informative for Bf or HLA (see Table 4 for the data base and affectedness assignments). Evidence for possible linkage was strengthened when Greenberg *et al.* increased the original sample of families to 33, 18 of whom were informative for Bf and four of whom were informative for HLA (28) (see Table 3). The maximum lod score obtained for this analysis was 3.78 ($\Theta m=f=0.01$) assuming autosomal dominant (AD) inheritance and 90 per cent penetrance. Assuming autosomal recessive inheritance (AR) with complete penetrance, the maximum lod score was 3.05 ($\Theta m=f=0.01$). This suggested that a juvenile myoclonic epilepsy locus was present in the 6p21.3 area (Greenberg *et al.*, 1991).

Since then, two independent studies, namely those of Weissbecker *et al.* (1990) and Durner et al. (1991), have observed similar observations. Weissbecker *et al.* (1990) used HLA serological markers, whereas Durner *et al.* (1991) used DNA markers in the HLA-DQ region, in analysing 143 family members of 25 Berlin pedigrees. In the studies of Durner *et al.* (1991), lod scores were 3.65 (0 to 0.1 and 0.5) when asymptomatic family members with abnormal EEGs were considered affected.

Table 3. Data base and basis for classifying affectedness during genetic linkage analysis

(a)		Normal by normal matings		
Original 11 families	Subsequent 33 families	Clinically affectedness	EEG affectedness	Family classification
4	14	Proband only	Normal EEGs on all non-proband members	Simplex by clinical & EEG
1†	7	Proband & sibling	Proband & one sibling by 3.5–6 Hz multispike wave complexes	Multiplex by clinical & specific EEG pattern
2	2	Proband only	Proband & one sibling by 3.5–6 Hz multispike wave complexes	Multiplex by specific EEG paroxysms only
0	3	Proband only	Proband & one sibling by non-specific epileptiform EEG paroxysms	Multiplex by non-specific EEG paroxysms only
(b)		Normal by affected matings		
Original 11 families	Subsequent 33 families*	Clinically affectedness	EEG affectedness	Family classification
1	3	Proband, one parent and/or sibling	Proband and sibling by 3.5–6 Hz multispike wave complexes	Multigenerational and multiplex by clinical and specific EEG paroxysms
3 (2‡)	4	Proband only	One parent has non-specific epileptiform EEG paroxysms	Multigenerational by non-specific EEG paroxysms

* These included the original 11 families. † Multiplex by clinical but other sibling(s) asymptomatic with epileptiform EEG patterns. ‡ Sibling(s) also has epileptiform non-specific patterns.

The different clinical subphenotypes of probands with juvenile myoclonic epilepsy and affected family members have already been reviewed in Table 1. Since other forms of idiopathic generalized epilepsies are observed in family members of patients with juvenile myoclonic epilepsy, as in subphenotypes III, IV and VII, does it mean that other generalized epilepsies, such as childhood absence and grand mal, have their genetic locus in chromosome 6p identical to the genetic locus of juvenile myoclonic epilepsy? Is there homogeneity within the primary generalized epilepsies? Is there homogeneity within juvenile myoclonic epilepsy? The answer to all three questions is *no*. There is no homogeneity within the common primary generalized epilepsies and there is no homogeneity within juvenile myoclonic epilepsy. Our latest studies using chromosome 6p reference DNA markers show that there are families with juvenile myoclonic epilepsy which do not genetically map to chromosome 6p (Liu et al., 1993). In fact, childhood absence with or without grand mal do not map to the same *EJM-1* locus (Serratosa et al., 1993). In the last year, Dr Serratosa, Dr Liu and Dr Delgado-Escueta have studied 207 family members of 12 patients with childhood absence. Results favour a locus for childhood absence outside the chromosome 6p locus for E-JM-1 and outside the E-PM-1 locus in chromosome 21.

In 1991 to 1992, we screened 12 juvenile myoclonic epilepsy families with DQa and eight other chromosome 6p reference markers above (D6105, D6S89, D6S109, F13A1) and below (D6S29, GL01, TCTE1, D6Z1) HLA. Juvenile myoclonic epilepsy was treated as an autosomal dominant trait with equal penetrance of 70 per cent for homozygotes and heterozygotes. The disease allele was given a frequency of 0.001 to account for his morbid risk in the population. Lod scores were negative when pairwise analyses between the nine loci located in chromosome 6p and juvenile myoclonic epilepsy were carried out. In the light of earlier studies, which suggested juvenile myoclonic epilepsy genetic linkage to HLA, our results could favour genotypic heterogeneity and a second locus for juvenile myoclonic epilepsy outside chromosome 6p must now be sought. Thus, the pathogenesis of juvenile myoclonic epilepsy in the Berlin families analysed by Weissbecker et al. (1990) and Durner et al. (1991) and other Los Angeles pedigrees studied by our group probably involves mutations at different chromosomal sites. At present, it seems there at least two loci which possibly lead to the same EEG and clinical phenotypes of juvenile myoclonic epilepsy.

The E-JM-1 locus and juvenile myoclonic epilepsy subpphentoypes I, IIA and IIb

At the June 1992 *Chromosome 6 Workshop* (Ann Arbor, Michigan), Michel Rees from Dr Gardiner's laboratory presented pairwise lod score for various chromosome 6 markers from HLA DQa to F13A in 25 juvenile myoclonic epilepsy familes from England and Sweden. Results excluded linkage of the above chromosome 6p markers.

Because of strong exclusionary evidence presented by the London group and our own juvenile myoclonic epilepsy families who do not show linkage to chromosome 6p markers (Liu et al., 1992), we reviewed the clinical subphenotypes of the original 11 juvenile myoclonic epilepsy families reported in 1987 to be informative for Bf or HLA. We are presently correlating the results of these HLA serologies with chromosome 6p DNA markers. Perhaps, most importantly, we are also comparing the subphenotypes of juvenile myoclonic epilepsy found in families that show positive lod scores, as in the original 1987 study, and those that show negative lod scores, as recently reported by Liu et al. It is important to understand that in these early studies on genetic linkage mapping of 22 Los Angeles juvenile myoclonic epilepsy families, reported in 1987, we rejected probands with childhood absence, pure grand mal, myoclonic absences, myoclonus absences and pathogenic epilepsies. Of 11 families informative for Bf or HLA, two juvenile myoclonic epilepsy families with unaffected parents were multiplex on account of 3.5 to 6 Hz multispike wave paroxysms and two other juvenile myoclonic epilepsy families were multiplex on account of nonspecific epileptiform patterns. Two other juvenile myoclonic epilepsy families were multiplex on account of a sibling affected with juvenile myoclonic epilepsy (see Table 4). In this early study, no siblings or parents had childhood absence. Three families were multigenerational by virtue of a parent with nonspecific epileptiform paroxysms. Thus, in six of 11 informative families, affectedness of family members was determined by the EEG. An early concern we had was whether genetic linkage was being suggested to the EEG trait or to both the EEG and clinical traits of juvenile myoclonic epilepsy.

Because of early suggestions of possible genetic linkage of juvenile myoclonic epilepsy subphenotypes I, IIa and IIb with Bf-HLA, and our more recent results showing exclusion of linkage between CAE and chromosome 6p markers, we have tightened up our rejection criteria, emphasizing rejection of any probands with absences only, or grand mal only or drop seizures as part of juvenile myoclonic epilepsy and the importance of rejecting juvenile myoclonic epilepsy families whose family members have early childhood, childhood or juvenile absences. In other words, we are now concentrating recruitment on the juvenile myoclonic epilepsy subphenotype I, IIa and IIb, listed in Table 1. This was the original group studied in 1987 with the exception of one patient who had adolescent drop attacks as part of the juvenile myoclonic epilepsy syndrome.

As a consequence of all the above developments, we have modified our strategy for locating the genetic loci of juvenile myoclonic epilepsy, childhood absence, early childhood familial myoclonic epilepsy and grand mal epilepsies. Figure 3 illustrates the flow of patients as they are screened first with chromosome 6p markers, chromosomes 20 and 21 markers (where loci for BFNC and PME are located) and then chromosomal sites homologous to mice spike–wave loci, (namely, chromosomes 2q, 8q, 11p, 12p, 15q, 16q). If all these studies do not favour genetic linkage, we proceed to screen the rest of the human genome. For these new approaches, we have recruited and are genotyping 17 large multiplex or multigenerational juvenile myoclonic epilepsy families from Mexico and one large family from Los Angeles and Belize. As mentioned above, we are also comparing results of HLA serology and chromosome 6p RFLP and PCR/microsatellite markers in families previously shown to have positive lod scores using Bf-HLA serology.

References

Delgado-Escueta, A.V. & Enrile Bacsal, F. (1984): Juvenile myclonic epilepsy. *Neurology* **34**, 285–294.

Delgado-Escueta, .V., Greenberg, D.A., Treiman, L., Liu, A., Sparkes, R.S., Park, M.S. & Terasaki, P.L. (1989): Mapping the gene for juvenile myoclonic epilepsy. *Epilepsia* **30**, S8–S18.

Delgado-Escueta, A.V., Greenberg, D.A., Weissbecker, K., Liu, A., Treiman, L., Sparkes, R.S., Prk, M.S., Barbetti, A. & Terasaki, P.L. (1990): Gene mapping in the idiopathic generalized epilepsies. Juvenile myoclonic epilepsy, childhood absence epilepsy, epilepsy with grand mal seizures, and early childhood myoclonic epilepsy. *Epilepsia* **21**, S19–S29.

Delgado-Escueta, A.V., Medina, M.T., Weissbecker, K., Gee, M., Serratosa, J.M., Maldonado, H., Abad-Herrera, P., Spellman, J. & Sparkes, R.X. (1993): Juvenile myoclonic epilepsy. Segregation analysis of clinical and EEG phenotypes. Submitted for publication.

Durner, M., Sander, T., Greenberg, D.A., Johnson, K. & Janz, D. (1991): Localization of idiopathic generalized epilepsy on chromosome 6p in families ascertained through juvenile epilepsy patients. *Neurology* **41**, 1651–1655.

Greenberg, D.A., Delgado-Escueta, A.V., Widelitz, H., Sparkes R.S., Treiman, L.J., Maldonado, H.M., Tarasaki, P.I. & Park, M.S. (1988): Juvenile myoclonic epilepsy (JME) may be linked to the BF and HLA loci in human chromosome 6. *Am. J. Med. Genet.* **31**, 185–192.

Liu, A.W.I., Delgado-Escueta, A.V., Zhao, H., Shi, G., Serratosa, J.M., Treiman, I.J. & Sparkes R.S. (1993): Juvenile myoclonic epilepsy and chromosome 6p markers. Negative linkage and evidence for a second autosomal EJM locus. To be submitted for publication.

Serratosa, J.M., Delgado-Escueta, A.V., Pascual-Castroviejo, I., Liu, A., Weber, J.L., Wang, S., Treiman, L.J., Pineda, G. & Sparkes R.S. (1993): Childhood absence epilepsy. Exclusion of genetic linkage to chromosome 6p markers. Submitted for presentation: *International Workshop on Idiopathic Generalized Epilepsies*, Strasbourg, Alsace, France.

Weber, J. & May, P. (1989): Abundant class of human DNA polymorphisms which can be typed using the polymerase chain reaction. *Am. J. Hum. Genet.* **44**, 388–396.

Weissbecker, K., Durner, M., Janz, D., Scaramelli, A., Sparkes, R.S. & Spence, M.A. (1991): Confirmation of linkage between the juvenile myoclonic epilepsy locus and the HLA region of chromosome 6. *Amer. J. Med. Genet.* **38**, 32–36.

Chapter 25

Phenotypic variability of idiopathic generalized epilepsies and refinement of the map position of EJM1 in JME families

D. Janz[*], G. Beck-Managetta[*], T. Hildman[†], T. Sander[‡] and H. Neitzel[†]

[*]*Klinikum Rudolph Virchow der Freien Universität, Abteilung für Neurologie, 14050 Berlin, Germany;* [†]*Klinikum Rudolph Virchow der Freien Universität, Psychiatrische Klinik, 14050 Berlin, Germany;* [‡]*Institut für Humangenetik, 1000 Berlin, Germany*

Phenotypic variability of idiopathic generalized epilepsies

Of all types of epilepsy, juvenile myoclonic epilepsy (JME) is considered to be especially suitable for genetic studies for the following reasons: the syndrome is easy to define and detect, it is frequent, it shows familial clustering and always occurs as idiopathic without any known or suspected underlying cause other than a possible hereditary predisposition. In addition under nosological aspects the position of juvenile myoclonic epilepsy seems rather clear within the classification system of idiopathic generalized epilepsy (IGE) as can be seen in Table 1. It shows the approximate frequency, the age of onset and the overlap of the four syndromes clinically and genetically closely related to each other.

But to prove to be an ideal candidate for genetic studies the syndrome is not uniform enough. Consistency refers to the occasional bilateral jerks of shoulders and arms mainly after awakening. All other signs are variable: in some case,s but not all, tonic–clonic seizures may occur, one-third of patients have additional absence seizures, half of the female patients with juvenile myoclonic epilepsy are photosensitive, male patients do not differ from probands with other types of IGEs in this respect. Age of onset clusters about the age of 15 years but earlier and later manifestations are not uncommon.

An extended list of what we would like to call 'juvenile myoclonic epilepsy plus symptoms' may contain questions concerning previous febrile convulsions (FC), the kinds of absence syndrome or the type of absence seizure like those that Panayiotopoulos (Ch. 9) intended to discriminate. Juvenile myoclonic epilepsy plus symptoms may refer to a subtle correlation ofthe different types of bilateral spike and wave discharges like those in the attempt of Waltz (Ch. 28). Such a sophisticated differentiation however cannot be *l'art pour l'art*, but should contribute to the solution of the problem of heterogeneity. The question therefore is: Is genetic heterogeneity expressed by the

Table 1. Juvenile myoclonic epilepsy (JME) plus symptoms

- Febrile convulsions
- Age of onset spectrum
- Absence syndrome
- Absence type
- Grand mal
- Interictal spike wave pattern
- Photosensitivity

variability of clinical symptoms or – to be more precise – is it possible that juvenile myoclonic epilepsy with or without absences, with or without photosensitivity or even more complex combinations of symptoms reflects different genetic mechanisms?

The approach to these questions will be from two sides: on one hand we will correlate the phenotypic variability in families of juvenile myoclonic epilepsy probands to criteria for homologous and heterologous transmission. On the other hand we intend to compare the occurence of clinical signs to positive or negative lod scores for linkage with the EJM1 locus. Both approaches – we may presume in advance – do not lead to clear-cut results. But nevertheless we do not hesitate to comment on this, because we consider our attempt to be a pilot study, which may prove to be suggestive with larger numbers and because we need stimulating and critical comments.

The clinical study comprises 25 pedigrees of multiplex and multigenerational families. From 108 close relatives of the 25 juvenile myoclonic epilepsy probands, clinical data including the results of EEG recording were available. Relatives without sufficient clinical information and/or EEG data were excluded from this study. In 11 families there was one additional family members besides the proband suffering from an epileptic manifestation, in eight families two, in two families four and in one family each five and six affected family members. Offspring younger than 15 years of age were excluded from the analysis, if clinically healthy and with a normal EEG. The kind of affectedness, that means the clinical type of the epileptic manifestation, is distributed in parents siblings and offspring in the following way (Table 2). These figures, referring to selective material, do not have any epidemiological relevance, but as the selection leads to a 'genetic condensation', it may nevertheless allow an interpretation with respect to genetic transmission. At first sight the present distribution does not seen to confirm the hypothesis of a tendency to homopheneous transmission. Among the affected relatives, the relative frequency of those with absence epilepsies and those with epilepsies with tonic–clonic seizures is equal to those with juvenile myoclonic epilepsy again. But these results need a critical clinical analysis, especially because the grand mal epilepsies do not share the same diagnostic quality as the other syndromes. Six cases have single (isolated) seizures only. These cases and the others, that could be classified as having typical grand mal on awakening, have not been investigated carefully enough to detect, for instance by means of video EEG recordings, additional absences or myoclonic jerks. We share the opinion of Delgado-Escueta of pure grand mal epilepsies being the rarer, the more carefully absences and jersks concomitant or introductory to grand mal are searched for. It may be presumed that, depending on the attention paid, some of the cases with grand mal epilepsies will turn out to have absence epilepsies or juvenile

Table 2. Prevalence of clinical forms among relatives of 25 probands with juvenile myoclonic epilepsy

	Febrile convulsions n = 9	Absence epilepsy n = 10	JME n = 10	GME n = 11	SW n = 8
Offspring; n = 25	12%	8%	4%	8%	16%
Siblings; n = 52	8%	10%	12%	14%	8%
Parents; n = 31	3%	10%	10%	7%	–

Table 3. Maximum lod score for model 2 (members with idiopathic generalized epilepsy are affected)

Family	lod score	Family	lod score
1	−0.067	19	−0.087
2	1.354	22	0.000
3	0.296	23	0.187
5	0.187	26	0.226
6	0.601	27	0.000
7	−0.258	28	0.187
9	0.374	29	0.000
10	−0.336	30	0.187
11	0.562	31	−0.032
13	0.449	32	0.260
14	0.446	34	0.338
16	−0.485	35	0.141
18	−0.149	38	0.487
		Total	4.869

Twenty-six families are tested under a (1) dominant mode of inheritance, (2) recombination fraction male/female = 0.0/0.0, (3) 70 per cent penetration.

myoclonic epilepsy. The equal frequency of absence epilepsies and juvenile myoclonic epilepsy does not represent a distribution of syndromes by chance. If that was the case, absence epilepsies should occur twice as often as juvenile myoclonic epilepsy. This knowledge may support a certain confirmation of homophenous transmission within JME families. This corresponds to the fact that in families of probands with absence epilepsies, juvenile myoclonic epilepsy is detected less frequently than absences in the affected family members (Janz 1992).

It seems worth mentioning the fact that offspring, and even siblings too, have a relatively frequent history of febrile convulsions. It seems noteworthy too, that in the EEG of offspring and siblings bilateral spike and wave could often be detected without signs of clinical manifestations. Whether there is a correlation on a genetic basis between these symptoms (febrile convulsions and bilateral spike–wave) and the juvenile myoclonic epilepsy syndrome needs to be clarified with more families and in comparison to other syndromes, for instance absence epilepsies.

In the second part of our attempt to detect clinical criteria for heterogeneity, we refer to the results

Table 4. Phenotypic variance in JME families with positive lod score (n = 16)

Rank	Pedigree	lod score	Idiopathic generalized epilepsies	Family size
1	2	1.354	JME (2), SS, GSW (2)	18
2	6	0.601	JME (2), JAE	5
3	11	0.562	JME, CAE, JAE, GMA, GSW	11
4	38	0.487	JME, OGM, LG	8
5	13	0.449	JME, CAE	8
6	14	0.446	JME, CAE	7
7	9	0.374	JME, JAE	9
8	34	0.338	JME, GMA, GM-status	7
9	3	0.296	JME (2), AE (2)	5
10	32	0.260	JME	7
11	26	0.226	JME	5
12	5	0.187	JME, GSW	8
13	23	0.187	JME, GSW	4
14	28	0.187	JME	4
15	30	0.187	JME (2)	3
16	35	0.141	JME, SS	4

Table 5. Phenotypic variance in JME families with zero or negative lod score lod score (n = 10)

Rank	Pedigree	Lod score	Idiopathic generalized epilepsies	Family size
17	22	0.00	JME, GMA	4
18	27	0.00	JME	4
19	29	0.00	JME	5
20	31	−0.032	JME (2), GM	5
21	1	−0.067	JME (2)	3
22	19	−0.087	JAE/JME	4
23	18	−0.149	JME	5
24	7	−0.258	JME	3
25	10	−0.336	CAE/JME, JAE	5
26	16	−0.485	JME, CAE	7

of the linkage analysis. Considering family members with IGE as affected, the lod score supporting linkage with a marker on chromosome 6 close to the HLA-region sums up to 4.9 under the assumption of a dominant mode of inheritance with 70 per cent penetrance (Table 3). Comparing the 16 families with a positive lod score to those with missing or negative lod scores it turns out, in concordance with expectations – that family size in 'positive' families exceeds that in negative families. On average the positive have 7.1 family members compared to 4.5 members in negative families (Tables 4 and 5). The relative frequency of affected members in positive families is greater (2.5 per family) than in negative families (1.6 per family). This corresponds to the fact that, among the families with negative lod scores, simplex families preponderate whereas this is the case for multiplex and multigenerational families in families with positive lod score. For further questions concerning clinical characteristics indicating genetic heterogeneity the average lod scores may be compared (Table 6).

Families with affected members with absence epilepsies show up with a remarkably higher lod score than families without absences either as an additional symptom in the proband or in affected members. The interpretation of these findings is limited by the fact that higher lod scores correspond to larger family size. This result is additionally confusing, as we will hear later in more detail because for families with absence epilepsies without combinations with juvenile myoclonic epilepsy there is no linkage to the HLA region.

As far clues can be drawn from comparing family lod scores, photosensitivty does not seem to be linked to the markers close to the HLA region. This can be reliably assumed because family size in both groups is mainly equal. If one or more family members suffer from juvenile myoclonic epilepsy besides the proband, the lod scores are higher, referring to equal family size, than in families without any further or different manifestation. This result may support the assumption of a homophenous transmission. The eight families with at least one additional member affected with juvenile myoclonic epilepsy sum up to a lod score of 3.1 which is considered a hint for linkage, whereas in the 11 families with a symptomatology other than juvenile myoclonic epilepsy the lod score is 1.7.

Table 6. Average family lod scores in clinical JME variants

Absence epilepsies	With (n = 11)	Without (n = 15)
	0.288 (f.s. = 6.5)	0.095 (f.s. = 5.1)
Photosensitivity	With (n = 16)	Without (n = 11)
	0.133 (f.s. = 5.8)	0.249 (f.s. = 5.1)
JME in relatives	With (n = 8)	Without (n = 11)
	0.385 (f.s. = 6.4)	0.156 (f.s. = 6.8)

f.s. = family size.

On the other hand the quote of the different clinical syndromes of IGE in families with positive and negative lod scores does not differ remarkably from each (Table 7). But it should be mentioned, that persons with clinically latent bilateral synchronous spike-and-waves all are members of families with a positive lod score. Even more remarkable is the fact that a history of febrile convulsions is often reported in families with a positive lod score than in those with a negative score. *Vice versa* photosensitivity is detected twice as often in negative families and this finding is in accordance with the low average lod score in families with photosensitive members.

Table 7. Epileptic manifestations in JME families with positive and negative lod scores

	Positive (n = 133)		Negative (n = 45)	
	n	%	n	%
JME (with absences)	20 (3)	18 (3)	12 (2)	27 (4)
Absence epilepsies	7	6	2	4
Grand mal epilepsies	1	6	2	4
Lennox–Gastaut	1	1	–	–
Generalized spike wave	5	4	–	–
Idiopathic generalized epilepsies	**40**	**35.4**	**16**	**35.5**
Febrile convulsions	9	8	1	2
Other seizure	2	2	1	2
Photosensitivity	12	11	11	24

Refinement of the map position of EJM1 in JME families

In linkage analysis between the HLA DQ A1 locus and IGEs in JME families, we found a lod score of 4.9 (Fig. 1). This lod score was reached under a dominant mode of inheritance; 70 per cent penetrance and a recombination fraction of 0.0. The lod scores for the single families are shown in Table 3. The combined lod score is composed of positive as well as negative scores in these single families. In 26 analysed families we have six that show negative lod score. These are families 1, 7, 10, 18, 19 and 31. This might be a hint for an existing genetic heterogeneity between our chosen families. However, within these families, clinically unaffected individuals having the same haplotype as the affected ones cause the negative lod scores, presumably due to the relatively high penetrance value of 70 per cent. If we decrease the penetrance value to 50 per cent the lod scores become positive.

To narrow the chromosomal region, in which the gene might be located, multipoint mapping with highly informative markers is necessary. The gene locus can be refined by identifying recombinations within the region of interest. To prove these key recombinations one needs multigeneration families with multiply affected IGE family members. Besides at least one recombination event, these families should show strong evidence for linkage between the HLA region and IGE. Family 2 fulfils this condition (Fig. 2). In this family, we got the highest lod score of 1.35 with the HLA DQ A1 marker, assuming patients with IGE as affected. Other tested markers gave lower lod scores (Table 8). The marker D6S88, around 17 cM telomeric from the HLA region has a maximum lod score of 0.05, the more informative marker D6S89 a maximum lod score of 0.1 and the most telomeric localized Factor 13 A1 gives only negative lod scores. Furthermore, we have clear recombinations, if we include clinically healthy family members with generalized spike–wave discharges in the EEG in our families. Using this suggestion, we get the following results. In our analysis a recombination occurs between the HLA region and the marker D6S88 in individuals 14 and 18. These persons have both the same alleles of D6S88 and D6S89. This means the disease predisposition is co-segregating with the telomeric part of this region. Individuals 15 and 17 have the same haplotype in this chromosomal region, but they are clinically unaffected. This could have two alternative explanations. Firstly, these two individuals, although they are carriers of the putative

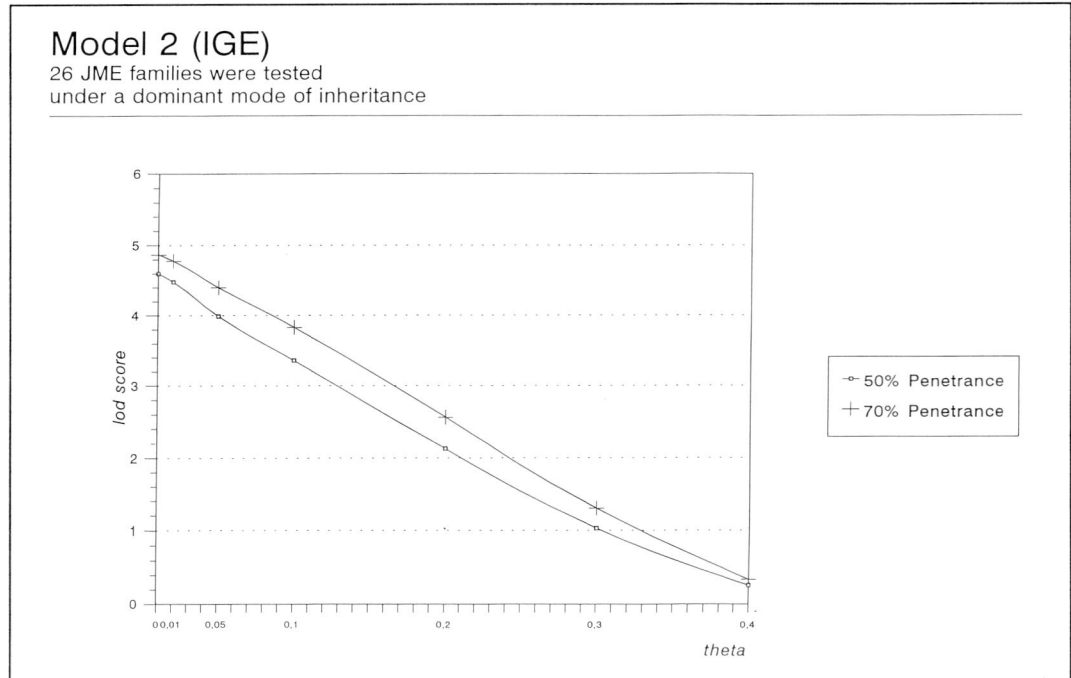

Fig. 1. Lod score values between juvenile myoclonic epilepsy and HLA DQ A1. Model 2 (members with idiopathic generalized epilepsy are affected). Dominant mode of inheritance. Recombination fraction male/female = 0.0/0.0.

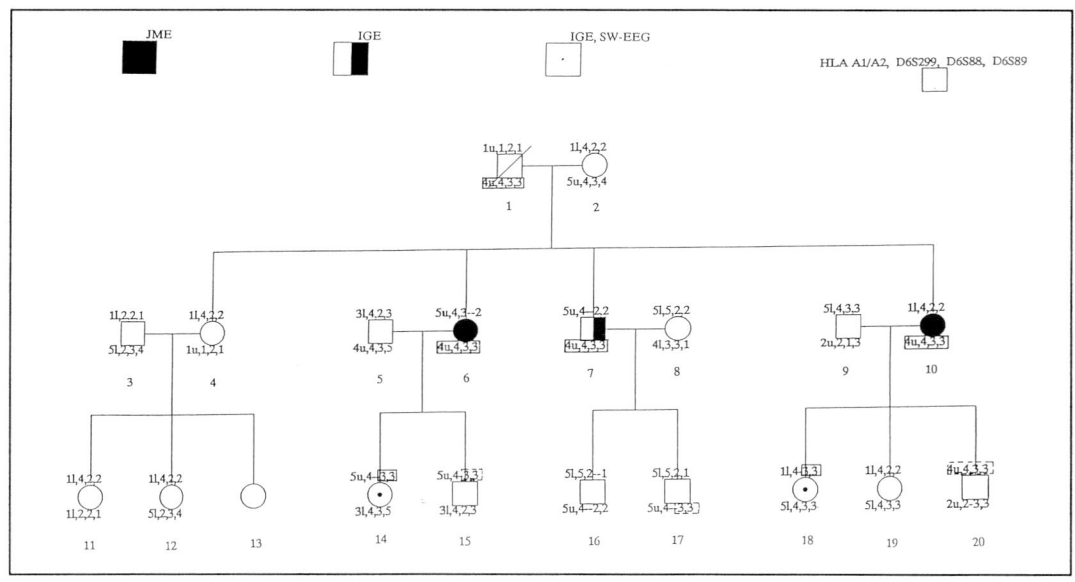

Fig. 2. Family tree of Family 2.

gene, are clinically unaffected because of the incomplete penetrance of EJM1.
Secondly, a recombination could occur between the putative gene locus of EJM1 and D6S88. From

Table 8. Lod score for family 2. Model 2 (members with idiopathic generalized epilepsy are affected); dominant mode of inheritance; recombination fraction male/female = 0.0/0.0; 70 per cent penetration (Ch 25 Janz)

Theta (Θ)	HLA DQ A1	D6S88	D6S89	F13A1
0.00	1.35	−0.03	−0.52	−5.31
0.01	1.33	−0.02	−0.42	−3.33
0.05	1.22	0.02	−0.17	−1.95
0.10	1.08	0.04	−0.02	−1.26
0.17		**0.05**		
0.20	0.76	0.05	0.09	−0.57
0.25			**0.10**	
0.30	0.41	0.03	0.09	−0.22
0.40	0.11	0.00	0.04	**−0.05**

this suggestion, this would determine the EJM1 gene locus between the flanking markers HLA DQ A1 and D6S88.

Conclusion

Following this preliminary and, in view of the small numbers, quite cautious report, we will speculate more as a hypothesis than as a solid statement on the results. Under clinical genetic as well as under molecular genetic aspects, some factors may be described as being in favour of linkage with EJM1 locus and some being not in favour with linkage (Table 9). Linkage is promoted by large family size and several affected relatives (that means in multiplex and multigenerational families) when other close family members also show juvenile myoclonic epilepsy and presumably by the additional occurence of absence epilepsies in the family. A history of febrile convulsions and the detection of clinical spike-and-wave discharges seems also to be supportive for linkage. The less frequent observation of linkage in simplex families may be conclusive because of the small family size on one hand and on the other due to sporadic cases. Other genes may interact in the occurrence of photosensitivity and be responsible for genetic heterogeneity in juvenile myoclonic epilepsy with photosensitivity.

Table 9. Factors in JME families in favour or not in favour of linkage with the EJM1 locus (Ch 25 Janz)

In favour	Not in favour
Multiplex/multigenerational family	Simplex family
JME in relatives	Photosensitivity
Absences in relatives	
Febrile convulsions	
Subclinical spike–waves	

Our linkage data lead to the following conclusions:
- the EJM1 locus seems to be located very near to the HLA region;
- additionally, the data from Family 2 support evidence for a key recombination that localizes EJM1 telomeric of the HLA region.

It is necessary to prove these results by analysing other families which fulfill the criteria of being a multigeneration family with many affected family members, including at least one recombination event and showing linkage to HLA.

Besides this, more markers flanking the interval of interest must be used, combined with a following multipoint analysis.

Part V
Photosensitivity

Chapter 26

Photosensitivity – a human 'model' of epilepsy

D.G.A. Kasteleijn-Nolst Trenité*, W. van Emde Boas* and C.D. Binnie[†]

Instituut voor Epilepsiebestrijding, Postbus 21, 2100 AA Heemstede, The Netherlands; [†]The Maudsley Hospital, Denmark Hill, London SE5 8AZ, UK

Introduction

Approximately 5 per cent of epileptic patients are found to be photosensitive (Jeavons & Harding, 1975; Kasteleijn-Nolst Trenité, 1989), i.e. they show generalized epileptiform discharges on intermittent photic stimulation (IPS) during an EEG registration. At least 60 per cent of those patients have a history of visually-induced seizures. Furthermore, during EEG investigations, a patient who is not receiving any anti-epileptic treatment and has a history of seizures induced by visual stimuli in daily life (such as sunlight shining through trees, sunlight on water, a television set, disco lights or an escalator), will nearly always show a photoparoxysmal response to IPS and/or pattern and television.

Dreifuss (1990), and the Commission on Classification and Terminology of the International League Against Epilepsy (1985), defined an epileptic syndrome as a cluster of signs and symptoms customarily occurring together. The syndrome is characterized by seizure type, family history, the presence or absence of abnormal neurological findings, a specific age-of-onset, a natural history with a predictable outcome and the patient's response to medication.

Although photosensitivity is associated with several mostly generalized epileptic syndromes, it could be considered a syndrome on its own: it constitutes a separate entity within the epilepsies both clinically and electro-neurophysiologically. Patients who are photosensitive have a specific clinical history of visually-evoked seizures. Most patients have a history of tonic–clonic and myoclonic seizures and suffer from an idiopathic generalized epilepsy (Jeavons & Harding, 1975; Kasteleijn-Nolst Trenité, 1989). In various studies (Wolf & Goosses, 1986; Jeavons & Harding, 1975; Kasteleijn-Nolst Trenité, 1989), there is a preponderance of females (60 per cent) and a peak-prevalence between the ages of 10 and 25 years of age.

This greater prevalence in women is independent of age, suggesting a genetic influence rather than changing hormonal influences. Follow-up studies show a general decline after the age of 25. Valproic acid is the drug of first choice in treating photosensitive patients. Thus, epileptic patients who show generalized epileptiform discharges on intermittent photic stimulation form a specific sub-group of epileptic patients and are therefore suitable, for example, for genetic studies.

Unlike most other epilepsies, photosensitive epilepsy is a reflex-epilepsy, and epileptiform discharges can be evoked at any time by intermittent photic stimulation in the laboratory. Furthermore, determination of a so-called sensitivity range (Jeavons & Harding, 1975) can be used as a measure of epileptogenesis. This range is related to liability to seizures in daily life, i.e. patients with a greater range have a higher likelihood of visually-induced seizures than those with a smaller range (Kasteleijn-Nolst Trenité, 1989). The photosensitivity range seems to be a reliable and reproducible measure of epileptogenesis in these patients. In 73 patients, photosensitivity ranges were determined over the course of a day, representing a total of 745 estimations; only five patients showed spontaneous and transitory disappearance of photosensitivity. The majority of photosensitive patients had remarkably stable ranges (Binnie *et al.*, 1986a). Determination of the range by intermittent photic stimulation can be repeated several times in the same patients in order to evaluate natural history and medication effects (Binnie *et al.*, 1985, 1986a,b). It can even help predict risk for recurrence of seizures after partial or complete withdrawal of medication (Overweg, 1985). Photosensitive children who have been treated successfully with valproic acid have a high likelihood of recurrence of seizures after withdrawal of medication (observed in practice and in publication: Matricardi *et al.*, 1989).

Technique

Establishing photosensitivity

A photic stimulator is required that produces no electrical interference and gives flashes of 0–60 Hz with about equal intensity levels. Unlike many industrial stroboscopes, the commercially available Grass PS22 or PS33-plus complies with these requirements. This stimulator with a diffuser should be used up to the intensity of 100 nits per flash with or without a grid (Jeavons & Harding, 1975). Although the grid superimposes a pattern stimulus, thus increasing the likelihood of evoking epileptiform discharges, we prefer stimulation with intermittent photic stimulation and pattern separately, in order to distinguish flicker from pattern sensitivity.

Intermittent photic stimulation is preferably performed with patients seated, and instructed to fixate on the centre of the photic stimulator, which is placed at a distance from the nasion of about 30 cm. The EEG technician has to check that fixation is maintained. Because many patients will show myoclonic jerks facially, especially eyelids, or movement of their arms, this can be recognized more easily when the patient is seated. Normal lighting conditions, between 250 and 750 lux, are appropriate; when using a stroboscope with a flash intensity of at least 10 lumen per s per square foot, the influence of background illumination is relatively minor.

Stimulation with increasing and decreasing flash frequencies until epileptiform discharges occur (for range see below) minimizes the risk of eliciting an epileptic seizure as stimulation is confined to frequencies at or outside the limits of the photosensitivity range (most often 10 to 30 Hz).

Furthermore, this procedure of 'approaching' the most epileptogenic frequencies makes it possible to discriminate spontaneous epileptiform discharges from those elicited by photic stimulation (false positive findings). Eye-closure during intermittent photic stimulation is the most provocative eye-condition, followed by eyes-closed and eyes-open (Kasteleijn-Nolst Trenité, 1989). Individual differences, however, can occur. All three eye conditions should be examined to detect any sensitivity to intermittent photic stimulation. Incomplete examination, insufficient flash intensity or inconsistent fixation on the centre of the lamp can result in false negative results.

Photosensitivity range

Trains of flashes at constant frequency are delivered for 4–6 s at three different eye-conditions. The intervals between the successive trains of flashes at a given frequency lasts at least 4 s. As soon as generalized epileptiform activity appears in the EEG, the stimulation at the frequency and state of eye condition in question is instantly terminated in order to prevent occurrence of seizures. At first the lower limit is established by starting with 2 Hz stimulation and testing successive increasing

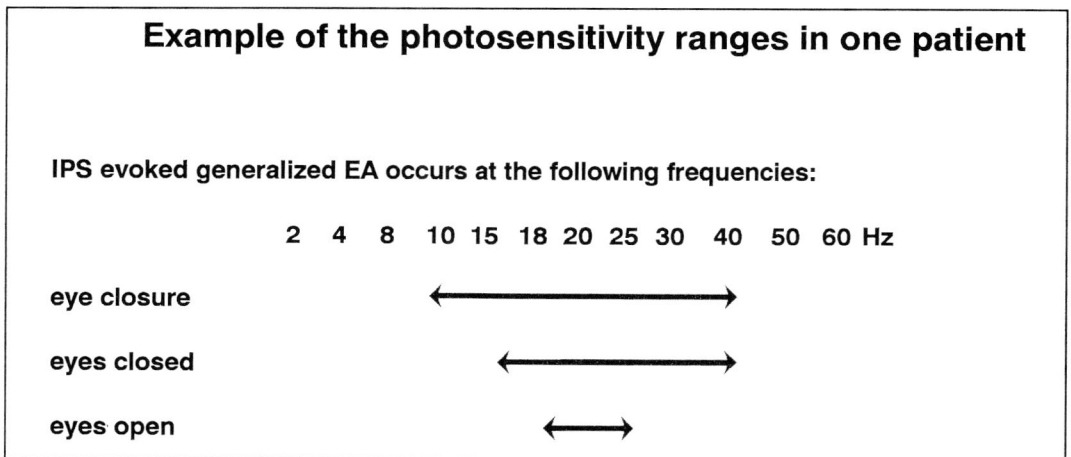

Fig. 1. An example of the photosensitivity ranges in one patient.

standard frequencies until epileptiform activity is elicited. Subsequently, the upper sensitivity limit is defined, beginning at 60 Hz and decreasing the flash frequency step-wise until, again, epileptiform activity is elicited. The following technique is suggested: the patient is asked to open the eyes; after 10 s of eyes-open the patient is asked to close the eyes and intermittent photic stimulation commences. The stimulus train lasts 4 s or is terminated immediately if a generalized epileptiform response is elicited. After a 4 s pause while the eyes remain closed, further bursts of intermittent photic stimulation with eyes-closed are continued for 4 s, or again until onset of photoparoxysmal response. The patient is asked to open the eyes and after a 4 s pause, again bursts of IPS with eyes-open, also lasting 4 s, are given or aborted if a photoparoxysmal response is elicited. After a photoparoxysmal response, a pause of 20 s is taken, or at least four times the length of the discharge before the procedure is continued.

The determination of the photosensitivity range in all the eye-conditions takes about 4 min per patient.

The ranges thus established represent a measure of the degree of photosensitivity and because the correlation with the clinical history is very apparent it can very well be used for monitoring the patient. An example of the ranges in a patient is given in Fig. 1.

Photosensitivity as model for acute anti-epileptic drug studies

Because the photosensitivity range represents a reliable and reproducible measure of epileptogenesis, it offers a unique model to study the effects of a single dose of an experimental antiepileptic drug in humans (in early phase II studies, so-called photosensitivity model (Binnie et al., 1986a). The model allows preliminary determination of acute anti-epileptic effect on photic-induced EEG discharges of single oral doses of the investigational drug. Furthermore, it is possible to determine the time of onset and the duration of this effect, to evaluate a dose-response relationship and to document plasma concentration-time profiles of the drug. Finally, some data with regard to tolerability could be compiled.

All major groups of anti-epileptic drugs have been shown to produce an acute reduction of photosensitivity in at least 50 per cent of subjects (Binnie et al., 1986a) and many experimental drugs have subsequently been studied in the photosensitivity model.

All drugs diminished or abolished photosensitivity in at least 50 per cent of patients e.g. progabide

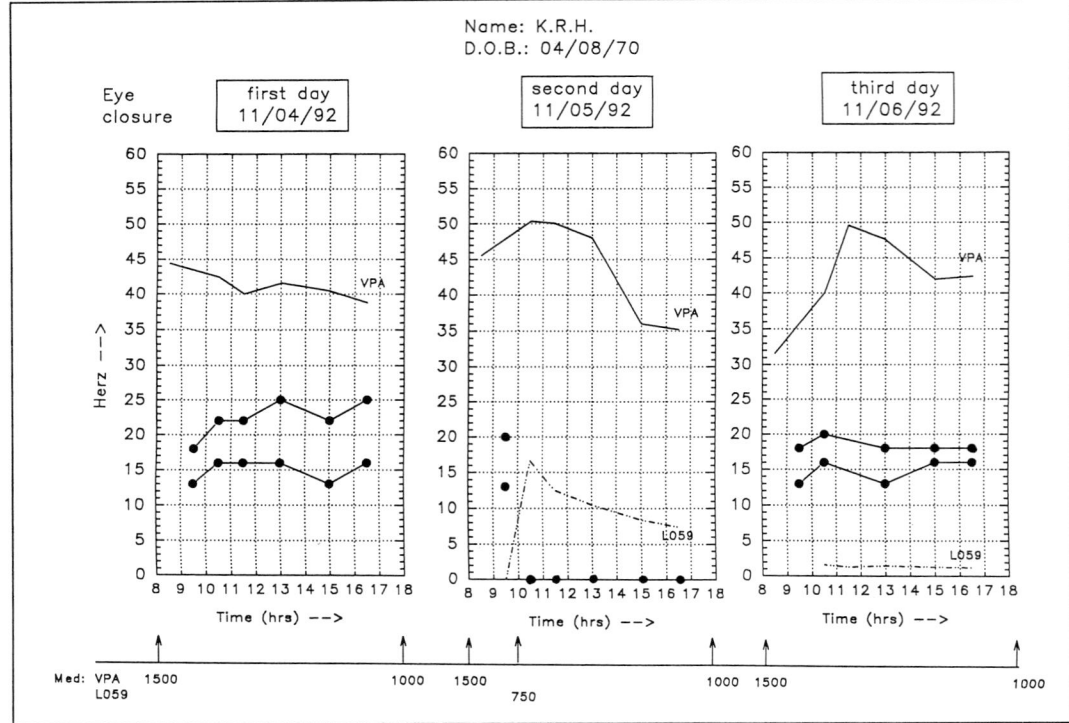

Fig. 2. Effect on the photosensitivity range after intake of a single oral dose on day 2 of the experimental antiepileptic drug LO59 ucb, a pyrolidine acetamide. Abolishment of the response in this patient is found half an hour after intake of 750 mg lasting about 24 h. There exists a clear relationship between the peak plasma level of LO59 and suppression of the photoparoxysmal response.

(Binnie et al., 1985), lamotrigine (Binnie et al., 1986b), flumazenil (in preparation), loreclezole (Overweg & De Beukelaar, 1990) and recently ucb LO59 (Fig. 2).

Org 6370 (Kasteleijn-Nolst Trenité et al., 1992) however, has demonstrated paradoxical enhancement of photo-sensitivity with provocation of myoclonic seizures (Fig. 3), while in animal experiments the drug proved to be anti-epileptic (Kasteleijn-Nolst Trenité et al., 1992). Further development of the drug was cancelled.

The outcome of these type of studies using reduction of the photosensitivity range as parameter, stress the importance of initial studies with a limited number of well-documented patients in which the subjects are under constant personal supervision, prior to the start of phase III trials.

Design

Standardized assessment of photosensitivity ranges as outlined above is carried out over three consecutive study days.

On study day 1 the patient is prepared for regular long-term EEG monitoring; after determination of the most sensitive and stable reaction to intermittent photic stimulation in a specific eye condition, i.e. eye-closure, eyes-closed or eyes-open, the determination of photosensitivity ranges is subsequently performed with that particular eye-condition. Patients serve as their own control, so day 1 is used to establish baseline values. At hourly intervals photosensitivity range determinations are taken, starting at 08:00 until 16:00 h. Subjects receiving regular antiepileptic medication con-

Chapter 26 Photosensitivity – a human 'model' of epilepsy

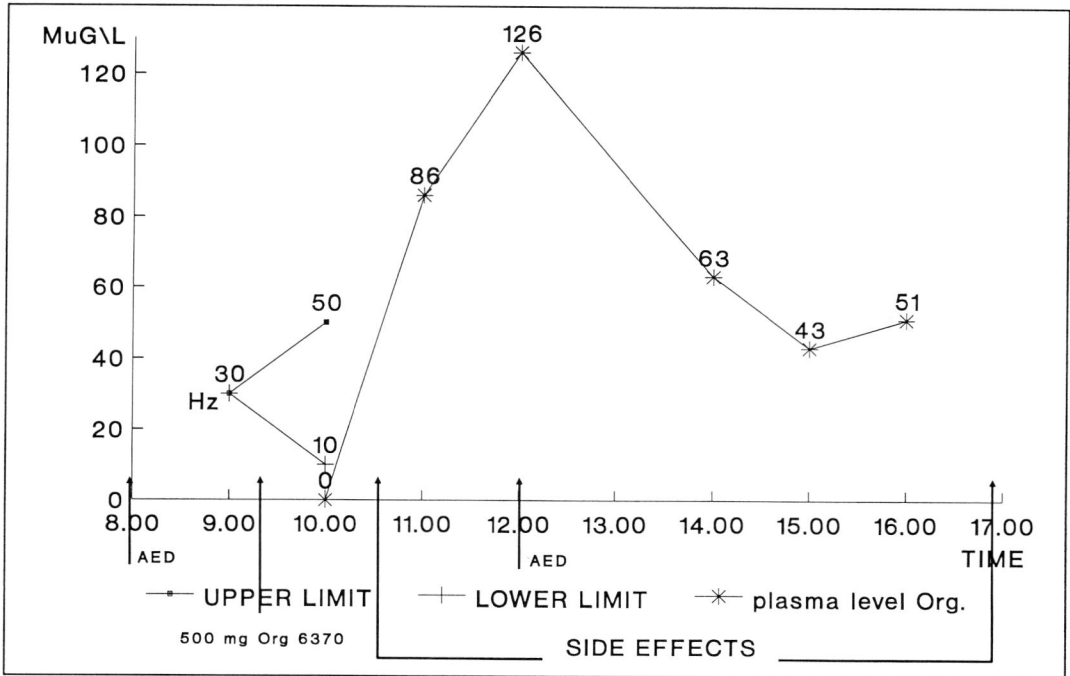

Fig. 3. Relationship between change in photosensitivity range, side effects, and Org 6370 serum levels, in µg/l, after oral intake of 500 mg Org 6370. Side-effects: dizziness, nausea, whole body myoclonus and at 11:55 h a spontaneous tonic–clonic convulsion; they disappeared at about 18:00 h. Because of the objective and subjective strong increase in photosensitivity, no further intermittent photic stimulation could be performed.

tinue to take it according to normal schedule, and blood samples are taken at hourly intervals immediately following each intermittent photic stimulation session.

On study day 2 the procedure is repeated but a single oral dose of the experimental drug is administered after the first IPS session. In patients with evidence of liver enzyme induction due to regular intake of antiepileptic drugs the single oral dose of the experimental drug may be increased. Blood samples of the experimental and concomitant drugs are taken shortly after the times of IPS determination (hourly) or more frequently, depending on the pharmacokinetics of the experimental drug.

The same test procedure as on day 1 is repeated on day 3 to investigate the duration of any observed effects and to document the eventual return to the approximate baseline values.

For the duration of the trial, patients are under continuous observation by skilled personnel and/or closed-circuit television. Additional EEG monitoring can be performed if patients show unexpected side effects. Each IPS section is recorded with standard 21-channel EEG equipment and the paper record of each session is coded. The photosensitivity range in each EEG record is then assessed independently by two investigators without knowledge of the sequence in which the record tracings were obtained. The topography and morphology of all responses, including sub-threshold reactions not meeting the criteria for a classical photoparoxysmal response, i.e. generalized spike-and-wave discharges outlasting the stimulus train, are noted to provide additional information on the profile of the new drug.

Finally, the results (changes in photosensitivity ranges) are compared within one patient, comparing day 1 with day 2 and 3. Furthermore, blood levels and adverse events are correlated in time with the IPS results. Statistical analysis is descriptive and individual patient data are listed with any abnormal findings highlighted and statistics are performed if meaningful.

Photosensitivity as a genetic marker

The prevalence of photosensitivity is greater in families with this phenomenon than in the general population. In 1956 Davidson & Watson reported several families with more than one photosensitive, epileptic patient. They considered 'stimulus sensitivity appearing as evoked cerebral electrical abnormalities with or without clinical seizures as a result of intermittent, retinal illumination as a manifestation of a genetically-determined disorder of central nervous system function'. Doose et al. (1969) carried out large scale EEG studies in siblings of photosensitive probands. According to this study, an abnormal response to intermittent photic stimulation should be regarded as a symptom of a genetically-determined photosensitivity. Furthermore, in 75 per cent of patients who show a generalised photoparoxysmal response outlasting the stimulus train, clinical signs can be seen during IPS, although 89 per cent of the IPS-evoked discharges have a duration of 3 s or less (Kasteleijn-Nolst Trenité et al., 1987). The evoked 'ictal' phenomena are predominantly myoclonic jerks in the eye lids, whole body, arms and shoulders. These subtle clinical signs are not noticed by about half of the patients, although many experience subjective symptoms such as pain or an awkward feeling in the eyes or dizziness. If a patient, however, experienced ictal phenomena these could always be seen. The evoked clinical signs and symptoms can be considered as 'ictal' events. Of additional interest is the fact that there exists an overlap between the syndrome of photosensitivity and juvenile myoclonic epilepsy, a syndrome which has been located on chromosome 6p (Delgado-Escueta et al., 1989).

With increasing age, the photosensitivity range diminishes and the reaction to intermittent photic stimulation becomes less generalized, remaining confined to the occipital areas. Although this localised occipital response has no clinical correlate in the sense of liability to seizures or, especially, visually-induced seizures, this minor response does indicate a genetic trait for photosensitivity. Doose and co-workers demonstrated again recently the value of this genetic trait (Waltz et al., 1992). The reaction to intermittent photic stimulation can be classified in four types; type 1: spikes within the occipital rhythm; type 2: parietal occipital spikes with bi-phasic, slow-wave; type 3: parietal occipital spikes with bi-phasic slow-wave and spreading to the frontal region; type 4: the occurrence of generalized poly spike and spike waves, consistently elicited by intermittent photic stimulation, not frequency-locked to the stimulus and outlasting the stimulus train at least by some 100 ms. Type 4 is the so-called classical photoparoxysmal response which correlates highly with a history of epilepsy and photosensitive epilepsy in particular.

Concluding remarks

The phenomenon of photosensitivity offers an interesting human model for the study of epilepsy. Photosensitive patients have a specific clinical history with an age-of-onset during late childhood and peak-prevalence at puberty. Seizure types are mainly tonic–clonic seizures, myoclonic seizures and absence seizures. Furthermore, there is a female predominance (60 per cent) independent of age and also familial occurrence. The EEG-correlate and the photoparoxysmal response is repeatable and relatively stable within a patient and can be considered as 'ictal'. Unlike in most animal models, the evoked paroxysmal epileptiform activity occurs in a natural situation and not as the result of lesions; the visual system in these patients functions completely normally up to the level of the visual cortex in the occipital lobes where the paroxysmal discharges originate. Photosensitivity can therefore offer a human 'model' of epilepsy.

Acknowledgement

We would like to thank all colleagues in our Institute for referring patients for investigation. We thank the EEG technicians for investigation, with special thanks to R.A. de Korte and E. Dekker. We would like to acknowledge help with preparing the text by A. Tierlier-Long. Study results are given from studies, sponsored by UCB Pharma SA, Belgium and Organon International BV, The Netherlands.

References

Binnie, C.D., Pestre, M., De Korte, R.A., Kasteleijn-Nolst Trenité, D.G.A., Loiseau, P. & Meijer, J.W.A. (1985): Acute effects of single-dose administration of progabide on human photosensitivity. In: *LERS Monographs 3: Epilepsy and GABA receptor agonists*, eds. G. Bartholini, L. Bossi & P. Morselli, pp. 311–319. New York: Raven Press.

Binnie, C.D., Kasteleijn-Nolst Trenité, D.G.A. & De Korte, R.A. (1986a): Photosensitivity as a model for acute anti-epileptic drug studies. *Electroencephalogr. Clin. Neurophysiol.* **63**, 35–41.

Binnie, C.D., Van Emde Boas, W., Kasteleijn-Nolst Trenité, D.G.A., De Korte, R.A., Meijer, J.W.A., Meinardi, H., Miller, A.A., Overweg, J., Peck, A.W. & Van Wieringen, A. (1986b): Acute effects of lamotrigine (BW430C) in persons with epilepsy. *Epilepsia* **27**, 248–254.

Commission on Classification and Terminology of the International League Against Epilepsy (1985): Proposal for classification of epilepsies and epileptic syndromes, *Epilepsia* **26**, 268–278.

Davidson, S. & Watson, C.W. (1956): Hereditary light sensitive epilepsy. *Neurology* **6**, 235–261.

Delgado-Escueta, A.V., Greenberg, D.A., Treiman, L., Liu, A., Sparkes, R.S, Berbetti, A., Park, M.S. & Tersaki, P.I. (1989): Mapping the gene for juvenile myoclonic epilepsy. *Epilepsia* **30**, S8–18.

Doose, H., Gerken, H., Hien-Völpel & Völzke, E. (1969): Genetics of photosensitive epilepsy. *Neuropädiatrie* **1,1** 56–73.

Dreifuss, F.E. (1990): The syndromes of generalized epilepsy. In: *Generalized epilepsy, neurobiological approaches*, eds. M. Avoli, P. Gloor, G. Kostopoulos & R. Naquet, pp. 19–29. Boston: Birkhäuser.

Jeavons, P.M., Harding, G.F.A. (1975): *Photosensitive epilepsy*. London: Heinemann.

Kasteleijn-Nolst Trenité, D.G.A., Binnie, C.D. & Meinardi, H. (1987): Photosensitive patients: symptoms and signs during intermittent photic stimulation and their relation to seizures in daily life. *J. Neurol. Neurosurg. Psychiatry* **50**, 1546–1549.

Kasteleijn-Nolst Trenité, D.G.A. (1989): Photosensitivity in epilepsy: electrophysiological and clinical correlates. *Acta Neurol. Scand.* **80 (Suppl. 125)** 1–149.

Kasteleijn-Nolst Trenité, D.G.A., Van Emde Boas, W., Groenhout, C.C. & Meinardi, H. (1992): Preliminary assessment of the efficacy of Org 6370 in photosensitivity and provocation of myoclonic seizures. *Epilepsia* **33**, 135–141.

Matricardi, M., Brinciotti, M. & Benedetti, P. (1989): Outcome after discontinuation of anti-epileptic drug therapy in children with epilepsy. *Epilepsia* **30**, 582–589.

Overweg, J. (1985): *Withdrawal of antiepileptic drugs in seizure-free adult patients*. Thesis: Amsterdam.

Overweg, J. & De Beukelaar, F. (1990): Single-dose efficacy evaluation of loreclezole in patients with photosensitive epilepsy. *Epilepsy Res.* **6**, 227–233.

Waltz, S., Christen, H.-J. & Doose, H. (1992): The different patterns of the photoparoxysmal response – a genetic study. *Electroencephalogr. Clin. Neurophysiol.* **83**, 138–145.

Wolf, P. & Goosses, R. (1986): Relation of photosensitivity to epileptic seizures. *J. Neurol. Neurosurg. Psychiatry* **49**, 1386–1391.

Chapter 27

Pathophysiological mechanisms of photosensitivity in IGEs

Takeo Takahashi

Division of Neuropsychiatry, Sendai City Hospital, 3–1, Shimizukoji, Wakabayashiku, Sendai 981, Japan

Introduction

Patients with photosensitive epilepsy are particularly sensitive to the full-field visual stimulus of a red flicker and/or a flickering geometric pattern, when a decreased luminance, such as 10–20 nits, is used as a light source of the stimulation (Takahashi, 1989). According to Matsuoka *et al.* (1989), as cited by Takahashi (1989), 61 out of 341 epileptic patients showed photoparoxysmal responses (PPRs) elicited by these stimuli. In that study, therefore, the incidence of photosensitivity in epileptics (18 per cent) is 3.6 times higher than that of the commonly accepted 5 per cent reported by Binnie & Jeavons (1992). Furthermore, among 61 patients, 45 were idiopathic generalized epilepsies (IGEs). The rate of 51 per cent (45 out of 88 patients) with IGEs is also higher than that of 25 per cent shown by Binnie & Jeavons (1992) as well. These results would suggest that detailed studies of photoparoxysmal responses elicited by a red flicker and/or a flickering geometric pattern may deepen our understanding of IGEs. To specifically elucidate EEG abnormalities in the cortical visual areas, EEG examinations with regional visual stimuli in patients with photosensitive epilepsy is considered to be useful (Takahashi, 1989, 1993). This is an EEG examination in which visual stimuli to the centre, periphery and each hemifield, in addition to the full-field stimulation, are given to patients during EEG recordings. In this study, a systematic EEG examination of 25 patients with photosensitive epilepsy was performed using regional visual stimulation.

Patients and methods

Table 1 shows clinical data of 25 patients (six male and 19 female) with photosensitive epilepsy. Their ages ranged from 10 to 32 years, with a mean age of 19.2 years. The patients were classified according to a proposal for revised classification of epilepsies and epileptic syndromes (Commission, 1989): 12 patients had generalized tonic–clonic seizures on awakening, six patients had juvenile myoclonic epilepsy, three had childhood absence epilepsy, two had temporal lobe epilepsy, and two had febrile convulsions. A stroboscope (LS-7000, Nihon Kohden, Tokyo) was placed 30 cm above the patient's eyes, and 15 Hz intermittent photic stimulation (IPS) for 21 s was successively given to the patients in a supine position. The first 7 s IPS was given to the patients with their eyes closed, the second with their eyes open, and the last with their eyes closed again.

Visual stimuli were then given to the patients by means of a visual stimulator (SLS-5100, Nihon Kohden, Tokyo) (Takahashi et al., 1980). The subject, in a sitting position, looked at a tangent screen set 25 cm from the eyes, and the stimuli were projected on a screen measuring 25 cm × 25 cm (53° × 53°). The maximal luminance of the white background of the black patterns and the red light stimuli was kept at 9.8 and 9.7 nits, respectively. Two kinds of dot and grating patterns were used: the visual angle of a single dot was 1.33° whereas that of a line was 0.41°. These stimuli were modulated sinusoidally at a frequency of 15 Hz, yielding a flickering pattern and a red flicker stimuli. Figure 1 demonstrates the filters used to provide the flickering dot pattern and the red flicker stimuli to the centre, periphery, centre plus periphery (full-field) and right hemifield by use of the same visual stimulator. The flickering dot pattern and the red flicker stimuli to the left, upper and lower hemifields were produced by rotating filters shown in the right tracings of Fig. 1. Regional visual stimuli by a grating pattern were produced as shown in this figure. When generalized photoparoxysmal responses were elicited by any of the full-field stimuli of the grating pattern, the flickering dot pattern and the red flicker, which were given for less than 7 s each in no specific order, regional visual stimuli by use of the effective stimulation were given to the patients. The regional visual stimuli, given in no specific order, was also presented for 7 s each with an interval of at least 30 s. If photoparoxysmal responses were elicited by any of them, including stroboscopic IPS, the stimulation was immediately terminated. When EEG examinations were performed, 21 patients were receiving anticonvulsants and four patients were not receiving any medication (see Table 1).

Results

EEG data obtained by regional visual stimuli of 25 patients are shown in Table 2.

Table 1. Clinical data of 25 patients with photosensitive epilepsy

Case	Age	Sex	Heredity	Past history	Diagnosis	Precipitating factors	CT scans	Antiepileptic drugs (mg/day)
1	16	F	–	–	GTCS on awakening	Television	Normal	–
2	18	F	Mother	–	GTCS on awakening	–	Normal	VPA (800), PHT (200)
3	19	F	–	–	GTCS on awakening	–	Normal	–
4	24	F	–	–	GTCS on awakening	Television	Normal	VPA (400)
5	30	M	Cousin	–	Juvenile myoclonic	Television	Normal	–
6	30	F	–	–	Juvenile myoclonic	–	Normal	VPA (500), PHT (50)
7	13	M	–	Febrile convulsions	Febrile convulsion	–	–	VPA (100)
8	21	F	–	–	Childhood absence	Flashing light	–	VPA (100)
9	32	F	–	–	GTCS on awakening	Television, pattern	Normal	VPA (400), PHT (100)
10	22	F	–	–	Juvenile myoclonic	Pattern, flashing light	Normal	VPA (600)
11	14	F	–	Febrile convulsions	Childhood absence	Television	–	VPA (300)
12	14	F	–	–	GTCS on awakening	Television	Normal	PHT (300)
13	15	F	–	–	GTCS on awakening	–	–	VPA (200)
14	21	F	Sister	Head trauma	Temporal lobe	–	Cyste (LT)	CBZ (300)
15	10	M	–	Vacuum extraction	Temporal lobe	–	Cavum vergae	VPA (100)
16	11	M	–	Vacuum extraction, febrile convulsions	Childhood absence	Television	Normal	–
17	17	M	–	Head trauma	Juvenile myoclonic	Television	Normal	VPA (400)
18	15	F	–	Vacuum extraction, febrile convulsions	Febrile convulsion	–	–	VPA (100)
19	12	F	–	Febrile convulsions	GTCS on awakening	–	Normal	VPA (100)
20	15	F	–	Febrile convulsions	GTCS on awakening	–	Normal	VPA (200)
21	17	F	–	–	Juvenile myoclonic	–	Normal	VPA (200)
22	16	F	–	Febrile convulsions	GTCS on awakening	Television	Normal	VPA (200)
23	24	M	–	–	Juvenile myoclonic	–	Normal	VPA (400)
24	27	F	–	–	GTCS on awakening	–	–	PHT (75)
25	27	F	–	Febrile convulsions	GTCS on awakening	–	Normal	VPA (200), PHT (50)

VPA: valproate; PHT: phenytoin; CBZ: carbamazepine.

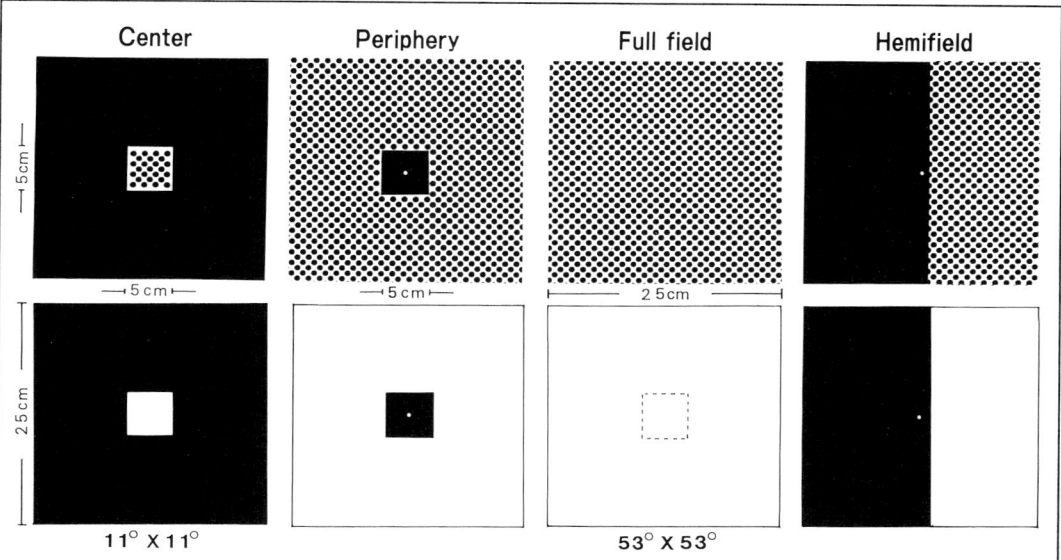

Fig. 1. Filters used to provide regional visual stimuli of flickering dot pattern (upper tracings) and red flicker (lower tracings) by the use of a visual stimulator (SLS-5100, Nihon Kohden). Hemifield stimuli were presented on one side of the screen and black on the other, with an 8 mm 2° gap between the edge of the black hemifield and the central fixation point.

Table 2. EEG data of 25 patients with photosensitive epilepsy

Case	Strobe IPS	Grating F	Flickering dot pattern* C	P	F	LH	Red flicker* C	P	F	LH	Hemifield flickering dot pattern Le	R	U	Lo	Hemifield red flicker Le	R	U	Lo
1	+	+	−	+	+	Equal	+	+	+	Equal	+	+	+	+	+	+	+	+
2	+	+	−	+	+	Equal	+	−	+	Equal	+	+	+	+	+	+	−	−
3	−	−	−	+	+	Equal	+	−	+	Equal	+	+	+	−	+	+	−	−
4	−	−	−	+	+	Equal	+	−	+	Equal	+	+	+	−	+	+	+	+
5	+	−	−	+	+	Equal	+	−	+	Equal	+	+	+	−	+	+	+	−
6	−	−	−	+	+	Equal	−	−	+	Equal	+	+	+	−	+	+	−	+
7	+	−	−	+	+	Equal	+	−	+	No	+	+	+	+	−	−	−	−
8	+	−	−	−	+	Equal	+	−	+	No	+	+	+	+	−	−	−	−
9	+	+	+	+	+	Equal	+	−	+	No	+	+	+	+	−	−	−	−
10	−	−	−	+	+	Equal			−		+	+	+	−				
11	−	−	−	+	+	No	+	−	+	Equal	−	−	−	−	+	+	−	−
12	+	−			−		+	+	+	Equal					+	+	−	+
13	+	−			−		−	−	+	Equal					+	+	−	−
14	−	−		+	+	Unequal			−		+	−	+	−				
15	+	−			−		+	−	+	Unequal					+	−	−	−
16	+	−			−		−	−	+	Unequal					+	−	−	−
17	−	−			−		−	−	+	Unequal					−	+	−	−
18	−	−	−	−	+	No	+	−	+	No	−	−	−	−	−	−	−	−
19	+	−	−	+	+	No			−		−	−	−	−				
20	−	−	−	+	+	No			−		−	−	−	−				
21	+	−	−	+	+	No			−		−	−	−	−				
22	−	−			−		−	−	+	No					−	−	−	−
23	−	−			−		−	−	+	No					−	−	−	−
24	−	−			−		+	−	+	No					−	−	−	−
25	−	−			−		−	−	+	No					−	−	−	−

*C: centre; P: periphery; F: full; LH: lateral hemifield; Le: left; R: right; U: upper; Lo: lower.

Full-field stimulation

Generalized photoparoxysmal responses were elicited from three patients by a grating pattern, a flickering dot pattern and a red flicker stimuli. Eight patients responded to a flickering dot pattern and a red flicker stimulus. The flickering dot pattern stimulation was effective with only five patients. In nine patients, generalized photoparoxysmal responses were induced by the red flicker stimulation alone (Table 3).

Table 3. Photoparoxysmal responses elicited by full-field visual stimuli

Grating	Flickering dot	Red flicker	No. of patients
+	+	+	3
−	+	+	8
−	+	−	5
−	−	+	9
Total			25

Stimulation of the centre and periphery

Grating pattern stimulation of the centre was effective with one patient, whereas that of the periphery was effective with two patients. Only one patient (6 per cent) responded to the flickering dot pattern stimulation of the centre but 14 patients (89 per cent) responded to that of the periphery. By contrast, the red flicker stimulation of the centre was effective with 13 patients (65 per cent) and that of the periphery showed a decrease down to two patients (10 per cent) (Table 4). These differences brought about by the flickering dot pattern and the red flicker stimuli to the centre and periphery were statistically significant ($\chi^2 = 16.21$, 1 df, $P < 0.01$). Figure 2 shows examples of generalized photoparoxysmal responses elicited by the red flicker stimulation of the centre and the flickering dot pattern stimulation of the periphery in a 13-year-old male patient with febrile convulsions (Case 7). Regarding mean latencies of photoparoxysmal responses elicited by the stimuli to the centre, periphery and full-field, all three mean latencies of photoparoxysmal responses elicited by full-field stimuli were the shortest, followed by those with stimuli to the periphery and centre. The difference in latencies of response to the red flicker stimuli of the centre and full-field was only statistically significant (Student's paired t-test, $P < 0.001$).

Table 4. Photoparoxysmal responses elicited by visual stimuli to the centre, periphery and full-field

Visual stimuli	No. of patients (%)			Mean latency (sec) ± SD		
	Centre	Periphery	Full	Centre	Periphery	Full
Grating	1	2	3	6.6	2.50 ± 0.14	2.35 ± 0.92
Flickering dot	1 (6)	14 (89)	16	6.8	3.49 ± 1.56	2.97 ± 1.56
Red flicker	13 (65)	2 (10)	20	3.35 ± 1.50	3.05 ± 0.49	1.70 ± 0.93

Hemifield stimulation

One of the three patients sensitive to the grating pattern stimulation to the full-field was also sensitive to the lateral hemifield stimulation but not to the stimuli to the upper and lower hemifields. Stimulation of the left, right, upper and lower hemifields with the flickering dot pattern elicited generalized photoparoxysmal responses in 11 (69 per cent), 10 (63 per cent), 11 (69 per cent) and five (31 per cent) patients, respectively. For the red flicker, generalized photoparoxysmal responses were elicited in 11 (55 per cent), 10 (50 per cent), three (15 per cent) and four (20 per cent) patients, respectively (Table 5). Stimulation of the upper and lower hemifields by the flickering dot pattern elicited more frequent photoparoxysmal responses than by the red flicker. For mean latencies of photoparoxysmal responses elicited by each hemifield stimulation by the use of both stimuli,

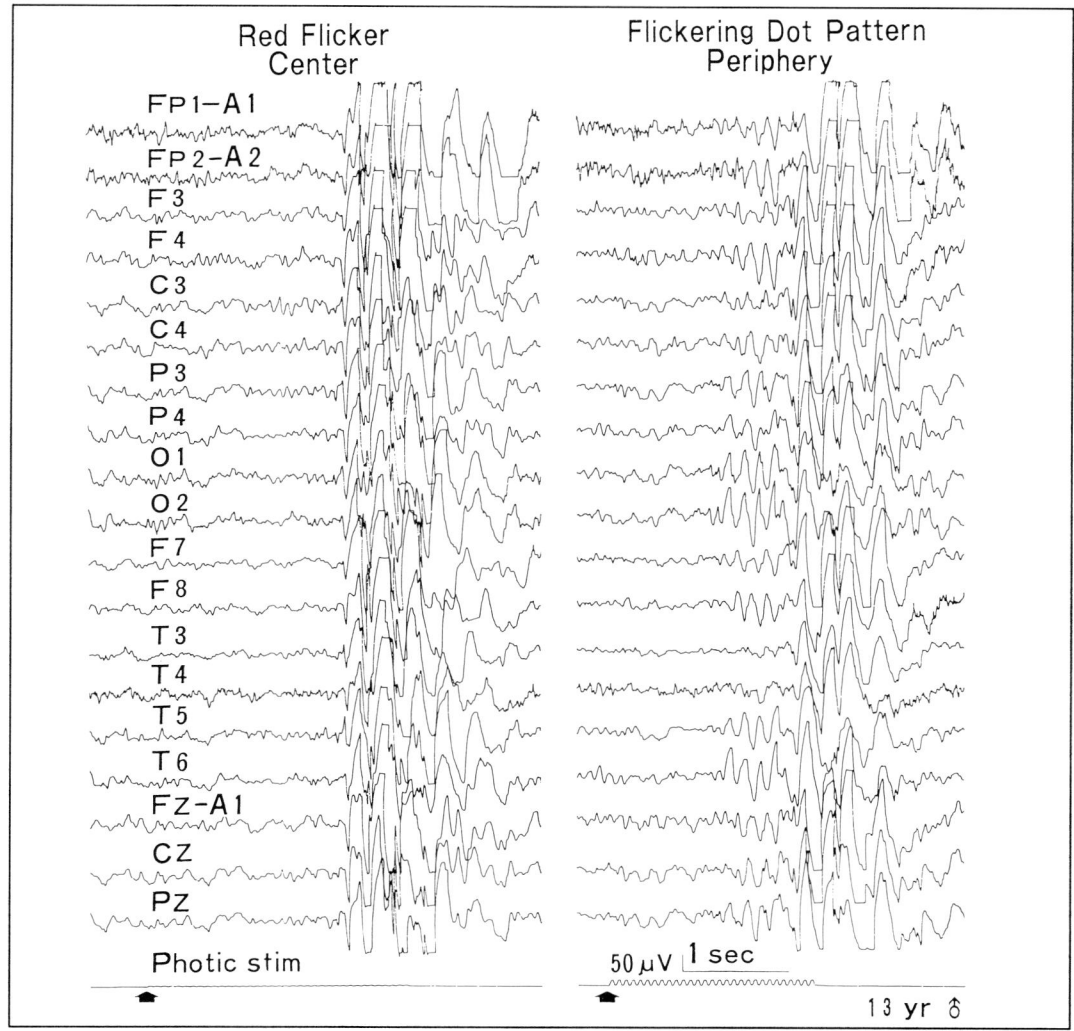

Fig. 2. Generalized photoparoxysmal responses elicited by red flicker stimulation of the centre and flickering dot pattern stimulation of the periphery in Case 7.

comparisons were made between (1) latencies in response to the stimuli to the full-field and each hemifield, and (2) latencies in response to the stimuli to the right and left hemifields; neither of them showed a statistically significant difference.

Table 5. Photoparoxysmal responses elicited by visual stimuli to each hemifield

Visual stimuli	No. of patients				Mean latency (s) ± SD			
	Left	Right	Upper	Lower	Left	Right	Upper	Lower
Grating pattern	1	1	0	0	2.60	3.00	–	–
Flickering dot	11	10	11	5	2.77 ± 1.28	3.49 ± 1.62	3.28 ± 1.49	3.82 ± 2.56
Red flicker	11	10	3	4	2.43 ± 1.53	1.75 ± 0.91	2.60 ± 0.40	3.95 ± 1.93

IDIOPATHIC GENERALIZED EPILEPSIES

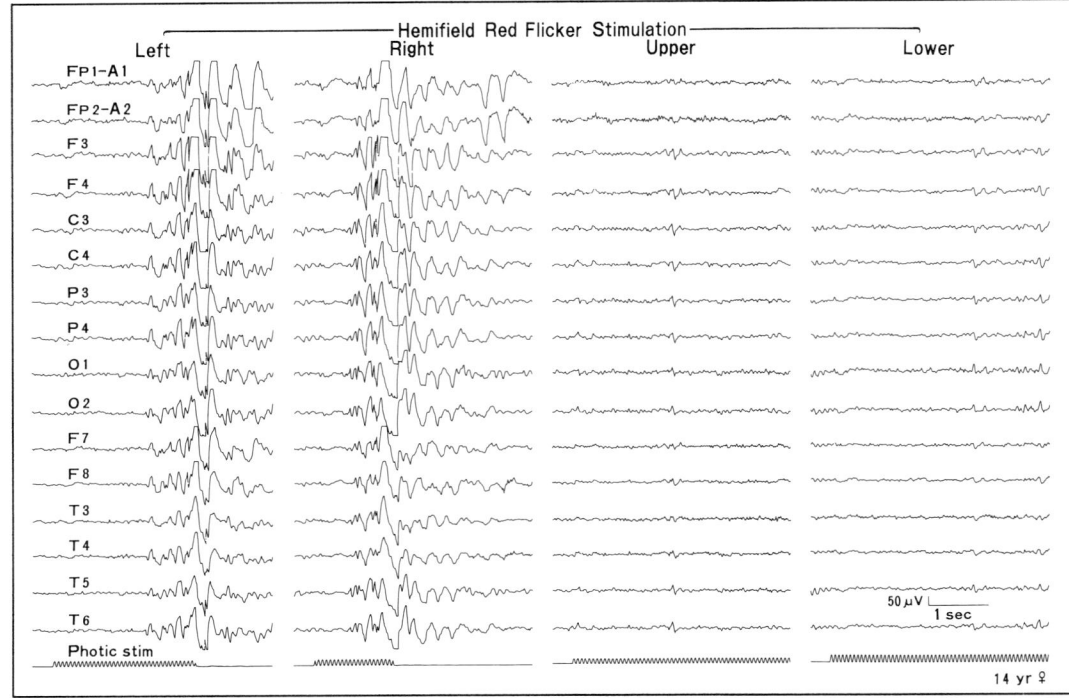

Fig. 3. EEG changes in response to each hemifield red flicker stimulation in case 12.

Lateral hemifield stimulation and three subgroups

Analysis of the results obtained by lateral hemifield stimulation gives us more clinically useful information than obtained by stimulation of the upper and lower hemifields. Attention was therefore paid only to the findings derived from the lateral hemifield stimulation (Table 6). In photosensitive individuals, EEG findings in response to lateral hemifield stimulation could be divided into three subgroups: equal, unequal and no photoparoxysmal responses (Takahashi, 1989, 1993).

Table 6. Lateral hemifield visual stimuli and clinical correlates

Subgroups	No. of patients (%)	Significant past histories (%)	Precipitating factors (%)
Equal response	13 (52)	0	8 (32)
Unequal response	4 (16)	4 (16)	2 (8)
No response	8 (32)	1 (4)	1 (4)
Total	25 (100)	5 (20)	11 (44)

Equal photoparoxysmal responses

Figure 3 shows an example of 'equal PPRs' in a 14-year-old female patient with epilepsy with grand mal seizures on awakening (Case 12). Generalized photoparoxysmal responses were immediately induced by lateral hemifield red flicker stimuli. This patient had no significant past history and genetic factors were presumed to have played an important role in the genesis of generalized PPRs.

Unequal photoparoxysmal responses

A 21-year-old patient with temporal lobe epilepsy (Case 14) has had complex partial seizures since

Chapter 27 Pathophysiological mechanisms of photosensitivity in IGEs

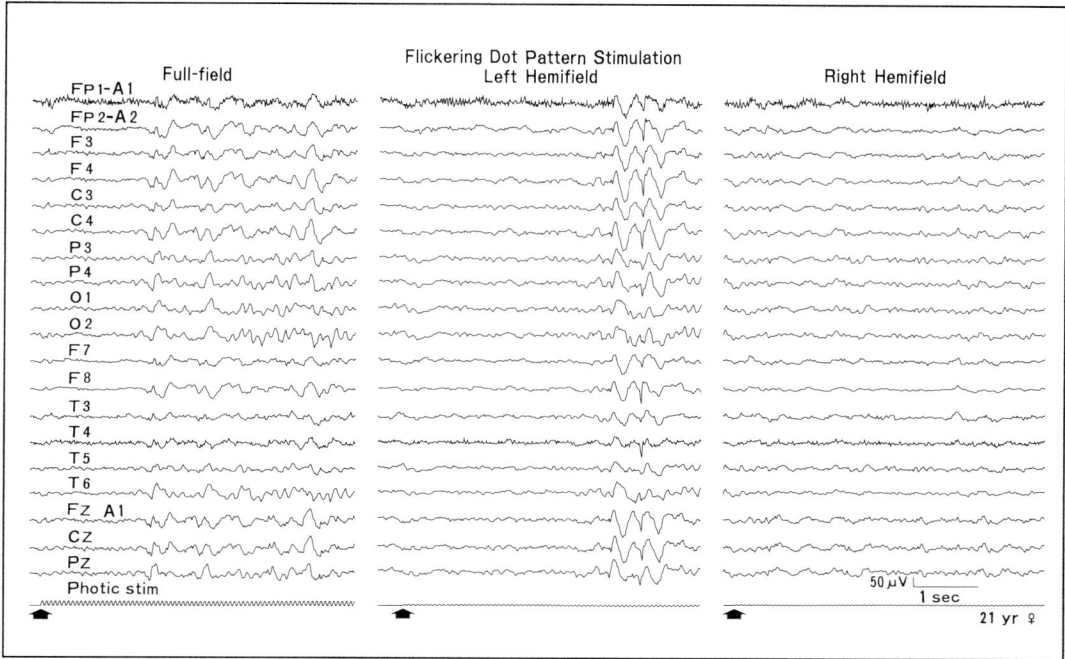

Fig. 4. EEG changes in response to full-field and lateral hemifield flickering dot pattern stimuli in Case 14.

the age of 15. Figure 4 shows the EEG findings produced by full-field and lateral hemifield the flickering dot pattern. Similar generalized photoparoxysmal responses elicited by the full-field stimulation were induced by the left hemifield stimulation; it was preceded by spikes over the posterior regions in the contralateral hemisphere. The right hemifield stimulation, however, was ineffective. A repeat examination showed the same findings. These EEG changes were designated 'unequal responses'. The left and right tracings in Fig. 5 demonstrate MRIs with T_1 and T_2 intensification, respectively, and disclosed a small cyst in the inner part of the left temporal lobe. Figure 6 shows SPECTs that reveal a hypoperfusion area in the inner part of the left temporal lobe.

No photoparoxysmal responses

In spite of showing sensitivity to the full-field stimuli, there was no provocation of photoparoxysmal responses. This is called 'no PPRs'. Table 6 shows results obtained by lateral hemifield stimulation in 25 photosensitive patients. Of four patients with unequal PPRs, two had previous histories of perinatal cerebral disturbance and two had suffered from head trauma. A total of 21 patients with equal PPRs and/or no PPRs revealed that seven and one patients had previous histories of febrile convulsions and perinatal cerebral disturbance, respectively. In other words, of the 21 patients, excluding those with febrile convulsions, only one patient (Case 18) showed a significant past history.

Lateral hemifield stimulation and visual precipitating factors

As shown in Table 6, of 17 patients with equal and unequal PPRs, 10 (40 per cent) had seizures with visual precipitating factors. On the contrary, visual precipitating factors were found in only one (4 per cent) out of eight patients with no PPRs.

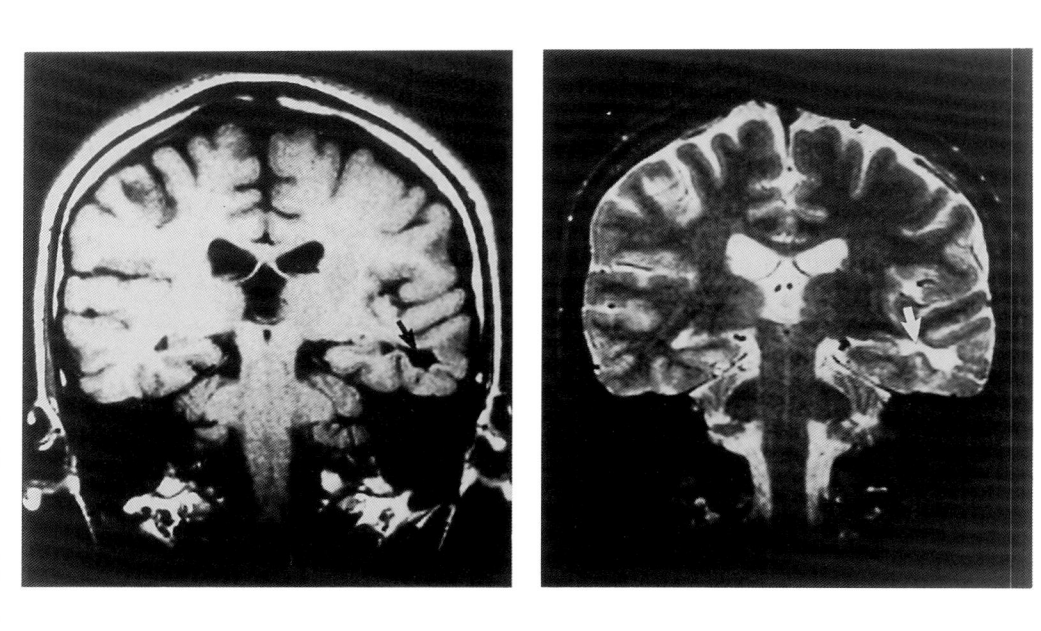

Fig. 5. MRI in Case 14. Coronal sections of T_1 (left tracing) and T_2 (right tracing) intensification. An arrow indicates a cyst in the left temporal lobe.

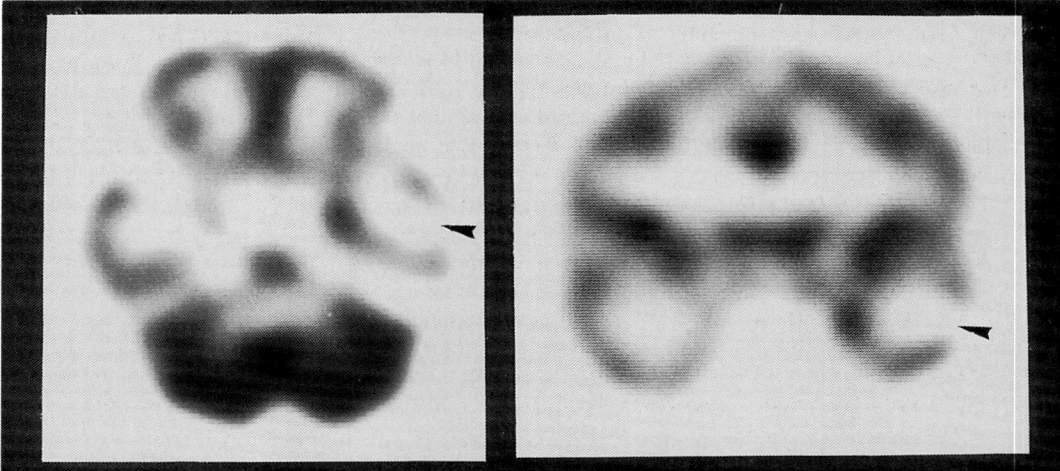

Fig. 6. 99Tc-HMPAO SPECT in Case 14. Transaxial (left tracing) and coronal (right tracing) sections. An arrow indicates a hypoperfusion area in the left temporal lobe.

Discussion

Since provocation of photoparoxysmal responses by a grating pattern stimulation to the full-field was observed in only three patients, discussion of the findings from regional visual stimuli will focus on those obtained by the flickering dot pattern and the red flicker stimuli.

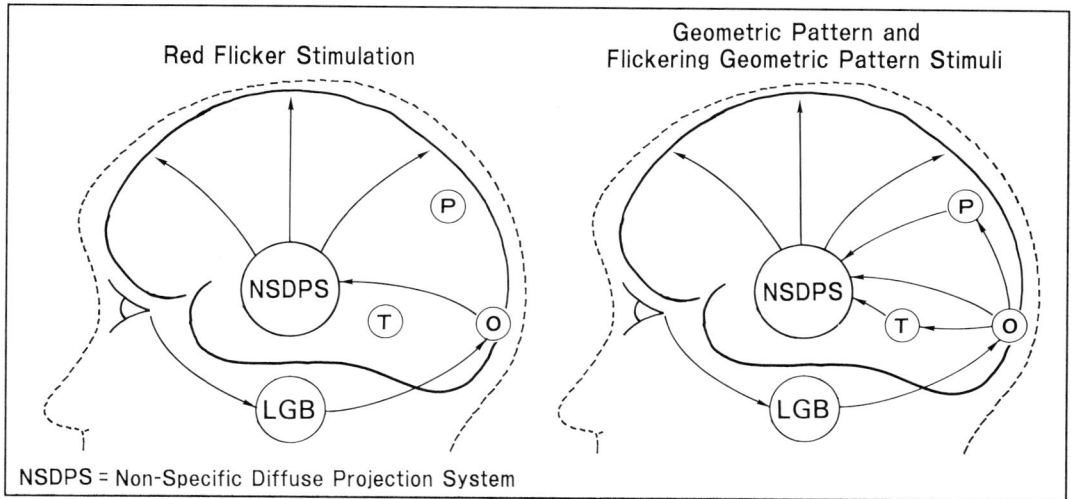

Fig. 7. Schematic representation of generalized photoparoxysmal responses elicited by the visual stimuli of red flicker, geometric patterns and flickering geometric patterns.

Stimulation to the centre and periphery

For generalized photoparoxysmal responses, our data indicate that red flicker stimulation of the centre is more effective than of the periphery, whereas flickering dot pattern stimulation of the periphery is more effective than of the centre. When the morphology of the photoparoxysmal responses elicited by the red flicker stimulation of the centre and the flickering dot pattern stimulation to the periphery is compared, as shown in Fig. 2, there appears to be a distinct difference between them: the simultaneous onset of photoparoxysmal responses from all areas of the brain was produced by red flicker stimulation of the centre, whereas its local onset from the posterior regions was produced by the flickering dot pattern stimulation of the periphery. Although each of the full-field stimuli was the most effective in eliciting photoparoxysmal responses, such a morphological difference of generalized photoparoxysmal responses became evident by the use of regional visual stimulation. Based on these findings, it may be assumed that the cortices primarily responsive to the red flicker and flickering geometric pattern stimuli are different. As reported earlier (Takahashi, 1989), when the retinotopic projection from the centre of the visual field onto the visual cortex is taken into consideration, the latter at the occipital pole is thought to be the most sensitive to red flicker stimulation. Similarly, the anterior portion of the striate cortex would be more sensitive to flickering geometric pattern stimulation. In addition to this area, parastriate cortices of areas 18 and 19 might also be hyperexcitable to flickering geometric pattern stimulation because the spikes of photoparoxysmal responses elicited by that stimulation always occur over the occipital, posterior–temporal, and parietal areas. Therefore, the patients sensitive to the red flicker and the flickering geometric pattern stimuli, for example, are thought to have hyperexcitable areas not only in the striate cortex but also in the parastriate cortices. As shown in Fig. 7, local photoparoxysmal responses in the striate cortex elicited by the red flicker stimulation would immediately transmit to the nonspecific diffuse projection system. This could give rise to generalized photoparoxysmal responses with their simultaneous occurrence over all the areas as distinguished from those elicited by the flickering geometric pattern stimulation. In the latter, initial local photoparoxysmal responses would seem to be produced in the striate cortex as well as in the parastriate cortices. These might produce different generalized photoparoxysmal responses, preceded by spikes over the posterior regions.

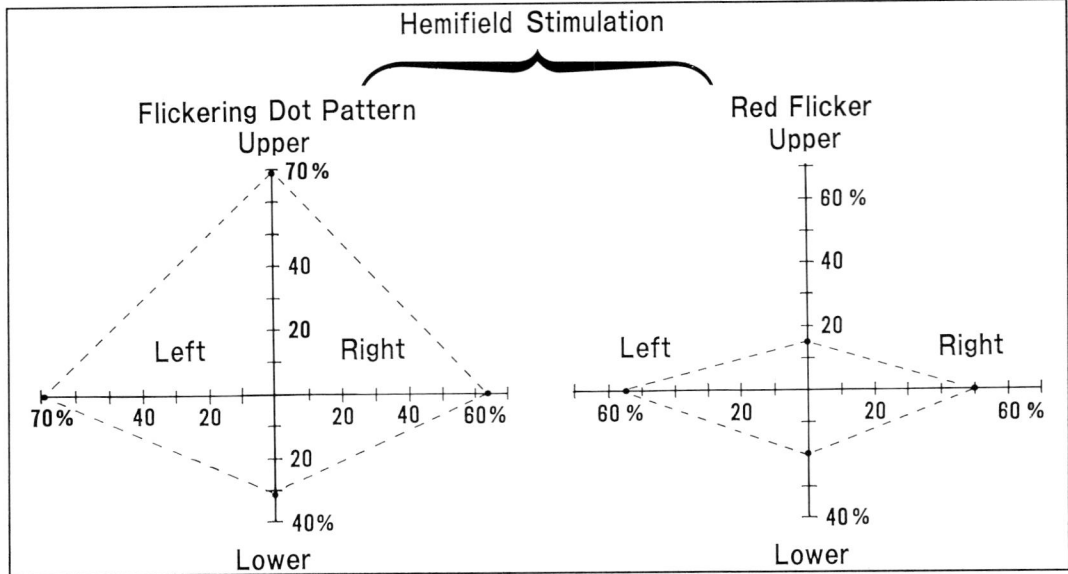

Fig. 8. *Effective visual fields by both stimuli in eliciting generalized photoparoxysmal responses in 25 patients with photosensitive epilepsy.*

Hemifield stimulation

Based on the results shown in Table 5, effective visual fields by both stimuli in eliciting generalized photoparoxysmal responses are schematically shown in Fig. 8. Those produced by the red flicker were narrow in the vertical direction compared to those produced by the flickering dot pattern; with regard to those produced by upper and lower hemifield flickering dot pattern, the upper hemifield was more potent than the lower one. Considering the retinotopic projection from these visual fields onto the visual cortex (Takahashi, 1984, 1993), our data in photosensitive patients would suggest the following: (1) hyperexcitable visual areas sensitive to a flickering dot pattern might be more widely spread in the lower than in the upper lips of the visual cortex, and (2) those sensitive to red flicker, the lower lips in particular, might be slightly more narrow than those sensitive to a flickering dot pattern. Owing to the EEG findings in response to lateral hemifield stimulation, photosensitive patients could be divided into three subgroups: (1) equal PPRs (sensitive to each lateral hemifield stimulation), (2) unequal PPRs (sensitive to either right or left hemifield stimulation), and (3) no PPRs (sensitive to neither right nor left hemifield stimulation). When these subgroups are considered from an aetiological viewpoint, our data suggest that unequal PPRs are significantly related to acquired factors, whereas equal PPRs and no PPRs probably have a closer link to genetic factors. Regarding the unequal PPRs of case 14, further explanation may be needed. In this patient, upper hemifield flickering dot pattern stimulation induced generalized PPRs similar to those induced by the full-field and left hemifield stimuli. These findings would suggest that the right lower lip of the visual cortex is the area most sensitive to that stimulation. It would also suggest that structural changes associated with lowered blood flow in the inner part of the left temporal lobe, as demonstrated in Figs. 5 and 6, might perhaps caused an insensitivity to the right hemifield stimulation. Precipitating factors were more often found in the groups with equal PPRs and unequal PPRs than in the group with no PPRs. All the results described above suggest that the EEG examination by regional visual stimuli in patients with photosensitive epilepsy is a clinically useful method that may provide valuable information for the understanding of IGEs as well. Additionally, we indicated that blue sunglasses are useful in the treatment of epilepsy patients who are sensitive to red flicker and/or flickering geometric pattern stimuli (Takahashi & Tsukahara, 1992). In a practical manner, occasionally wearing blue sunglasses while watching television and when confronted by a flickering light stimulus, in conjunction with antiepileptic drug therapy (e.g. valproate), has brought about good results in our experience.

Acknowledgement

The author wishes to thank Professor Yasuo Tsukahara for his discussions of the manuscript and Messrs Kazuya Kuriyagawa and Kazuyoshi Kataoka for their help in recording EEGs. The author is also very grateful for Dr Kiyoshi Ishii, who provided us with radiological data.

References

Binnie, C.D. & Jeavons, P.M. (1992): Photosensitive epilepsies. In: *Epileptic syndromes in infancy, childhood and adolescence*, eds. J. Roger, M. Burreau, Ch. Dravet, F.E. Dreifuss, A. Perret & P. Wolf, pp. 299–305. London: John Libbey.

Commission on Classification and Terminology of the International League against Epilepsy (1989): Proposal for classification of epilepsies and epileptic syndromes. *Epilepsia* **30,** 389–399.

Matsuoka, H., Saito, H., Fuse, Y., Matsue, K. & Sato, M. (1989): Subgroups of epilepsy and photosensitivity. *Jap. J. EEG EMG* **17,** 71.

Takahashi, T., Tsukahara, Y. & Kaneda, S. (1980): EEG activation by use of stroboscope and visual stimulator SLS-5100. *Tohoku J. Exp. Med.* **130,** 403–409.

Takahashi, T. (1984): Hemifield red flicker stimulation in a patient with pattern-sensitive epilepsy. *Epilepsia* **25,** 223–228.

Takahashi, T. (1989): Techniques of intermittent photic stimulation and paroxysmal responses. *Am. J. EEG Technol.* **29,** 205–218.

Takahashi, T. & Tsukahara, Y. (1992): Usefulness of blue sunglasses in photosensitive epilepsy. *Epilepsia* **33,** 517–521.

Takahashi, T. (1993): Activation methods. In: *Electroencephalography: basic principles, clinical applications, and related fields*, eds. E. Niedermeyer & F. Lopes da Silva, pp. 241–262. Baltimore: Williams & Wilkins.

Chapter 28

Photosensitivity and epilepsy: a genetic approach

Stephan Waltz

Neuropediatric Department, University of Kiel, Schwanenweg 20, D-24105 Kiel, Germany

Introduction

Photosensitivity is a frequent electroencephalographic finding in idiopathic generalized epilepsy. It is the most frequent environmental seizure precipitating mechanism in epilepsy (Kasteleijn-Nolst Trenité *et al.*, Ch. 26). Moreover, family studies showed that photosensitivity is a major factor in the multifactorial pathogenesis of epilepsy. Thus genetic studies of photosensitivity, appear to be an important contribution to the genetics of idiopathic generalized epilepsy. However, there still is no universally accepted definition of the photoparoxysmal response (PPR), the electroencephalographical correlate of photosensitivity and its mode of inheritance is difficult to assess. In a first step, an approach towards a rational definition of the photoparoxysmal response, valuable for genetic studies, is shown. In a second step, the role of photosensitivity in the pathogenesis of epilepsy will be reviewed. Third, current knowledge about genetics of photosensitivity will be reviewed, and evidence for the autosomal-dominant transmission of photosensitivity is presented.

Definition

Photosensitivity is defined by the occurrence of spikes or spikes and waves in response to intermittent light stimulation. It has carefully to be distinguished from generalized spikes and waves during rest and hyperventilation, which have been shown to be genetically different (Rabending & Klepel, 1970; Doose & Gerken, 1973).

The precise definition of the electroencephalographical correlate of photosensitivity has been discussed controversially for a long time. In their original description, Bickford *et al.* (1952) claimed, that exclusively *generalized* spikes and waves elicited by photic stimulation should be regarded as photosensitivity, because of their close relationship to epilepsy. This phenomen was called photoconvulsive reaction. Investigators who follow this definition in clinical studies consequently find a high correlation between photosensitivity and epilepsy (Jeavons & Harding, 1975; Binnie *et al.*, 1986; Kasteleijn-Nolst Trenité *et al.*, 1987; Obeid *et al.*, 1991; Binnie & Jeavons, 1992). An even stronger association with epilepsy was found by Reilly & Peters (1973), when 'self-limited' responses were disregarded and only generalized spikes and waves outlasting the duration of photic stimulation were accepted. Some authors (Binnie *et al.*, 1986; Kasteleijn-Nolst Trenité, 1989)

IDIOPATHIC GENERALIZED EPILEPSIES

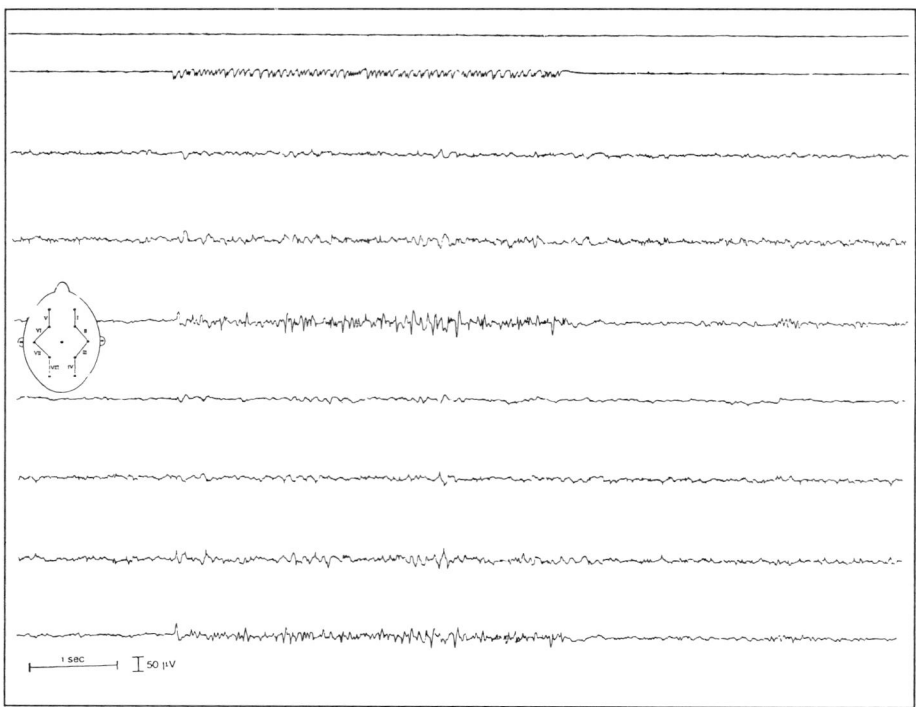

Fig. 1. Type 1: spikes within the occipital background activity.

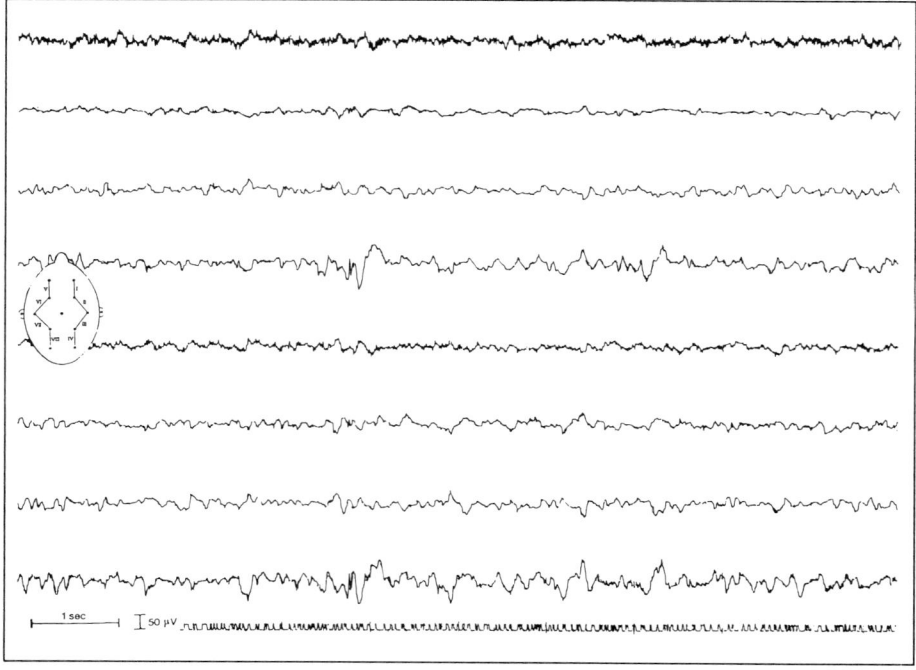

Fig. 2. Type 2: parieto-occipital spikes with a biphasic slow wave.

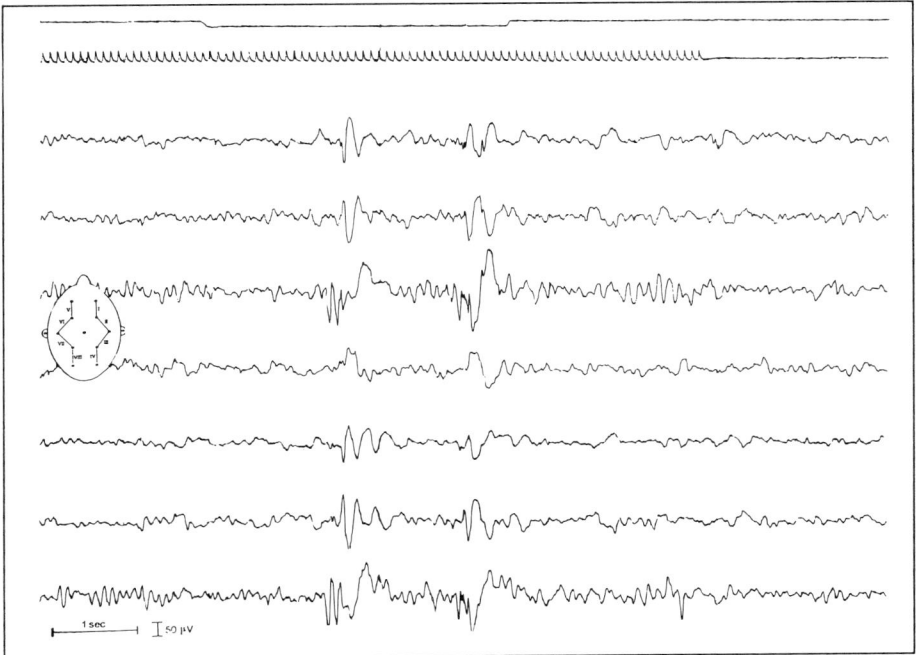

Fig. 3. Type 3: parieto-occipital with a biphasic slow wave and spread to the frontal region.

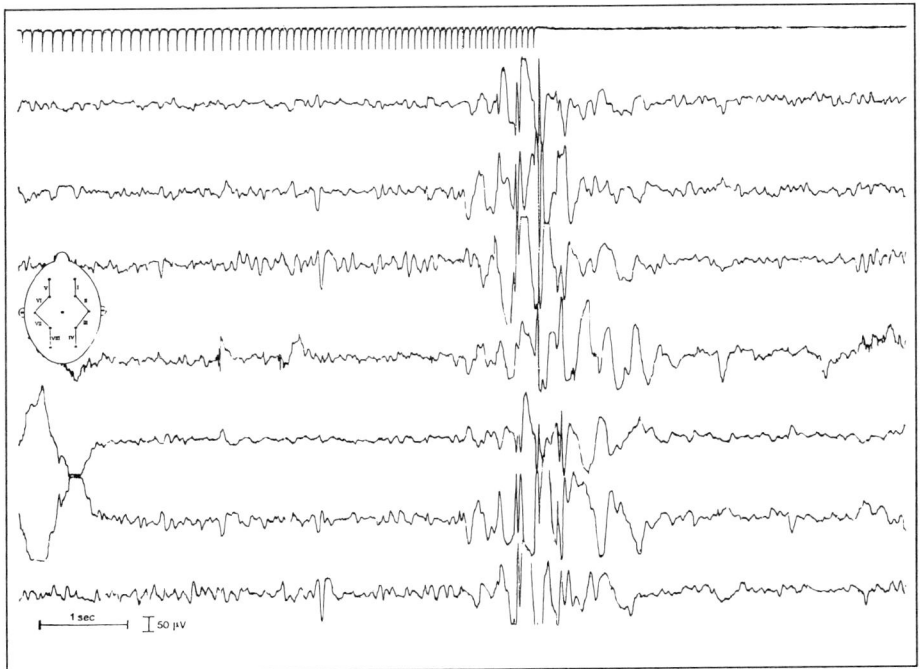

Fig. 4. Type 4: generalized spikes and waves.

consider responses as 'classical', if this criterion is fulfilled. However, the findings of Reilly & Peters (1973) were not confirmed in subsequent studies by So et al. (1993) and Jayakar & Chiappa (1990), who showed that the classification as prolonged or self-limited might merely depend on the time the technician takes to stop the stimulus after the discharge has appeared.

As it became evident that the 'photoconvulsive reaction' is not necessarily accompanied by clinical seizures, and that most seizures provoked by intermittent light stimulation are not convulsive, the term was abandoned and replaced by 'photoparoxysmal response' (Klass & Fischer-Williams, 1976).

A definition different to that of Bickford et al. (1952) was chosen by Doose and coworkers (Doose et al., 1969; Doose & Gerken, 1973) and Rabending & Klepel (1970) in genetic studies of photosensitivity. They also included discharges confined to the parieto-occipital region, if definite spikes were registered. In their studies, the photoparoxysmal response appears as a rather widespread condition with variable expression, occurring in 7.6 per cent of healthy children (Doose & Gerken, 1973).

To clarify the significance of the different responses to intermittent light stimulation and to obtain a rational definition of the photoparoxysmal response suitable for genetic studies, a family study in 135 photosensitive probands and 371 relatives was carried out (Waltz et al., 1992). In a categorial order, the photoparoxysmal response was subclassified into four different types according to the degree of generalization:

> Type 1: spikes within the occipital background activity (Fig. 1)
>
> Type 2: parieto-occipital spikes with a biphasic slow wave (Fig. 2)
>
> Type 3: parieto-occipital spikes with a biphasic slow wave and spread to the frontal region (Fig. 3)
>
> Type 4: generalized spikes and waves or polyspikes and waves (= photoconvulsive reaction of Bickford et al., 1952) (Fig. 4).

The incidence of photoparoxysmal response in siblings of probands with a Type 1–3 photoparoxysmal response was as high as in those of probands with a Type 4 photoparoxysmal response (= photoconvulsive reaction) (35 per cent and 38 per cent). Thus, the genetic impact of less expressive types of the photoparoxysmal response is the same as that of the generalized type of the photoparoxysmal response. The ensuing assumption, that generalized spikes and waves are just one of the phenotypical expressions of photosensitivity was endorsed by the significant age-dependency of the phenotypical expression of the photoparoxysmal response (Fig. 5): Type 4 discharges were the most frequent finding in relatives up to 10 years of age. The rate of Type 2 discharges was significantly higher in 11–15-year-old individuals than in younger or older ones. Finally Type 1 discharges occurred almost exclusively in relatives older than 15 years.

The marked age-dependency, the identical incidence rate in siblings of probands with Type 1–3 discharges compared to siblings of probands with Type 4 discharges and the occurrence of different types in the same patient strongly suggest that the diverse types of the photoparoxysmal response only represent different levels of expression of the same genetically determined trait. The photoconvulsive reaction as defined by Bickford et al. (1952) represents only a special case in this spectrum. For genetic studies however, the whole spectrum has to be considered.

Incidence

Incidence figures of photosensitivity given in the literature vary largely, depending on the definition of the photoparoxysmal response, the stimulation technique and the age of the studied population (for an overview, see Newmark & Penry (1979)). For genetic purpose, investigations of populations beyond the age of maximum penetrance are of limited value. The same applies for studies using the restrictive definition of Bickford et al. (1952) only, leading to an important bias towards underes-

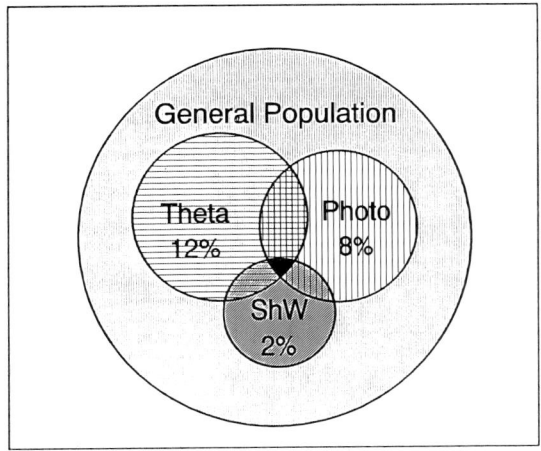

Fig. 5. Age-dependent expression of the photoparoxysmal response in affected relatives of photosensitive probands (N = 114). (From Waltz et al. 1992).

timation. In a standardized investigation of 662 healthy children between 1 and 16 years old, Doose & Gerken (1973) found a photoparoxysmal response in 7.6 per cent, considering the four types of the photoparoxysmal response. Only 2.9 per cent of the children showed generalized spikes and waves (Type 4). A similar result has been reported by Eeg-Olofsson et al. (1971), who found a photopar-oxysmal response in 8.3 per cent and generalized discharges in 2.1 per cent of healthy children under 15 years. In both studies, females were more often affected than males.

Although photosensitivity is not specific for epilepsy, its incidence in individuals with epilepsy is strikingly elevated. Photosensitivity is found in generalized and in focal epilepsy (Andermann, 1982b) as well as in idiopathic, cryptogenic and sympomatic epilepsies, but the highest incidence has been found in generalized epilepsy (Wolf & Goosses, 1986). In the study of Wolf & Goosses (1986), 13 per cent of patients with absence-epilepsies were photosensitive with a marked difference between childhood absence epilepsy (7.5 per cent) and juvenile absence epilepsy (18 per cent). This difference was not reduplicated by Waltz et al. (1990), who found an overall rate of photosensitivity of 18 per cent in both absence epilepsies. At age 10–14 years, 32 per cent were affected (Waltz, 1994). The overall rate of photosensitivity in patients with juvenile myoclonic epilepsy (JME) was found to be 30 to 38 per cent (Asconape & Penry, 1984; Wolf & Goosses, 1986; Obeid & Panayiotopoulos, 1988; Waltz et al., 1990). Juvenile myoclonic epilepsy patients without absences showed even a higher rate than those with absences (42 per cent vs 29 per cent (Waltz et al., 1990)). It is important to notice, that all these studies were done in mainly adult patients, who had mostly been treated with antiepileptic drugs. Thus, these figures are thought to represent only a minimum and not the real incidence (Wolf, 1992).

Photosensitivity in the multifactorial pathogenesis of epilepsy

Epilepsies are regarded as multifactorially determined disorders (Andermann, 1982a). There is evidence that multiple gene loci are involved in the pathogenesis of idiopathic generalized epilepsy (Greenberg et al., 1992). Genetic analysis of such disorders is extremely difficult (Anderson & Hauser, 1988). Studying the genetic basis of epilepsies, one may profit from the advantage that some of the involved pathogenetic factors can be visualized by the EEG. On the basis of large EEG studies, including patients with epilepsies and their relatives as well as healthy controls, Doose and coworkers showed that generalized spikes and waves at rest or hyperventilation, 4–7/s rhythms, benign focal sharp waves and photosensitivity can be regarded as markers of a genetically determined seizure liability (Doose & Gerken 1972, 1973; Gerken & Doose, 1973; Doose & Baier, 1987, 1989; Doose, 1989; Doose & Waltz, 1993).

The main conclusions from these studies will be summarized briefly. The EEG traits mentioned are independently transmitted and are remarkably widespread in the general population: 4–7/s (theta) rhythms were found in 12 per cent, benign focal sharp waves and generalized spikes and waves in 2 per cent each and a photoparoxysmal response in 8 per cent of healthy children. Only a small proportion of carriers of one of these traits will exhibit seizures. As these traits are inherited independently, coincidences will occur with calculable probability and consequently some individ-

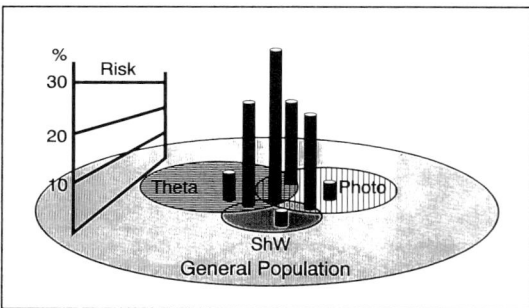

Fig. 6. *Distribution of genetic liabilities characterized by EEG markers in healthy children aged 2–15 years. (Theta = theta rhytm, Photo = photoparoxysmal response, Shw = focal sharp waves). (From Doose & Waltz, 1993.)*

uals will show two of these traits (Fig. 6). The seizure risk of carriers of one of these traits barely exceeds that of the general population (Fig. 7). For example, the seizure risk in individuals with a photoparoxysmal response alone is 2 per cent. By contrast, in combination with theta-rhythms, the seizure risk is significantly increased (Gundel & Doose, 1986; Baier & Doose, 1987) and higher than in carriers of only one of these traits (Fig. 7). Thus it is the coincidence of two different genetic traits, either of which has little clinical significance alone, which accounts for the increased seizure risk of the individual. The interaction of these EEG-traits has been reviewed in more detail by Doose & Gundel (1982) and Doose & Waltz (1993).

Several family studies have been undertaken to clarify the pathogenetic relations between photosensitivity and epilepsy. Two different types of studies can be distinguished: those investigating the incidence of photosensitivity in relatives of probands with photosensitivity and/or epilepsy (Rabending & Klepel, 1970; Waltz et al., 1992) and those investigating the influence of photosensitivity on the seizure risk (Doose et al., 1969; Hauser et al., 1983; Doose & Baier 1987; Waltz & Doose 1994).

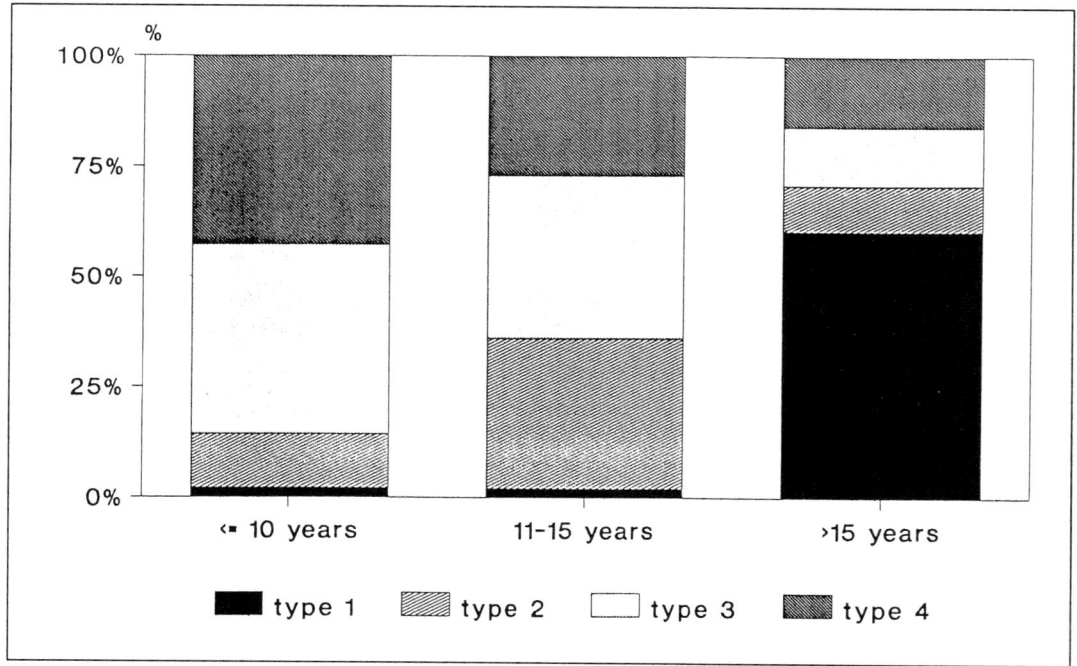

Fig. 7. *Seizure risk and interacting genetic liabilities. (From Doose & Waltz, 1993.)*

Photosensitivity in relatives of probands with photosensitivity and/or epilepsy

Rabeding & Klepel (1970) investigated the incidence of photosensitivity in relatives of photosensitive probands with heterogenous clinical conditions compared to relatives of patients with spike-and-wave absences without photosensitivity. A photoparoxysmal response was found significantly more often in siblings of photosensitive probands (22.0 per cent) than in siblings of probands with absences (7.8 per cent). Waltz et al. (1992) studied photosensitivity in relatives of photosensitive probands with and without epilepsy. The rate of photosensitivity was equal in both groups: siblings of probands with epilepsy showed the trait in 39 per cent, parents in 15 per cent; the respective figures in relatives of probands without epilepsy were 44 per cent and 18 per cent. Thus the incidence of photosensitivity is closely related to photosensitivity in the index case, but it does not depend on whether the proband has epilepsy or not.

Photosensitivity and seizure risk

Doose et al. (1969) reported that the seizure risk in relatives of photosensitive individuals with epilepsy was significantly higher (4.4 per cent) than in relatives of photosensitive probands without epilepsy (1.6 per cent). The authors concluded that photosensitivity alone, without an additional genetic impact towards epilepsy, does not lead to an increased seizure risk. This assumption is consistent with the results of three follow-up studies of initially non-epileptic photosensitive patients: less than 2 per cent developed seizures (Scollo-Lavizzari, 1971; Iwannek, 1979; So et al., 1993). In interaction with other genetic factors predisposing to epilepsy, however, photosensitivity produces an enhancing effect. This was confirmed by Hauser et al. (1983), who investigated siblings of seizure patients with different EEG findings. Siblings of patients with generalized spikes and waves (in rest or hyperventilation) alone, presented more often with seizures than siblings of probands who showed only photosensitivity in the EEG. The highest seizure risk was found in siblings of probands with both spikes and waves *and* photosensitivity.

In a recent study, the influence of a parental photosensitvity was studied in siblings of epileptic probands with one photosensitive parent (Waltz & Doose, 1994, unpublished data). The incidence of photoparoxysmal response and seizures in the siblings were determined and compared to that in siblings of photosensitive probands with epilepsy and both parents without photosensitivity. Out of 60 siblings of probands with one photosensitive parent, 18 per cent presented with seizures, compared to 4 per cent of 93 siblings of photosensitive probands whose parents were not photosensitive. The same significant difference was found when families with seizures in the parental generation were excluded. A similar finding was reported by Doose & Baier (1987) in a family study of patients with idiopathic generalized epilepsy. This is remarkable for two reasons. First, according to the above mentioned studies of Doose and coworkers and Rabending & Klepel (1970), photosensitivity alone can hardly explain the significantly increased seizure risk in offspring. Secondly, photosensitivity is a strongly age-dependent trait (Fig. 8) and is only exceptionally seen in healthy adults (Kasteleijn-Nolst Trenité, 1989; Doose & Waltz, 1993). By contrast, in adult patients with generalized epilepsy, photosensitivity is is found in up to 42 per cent (see above). Thus, the exceptional persistance of photosensitivity into adult age might be due to the interaction with other genetic factors predisposing to epilepsy, explaining the increased seizure risk in offspring.

In both groups, photosensitive siblings had a higher seizure risk than non-photosensitive siblings. The highest seizure risk was found in photosensitive siblings of probands with one photosensitive parent (33 per cent), only 9 per cent of non-photosensitive siblings had seizures. The same trend was found in the families without photosensitivity in parents, but the difference did not reach statistical significance (7 per cent *vs* 3 per cent).

Although the pathogenetic relations between photosensitivity and epilepsy have not been fully elicited yet, the following conclusions may be derived:

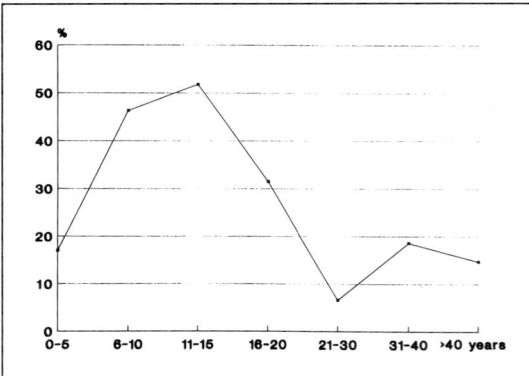

Fig. 8. Age-dependent penetrance of the photoparoxysmal response in relatives of photosensitive probands (n = 371). (From Waltz et al., 1992.)

The incidence of photosensitivity in relatives of photosensitive probands does not depend on whether the proband has epilepsy or not. By contrast, it is closely related to photosensitivity in the index case.

Photosensitivity alone does not necessarily indicate an increased seizure risk.

In the presence of other genetic factors predisposing to epilepsy, photosensitivity entails a substantial enhancing effect: the seizure risk in relatives of patients with epilepsy is increased, if photosensitivity is shown in the parental generation or in the individual itself.

Genetics

Family studies

Family studies provided ample evidence for genetic transmission of photosensitivity (Davidson & Watson, 1956; Doose et al., 1969; Rabending & Klepel, 1970; Doose & Gerken, 1973; Waltz et al., 1992; Waltz & Doose, 1992b) with age- and sex-dependent penetrance (for literature, see Newmark & Penry (1979)). The age of maximum penetrance is between 5 and 15 years of age (Fig. 8). Females are significantly more often affected than males. The overall incidence of PPR in siblings of unselected photosensitive probands in a paediatric population was 26.2 per cent (Doose et al., 1969), 22.0 per cent (Rabending & Klepel, 1970) and 22.9 per cent (Doose & Gerken, 1973). At the age of maximum penetrance, up to 40 per cent of siblings showed the trait (Doose et al., 1969; Doose & Gerken, 1973). Parents were found to be affected in 10.3 per cent (Rabending & Klepel, 1970) and in 16.1 per cent (Waltz et al., 1992). The only investigation in offspring of photosensitive probands was done by Watson & Marcus (1962), who found 32 per cent to be photosensitive. However, the authors mentioned neither number nor age of offspring.

Twin studies

A systematic study on photosensitive twins has not yet been published. In 11 pairs of monozygotic twins reported in the literature (Newmark & Penry, 1979), 10 were shown to be concordant for photosensitivity. The only discordant pair of identical twins were two boys who showed physical differences in height and weight (Jeavons & Harding, 1975). We observed one pair of monozygotic twins, which was concordant not only for photosensitivity, but also for the phenotypical expression of the photoparoxysmal response and the frequency of photic stimulation at which the responses were obtained. As no data on dizygotic twins for comparison are available, the high concordance rate in monozygotic twins is suggestive of an important genetic influence but cannot be used to determine a specific pattern of inheritance.

Mode of inheritance

The large family studies were confined to siblings (Doose et al., 1969; Doose & Gerken, 1973) or siblings and parents of photosensitive probands (Rabending & Klepel, 1970) and failed to reveal a defined pattern of inheritance. The major problem in assessing the mode of inheritance of photosensitivity is the age-dependent penetrance with the ensuing difficulty to ascertain photosensitivity in adults. Photic stimulation with a negative result in an adult does not necessarily mean that he is not affected, as he might have shown the trait at a younger age. As a consequence, in adults, the affection status can only be accurately defined in photosensitive subjects. Therefore our EEG study on the mode of transmission of the photoparoxysmal response was carried out in siblings of mostly epileptic patients with one photosensitive parent (Waltz & Doose, 1992a). The incidence of the photoparoxysmal response in the siblings of the probands was compared to that in siblings of photosensitive probands with both parents being unaffected. The incidence of the photoparoxysmal response in all 83 siblings of probands with one photosensitive parent was 39 per cent. At the age of maximum penetrance (5–15 years), 49 per cent of the remaining 51 siblings were carriers of photoparoxysmal response. In the control families with both parents being unaffected only 15 per cent of 82 siblings showed the trait. Girls were slightly more often affected than boys. These data indicate that a photoparoxysmal response in parents is a major determinant for the risk of photoparoxysmal response in offspring and are strongly suggestive of an autosomal-dominant mode of inheritance with sex- and age-dependent penetrance. As it appears reasonable to admit that some of the parents in the control families, which were classified as non-photosensitive after investigation at adult age, had been photosensitive in childhood, there might be autosomal-dominant transmission in some of these families, while the photosensitive probands of the remaining families might be sporadic cases. No evidence for sex-linked or mitochondrial transmission was found. The assumption of a single locus mendelian mode of inheritance is supported by several published pedigrees (Watson & Davidson, 1957; Watson & Marcus, 1962; Jeavons & Harding, 1987) and case histories (Haneke, 1963; Delgado-Escueta et al., 1975) consistent with autosomal-dominant transmission. However, an autosomal-recessive mode of inheritance cannot be ruled out in the control families of our study and genetic heterogeneity has to be considered. Confirmation of our data through investigation of offspring of grown-up patients who were photosensitive in childhood or adolescence is desirable, but will be difficult to obtain.

Molecular genetic approach

In view of the conflicting results obtained in molecular genetic studies of clinically defined syndromes (Whitehouse et al., 1993; Serratosa et al., 1993; Delgado-Escueta et al., Ch. 24; Janz et al., Ch. 25), genetic analysis of the underlying pathogenetic factors, as shown in the EEG, appears to be a promising alternative. In this context, the photoparoxysmal response is a suitable candidate for linkage analysis: it is a frequent and well defined EEG trait and its incidence in idiopathic generalized epilepsy is strikingly elevated. It is easily detectable and reproducible in an adequate recording and evidence for a mendelian mode of inheritance is given. Before performing molecular genetic studies of EEG traits involved in the pathogenesis of epilepsy, systematic EEG studies in families of affected probands have to be done in order to obtain a sufficient number of multiplex families. Furthermore, all EEG traits associated with epilepsy are strongly age dependent. Thus, a maximum of family members should be investigated at the age of maximum penetrance. In the neuropediatric department in Kiel, family EEG studies have been performed since 1969. Out of this large data pool, 15 multiplex families suitable for linkage analysis have been selected and blood samples for DNA extraction have been collected. Before screening the entire human genome with microsatellites, the hypothesis of linkage to known loci of disorders associated with photosensitivity will be tested.

Juvenile myoclonic epilepsy (JME)

A gene locus for juvenile myoclonic epilepsy has been mapped to chromosome 6p on the basis of linkage to the BF and HLA-loci (Greenberg et al., 1987; Durner et al., 1991) applying a variable phenotype definition of affected relatives. In six of 11 families in the study of Greenberg et al. (1987) affectedness of a family member was not determined by clinical epilepsy, but exclusively by a 'epileptiform' EEG-pattern (Delgado-Escueta et al., 1994). In Durner's study, the lod-score in favour of linkage was higher, when healthy relatives with generalized spikes and waves in the EEG were included. In neither of the studies it was mentioned whether these EEG-changes occurred spontaneously or during photic stimulation. Thus the HLA-region on chromosome 6p is an interesting candidate locus for photosensitivity.

Progressive myoclonus epilepsy (PME) Unverricht–Lundborg

Progressive myoclonus epilepsy Unverricht–Lundborg is transmitted by an autosomal-recessive mode of inheritance. Photosensitivity is found in almost 90 per cent of patients with this type of progressive myoclonus epilepsy (Roger *et al.*, 1992). Despite its progressive course it shares some clinical and electroencephalographical features with idiopathic generalized epilepsy (Koskiniemi *et al.*, 1974a, b): age of onset is between 5 and 16 years, myoclonic seizures and generalized tonic–clonic seizures occur mostly on awakening. EEG recordings show generalized spikes and waves. Localization of the gene to chromosome 21 (21q22.3) was reported by Lehesjoki *et al.* (1991), and Malafosse *et al.* (1992) showed that the Mediterranean type of progressive myoclonus epilepsy maps to the same locus.

Gaucher's disease

Type 3 (juvenile form) is a rare subtype of Gaucher's disease and may present as progressive myoclonus epilepsy with onset in childhood or adolescence. Photosensitivity is a frequent EEG finding. The gene for the deficient enzyme glucocerebrosidase has been mapped to q21–q31 of chromosome 1 (Barnveld *et al.*, 1983).

Acknowledgements

I am very much indebted to Professor H. Doose for help and suggestions while preparing this paper. A part of the work was supported by the Wellcome-Stipendium für klinische Epilepsieforschung.

References

Andermann, E. (1982a): Multifactorial inheritance in generalized and focal epilepsy. In: *Genetic basis of the epilepsies*, eds. V.E. Anderson, W.A., Hauser, J.K. Penry & C.F. Sing, pp. 355–374. New York: Raven Press.

Andermann, E. (1982b): Family studies on epileptiform EEG abnormalities and photosensitivity in focal epilepsy. In: *Advances of epileptology: XIIIth Epilepsy international symposium*, eds. H. Akimoto, H. Kazamatsuri, M. Seino & A. Ward, pp. 105–112. New York: Raven Press.

Anderson, V.E. & Hauser, W.A. (1988): Genetics. In: *A textbook of epilepsy*, eds. J. Laidlaw, A. Richens & J. Oxley, pp. 49–77. Edinburgh: Churchill Livingstone.

Asconapé, J. & Penry, J.K. (1984): Some clinical and EEG aspects of benign juvenile myoclonic epilepsy. *Epilepsia* **25**, 108–114.

Baier, W.K. & Doose, H. (1987): Interdependence of different genetic EEG patterns in siblings of epileptic patients. *Electroencephalogr. Clin. Neurophysiol.* **66**, 483–488.

Barnveld, R.A., Kiejzer, U. Tegelders, F. et al. (1983): Assignment of the gene for human b-glucocoebrosidase to the region of g21-g31 of chromosome 1 using monoclonal antibodies. *Hum. Genet.* **64**, 227–231.

Bickford, R.G., Sem-Jacobsen, C.W., White, P.T. & Daly, D. (1952): Some observations on the mechanism of photic and photometrazol activation. *Electroencephalogr. Clin. Neurophysiol.* **4**, 275–282.

Binnie, C.D., Kasteleijn-Nolst Trenité, D.G.A. & De Korte, R. (1986): Photosensitivity as a model for acute antiepileptic drug studies. *Electroencephalogr. Clin. Neurophysiol.* **63**, 35–41.

Binnie, C. & Jeavons, P. (1992): Photosensitive epilepsies. In: *Epileptic syndromes in infancy, childhood and adolescence*, 2nd edn, eds. J. Roger, C. Dravet, M. Bureau, F. Dreifuss & P. Wolf, pp. 299–305. London: John Libbey.

Davidson S. & Watson C.W. (1956): Hereditary light sensitive epilepsy. *Neurology (Minneap.)* **6**, 235–261.

Delgado-Escueta A.V., Abad Herrera P., Treiman L., Maldonado H., Greenberg, D.A. & Schwartz B.E. (1987): Clinical and EEG phenotypes of early childhood photic and self-induced epilepsy: five generations in one pedigree. *Epilepsia* **28**, 584–585.

Delgado-Escueta, A.V., Serratosa, J.M., Liu, A. et al. (1994): Progress in mapping human epilepsy genes. *Epilepsia* **35(Suppl. 1)**, S29–S40.

Doose, H., Gerken H., Hien-Voelpel, K.F. & Voelzke, E. (1969): Genetics of photosensitive epilepsy. *Neuropaediatrie* **1**, 56–73.

Doose, H., Gerken, H. & Völzke, E. (1972): On the genetics of EEG-anomalies in childhood. I. Abnormal theta rhythms. *Neuropaediatrie* **3**, 386–401.

Doose, H. & Gerken, H. (1973): On the genetics of EEG-anomalies in childhood. IV. Photoconvulsive reaction. *Neuropaediatrie* **4**, 162–171.

Doose, H. & Gundel, A. (1982): 4 to 7 CPS rhythms in the childhood EEG. In: *Genetic basis of the epilepsies*, eds. V.E. Anderson, W.A. Hauser, J.K. Penry & C.F. Sing, pp. 83–92, New York: Raven Press.

Doose, H. & Baier, W.K. (1987): Genetic factors in epilepsies with primarily generalized minor seizures. *Neuropediatrics* **18(Suppl. I)**, 1–64.

Doose, H. (1989): Generalized spikes and waves. In: *Genetics of the epilepsies*, G. Beck-Managetta, V.E. Anderson, H. Doose & D. Janz, pp. 95–103. New York, Heidelberg: Springer Verlag.

Doose, H. & Baier, W.K. (1989): Benign partial epilepsies and related syndromes – multifactorial pathogenesis with hereditary impairment of brain maturation. *Eur. J. Pediatr.* **149**, 152–158.

Doose, H. & Waltz, S. (1993): Photosensitivity: genetics and clinical significance. *Neuropediatrics* **24**, 250–255.

Durner, M., Sander, T., Greenberg, D.A., Johnson, K., Beck-Managetta, G. & Janz, D. (1991): Localization of idiopathic generalized epilepsy on chromosome 6p in families of juvenile myoclonic epilepsy patients. *Neurology* **41**, 1651–1655.

Eeg-Olofsson, O., Petersén, I. & Selldén, U. (1971): The development of the electroencephalogram im normal children from the age of 1 through 15 years. *Neuropädiatrie* **2**, 375–404.

Gerken, H. & Doose, H. (1973): On the genetics of EEG-anomalies in childhood. III. Spikes and waves. *Neuropädiatrie* **4**, 88–97.

Greenberg, D.A., Delgado-Escueta, A.V., Widelitz, H. et al. (1987): A locus involved in the expression of juvenile myoclonic epilepsy and of an associated EEG trait may be linked to HLA and Bf. *Cytogenet. Cell. Genet.* **46**, 623.

Greenberg, D., Durner, M. & Delgado-Escueta, A. (1992): Evidence for multiple gene loci in the expression of the common generalized epilepsies. *Neurology* **42(Suppl. 5)**, 56–62.

Hauser, W.A., Anderson, V.E. & Rich, S.S. (1983): Effect of photoconvulsive response (PCR) on the occurence of generalized EEG patterns in siblings of generalized spike and wave (GSW) probands. *Electroencephalogr. Clin. Neurophysiol.* **56**, 27p.

Gundel, A. & Doose, H. (1986): Genetic EEG pattern in febrile convulsions – a multivariate analysis. *Neuropediatrics* **17**, 3–6.

Haneke, K. (1963): Über drei Fälle latenter und manifester photogener Epilepsie in einer Familie. *Kinderaerztl. Prax.* **31**, 149–156.

Iwannek, K.W. (1979): Verlaufsuntersuchungen von photosensiblen nicht epileptischen Kindern. Dissertation, Universität Kiel.

Jayakar, P. & Chiappa, K.H. (1990): Clinical correlates of photoparoxysmal responses. *Electroenceph. Clin. Neurophysiol.* **75**, 251–254.

Jeavons, P.M. & Harding, G.F.A. (1975): *Photosensitive epilepsy*. London: Heinemann.

Kasteleijn-Nolst Trenité, D.G.A., Binnie, C.D. & Meinardi, H. (1987): Photosensitive patients: symptoms and signs during intermittent light stimulation and their relation to seizures in daily live. *J. Neurol. Neurosurg. Psychiatry* **50**, 1546–1549.

Kasteleijn-Nolst Trenité, D.G.A. (1989): Photosensitivity in epilepsy. Electrophysiological and clinical correlates. *Acta Neurol. Scand.* **80**, Suppl. 125.

Klass, D.W. & Fischer-Williams, M. (1976): Sensory stimulation, sleep and sleep deprivation. In: *Handbook of EEG*, Vol. 1b, ed. A. Rimond, pp. 5–73. Amsterdam: Elsevier.

Koskiniemi, M., Donner, M., Majuri, H., Haltia, M. & Norio, R. (1974a): Progressive myoclonus epilepsy: a clinical and histopathological study. *Acta Neurol. Scand.* **50**, 307–332.

Koskiniemi, M., Tovakka, E. & Donner, M. (1974b): Progressive myoclonus epilepsy: electroencephalographic findings. *Acta Neurol. Scand.* **50**, 333–359.

Lehesjoki, A.E., Koskiniemi, M., Sistonen, P., Miao, J., Hästbacka, J., Norio, R. & de la Chapelle, A. (1991): Localisation of a gene for progressive myoclonus epilepsy to chromosome 21q22. *Proc. Natl. Acad. Sci. USA* **88**, 3696–3699.

Malafosse, A., Lehesjoki, A., Genton, P. *et al.* (1992): Identical genetic locus for Baltic and Mediterranean myoclonus. *Lancet* **339**, 1080–1081.

Newmark, M.E. & Penry, J.K. (1979): *Photosensitivity and epilepsy: a review.* New York: Raven Press.

Obeid, T. & Panayiotopoulos, C.P. (1988): Juvenile myoclonic epilepsy: a study in Saudi Arabia. *Epilepsia* **29**, 280–282.

Obeid, T., Daif, A.K., Waheed, G., Yaqub, B., Panayiotopoulos, C.P., Tahan, A.R. & Shamena, A. (1991): Photosensitivity and photoconvulsive responses in Arabs. *Epilepsia* **32**, 77–81.

Rabending, K. & Klepel, H. (1970): Fotokonvulsivreaktion und Fotomyoklonus. Altersabhängige genetisch determinierte Varianten der gesteigerten Fotosensibilität. *Neuropaediatrie* **2**, 164–172.

Reilly, L.R. & Peters, J.F. (1973): Relationship of some varieties of electroencephalographic photosensitivity to clinical convulsive disorders. *Neurology* **23**, 1050–1057.

Roger, J., Genton, P., Bureau, M. & Dravet, C. (1992): Progressive myoclonus epilepsies in childhood and adolescence. In: *Epileptic syndromes in infancy, childhood and adolescence*, 2nd edn, eds. J. Roger, C. Dravet, M. Bureau, F. Dreifuss & P. Wolf, pp. 381–400. London: John Libbey.

Scollo-Lavizzari, G. (1971): Prognostic significance of 'epileptiform' discharges in the EEG of non-epileptic subjects during photic stimulation. *Electroencephalogr. Clin. Neurophysiol.* **31**, 174.

Serratosa, J.M., Delgado-Escueta, A.V., Pascual-Castroviejo, I. *et al.* (1993): Childhood absence epilepsy: exclusion of genetic linkage to chromosome 6p markers. *Epilepsia* **34**(Suppl. 2), S149.

So, E.L., Ruggles, U.H., Ahmann, P.A. & Olson, U.A. (1993): Prognosis of photoparoxysmal response in nonepileptic patients. *Neurology* **43**, 1713–1722.

Tsuji, S., Choudary, P.V., Martin, B.M. *et al.* (1987): A mutation in the human glucocerebrosidase gene in neuronopathic Gaucher's disease. *N. Engl. J. Med.* **316**, 570–575.

Waltz, S., Beck-Mannagetta, G. & Janz, D. (1990): Are there syndrome-related genetically determined spike and wave patterns? A comparison between syndromes of generalized epilepsies. *Epilepsia* **31**, 819.

Waltz, S., Christen, H.-J. & Doose, H. (1992): The different patterns of the photoparoxysmal response – a genetic study. *Electroencephalogr. Clin. Neurophysiol.* **83**, 138–145.

Waltz, S. & Doose, H. (1992a): Photosensibilität – neue genetische Aspekte. In: *Epilepsie 1991*, ed. D. Scheffner, pp. 41–45. Reinbek: Einhorn Presse Verlag.

Waltz, S. & Doose, H. (1992b): Photosensitivity is an autosomal-dominant trait. *J. Neurol.* **239**(Suppl. 2), S35.

Waltz, S. (1994): Elektroencephalographische Befunde bei der Epilepsie mit pyknoleptischen Absencen und der juvenilen Absencen-Epilepsie. Dissertation. Freie Universität, Berlin.

Whitehouse, W., Rees, M., Curtis, D. *et al.* (1993): Linkage analysis of idiopathic generalized epilepsy (IGE) and marker loci in families of patients with juvenile myoclonic epilepsy: no evidence for an epilepsy locus in the HLA-region. *Am. J. Hum. Genet.* **55**, 652–662.

Watson, C. & Davidson, S. (1957): The pattern of inheritance of cerebral light sensitivity. *Electroencephalogr. Clin. Neurophysiol.* **9**, 378.

Watson, C.W. & Marcus, E.M. (1962): The genetics and clinical significance of photogenic cerebral electrical abnormalities, myoclonus and seizures. *Trans. Am. Neurol. Assoc.* **87**, 251–253.

Wolf, P. & Goosses, R. (1986): Relation of photosensitivity to epileptic syndromes. *J. Neurol. Neurosurg. Psychiatry* **49**, 1386–1391.

Wolf, P. (1992): Juvenile myoclonic epilepsy. In: *Epileptic syndromes in infancy, childhood and adolescence*, 2nd edn, eds. J. Roger, C. Dravet, M. Bureau, F. Dreifuss & P. Wolf, pp. 313–327. London: John Libbey.

Part VI
Pathophysiology of convulsive seizures

Chapter 29

The epileptic and nonepileptic generalized myoclonus of the *Papio papio* baboon

C. Menini, C. Silva-Barrat and R. Naquet

Institut Alfred Fessard. C.N.R.S., 91198 Gif-sur-Yvette Cedex, France

Introduction

The photosensitive epilepsy of *Papio papio* baboons is characterized by the appearance, when animals are submitted to intermittent light stimulation (ILS), of reflex paroxysmal electrographic discharges which are always bilateral and synchronous and occupy large cortical territories (Killam et al., 1966a, 1967a). These paroxysmal discharges first appear in the frontal cortical regions (Fischer-Williams et al., 1968) and are associated with clinical epileptic manifestations (bilateral and synchronous myoclonic jerks) initially involving the eyelids and the face. The photically induced epileptic manifestations can be followed by generalized convulsive seizures resembling grand mal seizures of human patients. This form of epilepsy can be considered as a 'primary generalized epilepsy' as in epileptic patients for whom no neurological deficit and no obvious aetiological factors can be identified (Gastaut, 1973).

It was then discovered that some *Papio papio* baboons may naturally present a second kind of myoclonus with characteristics completely different from those of ILS-induced myoclonus (Fig. 1). These myoclonia are spontaneous, symmetrical and synchronous jerks mainly involving the trunk musculature and resembling a startle response. Their appearance is facilitated by active movements of the animals or by proprioceptive stimulations such as those caused by pressure on the sternum or by tension applied to a limb. In contrast, these reflex myoclonic jerks disappear completely when the animal is motionless or in the first stages of sleep. This second type of myoclonus was described for the first time in 1978 (Brailowsky et al., 1978) in animals in which the cerebellar vermis had been ablated to explore the possible effects on photosensitive epilepsy. The cerebellar lesion induced atonia and postural disturbances lasting for 2–3 weeks and then disappearing. The spontaneous myoclonus appeared from days to weeks after surgery and persisted throughout the survival time of the animal. More recently, it has been observed that benzodiazepines, which block epileptic jerks induced by intermittent light stimulation in photosensitive baboons, facilitate the appearance of a spontaneous myoclonus similar to the one observed after cerebellar lesion (Cepeda et al., 1982; Valin et al., 1981, 1983; Naquet et al., 1985). Given that it is never preceded or accompanied by any sign of paroxysmal activity at the EEG level and that it never evolves into seizures, this

IDIOPATHIC GENERALIZED EPILEPSIES

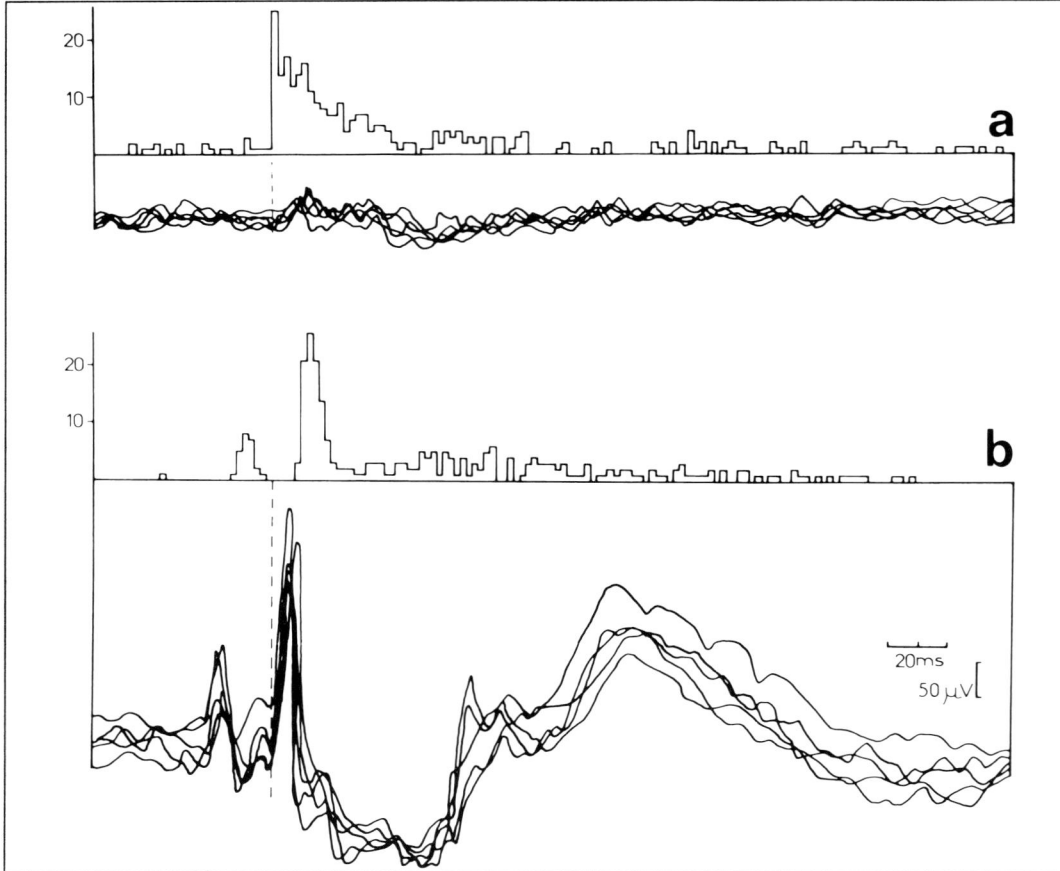

Fig. 1. *Comparison, in one baboon, of the spontaneous myoclonus (A) and of the ILS-induced myoclonus (B) In both cases, the upper trace is the EMG of the trapezius muscle, and the lower trace is the fronto-central EEG. In (A), the EMG onset, marked by a dashed line, precedes a small evoked potential. In (B), the onset of the cortical paroxystic spike, marked by a dashed line, precedes the EMG discharge.*

myoclonus was considered as 'nonepileptic' (Menini & Naquet, 1986) even though the actual nonepileptic nature of this myoclonus can be questioned (see 'Conclusions'). Nevertheless, it has been recognized that this myoclonus can occur spontaneously in intact baboons whether photosensitive or not. Therefore, the *Papio papio* baboon is now considered to be naturally predisposed to the nonepileptic myoclonus (Menini & Naquet, 1986; Rektor *et al.*, 1986).

Comparison of clinical and EEG manifestations accompanying both types of myoclonus

ILS-induced myoclonus

In predisposed animals, intermittent light stimulation at 25 Hz frequency induces clinical manifestations composed of myoclonus of four levels of severity (Killam *et al.*, 1966b; Meldrum *et al.*, 1970a).

1 = Palpebral myoclonus

2 = Palpebral myoclonus radiating to the face and head

3 = Palpebral and head myoclonus secondarily involving the entire body and thus appearing to be a massive, bilateral, and synchronous myoclonus similar to that described in human photosensitive patients (Gastaut et al., 1958). This myoclonus may occur isolated or grouped in bursts and stops when intermittent light stimulation is stopped.

4 = In the most sensitive animals, generalized myoclonus such as in level 3 continues after cessation of intermittent light stimulation and appears as either a more or less prolonged postdischarge which predominates in the two fronto–rolandic areas, or a tonic–clonic grand mal seizure similar to grand mal seizures in humans.

The main characteristics of the ILS-induced myoclonus is that it is always accompanied by paroxysmal discharges (PDs) constituted of spike-waves or polyspike-waves which first appear in the fronto-rolandic (FR) cortical regions (areas 4 and 6). When intermittent light stimulation is pursued and myoclonus of increasing severity develops, paroxysmal discharges irradiate to the anterior cortical areas and to some subcortical regions such as internal capsule, pons, and brain-stem, and finally invade all the subcortical structures except the rhinencephalon (Fischer-Williams et al., 1968). The initiation of paroxysmal discharges in the fronto-rolandic cortex is constant, and paroxysmal discharges initiated in other cerebral regions have never been observed, either in the occipital areas (even though occipital spike-waves could occur in some photosensitive human patients) or in the brain-stem.

A constant relationship exists between paroxysmal discharges and myoclonic discharges: the spike of a spike-wave is followed, a few milliseconds later, by a burst of electromyographic discharge while the wave is correlated to a muscular inactivation (Naquet et al., 1983) (Fig. 1). Moreover, the amplitudes of paroxysmal discharges and of muscular jerks are directly correlated: the higher the voltage of the cortical spike the greater the muscular discharge. From these characteristics, the ILS-induced myoclonus of baboons can be considered as a 'pyramidal' or 'cortical' myoclonus according to several authors who have attempted to classify the different types of myoclonus (Hallett et al., 1979; Marsden et al., 1982).

The constant relationship seen in baboons between EEG cortical spikes and myoclonic jerks differs from that seen in photosensitive human subjects in whom two types of manifestations are described (see the review by Naquet & Poncet-Ramade, 1982): (1) The frontopolar or oculoclonic response, manifested by myoclonic twitches of the eyelids, is generally not associated with epilepsy and is caused by an abnormal reactivity of brain-stem motor neuronal structures to flickering light. However recently, artieda and Obeso (1993) have shown that the fronto-rolandic cortex plays an important role in the oculo-clonic manifestations of human patients; (2) The frontocentral or photoconvulsive response is manifested by generalized myoclonic jerks which can be followed by grand mal seizures; this response is found in patients in whom epilepsy is either proven or strongly suspected. From this description, the baboon's ILS-induced manifestations can be considered as a constant association of oculoclonic and photoconvulsive responses while, in man, this association is observed only in some particularly photosensitive patients.

The degree of photosensitivity of baboons varies with age, sex, geographical origin, and species (Killam et al., 1967b, 1969; Balzamo et al., 1975). Young *Papio papio* baboons between 9 months and 4 years of age are generally more photosensitive than adults, while baboons less than 7–9 months old never show EEG or clinical symptoms when submitted to intermittent light stimulation. Females are more frequently photosensitive than males. Photosensitive epilepsy is found most frequently in the *Papio papio* from western Africa and more precisely from the Casamance region of Senegal (50–60 per cent of the baboon population show photosensitivity levels 3 or 4), while animals living in the southeastern regions (Niokolokoba Park) are less frequently photosensitive (20–25 per cent). Photosensitivity is also found in other baboons such as *Papio anubis* and *Papio hamadryas*, but the proportion of light-sensitive individuals does not exceed 10 per cent.

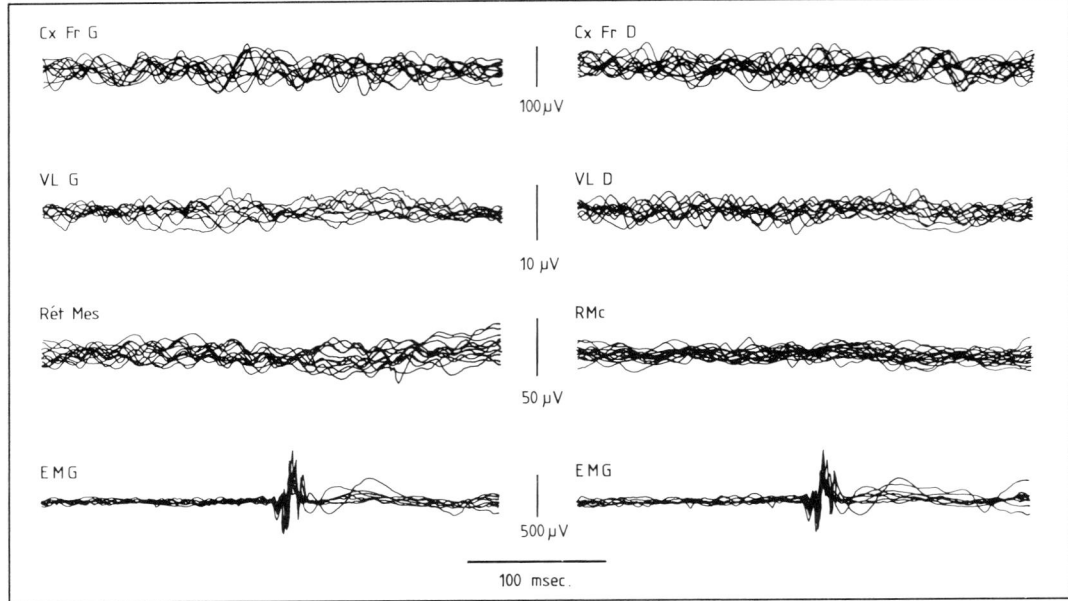

Fig. 2. Spontaneous myoclonus after benzodiazepine (lorazepam) in a nonphotosensitive baboon. Bottom traces: superposition of EMG discharges in the triceps muscle. Upper traces: recordings in the left and right frontal cortex (Cx Fr), the left and right ventral lateral thalamic nuclei (VL), the left mesencephalic reticular formation (Ret Mes) and the right reticular magnocellular nucleus (RMc). Note the absence of paroxysmal activity in all the recorded structures.

Nonepileptic myoclonus

The nonepileptic myoclonus may occur spontaneously in some predisposed baboons, either photosensitive or not. Its appearance is facilitated by activation of somatosensory afferents or by injection of compounds such as benzodiazepines or atropine. This myoclonus involves mainly the neck, shoulder and trunk musculature. Electromyographic recordings have shown that the myoclonus corresponds to brief contractions of the concerned muscles, lasting 30 ms on average, and occurring bilaterally and symmetrically. The trapezius is one of the first muscles involved in this myoclonus. At the EEG level, the nonepileptic myoclonus is never preceded or accompanied by any sign of paroxysmal activity in all the cortical structures. By using the back-averaging technique, any low-voltage signal preceding the jerk was detected, and only a somatic evoked potential occurring in the fronto-parietal cortex 10 to 15 ms after the beginning of the myoclonic jerk was detected. Numerous subcortical structures at the thalamic or the brain-stem levels were also recorded without any success (Fig. 2).

The nonepileptic myoclonus, which seems analogous to 'startle disease', appears as an exaggerated startle response corresponding to the myoclonic jerks ('secousses myocloniques') of Gastaut (1968) in human patients. Clinically, it also resembles the human action myoclonus described by Lance & Adams (1963) and the human reticular reflex myoclonus as defined by Hallett et al. (1977). Since it is facilitated after lesion of the cerebellar vermis, the baboon's nonepileptic myoclonus can be compared to the myoclonus induced by movement in human patients who present degenerative cerebellar syndromes generally associated with epilepsy (Bradshaw, 1954). These patients may also present ILS-induced myoclonus associated with either oculoclonic or photoconvulsive response.

In a photosensitive baboon, the nonepileptic myoclonus does not modify that induced by intermittent light stimulation, both types of myoclonus being easily distinguishable by their clinical and electrographic manifestations as well as by their mode of induction.

Pharmacological reactivity of the baboon's epileptic and nonepileptic myoclonus

ILS-induced myoclonus

In photosensitive baboons, inhibitory and excitatory mechanisms play an important role as revealed by the powerful action of drugs acting on both GABAergic and NMDA metabolisms.

Cerebrospinal fluid levels of GABA metabolites correlate inversely with the degree of photosensitivity in baboons (Lloyd et al., 1986). In addition, it has been widely described that drugs favouring GABAergic neurotransmission have a powerful anticonvulsant action on baboon photosensitive epilepsy. This is the case for drugs that increase the level of GABA by inhibiting GABA transaminase, such as amino-oxyacetic acid and gamma-vinyl GABA (Meldrum & Horton, 1978). This is also the case for agonists of GABA receptors, such as benzodiazepines (diazepam, clonazepam, see Fig. 3), barbiturates (phenobarbital) (Stark et al., 1970; Killam et al., 1966c, 1973), progabide (Cepeda et al., 1982; Naquet et al., 1985), and baclofen (Meldrum & Horton, 1974). Surprisingly, drugs that bind specifically to the post-synaptic GABA receptors (muscimol, THIP) do not suppress ILS-induced paroxysmal discharges in baboons but favour the occurrence of spontaneous paroxysmal discharges (Meldrum et al., 1975; Pedley et al., 1979; Meldrum & Horton, 1980).

Drugs that inhibit GABAergic neurotransmission have a powerful convulsant action and induce spontaneous seizures in various species, including baboons. This is the case for drugs that impair the GABA synthesis by blocking the activity of glutamic acid decarboxylase, such as isoniazid, thiosemicarbazide and 4-deoxypyridoxine (Meldrum et al., 1970a). Of special interest is DL-allyl-glycine, a pyridoxal phosphate antagonist that inhibits glutamic acid decarboxylase and consequently decreases the level of cerebral GABA. When given intravenously at appropriate doses, DL-allylglycine only decreases the threshold of epileptogenic responsiveness of baboons (Horton & Meldrum, 1973; Menini et al., 1977). When given at high doses, allylglycine may provoke the appearance of spontaneous paroxysmal discharges and seizures having an occipital localization which is never the case in naturally photosensitive baboons. Specific antagonists of benzodiazepine receptors (beta-carboline 3-carboxylic acid) are also potent convulsants in the baboon and at low doses facilitate the induction of myoclonic responses (Cepeda et al., 1981; Croucher et al., 1980, 1984; Valin et al., 1982).

Drugs that selectively block the excitation produced by N-methyl-D-aspartate (NMDA) have proved to be potent anticonvulsants in baboons, as well as in many other animal models of epilepsy (Meldrum, 1984). This is the case for compounds such as tizanidine which impairs the synaptic release of excitatory aminoacids (De Sarro et al., 1984), 2-amino-phosphono valeric acid, and 2-amino-phosphono heptanoic acid which selectively block the post-synaptic NMDA receptors (Meldrum et al., 1983). It is also interesting to observe that substances able to decrease the influx of calcium ions by acting directly on calcium channels possess significant anticonvulsant action in the photosensitive baboon (De Sarro et al., 1986) as well as in human epileptic patients (Binnie, 1989).

Other neurotransmitter systems seem either not to be involved, such as acetylcholine (Meldrum et al., 1970b) and opiates (Meldrum et al., 1979; Meldrum & Menini, 1981), or play only an indirect role, such as norepinephrine (Meldrum & Balzamo, 1971), dopamine (Meldrum et al., 1975; Altshuler et al., 1976; Anlezark et al., 1981, 1983) and serotonin (Wada et al., 1972).

Nonepileptic myoclonus

Testing the anticonvulsant effects of benzodiazepines (diazepam and lorazepam) on ILS-induced epileptic myoclonus (Valin et al., 1981) observed that these drugs blocked the ILS-induced epileptic manifestations and facilitated the occurrence of a nonepileptic myoclonus at the same time (Fig. 3).

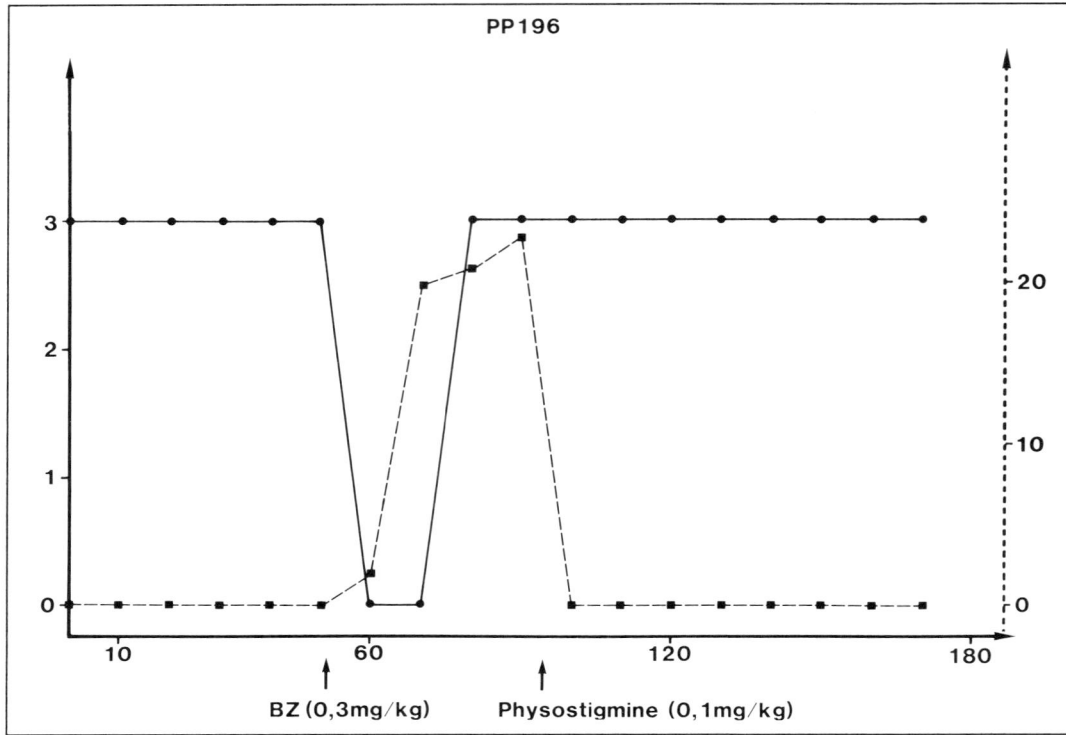

Fig. 3. Differential reactivity of the two types of myoclonus in a photosensitive baboon. Left ordinate: photosensitivity level evaluated as indicated in the text. Right ordinate: amount of nonepileptic myoclonus counted by 10 min epochs (abscissa). Clonazepam temporarily blocks the ILS-induced epileptic myoclonus (solid line) and facilitates the appearance of the nonepileptic myoclonus (interrupted line), the two phenomena having different timings. Subsequent administration of physostigmine suppresses the nonepileptic myoclonus without affecting photosensitivity.

Interestingly, these two effects had different temporal evolutions. After intravenous injection, the antiepileptic effect occurred in a few seconds, reached a maximum at 2 min and lasted for approximately 2 h, while the nonepileptic myoclonus occurred after a delay of 30–40 min and lasted for 3–5 h in such a way that there was a period during which the two myoclonia could be induced alternatively. The nonepileptic myoclonus was similarly facilitated when the drugs were administered to nonphotosensitive baboons. These effects of benzodiazepines are not GABA mediated, since drugs acting directly on GABA receptors have no effect on the nonepileptic myoclonus (Rektor et al., 1990, 1991a).

Pharmacological studies have demonstrated that the cholinergic system is involved in the generation of the nonepileptic myoclonus, and the facilitating action of benzodiazepines appears in fact to result from an indirect action of benzodiazepines on the cholinergic system (Rektor et al., 1986, 1990). Benzodiazepine-induced myoclonus is blocked by physostigmine, a substance which blocks acetylcholine esterase and increases the cerebral level of acetylcholine, while it is potentiated by atropine (Rektor et al., 1984), an anticholinergic drug. In most baboons, atropine alone facilitates the appearance of a nonepileptic myoclonus for several hours. The atropine-induced myoclonus, which was suppressed after physostigmine, was similar to the one observed in vermisectomized baboons or in baboons administered with benzodiazepines. Quinuclidinyl benzylate, a specific antagonist of central muscarinic receptors, induced nonepileptic myoclonus while this was not the

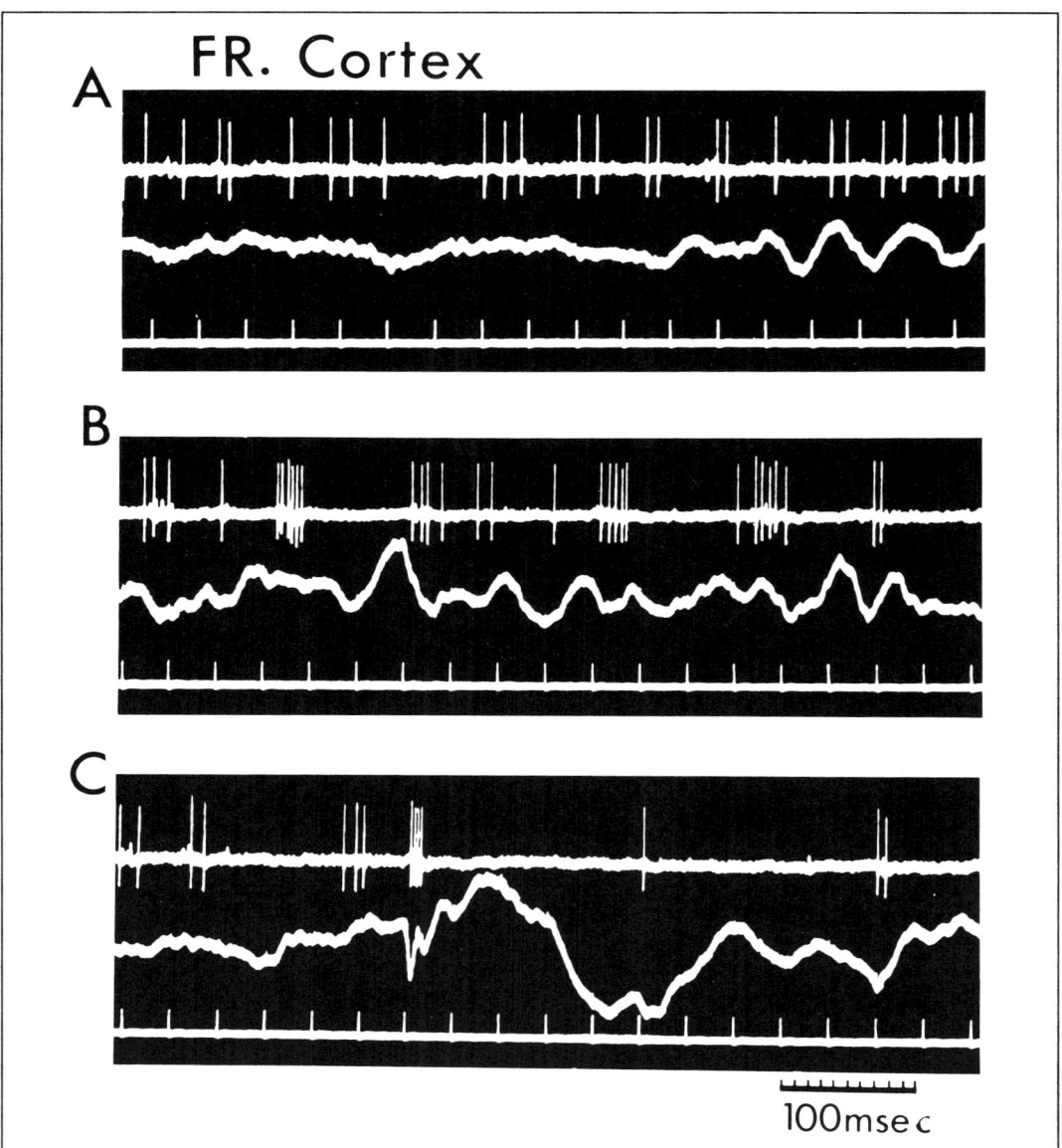

Fig. 4. Patterns of unit activity in the frontal cortex during light stimulation in a photosensitive baboon. Top trace: extracellular recording in the frontal cortex. Middle trace: EEG recording of the frontal cortex. Bottom trace: light stimulation. (A) At the beginning of the stimulation, the cell discharges with a pattern similar to spontaneous activity. (B) After a series of stimulations, bursts occur in the absence of EEG paroxysmal activity. (C) Later, paroxysmal discharges appear, and neuronal bursts are synchronous with the spike of the cortical PD.

case for methyl-quinuclidinyl benzylate, a methylated derivative which does not cross the blood–brain barrier and acts only on peripheral receptors. The benzodiazepine-induced myoclonus was abolished after injection of Ro15-1788 (Valin et al., 1983), a specific antagonist of benzodiazepine receptors. However, this drug had no effect on the atropine-induced myoclonus or on the nonepi-

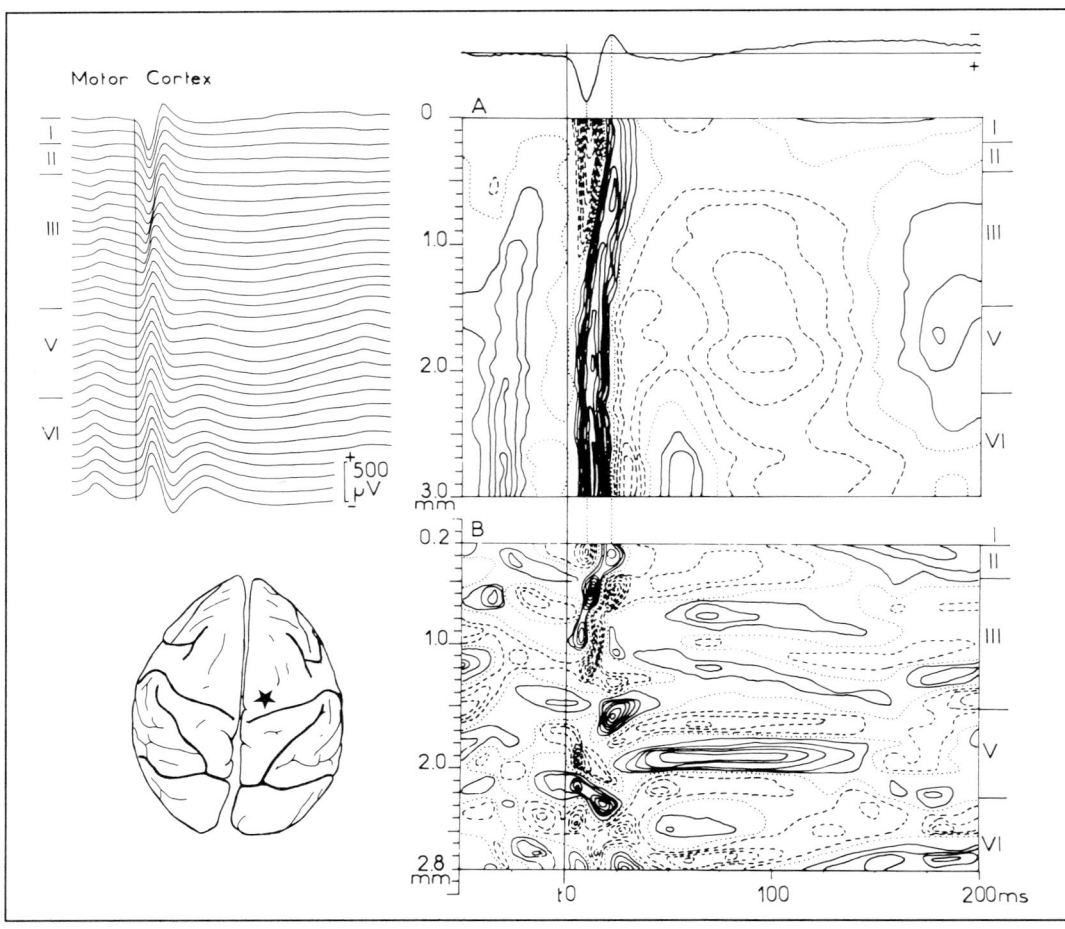

Fig. 5. Current source density study of ILS-induced paroxysmal discharges in the motor cortex, at the location indicated by a star. Recordings of paroxysmal discharges were performed at constant intervals in the depth of the motor cortex (upper left). Cortical layers are indicated by Roman numerals. From these intracortical laminar recordings, a map of field potentials (upper right) and then a map of current density (bottom) were calculated with respect to time (abscissa) and cortical depth (ordinate). Solid contour lines represent current sinks (meaning activated or depolarized zones) and dashed lines represent current sources (meaning inactivated or hyperpolarized zones).

leptic myoclonus which occurs naturally in some predisposed baboons and which can nevertheless be blocked by physostigmine.

These observations are in accordance with data in the literature, suggesting an interaction between benzodiazepines and the cholinergic system: physostigmine is utilized for the treatment of benzodiazepine intoxications (Vogel, 1977); benzodiazepines are part of the therapy against intoxication by organophosphates (Rump & Faff, 1976).

Other neurotransmitter systems such as the noradrenergic and the dopaminergic systems may influence the nonepileptic myoclonus, but inconsistently (Rektor et al., 1989, 1991b).

Differential role of the frontal cortex in epileptic and non epileptic myoclonus

ILS-induced myoclonus and seizures

The data which are summarized hereafter demonstrate that the ILS-induced manifestations of photosensitive baboons are corticofrontal in origin.

Under ILS, the frontal cortical neurons are progressively activated in bursts of action potentials. Bursting activity initially occurs when paroxysmal discharges cannot be distinguished in the surface EEG recordings. Then, when paroxysmal discharges are constituted, each burst is synchronous of a paroxysmal discharge spike while the paroxysmal discharge wave corresponds to a cellular inactivation (Menini et al., 1981) (Fig. 4). In other cerebral structures, neuronal activation either is not correlated to paroxysmal discharges, or appears secondarily to the frontal bursting activity when paroxysmal discharges have reached a sufficient amplitude (Menini et al., 1981; Silva-Barrat et al., 1986).

The demonstration that generators of paroxysmal discharges are localized in the frontal cortex was achieved by performing a current source density study in areas 4 and 6 in photosensitive baboons submitted to intermittent light stimulation (Silva-Barrat et al., 1988a) (Fig. 5). Data show that area 4 is the first involved, and that paroxysmal discharges result from the activation of this area at two levels: neurons in layer III are activated by corticocortical afferents coming indirectly from the occipital areas and ending at this level; pyramidal cells in layers V and VI are activated by thalamocortical afferents which end at this level. However, since subcortical structures are involved only secondarily, it appears that visual afferents arriving in the motor cortex from the occipital lobe play a determinant role in photosensitive epilepsy by triggering the cortical generators of paroxysmal discharges. This was confirmed by the observation of baboons with corpus callosum section or with prolonged infusions of GABA in different cerebral structures.

The hemispheric synchronization of ILS-induced paroxysmal discharges and seizures is disrupted after section of the corpus callosum (Catier et al., 1970; Naquet et al., 1972). When the corpus callosum section is associated with a unilateral motor cortical lesion, ILS-induced seizures occur only on the nonlesioned side (Naquet et al., 1972). When the sectioning of the corpus callosum is associated with a temporal hemiretina lesion in one eye (see above), the monocular visual stimulation of the operated eye triggers seizures which occur uniquely in the contralateral hemisphere (Fukuda et al., 1989). Immediately after such a seizure, visual stimulation of the nonoperated eye can trigger a seizure on the other hemisphere, even during the post-ictal period of the previous seizure. These observations indicate, first, that visual afferents are necessary to trigger paroxysmal discharges and seizures, second, that the epileptogenic reactivity of one hemisphere is independent of the other, and third, that the corpus callosum is the only structure responsible for the bilateral synchronization of paroxysmal discharges and seizures: a unilateral seizure cannot cross to the contralateral side in the absence of functional callosal connections.

Prolonged GABA infusions were performed in different cerebral structures in order to test their involvement in ILS-induced epileptic manifestations (Brailowsky et al., 1987, 1989; Silva-Barrat et al., 1988b). Chronic (7 days) GABA infusions directed to the motor as well as the occipital cortex completely blocked the ILS-induced EEG and clinical epileptic manifestations during the entire infusion period. Similar infusions directed to the premotor or prefrontal cortex (areas 6 and 8) had no effect on photosensitivity. These observations demonstrate that the motor and occipital cortical areas are key structures for photosensitive epilepsy, the first one because neuronal generators of paroxysmal discharges are located there, and the second because it is the origin of visual afferents necessary to trigger the paroxysmal discharge generators. These observations also demonstrate that the GABAergic system plays, at the level of discrete cortical areas, an important role in photosensitive epilepsy.

By using ion-sensitive electrodes, it was possible to measure the changes in extracellular Ca^{2+} concentration in the baboon's frontal cortex during ILS-induced seizures. It was shown that the seizure onset is preceded and accompanied by a strong reduction in extracellular Ca^{2+} concentration, from 1.3 to 0.1 mM (Pumain *et al.*, 1985), a level which is maintained throughout the seizure. This level is so low that it is incompatible with chemical synaptic transmission (Dingledine & Somjen, 1981), in such a way that the perseveration of the seizure is probably due to nonsynaptic mechanisms. These phenomena occurring in the frontal cortex at the beginning of the seizures seem to be a prerequisite for the subsequent development of any other ictal manifestations, especially those involving the subcortical structures (see below).

Nonepileptic myoclonus

The origin of this myoclonus remains unknown, but a cortical origin is unlikely for several reasons. First, the myoclonus is never accompanied by any EEG discharge. Second, since benzodiazepines induce the myoclonus, they should at the same time block an EEG discharge if it existed anywhere in the cortex. Third, in some photosensitive baboons, the nonepileptic myoclonus occurs in the absence of any abnormal EEG discharge even though the cortex of these animals is hyperexcitable and able to develop paroxysmal discharges under intermittent light stimulation and spontaneously during sleepiness (Menini & Naquet, 1986).

Roles played by subcortical structures in epileptic and non epileptic myoclonus

ILS-induced myoclonus and seizures

Subcortical structures seem to play only a secondary role in the mechanisms reponsible for ILS-induced paroxysmal discharges and a more important role in seizures.

The study of multiunitary activities in different subcortical structures (Silva-Barrat *et al.*, 1986) has shown that, during the induction of paroxysmal discharges by intermittent light stimulation, pontine and mesencephalic reticular formations and the facial nuclei were activated only after the fronto-rolandic paroxysmal discharges had reached a certain amplitude (greater than 200 µV). The thalamic nuclei (ventralis lateralis, centrum medianum, lateralis posterior) were activated later, only when the fronto-rolandic paroxysmal discharges had reached an even greater amplitude (more than 400 µV). The secondary pontine and mesencephalic activations could thus reinforce those of the fronto-rolandic cortex and then the thalamus. The different roles played by the brain-stem reticular formation in paroxysmal discharge and seizure mechanisms were confirmed by the effects of local chronic infusions of GABA which were able to diminish the frequency of cortical paroxysmal discharges (–20 per cent) but not to suppress them (Silva-Barrat *et al.*, 1988b), while the main effect was to almost completely block the appearance of seizures.

The beginning of a grand mal seizure in baboons is characterized by the disappearance of EEG polyspike-waves and the appearance of rapid EEG rhythms of low voltage. Clinically, this episode corresponds to the tonic phase of the seizure which lasts for a few seconds. During this period, the activity of fronto-rolandic neurons is weak and the correlation between unitary activity and EEG disappears. At this point, the discharge of the fronto-rolandic cortical neurons is diminished compared to the pre-ictal period during which fronto-rolandic neuronal bursts are correlated with paroxysmal discharges. Simultaneously, most of the deep structures are strongly activated with the reticular (pontine and mesencephalic) formations showing the highest activation level (Silva-Barrat *et al.*, 1986). This powerful tonic reticular activation precedes the occurrence of a seizure and may be responsible for cerebral and extracerebral vascular changes which, in turn, may modify the cerebral excitability and participate in the appearance of the seizure. More precisely, the seizure onset is preceded and accompanied by tachycardia, hypertension (+38 per cent) and changes in blood pressure and regional blood volumes: the hepatic and nasal blood volumes are reduced (–27 per cent and –22 per cent respectively), and the cerebral blood volume is increased by +30 per cent (Ancri *et al.*, 1981). These changes provide an indication for the early involvement of cerebrovascular centres and of the reticular formation where these centres are situated.

Even if it precedes the seizure onset, the reticular activation depends on pre-existing fronto-rolandic paroxysmal discharges and on the occurrence of cortical ionic changes. These ionic changes are incompatible with chemical synaptic transmission in such a way that strong activation of brain-stem reticular structures can be interpreted as resulting from the loss of the control exerted by the cortex on the deep structures, consecutive to the intense activation of these structures during paroxysmal discharges (Silva-Barrat et al., 1986).

Nonepileptic myoclonus

Until the present time, direct subcortical recordings have not allowed the determination of which brain-stem structure is involved in the genesis of the nonepileptic myoclonus (Fig. 2). The facilitation of this myoclonus after ablation of the cerebellar vermis favours the hypothesis that it originates in the brain-stem, and more probably in the reticular formation (Rektor et al., 1993), as also suggested for the myoclonus observed in macaques after bilateral hemispherectomy (Denny-Brown, 1968). This hypothesis is in accordance with the clinical characteristics of the myoclonus which concerns the proximal musculature: proximal musculature is mainly involved during activation of the reticulo–spinal motor system while distal musculature is mainly involved during activation of the pyramidal system. Moreover, this hypothesis is in accordance with the presence, in the lower brain-stem, of reflex centres (responsible for the spino–bulbo–spinal reflexes observed in cats and monkeys under chloralose (Shimamura & Livingston, 1963; Shimamura et al., 1964)) which can constitute the functional substrate responsible for the nonepileptic myoclonus. Finally, this hypothesis is not in contradiction with the involvement of the cholinergic system since several cholinergic neuronal populations have been described in the brain-stem of baboons by using immunocytochemical techniques (Riche et al., 1987). In other species, it has been demonstrated that muscarinic receptors at this level present a very high affinity for ligands such as atropine or quinuclidinyl benzylate (Dawson & Poretski, 1983).

In rodents, a myoclonus not associated with cortical paroxysmal discharges can be induced by 5-HTP, a serotonin precursor, and transitorily blocked by methysergide, a serotonergic antagonist (Luscombe et al., 1982). The origin of this myoclonus is probably in the brain-stem where most of the serotonergic neurons are located. In *Papio papio*, the serotonergic system does not play an important role in the nonepileptic myoclonus since it is neither suppressed nor facilitated by methysergide (Valin et al., 1983).

Hypotheses on the mechanisms involved in epileptic and nonepileptic myoclonus

ILS-induced myoclonus

The photosensitive epilepsy of baboons is genetically transmitted (Balzamo et al., 1975), and is manifested in the absence of any convulsant drug. As with human photosensitive epileptic patients, the brain of photosensitive baboons has revealed no morphological or histological lesion allowing one to consider this animal a model for the study of 'idiopathic' generalized epilepsy (Gastaut, 1973). If it exists, the dysfunction underlying the epileptogenic reactivity of baboons is minimal, with no apparent manifestation in the absence of adequate stimulation: seizures occurring spontaneously have very rarely been observed, even in very photosensitive baboons. In the absence of intermittent photic stimulation, the electroencephalographic and neuronal activities in the frontal cortex of photosensitive baboons appear normal during wakefulness.

Given the data which are presented in this paper and which demonstrate the critical role played by the motor cortex in paroxysmal discharge genesis and seizure mechanisms, the functional abnormality underlying the epileptogenic reactivity of baboons very likely concerns this area. This dysfunction most probably results from an imbalance of the inhibitory and excitatory systems, as suggested by the results of dosage of amino acids in the cerebrospinal fluid which evidenced both a decrease in inhibitory neurotransmission (GABA and taurine) and an increase in excitatory mechanisms (aspartate) in photosensitive animals (Lloyd et al., 1986). In addition, the motor cortex of baboons seems to be characterized by a failure of Ca^{2+} regulation mechanisms since the decrease in extracellular calcium concentration observed at the beginning of seizures is much more important than that observed in other experimental epilepsy models (Pumain et al., 1985).

Can the minimal dysfunction underlying the epileptogenic reactivity of baboons be explained by the presence of microscopic neuroanatomic abnormalities with synaptic dysgenesis? This situation can occur when developmental disturbances of the cerebral organization, such as those due to neuronal migration disorders, occur during embryogenesis. Young neurons, guided by radial glial fibres, migrate to the cortical plate between 7 and 16 weeks of gestational age in the normal human brain. Under the effects of genetically determined dysfunctions which impair migration processes, neurons can be arrested while moving from the periventricular zone to the cortex, and they can constitute dystopic neurons scattered in the white matter of the adult brain (Rakic, 1975; Barth, 1987; Becker, 1991). These dystopic neurons are not only arrested at a wrong place, cannot establish a normal synaptic connectivity, and are at risk of early death, but they also are missing in the cortical area they should have reached. This could result in excitational disturbances of the cortex.

Mild cortical malformations could be a cause of epilepsy, as suggested from the anatomical examination of the brains of epileptic patients (Nordborg et al., 1987; Meencke & Janz, 1985). More specifically, the brains of patients with primary generalized epilepsy may present microdysgenesies which consist of dystopic neurons in the stratum moleculare of the neocortex, the white matter, the hippocampus and the cerebellar cortex (Meencke, 1983). In fact, dystopic neurons also exist in the brains of nonepileptic patients but at a density significantly lower than that found in subjects with primary generalized epilepsy and even in subjects with traumatic epilepsy (Meencke, 1983). In human patients, dystopic neurons frequently accompany less subtle microdysgenesies such as microgyrias or band heterotopias. In baboons, no similar histological abnormality has been revealed, and the hypothetical microdysgenesis underlying photosensitivity should better correspond to abnormalities at the subcellular or molecular level.

Among the underlying biochemical mechanisms, calcium channels, NMDA receptors and GABA are relevant. Calcium channels, which have been predominantly associated with neurotransmitter release, are involved in neuronal bursting activity and epileptogenesis especially in the baboon's ILS-induced seizures (see above). It was demonstrated recently that calcium channels play a transient but specific developmental role in directed migration of immature neurons before the establishment of their synaptic circuits (Komuro & Rakic, 1992). Moreover, these phenomena are modulated by NMDA receptors (Komuro & Rakic, 1993) which also play a role in controlling the neuronal excitability and epileptogenesis in the adult brain. Functions of GABA in the nervous system are also manifold. Apart from its role as the major inhibitory transmitter, another function of GABA is to influence neuronal development and synaptogenesis by different ways. GABA may act as a trophic agent during development as well as during synaptic reorganization in the adult nervous system (Wolff et al., 1993). GABA also has been demonstrated to influence the neonatal cerebellar and cortical development by enhancing the maturation of the N-CAM expression pattern (Meier et al., 1987) and by producing an increase in intracellular calcium (Cherubini et al., 1991). From these data, it can be hypothesized that an abnormal expression of genes coding for calcium channels, NMDA receptors or GABA very early during embryogenesis may not only affect the neuron's morphology and synaptic connectivity but also be responsible for an abnormal reactivity of neurons in the adult brain.

Nonepileptic myoclonus

Similar to that suggested for the ILS-induced myoclonus, it can be hypothesized that baboons predisposed to the nonepileptic myoclonus may present microscopic abnormalities with synaptic dysgenesis in the lower brain-stem, for example of a certain class of cholinergic neurons. In mice, several mutations (weaver, reeler, staggerer) impair the cerebellar and brain-stem development and are accompanied by myoclonic manifestations (Seyfried & Glaser, 1985). In man, neuronal migration disorders at the cerebellar and brain-stem levels are frequently associated with diffuse abnormalities, epilepsy and mental retardation. This is the case for numerous neurological syndromes such as fragile X syndrome (Musumeci *et al.*, 1991), autism (Bauman & Kemper, 1988) and Down's syndrome (Becker, 1991).

In baboons predisposed to the nonepileptic myoclonus, cellular or molecular abnormalities have not yet been demonstrated in the lower brain-stem, but their hypothetical presence could cause synaptic dysfunctions and explain abnormal reactivity. In that case, the activation of the brain-stem reticular formation during agitation periods would produce, in the absence of sufficient inhibitory influx coming from upper cerebral structures, a diffuse facilitation of spinal motoneurons, and finally the appearance of the nonepileptic myoclonus. Given that no histological abnormality has never been shown in the brain-stem of baboons with nonepileptic myoclonus, the hypothetical microdysgenesies, if they exist, should correspond to subcellular or molecular abnormalities (possibly at eceptor level) rather than dysplasias as classically defined (Sarnat, 1991).

The question as to whether or not the epileptic and nonepileptic myoclonus of baboons are linked remains open. Of 106 baboons tested for this purpose, 41 (39 per cent) were photosensitive, of which six also displayed the nonepileptic myoclonus. Of the remaining 65 baboons, four had nonepileptic myoclonus (unpublished observations). Statistical analysis of these data indicated that epileptic and nonepileptic myoclonus are independent of each other. It is thus probable that brain-stem abormalities, even if they are suspected in both cases, should implicate different areas and different mechanisms and occur independently in the two pathologies.

Conclusions

Papio papio baboons can present two different pathologies which can coexist in a given animal and which are completely independent: a genetically transmitted predisposition to a secondarily generalized photosensitive epilepsy with ILS-induced myoclonus, and a natural predisposition to a second kind of myoclonus not accompanied by any cortical paroxysmal discharge and never followed by seizures and thus named 'nonepileptic myoclonus'.

The baboon's photosensitive epilepsy remains, with the epileptic fowl (see Guy *et al.*, Ch. 31), one of the best models for the study of human photosensitive epilepsy. In baboons as well as in man, photosensitivity appears to be a generalized form of epilepsy with bilateral and synchronous PDs, and clinical observations or EEG recordings do not give any sign of a localized origin of the epileptogenic processes. Moreover, in both cases, seizures also occur bilaterally and synchronously in large cortical territories, as if they were triggered from a median structure with diffuse cortical projections. However, data reported in photosensitive baboons demonstrate that the origin of paroxysmal discharges and seizures is in the motor cortex. Their bilateralization and interhemispheric synchronization result from the involvement of the corpus callosum and do not need the implication of any 'centrencephalic' structure as initially suggested (Penfield & Jasper, 1954). Nevertheless, the brain-stem reticular formation plays a minor role in the induction of cortical paroxysmal discharges since facilitation of the GABAergic system at the reticular level is able to reduce the frequency of appearance of paroxysmal discharges. On the contrary, this structure plays a more important role in the mechanisms of generalized seizures. In man, in addition to the fronto-rolandic areas, the occipital territories also play an important role in the mechanisms of photosensitive epilepsy since paroxysmal discharges and seizures may start and sometimes remain localized in the occipital region (Naquet *et al.*, 1960).

It is not known whether the functional disturbance reponsible for the epileptogenic reactivity of baboons results from abnormalities in the synthesis of neurotransmitters or from the number and properties of their receptors. The obtained experimental data suggest that such abnormalities exist in the motor cortex where paroxysmal discharges are generated. No data suggest that similar abnormalities may also exist either in the visual cortex which sends an excess of afferents to the motor cortex, or in the reticular formation which is involved in the mechanisms of generalized seizures. Neuronal migration disorders, which result in microdysgenesies and which are associated with primary generalized epilepsy in some human patients, would explain the inherited hyperexcitability of the baboon's motor cortex; anatomical investigations must be performed in order to disclose if such microdysgenesies exist. In photosensitive human patients, the cortical hyperexcitability is more diffuse since it involves both the fronto-rolandic and the occipital areas.

The baboon's nonepileptic myoclonus may result from a natural abnormality of some muscarinic receptors on neurones at a place which is still undertermined but most probably located in the lower brain-stem. The exact nature of this myoclonus can be questioned. It was named 'nonepileptic' since it is never accompanied by EEG paroxysmal discharges and since the cerebral neocortex seems to play only a secondary role in their mechanisms. However, these characteristics also concern other well-known experimental epilepsy models such as audiogenic seizures in rodents and convulsions induced in rats by electrical stimulation of the brain-stem reticular formation (Kreindler *et al.*, 1958; Hirsch *et al.*, Ch. 34). The ability to develop epileptiform discharges in the absence of convulsant drugs result from the intrinsic organization of the neuronal network in some structures such as the neocortex or hippocampus. In the models cited above, the absence of paroxysmal discharges could result from a different organization in the neuronal network of the structures involved and particularly of the reticular formation. Given these various observations, the 'nonepileptic myoclonus' of baboons should better be named 'myoclonus without any cortical paroxysmal discharge' since its paroxysmal or epileptic nature is neither proven nor eliminated.

References

Altshuler, L., Killam, E.K. & Killam, K.F. (1976): Biogenic amines and the photomyoclonic syndrome in the baboon, *Papio papio. J. Pharmacol. Exp. Ther.* **196**, 156–166.

Ancri, D., Naquet, R., Menini, Ch., Meldrum, B.S., Stutzmann, J.M. & Basset, J.Y. (1981): Cerebral and extra-cerebral blood volume in generalized seizures in the baboon *Papio papio. Electroencephalogr. Clin. Neurophysiol.* **51**, 91–103.

Anlezark, G.M., Blackwood, D.H., Meldrum, B.S., Ram, V.J. & Neumeyer, J.L. (1983): Comparative assessment of dopamine agonist aporphines as anticonvulsants in two models of reflex epilepsy. *Psychopharmacology* **81**, 135–139.

Anlezark, G.M., Marrosu, F. & Meldrum, B.S. (1981): Dopamine agonists in reflex epilepsy. In: *Neurotransmitters, seizures and epilepsy*, eds. P.L. Morselli, K.G. Lloyd, W. Löscher, B.S. Meldrum & H. Reynolds. Raven Press: New York.

Artieda, J. & Obeso, J.A. (1993): The pathophysiology and pharmacology of photic cortical reflex myoclonus. *Ann. Neurol.* **34**, 175–184.

Balzamo, E., Bert, J., Menini, Ch. & Naquet, R. (1975): Excessive light sensitivity in *Papio papio*, its variations with age, sex and geographic origin. *Epilepsia* **16**, 269–276.

Barth, P.G. (1987): Disorders of neuronal migration. *Can. J. Neurol. Sci.* **14**, 1–16.

Bauman, M.L. & Kemper, L. (1988): Limbic and cerebellar abnormalities: consistent findings in infantile autism. *J. Neuropathol. Exp. Neurol* **47**, 369.

Becker, L.E. (1991): Synaptic dysgenesis. *Can. J. Neurol. Sci.* **18**, 170–180.

Binnie, C.D. (1989): Potential antiepileptic drugs flunarizine and other calcium entry blockers. In: *Antiepileptic drugs*, 3rd edn. eds. R. Levy, R. Mattson, B.S. Meldrum, J.K. Penry & F.E. Dreifuss, pp. 971–982. New York; Raven Press.

Bradshaw, J. (1954): A study of myoclonus. *Brain* **77**, 138–157.

Brailowsky, S., Menini, Ch. & Naquet, R. (1978): Myoclonus developing after vermisectomy in photosensitive *Papio papio. Electroencephalogr. Clin. Neurophysiol.* **45**, 82–89.

Brailowsky, S., Menini, Ch., Silva-Barrat, C. & Naquet, R. (1987): Epileptogenic gamma-aminobutyric acid-withdrawal syndrome after chronic, intracortical infusion in baboons. *Neurosci. Lett.* **74**, 75–80.

Brailowsky, S., Silva-Barrat, C., Menini, Ch., Riche, D. & Naquet, R. (1989): Effects of localized, chronic GABA infusions into different cortical areas of the photosensitive baboon, *Papio papio*. *Electroencephalogr. Clin. Neurophysiol.* **72**, 147–156.

Catier, J., Choux, M., Cordeau, J.P., Dimov, S., Riche, D., Eberhard, A. & Naquet, R. (1970): Résultats préliminaires des effets électrographiques de la section du corps calleux chez le *Papio papio* photosensible. *Rev. Neurol. (Paris)* **122**, 521–522.

Cepeda, C., Tanaka, T., Besselievre, R., Potier, P., Naquet, R. & Rossier, J. (1981): Proconvulsant effects in baboons of beta-carboline, a putative endogenous ligand for benzodiazepine receptors. *Neurosci. Lett.* **24**, 53–57.

Cepeda, C., Worms, P., Lloyd, K.G. & Naquet, R. (1982): Action of progabide in the photosensitive baboon *Papio papio*. *Epilepsia* **23**, 463–470.

Cherubini, E., Gaiarsa, J.L. & Ben-Ari, Y. (1991): GABA: an excitatory transmitter in early postnatal life. *Trends Neurosci.* **14**, 515–519.

Croucher, M.J., De Sarro, G.B., Jensen, L.H. & Meldrum, B.S. (1980): Behavioural and convulsant actions of two methyl esters of beta-carboline carboxylic acid in photosensitive baboons and in DBA/2 mice. *Eur. J. Pharmacol.* **104**, 55–60.

Croucher, M.J., Meldrum, B.S. & Collins, J.F. (1984): Anticonvulsant and proconvulsant properties of a series of structural isomers of piperidine dicarboxylic acid. *Neuropharmacology* **23**, 467–472.

Dawson, R.M. & Poretski, M. (1983): A comparison of the muscarinic cholinoceptors and benzodiazepine receptors of guinea-pig brain and rat brain. *Neurochem. Int.* **5**, 369–374.

Denny-Brown, D. (1968): Quelques aspects physiologiques des myoclonies. *Rev. Neurol. (Paris)* **119**, 121–129.

De Sarro, G.B., Croucher, M.J. & Meldrum, B.S. (1984): Anticonvulsant actions of DS 103–282: pharmacological studies in rodents and the baboon, *Papio papio*. *Neuropharmacology* **23**, 525–530.

De Sarro, G.B., Nistico, G. & Meldrum, B.S. (1986): Anticonvulsant properties of flunarizine on reflex and generalized models of epilepsy. *Neuropharmacology* **25**, 695.

Dingledine, R. & Somjen, G. (1981): Calcium dependence of synaptic transmission in the hippocampal slice. *Brain Res.* **207**, 218–222.

Fischer-Williams, M., Poncet, M., Riche, D. & Naquet, R. (1968): Light-induced epilepsy in the baboon *Papio papio*: cortical and depth recordings. *Electroencephalogr. Clin. Neurophysiol.* **25**, 557–569.

Fukuda, H., Valin, A., Menini, Ch., Boscher, C., De La Sayette, V., Riche, D., Kunimoto, M., Wada, J.A. & Naquet, R. (1989): Effect of macular and peripheral retina coagulation on photosensitive epilepsy in the forebrain bisected baboon *Papio papio*. *Epilepsia* **30**, 623–625.

Gastaut, H. (1968): Séméiologie des myoclonies et nosologie analytique des syndromes myocloniques. *Rev. Neurol. (Paris)* **119**, 1–30.

Gastaut, H. (1973): *Dictionnaire de l'épilepsie*. Geneva: OMS.

Gastaut, H., Trevisan, C. & Naquet, R. (1958): Diagnostic value of electroencephalographic abnormalities provoked by intermittent photic stimulation. *Electroencephalogr. Clin. Neurophysiol.* **10**, 194–195.

Hallett, M., Chadwick, D., Adam, J. & Marsden, C.D. (1977): Reticular myoclonus: a physiological type of human post-hypoxic myoclonus. *J. Neurol. Neurosurg. Psychiatry* **40**, 253–264.

Hallett, M., Chadwick, D. & Marsden, C.D. (1979): Cortical reflex myoclonus. *Neurology* **29**, 1107–1125.

Horton, R.W. & Meldrum, B.S. (1973): Seizures induced by allylglycine, 3-mercaptopropionic acid and 4-deoxypyridoxin in mice and photosensitive baboons & different modes of inhibition of cerebral glutamic acid decarboxylase. *Br. J. Pharmacol.* **49**, 52–63.

Killam, K.F., Joy, R.M., Killam, E.K. & Stark, L.G. (1969): Genetic models of epilepsy with special reference to the syndrome of the *Papio papio*. *Epilepsia* **10**, 229–238.

Killam, K.F., Killam, E.K. & Naquet, R. (1966a): Mise en évidence chez certains singes d'un syndrome myoclonique. *C.R. Acad. Sci. (Paris)* **262**, 1010–1012.

Killam, K.F., Killam, E.K. & Naquet, R. (1966c): Etudes pharmacologiques réalisées chez des singes présentant une activité EEG paroxystique particulière à la stimulation lumineuse intermittente. *J. Physiol. (Paris)* **58**, 543.

Killam, K.F., Killam, E.K. & Naquet, R. (1967a): An animal model of light sensitive epilepsy. *Electroencephalogr. Clin. Neurophysiol.* **22**, 497–513.

Killam, E.K., Matsuzaki, M. & Killam, K.F. (1973): Effects of chronic administration of benzodiazepines on epileptic seizures and brain electrical activity in *Papio papio*. In: *The benzodiazepines*, eds. S. Garattini, E. Mussini & L.O. Randall, pp. 443–460. New York: Raven Press.

Killam, K.F., Naquet, R. & Bert, J. (1966b): Paroxysmal responses to intermittent light stimulation in a population of baboons (*Papio papio*). *Epilespia* **7**, 215–219.

Killam, E.K., Stark, L. & Killam, K.F. (1967b): Photic stimulation of three species of baboons. *Life Sci.* **6**, 1569–1574.

Komuro, H. & Rakic, P. (1992): Selective role of N-type calcium channels in neuronal migration. *Science* **257**, 806–809.

Komuro, H. & Rakic, P. (1993): Modulation of neuronal migration by NMDA receptors. *Science* **260**, 95–97.

Kreindler, A., Zuckerman, E., Steriade, M. & Chimion, D. (1958): Electroclinical features of convulsions induced by stimulation of brain-stem. *J. Neurophysiol.* **21**, 430–436.

Lance, J.W. & Adams, R.D. (1963): The syndrome of intention or action myoclonus as a sequel to hypoxic encephalopathy. *Brain* **86**, 111–136.

Lloyd, K.G., Scatton, B., Voltz, C., Bryere, P., Valin, A. & Naquet, R. (1986): Cerebrospinal fluid amino acid and monoamine metabolite levels of *Papio papio*: correlation with photosensitivity. *Brain Res.* **363**, 390–394.

Luscombe, G., Jenner, P. & Marsden, C.D. (1982): Myoclonus in guinea pigs is induced by indole-containing but not piperazine-containing 5HT agonists. *Life Sci.* **30**, 1487–1494.

Marsden, C.D., Hallett, M. & Fahn, S. (1982): The nosology and pathophysiology of myoclonus. In: *Movement disorders*, eds. C.D. Marsden & S. Fahn, pp. 196–248. London: Butterworth.

Meencke, H.J. (1983): The density of dystopic neurons in the white matter of the gyrus frontalis inferior in epilepsies. *J. Neurol.* **230**, 171–181.

Meencke, H.J. & Janz, D. (1985): The significance of microdysgenesia in primary generalized epilepsy: an answer to the considerations of Lyon and Gastaut. *Epilepsia* **26**, 368–371.

Meier, E., Belhage, B., Drejer, J. & Schousboe, A. (1987): The expression of GABA receptors on cultured cerebellar granule cells is influenced by GABA. In: *Neurotrophic activity of GABA during development*, eds. D.A. Redburn & A. Schousboe, pp. 139–159. New York: Alan Liss.

Meldrum, B.S. (1984): Amino acid neurotransmitters and new approaches to anticonvulsant drug action. *Epilepsia* **25**(Suppl. 2), S140–S149.

Meldrum, B.S. & Balzamo, E. (1971): Etude des effets de l'α-méthylparatyrosine chez le *Papio papio*. *C.R. Soc. Biol. (Paris)* **165**, 2379–2381.

Meldrum, B.S., Balzamo, E., Gadea, M. & Naquet, R. (1970a): Photic and drug induced epilepsy in the baboon (*Papio papio*). The effect of isoniazid, thiosemicarbazide, pyridoxine and amino-oxyacetic acid. *Electroencephalogr. Clin. Neurophysiol.* **29**, 343–347.

Meldrum, B.S., Croucher, M.J., Badman, G. & Collins, J.F. (1983): Antiepileptic action of excitatory amino acid antagonists in the photosensitive baboon, *Papio papio*. *Neurosci. Lett.* **39**, 101–104.

Meldrum, B.S. & Horton, R.W. (1974): Neuronal inhibition mediated by GABA and patterns of convulsions in baboons with photosensitive epilepsy (*Papio papio*). In: *The natural history and management of epilepsy*, eds. P. Harris & C. Mawdsley, pp. 55–64. Edinburgh: Livingstone.

Meldrum, B.S. & Horton, R.W. (1978): Blockade of epileptic responses in the photosensitive baboon, *Papio papio*, by two irreversible inhibitors of GABA-transaminase γ-acetylenic GABA (4-amino-hex-5-ynoic acid) and γ-vinyl GABA (4-amino-hex-5-enoic acid). *Psychopharmacology* **69**, 47–50.

Meldrum, B.S. & Horton, R.W. (1980): Effects of the bicyclic GABA agonist, THIP, on myoclonic and seizure responses in mice and baboons with reflex epilepsy. *Eur. J. Pharmacol.* **61**, 231–237.

Meldrum, B.S., Horton, R.W. & Toseland, P.A. (1975): A primate model for testing anticonvulsant drugs. *Arch. Neurol.* **32**, 289–294.

Meldrum, B.S. & Menini, Ch. (1981): Effect of morphine, enkephalins, beta-endorphin and related compounds on seizure thresholds. In: *Neurotransmitters, seizures & epilepsy*, eds. P.L. Morselli *et al.*, pp. 185–194. New York: Raven Press.

Meldrum, B.S., Menini, Ch., Stutzmann, J.M. & Naquet, R. (1979): Effects of opiate-like peptides, morphine and naloxone in the photosensitive baboon *Papio papio. Brain Res.* **170**, 333–348.

Meldrum, B.S., Naquet, R. & Balzano, E. (1970b): Effects of atropine and eserine on the electroencephalogram, on behaviour and on light induced epilepsy in the adolescent baboon *Papio papio. Electroencephalogr. Clin. Neurophysiol.* **28**, 449–458.

Menini, Ch. & Naquet, R. (1986): Les myoclonies. Des myoclonies du *Papio papio* à certaines myoclonies humaines. *Rev. Neurol. (Paris)* **142**, 3–28.

Menini, Ch., Stutzmann, J.M., Laurent, H. & Valin, A. (1977): Les crises induites – ou non-par la stimulation lumineuse intermittente chez le *Papio papio* après injection d'allylglycine. *Rev. EEG Neurophysiol.* **7**, 232–238.

Menini, Ch., Silva-Comte, C., Stutzmann, J.M. & Dimov, S. (1981): Cortical unit discharges during photic intermittent stimulation in the *Papio papio*. Relationships with paroxysmal fronto-rolandic activity. *Electroencephalogr. Clin. Neurophysiol.* **52**, 42–49.

Musumeci, S.A., Ferri, R., Elia, M., Colognola, R.M., Bergonzi, P. & Tassinari, C.A. (1991): Epilepsy and fragile X syndrome: a follow-up study. *Am. J. Med. Genet.* **38**, 511–513.

Naquet, R., Fegersten, L. & Bert, J. (1960): Seizure discharges localized to the posterior cerebral regions in man, provoked by intermittent photic stimulation. *Electroencephalogr. Clin. Neurophysiol.* **12**, 305–316.

Naquet, R., Menini, Ch. & Catier, J. (1972): Photically induced epilepsy in *Papio papio*. The initiation of discharges and the role of the frontal cortex and of the corpus callosum. In: *Synchronization of the EEG in the epilepsies*, eds. H. Petsche & M.A.B. Brazier, pp. 347–367. Vienna: Springer-Verlag.

Naquet, R. & Poncet-Ramade, M. (1982): Paroxysmal discharges induced by intermittent light stimulation. *Electroencephalogr. Clin. Neurophysiol.* **35(Suppl.)**, 333–344.

Naquet, R., Silva-Comte, C. & Menini, Ch. (1983): Implication of the frontal cortex in paroxysmal manifestations (EEG and EMG) induced by light stimulation in the *Papio papio*. In: *Epilepsy and motor system*, eds. E. Speckmann & C. Elger, pp. 220–227. Munich: Urban and Schwarzenberg.

Naquet, R., Valin, A. & Bryere, P. (1985): Progabide, benzodiazepines and myoclonus in *Papio papio*. In: *Epilepsy and GABA receptor agonists. Basic and therapeutic research*, LERS Vol. 3, eds. G. Bartholini, L. Bossi, K.G. Lloyd & P.L. Morselli, pp. 159–171. New York: Raven Press.

Nordborg, C., Sourander, P., Silfvenius, H., Blom, S. & Zetterlund, B. (1987): Mild cortical dysplasia in patients with intractable partial seizures: a histological study. In: *Advances in epileptology*, Vol. 16, eds. P. Wolf, M. Dam, D. Janz & F.E. Dreyfuss, pp. 29–33. New York: Raven Press.

Pedley, T.A., Horton, R.W. & Meldrum, B.S. (1979): Electroencephalographic and behavioural effects of a GABA agonist (muscimol) on photosensitive epilepsy in the baboon *Papio papio. Epilepsia* **20**, 409–416.

Penfield, W. & Jasper, H.H. (1954): *Epilepsy and the functional anatomy of the human brain*. Boston: Little, Brown.

Pumain, R., Menini, C., Heinemann, U., Louvel, J. & Silva-Barrat, C. (1985): Chemical synaptic transmission is not necessary for epileptic seizures to persist in the baboon *Papio papio. Exp. Neurol.* **89**, 250–258.

Rakic, P. (1975): Cell migration and neuronal ectopias in the brain. *Birth Defects* **11**, 95–129.

Rektor, I., Bryere, P., Silva-Barrat, C. & Menini, Ch. (1986): Stimulus-sensitive myoclonus in the baboon *Papio papio*: pharmacological studies reveal interactions between benzodiazepines and the central cholinergic system. *Exp. Neurol.* **91**, 13–22.

Rektor, I., Bryere, P., Valin, A., Silva-Barrat, C., Naquet, R. & Menini, Ch. (1984): Physostigmine antagonizes the benzodiazepine-induced myoclonus in the baboon *Papio papio. Neurosci. Lett.* **52**, 91–96.

Rektor, I., Silva-Barrat, C., Barthuel, P. & Menini, Ch. (1991a): Drugs influencing the GABAergic neurotransmission have no effect on the non-epileptic myoclonus of baboons. *Electroencephalogr. Clin. Neurophysiol.* **79**, 148–152.

Rektor, I., Silva-Barrat, C., Barthuel, P. & Menini, Ch. (1990): Benzodiazepines: possible anticholinergic action independent on GABA. *Act. Nerv. Super.* **32**, 221–222.

Rektor, I., Svejdova, M., Silva-Barrat, C., Barthuel, P. & Menini, Ch. (1991b): Effects of drugs influencing the noradrenergic neurotransmission on nonepileptic myoclonus of *Papio papio* baboon. *Homeostasis* **33**, 164–165.

Rektor, I., Svejdova, M., Silva-Barrat, C. & Menini, Ch. (1989): Dopaminergic-cholinergic interaction in a myoclonus of *Papio papio* baboon. *Act. Nerv. Super.* **31**, 271–272.

Rektor, I., Svejdova, M., Silva-Barrat, C. & Menini, Ch. (1993): The cholinergic system-dependent myoclonus of the baboon *Papio papio* is a reticular reflex myoclonus. *Mov. Dis.* **8**, 28–32.

Riche, D., Condé, F., Silva-Barrat, C. & Menini, Ch. (1987): Morphology of different cholinergic groups of neurones in the hindbrain of the baboon. *Neuroscience* **22**, S784.

Rump, F. & Faff, J. (1976): Limitations of pharmacotherapy in organophosphate intoxications. In: *Medical protection against chemical warfare agents*, Ch. 10, eds. Sipri & Almquist. Stockholm: Wicksell International.

Sarnat, H.B. (1991): Cerebral dysplasias as expressions of altered maturational processes. *Can. J. Neurol. Sci.* **18**, 196–204.

Seyfried, T.N. & Glaser, G.H. (1985): A review of mouse mutants as genetic models of epilepsy. *Epilepsia* **26**, 143–150.

Shimamura, M. & Livingston, R.B. (1963): Longitudinal conduction systems serving spinal and brain-stem coordination. *J. Neurophysiol.* **26**, 258–272.

Shimamura, M., Mori, S., Matsushima, S. & Fujimori, B. (1964): On the spino–bulbo–spinal reflex in dogs, monkeys and man. *Jap. J. Physiol.* **14**, 411–421.

Silva-Barrat, C., Menini, Ch., Bryere, P. & Naquet, R. (1986): Multiunitary analysis of cortical and subcortical structures in paroxysmal discharges and grand mal seizures in photosensitive baboons. *Electroencephalogr. Clin. Neurophysiol.* **64**, 455–468.

Silva-Barrat, C., Brailowsky, S., Levesque, G. & Menini, Ch. (1988a): Epileptic discharges induced by intermittent light stimulation in photosensitive baboons: a current source density study. *Epilepsy Res.* **2**, 1–8.

Silva-Barrat, C., Brailowsky, S., Riche, D. & Menini, Ch. (1988b): Anticonvulsant effects of localized chronic infusions of GABA in cortical and reticular structures of baboons. *Exp. Neurol.* **101**, 418–427.

Stark, L.G., Killam, K.F. & Killam, E.K. (1970): The anticonvulsant effects of phenobarbital, diphenylhydantoin and two benzodiazepines in the baboon, *Papio papio*. *J. Pharmacol. Exp. Ther.* **173**, 125–132.

Valin, A., Dodd, R.H., Liston, D.R., Potier, P. & Rossier, J. (1982): Methyl-β-carboline induced convulsions are antagonized by Ro 15-1788 and propyl-β-carboline. *Eur. J. Pharmacol.* **85**, 93–97.

Valin, A., Cepeda, C., Rey, E. & Naquet, R. (1981): Opposite effects of lorazepam on two kinds of myoclonus in the photosensitive *Papio papio*. *Electroencephalogr. Clin. Neurophysiol.* **52**, 647–651.

Valin, A., Kaijima, M., Bryere, P. & Naquet, R. (1983): Differential effect of the benzodiazepine antagonist Ro15-1788 on two types of myoclonus in baboon *Papio papio*. *Neurosci. Lett.* **38**, 79–84.

Vogel, H.L. (1977): Intravenous use of physostigmine in the management of acute diazepam intoxication. *J. Am. Osteopath. Ass.* **76**, 349–351.

Wada, J.A., Terao, A. & Booker, H.E. (1972): Longitudinal correlative analysis of epileptic baboon *Papio papio*. *Neurology (Minneap.)* **22**, 1272–1285.

Wolff, J.R., Joo, F. & Kasa, P. (1993): Modulation by GABA of neuroplasticity in the central and peripheral nervous system. *Neurochem. Res.* **18**, 453–461.

Chapter 30

Forebrain convulsive mechanisms examined in the primate model of generalized epilepsy: emphasis on the claustrum

Juhn A. Wada

Divisions of Neurosciences and Neurology, University of British Columbia, Vancouver, BC, Canada V6T 2A1

Introduction

In idiopathic generalized epilepsy, the concurrence of non-convulsive and convulsive seizures is well recognized. Since both seizures share the unique electroclinical characteristics of being bisymmetrical and bisynchronous in onset, the centrencephalic theory with a hypothetical midline subcortical mechanism capable of ictally engaging both cerebral hemispheres was intuitively attractive. However, over the past decades, the theory has not received strong support, either experimentally or clinically. A striking feature of this theory was its absence of the massive forebrain commissures, particularly the corpus callosum. This is intriguing since the knowledge of the important role played by the corpus callosum for bilateralization of epileptic seizure in primates was already at hand in Montreal at the time when the theory was being formulated (Erickson, 1940). While the significance of the corpus callosum for seizure generalization and generalized seizure subsequently became established experimentally and clinically (Wada, 1980; Wada & Moyes, 1982; Marcus, 1985; Wada & Komai, 1985; Wada, 1987), the centrencephalic theory also underwent revision to assign a more appropriate role to the cerebral cortex, supported by extensive experimental exploitation of the feline model of generalized penicillin epilepsy (Gloor, 1969, 1978). In this animal model of generalized spike-and-wave discharge, the occasional occurrence of sustained tonic–clonic generalized spike discharge was also noted, but the underlying mechanism for this transformation remains obscure.

One major obstacle for the study of convulsive seizure has been the lack of an appropriate or valid animal model. Although generalized convulsive seizure can be acutely induced in normal animals by a variety of means, suggesting the capacity of the normal brain to produce electroclinical epileptic manifestations, it does not provide us with an insight as to the mechanisms underlying the chronic seizure recurrence which characterizes epilepsy.

In an ideal experimental model of epilepsy, in general, there should be: precise experimental control over the anatomy in terms of the area as well as the size of the epileptogenic lesion to be created

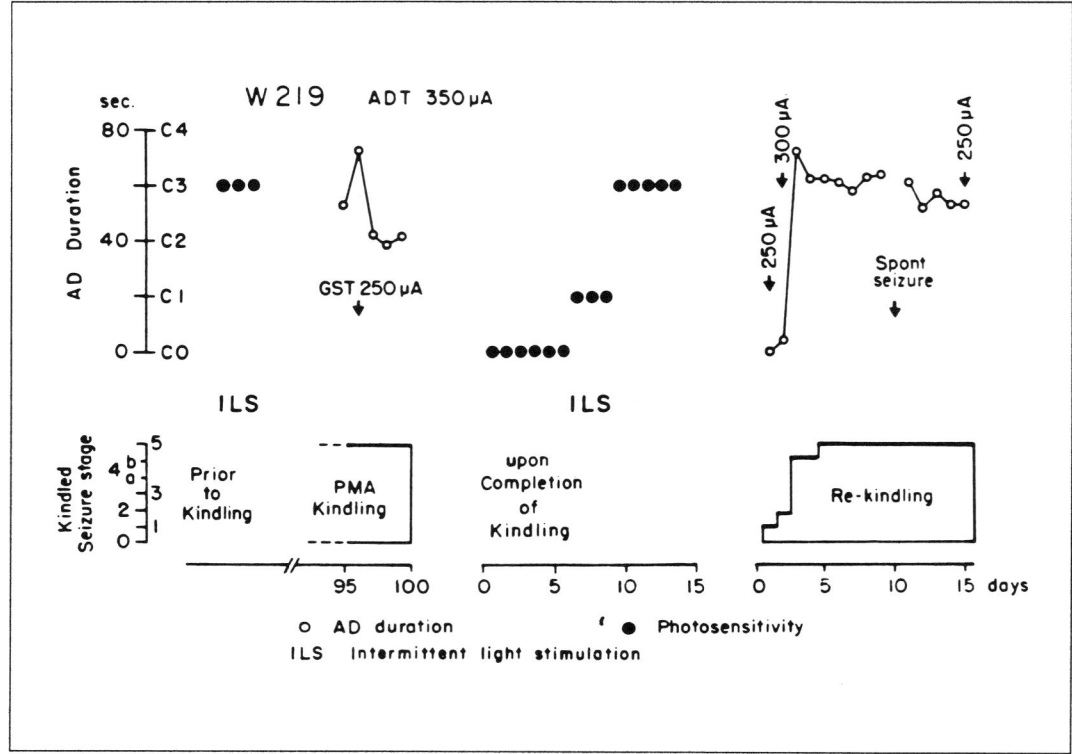

Fig. 1. Reciprocal susceptibility to premotor area (PMA) kindling and intermittent light stimulation in photosensitive baboon, Papio papio W219. Note transient decrease of photosensitivity following completion of PMA kindling and transient erosion of kindled seizure after repeated ILS-induced convulsions.

without introducing destructive pathology, accurate experimental control over the chronology of seizure development, ready precipitation of seizure by a discrete and identifiable experimental event, eventual development of a spontaneous recurrent seizure state and evidence in the model of persistence, progression or remission of the underlying pathophysiology, as in the case of some human epilepsies when untreated.

In this regard, a new era for the study of generalized convulsive seizure began in the mid-1960s with the concurrent discovery of two striking animal models of generalized convulsive seizure. One model is the Senegalese baboon, *Papio papio*, with genetically dictated photosensitivity (Killam et al., 1967; Naquet & Meldrum, 1972) and spontaneous recurrent generalized convulsion (Wada, 1971), regarded as a model of epilepsy with primary generalized convulsion. The other is the kindling model (Goddard, 1967; Goddard et al., 1969), capable of emitting spontaneous recurrent generalized convulsive seizure (Wada et al., 1974, 1975; Wada & Osawa, 1976; Pinell, 1981; Corcoran et al., 1984) and regarded as a model of epilepsy with partial onset secondarily generalized convulsion. These models meet most, if not all, the criteria enumerated above.

This paper will selectively review findings obtained in our laboratory with the *Papio papio* and kindling models over the past 25 years, with the emphasis on the forebrain mechanisms of generalized convulsive seizures.

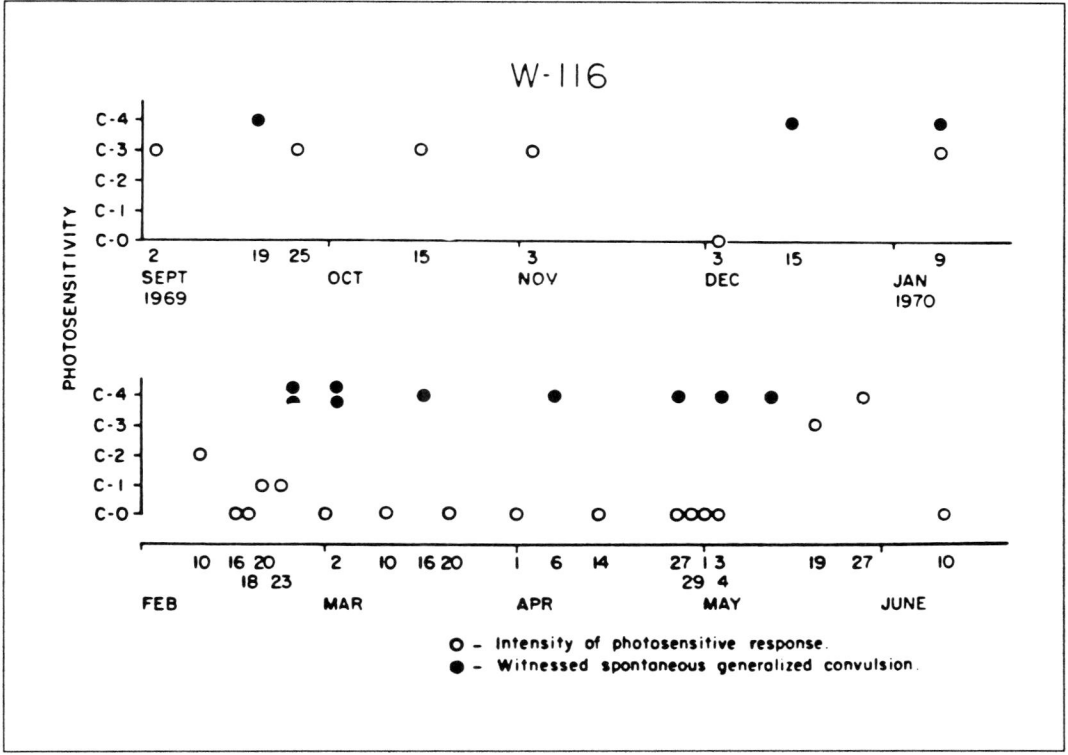

Fig. 2. Chronological reciprocity between degree of photosensitivity and spontaneous recurrent generalized convulsion in photosensitive baboon, Papio papio W116.

Generalized convulsive seizure induced by kindling or intermittent light stimulation (ILS) in primates

Kindling refers to repeated application of low intensity, initially ineffective, electrical stimulation to a localized brain area causing a progressive electroclinical seizure development culminating in a generalized convulsion (Goddard et al., 1969). The kindling effect is considered to be permanent and is due to widespread trans-synaptic change associated with certain morphological change (Sutula et al., 1988). It is an experimental model of partial onset secondarily generalized convulsions. Because of the relative ease with which kindling is accomplished, the amygdala (AM) has been the preferred site of stimulation in a number of animal species including four different primates (Wada & Sato, 1974; Wada & Osawa, 1976; Wada et al., 1978; Uemura & Wada, 1981; Corcoran et al., 1984). In addition, a number of different cortical sites have been subjected to kindling in primates in this laboratory. Despite the fact that all the primates at every brain site explored (except for the orbital site) developed asymmetrical generalization (stage 4 seizure), only some baboons (*Papio papio* and *Papio cynocephalus*) progressed to a final bisymmetrical and bisynchronous generalized convulsion (stage 5 seizure) which subsequently recurred spontaneously. The electroclinical manifestation of a kindled stage 5 seizure was indistinguishable from that of generalized convulsions induced by intermittent light stimulation (ILS) in *Papio papio*. The fact that the stage 5 seizure and the ILS-induced seizure mutually interact (Fig. 1) suggests that they are likely to share the same underlying mechanisms (Baba & Wada, 1987). This is further supported by our findings of the identical effect of callosal bisection in both amygdala-kindled and ILS-in-

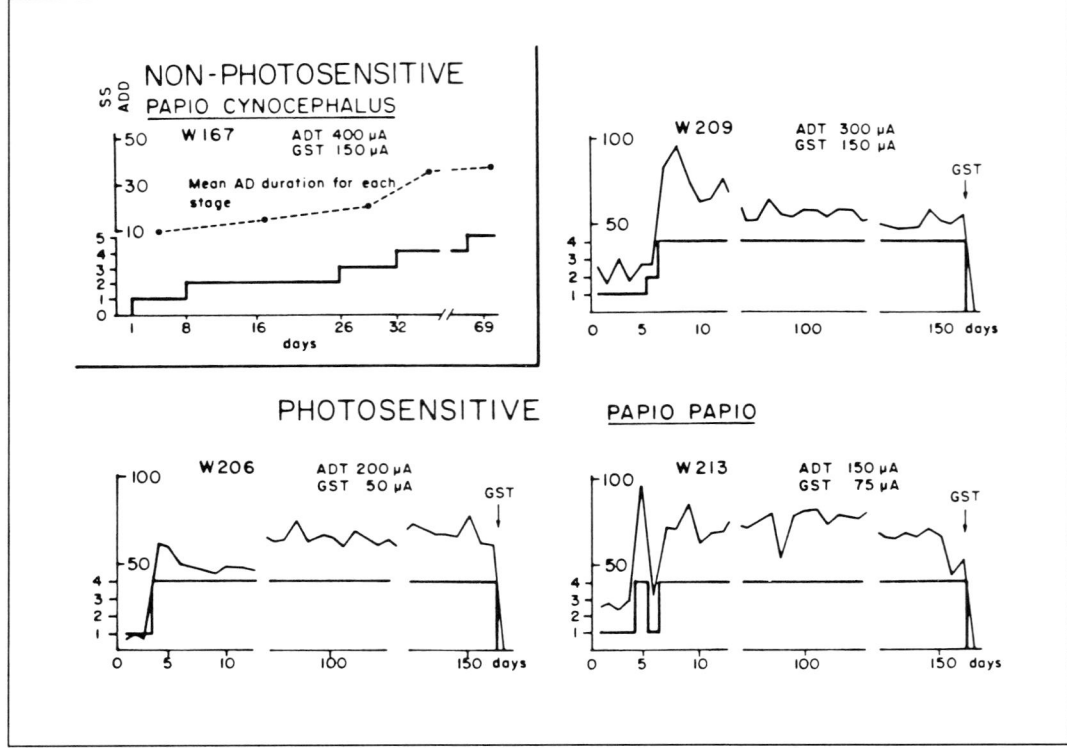

Fig. 3. Ultimate pattern of amygdaloid-kindled seizure. Note non-sensitive Papio cynocephalus *reaching stage 5 bisymmetrical convulsive state while sensitive* Papio papio *remains at stage 4 asymmetrical convulsive state.*

duced generalized convulsion in *Papio papio* to be described below. Similarly, some reciprocal tendency exists between the degree of photosensitivity and the timing of spontaneous emission of generalized convulsion in *Papio papio* (Fig. 2). However, stage 5 seizure may develop in some non-photosensitive baboons while some sensitive animals may remain at the stage 4 asymmetrical convulsive seizure stage (Fig. 3). Therefore, no precise relationship between the degree of photosensitivity and development of stage 5 bisymmetrical convulsive seizures by kindling can be established.

One of the striking features of stage 5 seizures was the development of early bilateral brain-stem discharge at the outset of the seizure whether it was kindling induced or spontaneously emitted. This discharge in the midbrain, pontine and bulbar reticular formation was coincident with that of the fronto-rolandic area. Such a discharge was not observed during the stage 4 secondarily generalized seizure state. It is interesting that the same brain-stem structures, particularly the pontine reticular formation, display repetitive spike discharges in the sensitive *Papio papio* upon intermittent light stimulation (Wada & Sato, 1973).

Senegalese baboons kindle in about 2 months, eventually developing stage 5 bisymmetrical and bisynchronous convulsions, indistinguishable from their spontaneously emitted or ILS-induced ones, which subsequently recur spontaneously. Motor seizure development and its bilateralization and generalization are all extremely rapid in this species (Wada & Osawa, 1976). In striking contrast, rhesus monkeys under the same kindling paradigm show difficulty in developing secondarily generalized convulsions even after over 1 year of daily stimulation. Thus, in rhesus monkeys, development of motor seizure, its bilateralization and generalization are extremely slow (Wada *et al.*, 1978). This difference suggests a genetic difference between these two species in the functional properties of the anatomical substrate underlying convulsive seizure development and its secondary generalization.

Search for the anatomical substratum for kindling induced convulsive seizure development

Our search for the anatomical substratum underlying convulsive seizure development in amygdala kindling was guided by two interrelated questions, i.e. how non-convulsive partial seizure originating in the amygdala becomes convulsive and how partial convulsive seizure becomes bilateral and generalized. We have investigated the substantia innominata for the former and both the corpus callosum and the midline thalamus for the latter.

Role of the substantia innominata (SI) for convulsive seizure development

The substantia innominata receives input from the mid- and lower brain-stem structures, including both dopaminergic and noradrenergic neurons, and projects widely and diffusely to the cerebral cortex. On the other hand, the ventral amygdaloid pathway, containing both the amygdalofugal and the amygdalopetal fibres, appears to have reciprocal connections between the basolateral nucleus and the substantia innominata. Based on our initial assessments (Kaneko *et al.*, 1981; Kimura *et al.*, 1981), we postulated that the substantia innominata plays a role in the expression of motor manifestations of amygdala-kindled seizures. Since the substantia innominata has high glutamic acid decarboxylase activity it was further postulated that GABAergic transmission in the substantia innominata exerts an inhibitory action on amygdala-kindled convulsions. Indeed, ipsilateral intra-SI injection of GABA mimetic drugs selectively suppresses the convulsive component of the amygdala kindled seizures while intra-amygdala injection of the same elevates the after-discharge threshold, indicating that the pharmacological enhancement of GABAergic transmission in the substantia innominata interferes with the process of convulsive seizure development, while the same in the amygdala reduces amygdala neuronal excitability (Okamoto & Wada, 1984). These findings have now been confirmed in cats (Morita *et al.*; 1985; Okamoto *et al.*, 1986) and *Papio papio* (Sakai & Wada, 1987).

Similar selective suppression of amygdala-kindled convulsion has been obtained by intra-SI injection of 2-amino-7-phosphoheptanoic acid (2-APH), a selective antagonist for N-methyl-D-aspartate (NMDA) receptors, or procaine (Mori & Wada, 1989; Mori *et al.*, 1993). Since both complete suppression and re-emergence of kindled convulsion was associated with prolonged delay of convulsive onset, it was postulated that the substantia innominata by itself does not directly participate in the expression of amygdala-kindled convulsion.

In *Papio papio*, intra-SI injection of gabaculine caused ipsilateral dominant but bilateral EEG slowing. When unilateral intra-SI gabaculine injection was made in animals with bisected forebrain commissures, however, EEG slowing was lateralized to the side of the injection (Sakai & Wada, unpublished data). This finding is consistent with our observation in *Papio papio* that intra-SI gabaculine eliminates generalized convulsions when injected ipsilateral to amygdala stimulation but causes contralateral hemiconvulsion when injected contralateral to amygdala stimulation. Therefore, amygdala-kindled seizure in *Papio papio* is due to secondary generalization of partial onset hemiconvulsive seizures despite bisymmetrical and bisynchronous presentation. When supplementary motor-cortex-kindled *Papio papio* were subjected to ipsilateral intra-SI gabaculine injection, kindled seizure was not only suppressed but also after-discharge could not be induced at the kindled cortical site despite a 20-fold increase in stimulus intensity (Fig. 4). This is in contrast to the same injection in amygdala-kindled baboons in which amygdala stimulation readily produced after-discharge (Sakai & Wada, 1987). These findings further suggest that the seizure suppressive effect observed is due to the reduced cerebral excitability of both cortical and subcortical motor mechanisms responsible for convulsive seizure.

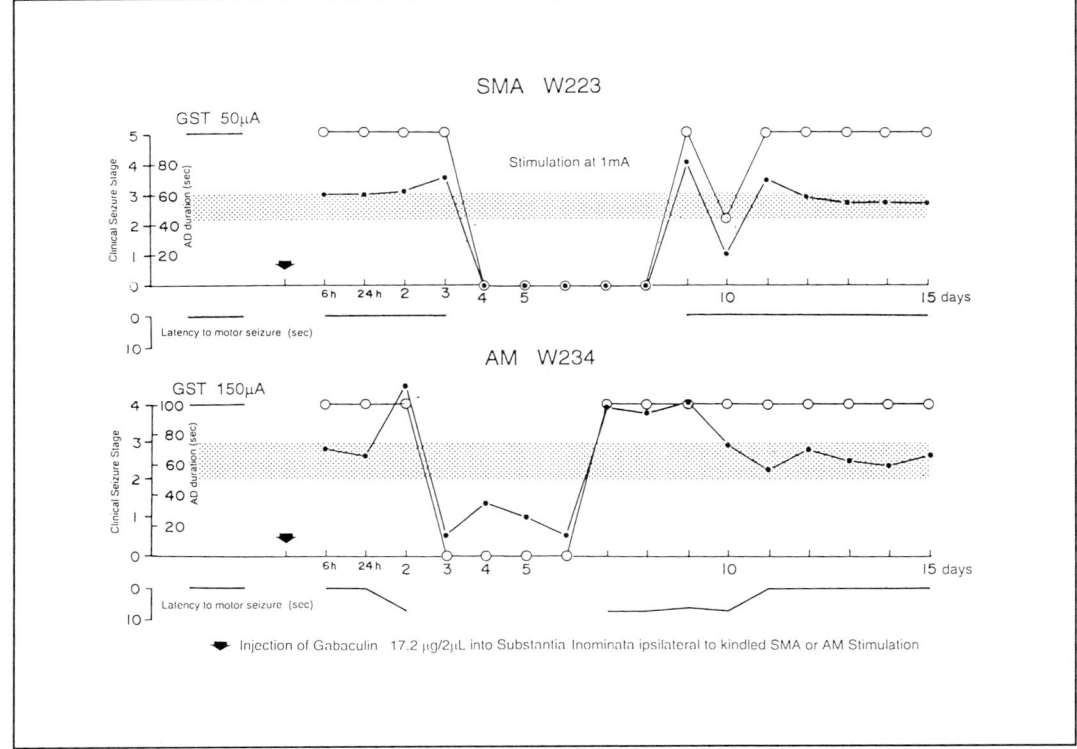

Fig. 4. *Differential effect of gabaculin injection into the substantia innominata in amygdaloid (AM) and supplementary motor area (SMA) kindled convulsion. Note kindled convulsion was eliminated in both animals. However, limbic seizure continues in amygdala-kindled animal while after-discharge cannot be induced despite increased stimulus intensity at the kindled SMA site.*

Role of subcortical midline structures for convulsive seizure bilateralization and generalization

Corpus callosum

In our studies of amygdala kindling in both *Papio papio* and the rhesus monkey with prior bisection of the corpus callosum, generalization of convulsive seizures was extremely difficult but some degree of bilateralization did occur when daily stimulation was applied persistently (Wada et al., 1981; Wada & Mizoguchi, 1984). On the other hand, when the amygdala-kindled *Papio papio* with stage 5 seizures underwent callosal bisection, kindled seizure became lateralized to the side contralateral to the amygdala stimulation (Wada & Komai, 1985). When the contralateral amygdala was subsequently subjected to kindling, only lateralized convulsive seizures developed. Furthermore, systemic pharmacological activation with Bemegride in these kindled but bisected animals resulted in a lateralized convulsive seizure. This is in contrast to the ready precipitation of bisymmetrical bisynchronous generalized convulsive seizures in the intact or kindled *Papio papio* undergoing similar pharmacological treatment. We found that the anterior two-thirds of the corpus callosum is the major anatomical substratum for both bilateralization of convulsive seizure and maintenance of an established pattern of generalized convulsion (Wada et al., 1981; Wada & Komai, 1985).

Although both *Papio papio* and rhesus monkey share the same anatomical substratum in this regard, there is a significant qualitative difference in the callosal bisection effect. Thus, only bisected rhesus monkeys show an accelerated rate of motor seizure development and the speed of the ictal motor

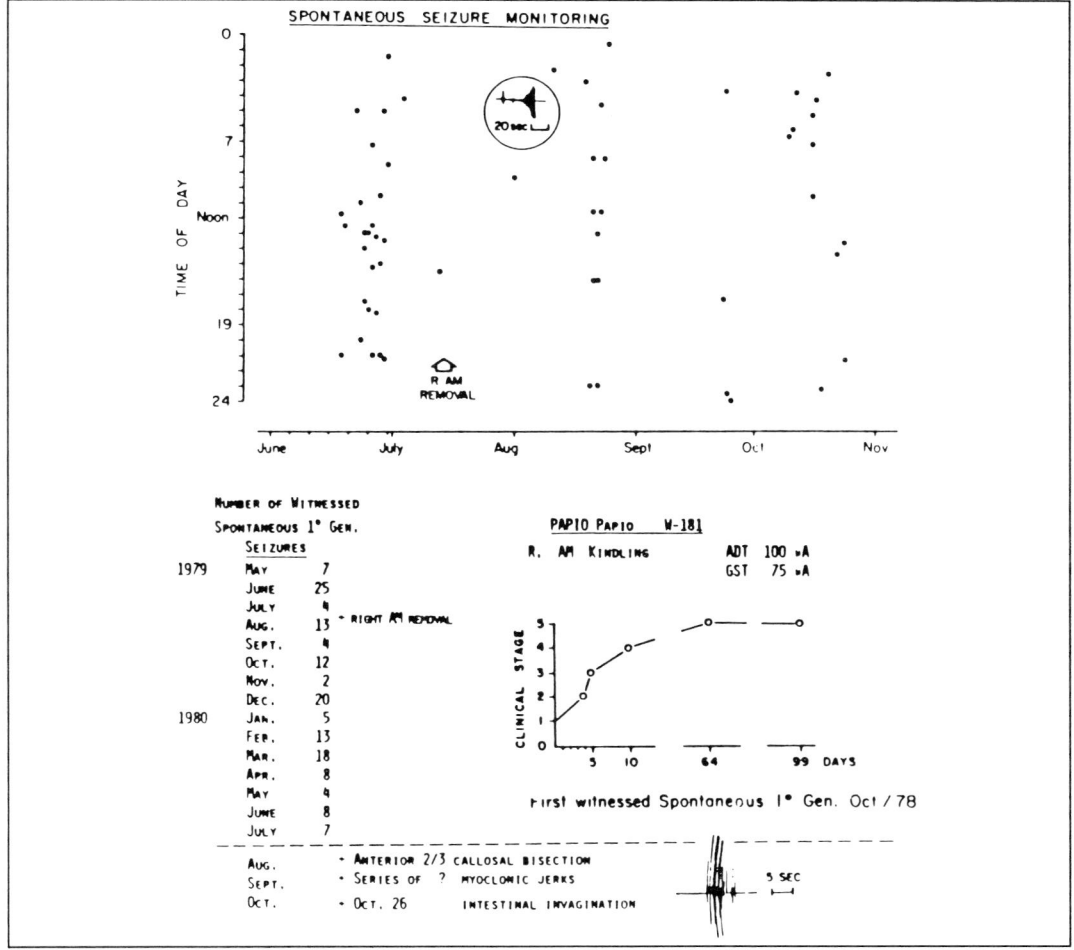

Fig. 5. Spontaneous recurrent generalized convulsion in right amygdaloid kindled Papio papio W181 is eliminated by anterior two-thirds callosal bisection (lower half) but not by suction removal of the kindled amygdala (upper half).

march within an individual hemiconvulsive seizure (stage 3) is nearly twice as fast as it is in nonbisected monkeys. Such acceleration is not observed in bisected *Papio papio*. These findings suggest that a facilitation (or the lack of inhibition) characterizes a function of the corpus callosum in *Papio papio*, and, therefore dysfunction of the corpus callosum may underlie aspects of predisposed seizure susceptibility in this species. This is consistent with our notion that the corpus callosum is involved in a more dynamic aspect of seizure generation in amygdala kindled *Papio papio* since spontaneous recurrent generalized convulsive seizure can be completely eliminated following anterior two-thirds callosal bisection (Fig. 5).

Finally, it should be noted that generalized convulsive seizure and complete forebrain bisection can occur in a baboon with hippocampal kindling (Wada & Mizoguchi, 1984), and secondary asymmetrical generalization does occur in bisected rhesus monkeys following kindled hemispheric onset convulsion with Bemegride. These findings suggest that a higher threshold alternative subcortical route in the brain-stem is available for seizure bilateralization in primates.

Midline thalamus-massa intermedia (MI)

The massa intermedia is a massive anatomical structure in all subhuman mammalian brains and is a part of the nonspecific medial thalamus to which prominent neurophysiological significance is attached for regulation of widespread cortical activity. Anatomically, the precentral motor cortex is known to project to the contralateral hemisphere through the massa intermedia in primates. Furthermore, evidence of ictal invasion from one hemisphere to another through the midline thalamus has been reported (Kusske & Rush, 1978; Ono et al., 1986). In human brain, the massa intermedia is small and often absent. However, since the difference in anatomy implies a difference in function, and our basic knowledge of the mechanism of epilepsy depends on the study of animal models, characterization of the functional significance of this structure in subhuman mammals is important for interpretation and interpolation of animal findings. Therefore, the possible role of the massa intermedia was examined by either stimulation of the massa intermedia in rat and cats (Ehara & Wada, 1989; Mori & Wada, 1992; Hirayasu & Wada, 1992, 1993) or selective midline section or lesioning of the massa intermedia in cats (Hiyoshi & Wada, 1988a,b; Ehara & Wada, 1990; Ishibashi & Wada, 1990).

The results obtained suggest that: (a) the massa intermedia is not essential for the development or maintenance of kindling-induced generalized convulsive seizure; (b) the horizontal pathway contained in the massa intermedia appears to participate in some aspect of bilateral patterning of secondarily generalized convulsion, and (c) perikarya in the MI and the intrahemispheric vertically organized neuronal network are important for the transhemispheric positive transfer effect in amygdala kindling.

A comparable amygdala kindling study in *Papio papio* with selective and complete midsagittal bisection of the massa intermedia confirmed the above (Sakai & Wada, unpublished data). Results of an electrolytic lesioning study were inconclusive, however, due to the unexpectedly limited nature of the lesion which involved only the anterodorsal portion of the massa intermedia.

If the massa intermedia is important for the development of generalized convulsion due to its strategic anatomical location, one might expect a rather rapid evolution of convulsive seizure from this site. However, results of massa intermedia kindling showed it to be slow, although following its completion a positive transfer effect was found at the amygdala (Mori & Wada, 1992). Additional studies in both cats and rats with intra-MI injection of N-methyl-D-aspartate (NMDA) indicated that the NMDA receptor in the massa intermedia is involved in modulation of temporal limbic excitability (Ehara & Wada, 1989; Hirayasu & Wada, 1992, 1993). These and other studies to this date (Wada, in press) suggest that the massa intermedia participates in modulation of temporal limbic excitability and is an integral part of the amygdala-kindled vertically oriented neurocircuitry extending from the cerebral cortex to the brain-stem.

Summary

Our findings obtained in kindling and kindled generalized convulsive seizure suggested that:

(i) The substantia innominata is critical for strengthening the linkage between the amygdala and the motor mechanism responsible for convulsive seizure development through modulation of cerebral motor excitability.

(ii) The corpus callosum is the major, if not exclusive, anatomical substratum for convulsive seizure bilateralization and maintenance of a generalized convulsive seizure state, although a high-threshold alternative pathway is available in the brain-stem.

(iii) The predominantly facilitatory (or disinhibitory) role of the corpus callosum is likely to be involved in a more dynamic process of seizure generation as an aspect of pathophysiology of the epileptic baboon, *Papio papio*,

(iv) The midline interthalamic connection participates in some aspect of bilateral patterning of

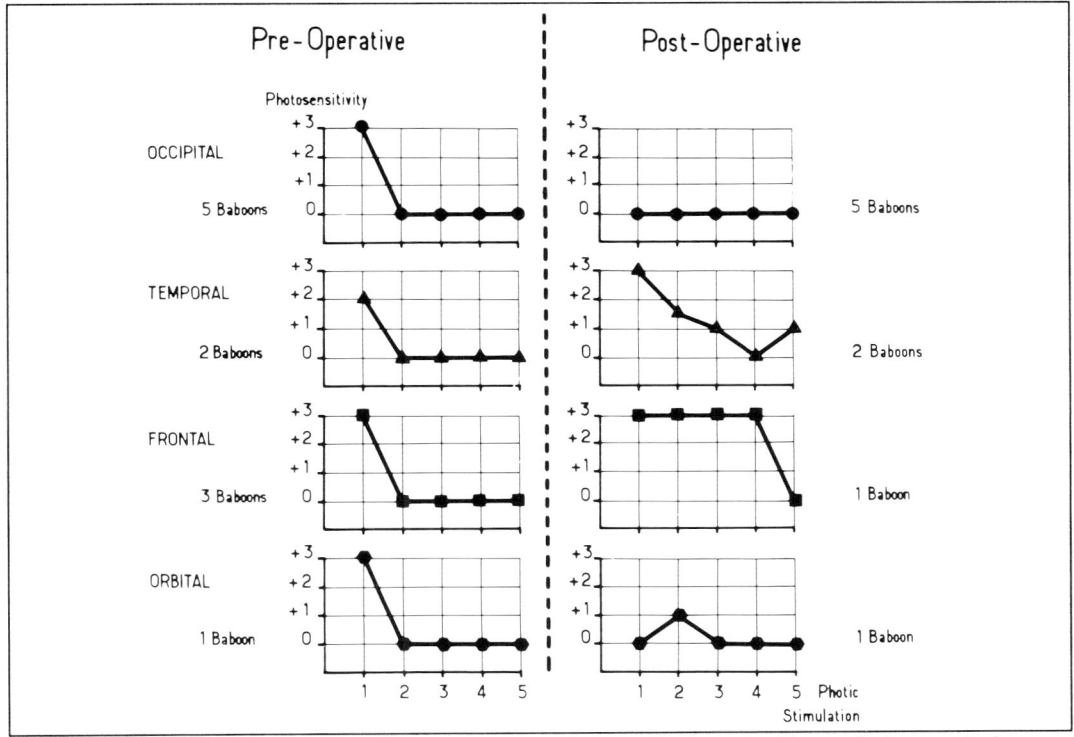

Fig. 6. Effect of bilateral corticectomy on photosensitive baboon, Papio papio. *Note only the occipital group lost photosensitivity.*

secondary generalization, but is not essential for the development and maintenance of generalized convulsive seizure.

(v) The perikarya in the midline thalamus is involved in both modulation of limbic excitability and transhemispheric positive transfer effect and thus participates in the mechanism of generation and expression of generalized convulsive seizure.

Search for the anatomical substratum for development of intermittent light stimulation (ILS) induced generalized convulsive seizure

The Senegalese baboon *Papio papio* is a natural primate model susceptible to specific external stimulus analogous to man for seizure precipitation. Despite some differences between this model and human generalized epilepsy, the bisynchronous and bisymmetrical nature of electroclinical convulsive seizure induced by intermittent light stimulation in this species provides us with an opportunity to systematically examine mechanisms underlying photosensitivity and generalized convulsive seizure. The importance of this animal model was underscored by the disclosure that some of this species has recurrent spontaneous generalized convulsive seizure as well (Wada, 1971; Wada et al., 1972).

The obvious importance of intermittent light stimulation in precipitation of generalized convulsive seizure in this species led us to a series of lesioning studies to define the cerebral structures which may be critically involved in the initiation and development of generalized convulsive seizure.

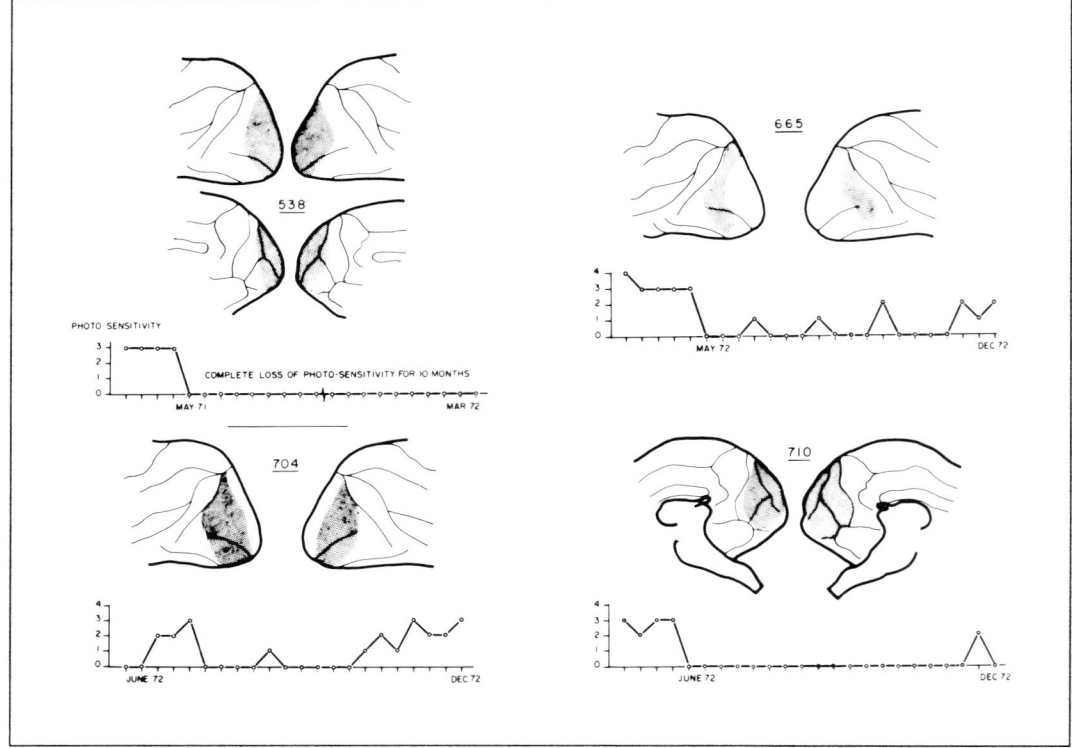

Fig. 7. Extent of bilateral occipital corticectomy abolishing photosensitive response in Papio papio. *Note complete loss of photosensitivity following mesial and lateral corticectomy in W538.*

Role of the superior colliculus

Since audiogenic seizure susceptibility in rodents was eliminated by destruction of the inferior colliculi (Wada et al., 1970), it was hypothesized that the superior colliculus may be involved in precipitation of photogenic seizure in this species. However, bilateral suction removal of the superior colliculus in two photosensitive baboons had no effect on ILS-induced seizure susceptibility (Wada et al., 1972).

Role of the occipital cortex and its projection

Subsequent studies involved either bilateral cortical resection or interruption of the occipito-frontal connection. All these animals possessed a strong and stable photosensitivity as verified by longitudinal study prior to surgery and were followed for 6 to 10 months postoperatively (Wada, 1971; Wada & Nacquet, 1972; Wada et al., 1973).

Bilateral corticectomy

Eleven animals were subjected to bilateral corticectomy involving the occipital (n = 4), frontal-orbital (n = 4) and mesial temporal (n = 3) regions. Only those animals with occipital corticectomy showed lasting loss of photosensitivity (Fig. 6). Subsequently, a new group of animals underwent bilateral occipital corticetomy involving exclusively lateral (n = 4), exclusively mesial (n = 4) and both mesial and lateral (n = 4) areas. As shown in Fig. 7, some effect was noted in all the animals but only the group with both mesial and lateral occipital resection showed persistent loss of photosensitivity.

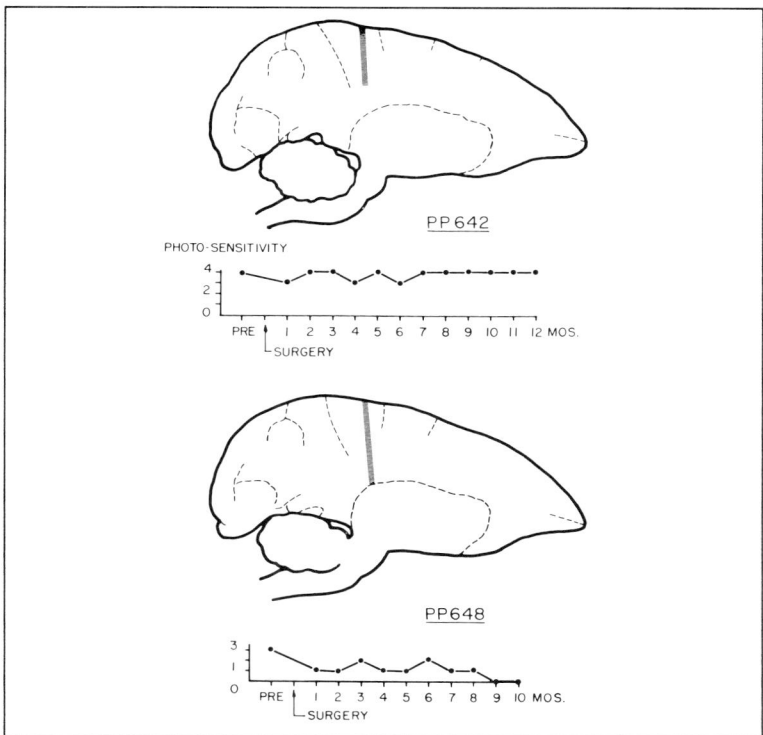

Fig. 8. Effect of suprasylvian anteroposterior division of both cerebral hemispheres on photosensitive baboon, Papio papio. *Note deeper division reduces but does not eliminate photosensitivity.*

Bilateral disruption of the occipito-frontal connection

The above findings have conclusively shown that the geniculo-occipital system is critical for a photosensitive response to occur. Since such afferents must access motor mechanisms before photosensitive seizures and since the frontorolandic cortex was identified as the site of major neurophysiological abnormality in this species, it was hypothesized that the longitudinal association fibres between the occipital and frontal cortical areas are involved in clinical photosensitive response (Wada *et al.*, 1973). In order to test this hypothesis, seven animals were subjected to anteroposterior division of the cerebral hemispheres. Bilateral division in the parietal region was carried out subpially and subcortically so that contiguity of the cortical and white matter was anteroposteriorly divided, thus largely if not completely interrupting the occipitofrontal connections above the sylvian fissure. Weekly examination of photosensitivity following the surgery showed a transient reduction in three animals from a mean of stable C +3.5 to C +2 with intermittent recurrence of C +1 to C +3 response during 10 months follow-up. In the remaining four animals, no significant change in the degree of photosensitivity was noted. Subsequent histological examination showed that the extent of the disruption was deeper in the three former animals, reaching the thalamus, while it was much shallower in the four latter animals (Fig. 8). These findings suggested that the occipitofugal pathway to an as yet unidentified subcortical site may be involved in the development of ILS-induced seizures.

Role of the corpus callosum

Based on our observation that (a) kindled and ILS-induced generalized convulsions share identical electroclinical phenomenology, and (b) kindled convulsions can be lateralized by callosal bisection, a series of studies in *Papio papio* examining the effect of selective stereotaxic callosal bisection was initiated in 1984 while the author was on sabbatical leave at Gif-sur-Yvette. Photosensitivity induced by either binocular/monocular or hemiretinal intermittent light stimulation confirmed the lateralizing effect of callosal bisection and indicated an independent seizure susceptibility of each hemisphere, with the corpus callosum playing a critical role for bisymmetrical and bisynchronous patterning of ILS-induced convulsive seizure in this species (Naquet & Wada, 1992; Fukuda *et al.*, 1988, 1989: Menini *et al.*, Ch. 29). Our findings further confirmed that kindled and ILS-induced generalized convulsions share the same callosal mechanism.

Summary

Our findings on ILS-induced generalized convulsive seizures in *Papio papio* suggested that:

(i) The primary visual receiving area in the occipital cortex and its projections, probably both the cortical and subcortical but not the superior colliculus, are critically involved.

(ii) Each cerebral hemisphere has independent photosensitive susceptibility. The corpus callosum is essential for bilateralization and generalization of hemispheric convulsive response.

(iii) The callosal mechanism is shared by both ILS-induced and kindled generalized convulsive seizures.

Search for the anatomical substratum for transformation of intermittent light stimulation or nonmotor seizures into convulsive seizures

How partial onset nonmotor seizure or visual afferents transforms into convulsive ones before secondary generalization remains unknown. As discussed earlier, our study on the substantia innominata suggested that it indirectly participates in the evolution of a partial nonmotor seizure to a hemiconvulsive one through modulation of excitability of the hemispheric motor mechanism responsible for convulsive seizure. However, the question of whether there is a specific pathway for a partial onset seizure to access the hemispheric motor mechanism remains unknown. As discussed above (*Midline thalamus-massa intermedia (MI)*, p. 356), results of our study of bihemispheric transection in photosensitive baboons suggested that occipitofugal projection to an as yet unidentified subcortical site may be involved in the mechanism of ILS-induced convulsive seizure. Among a number of potential candidate sites, the claustrum appears strategically located since it has widespread reciprocal connections with the neocortex (Riche & Lanoir, 1978; Sloniewski & Pilgrim, 1984; Druga, 1984).

The claustrum is partially continuous with the amygdala and has reciprocal connections with it (Kretteck & Price, 1978) as well as with the basal ganglia (Ishikawa *et al.*, 1969; Andersen, 1968). Reciprocal bilateral connections were also found between the claustrum and the cingulate cortex (Markowitsch *et al.*, 1984; Witter *et al.*, 1988). For bilateral claustral connections, the anterior commissure and the corpus callosum appear to participate for the basal ganglia (Andersen, 1968) and cortical areas (Macchi *et al.*, 1981), respectively. In addition, the massa intermedia participates for bilateral projection from the precentral cortex to the claustrum (Kuenzle, 1976).

In order to test the hypothesis that the claustrum is critically involved in the transformation of ILS-induced visual afferents or partial nonmotor seizure to a convulsive one, a series of studies has been performed in our laboratory. Results of our studies are selectively reviewed below.

Feline studies

Effect of unilateral claustral lesioning on ILS-induced generalized seizure following Systemic d,l-allylglycine (T. Kudo & J.A. Wada, unpublished data)

Fourteen adult male cats were used. The amount of D,L-allylglycine required to induce a photosensitive response (Meldrum et al., 1979) was a mean of 31.5 mg/kg (range 25–40 mg) for generalized myoclonic jerking and a mean of 34.0 mg/kg (range 25–40 mg) for bisymmetrical bisynchronous generalized convulsive seizures, respectively. Myoclonic jerking was associated with generalized spike, polyspikes and waves primarily in the subcortical structures, while the generalized convulsion was coincident with the bisymmetrical development of incremental sustained spike discharge in the motor cortices.-

Unilateral electrolytic lesioning of the claustrum by multiple stereotaxic penetrations through A 8.5–19.3 (Berman & Jones, 1982) caused no readily identifiable neurological deficit. Subsequent to the lesioning, the amount of d,l-allylglycine required was a mean of 35 mg/kg (range 25–45 mg) for the development of generalized myoclonic jerking and a mean of 39 mg/kg (range 25–45 kg) for generalized convulsions. These values were not significantly different from those of prelesioning and the electroclinical feature of the myoclonic jerking remained unchanged. However, when the convulsive seizure occurred, it showed a striking transformation from a bisymmetrical seizure to one of partial onset with ipsilateral tonic forelimb flexion, head and body turning, repeated axial rotation followed by ipsilateral hemiconvulsive seizure eventually evolving into a secondarily generalized one. This partial onset seizure was coincident with EEG seizure discharge commencing in the cortical motor area of the nonlesioned hemisphere. The specificity of this lesioning effect was supported by the development in one animal (whose lesion involved the caudate, putamen and internal capsule but not the claustrum) of bisymmetrical bisynchronous generalized convulsion identical to that of prelesioning.

Effect of unilateral claustral lesioning on amygdala-kindled generalized convulsion (Kudo & Wada, 1990)

Seven adult male cats, kindled from both the primary and secondary site amygdala, were used. The stability of the kindled seizure at both the primary and secondary sites was well established prior to unilateral electrolytic claustral lesioning. The lesioning was made by multiple stereotaxic penetrations through A 13.7–19.3. One animal had a unilateral lesion in the ectosylvian gyrus with an intact claustrum.

Amygdala stimulation at the established generalized seizure triggering threshold contralateral to the claustral lesioning readily reproduced kindled electroclinical seizure. Amygdala stimulation ipsilateral to the ectosylvian lesioning also reproduced the kindled generalized convulsion. In contrast, amygdala stimulation ipsilateral to the claustral lesioning caused a significant delay of convulsive seizure onset with a striking electroclinical modification having a mirror-image presentation of the kindled seizure, i.e., ipsilateral head turning, circling and axial rotation evolving into ipsilateral hemiconvulsion before progressing to a generalized one. EEG discharge associated with this mirror-image seizure began in the cortical motor area in the hemisphere contralateral to both the amygdala stimulation and the claustral lesioning.

These findings suggested that the claustrum ipsilateral to the kindled amygdala is critical for the development of convulsive seizures. The fact that amygdala stimulation contralateral to the claustral lesioning had no effect suggests that the claustrum is not critical for the mechanism of convulsive seizure generalization. Furthermore, the fact that ipsilateral claustral lesioning strikingly modified the kindled convulsive seizure to a mirror-image seizure initially involving the contralateral hemisphere, suggests that the amygdala onset seizure, when deprived of access to the ipsilateral claustrum, can access the contralateral hemispheric motor mechanism by way of an as yet unidentified transhemispheric pathway. Since these animals were already kindled at both the primary and secondary site amygdala prior to the claustral lesioning, it is possible that the mirror-image convulsive seizure development was due to prior kindling of the contralateral amygdala. Since the mechanism of kindling seizure development is not the same for the maintenance of kindled generalized seizure, the possibility exists that in the absence of the claustrum, amygdala kindling can access the ipsilateral hemispheric motor mechanism through an alternative route of seizure propagation.

Therefore, further study was undertaken in naive animals with lesioning of the unilateral claustrum prior to amygdala kindling.

Effect of unilateral claustral lesioning on amygdala convulsive seizure development (Kudo & Wada, 1990)

Nine naive adult male cats received unilateral electrolytic claustral lesioning which caused no overtly apparent neurological deficit. When these animals were subjected to ipsilateral amygdala kindling, significant modification of both the speed and pattern of seizure development was noted. Thus, the number of daily amygdala stimulations required for stage 4 contralateral head turning and circling was a mean of 29 (against 16 in the controls), and for the final stage 6 generalized convulsion, a mean of 37 (against 27 in the controls) was required. Furthermore, the pattern of both stage 4 aversive seizure and stage 6 generalized convulsive seizure became a mirror image of the expected pattern when they emerged. Thus, the animals showed initial ipsilateral head turning, circling and axial rotation, followed by ipsilateral clonic convulsion before becoming secondarily generalized. This pattern was coincident with the development of sustained EEG discharge in the cortical motor area of the contralateral nonlesioned hemisphere.

Summary

The above findings suggested that:

(i) The claustrum plays an important role in accession of visual afferents to the ipsilateral cortical motor mechanism for hemiconvulsive seizure development prior to its secondary generalization,

(ii) The claustrum ipsilateral to amygdala kindling is critical for accession of amygdala onset nonmotor seizure to the ipsilateral hemispheric motor mechanism before eventual convulsive seizure generalization, and

(iii) An as yet unidentified transhemispheric route is available for amygdala onset partial seizure to become secondarily generalized through the contralateral hemisphere motor mechanism.

Primate studies (Wada & Tsuchimochi, 1992)

In order to test our hypothesis that the claustrum plays a critical role in the evolution of convulsive response to both intermittent light stimulation and kindling of nonmotor structures in primates, the Senegalese baboon, *Papio papio* was used in the following studies. Electrolytic claustral lesioning was made stereotaxically on the left side in all the series. There was a transient clumsiness of the right arm lasting for a few days only. The extent of the lesions is shown in Fig. 9. At least 3–4 weeks elapsed before intermittent light stimulation or kindling stimulation was applied.

Effect of unilateral claustral lesioning on ILS-induced generalized convulsive seizure

Six baboons (one intact, three amygdala kindled and two cingulate kindled) underwent systemic d,l-allylglycine treatment. Intravenous administration of this compound in the range of 150–200 mg/kg made all the animals photosensitive when tested by 25 Hz intermittent light stimulation on an hourly basis. Results of intermittent light stimulation prior to the claustral lesioning showed no difference in either the dose of d,l-allylglycine or the pattern of photoconvulsive response among intact, amygdala or cingulate kindled animals. Therefore, the results were collapsed.

Prior to the lesioning, the intermittent light stimulation response progressed from bilateral eyelid twitching to generalized myoclonic jerking and bisymmetrical generalized convulsive seizures. The latter response began about 3–4 h after the drug treatment and lasted for 3–6 h when it was suppressed with i.v. diazepam.

Subsequent to the claustral lesioning, there was a remarkable change in the ILS-induced seizure pattern. The convulsive response began with an initial conjugate eye/head deviation and body turning to the left (ipsilateral to the claustral lesioning) and developed into a left hemiconvulsive seizure that gradually evolved into an asymmetrical generalized tonic–clonic convulsion. EEG

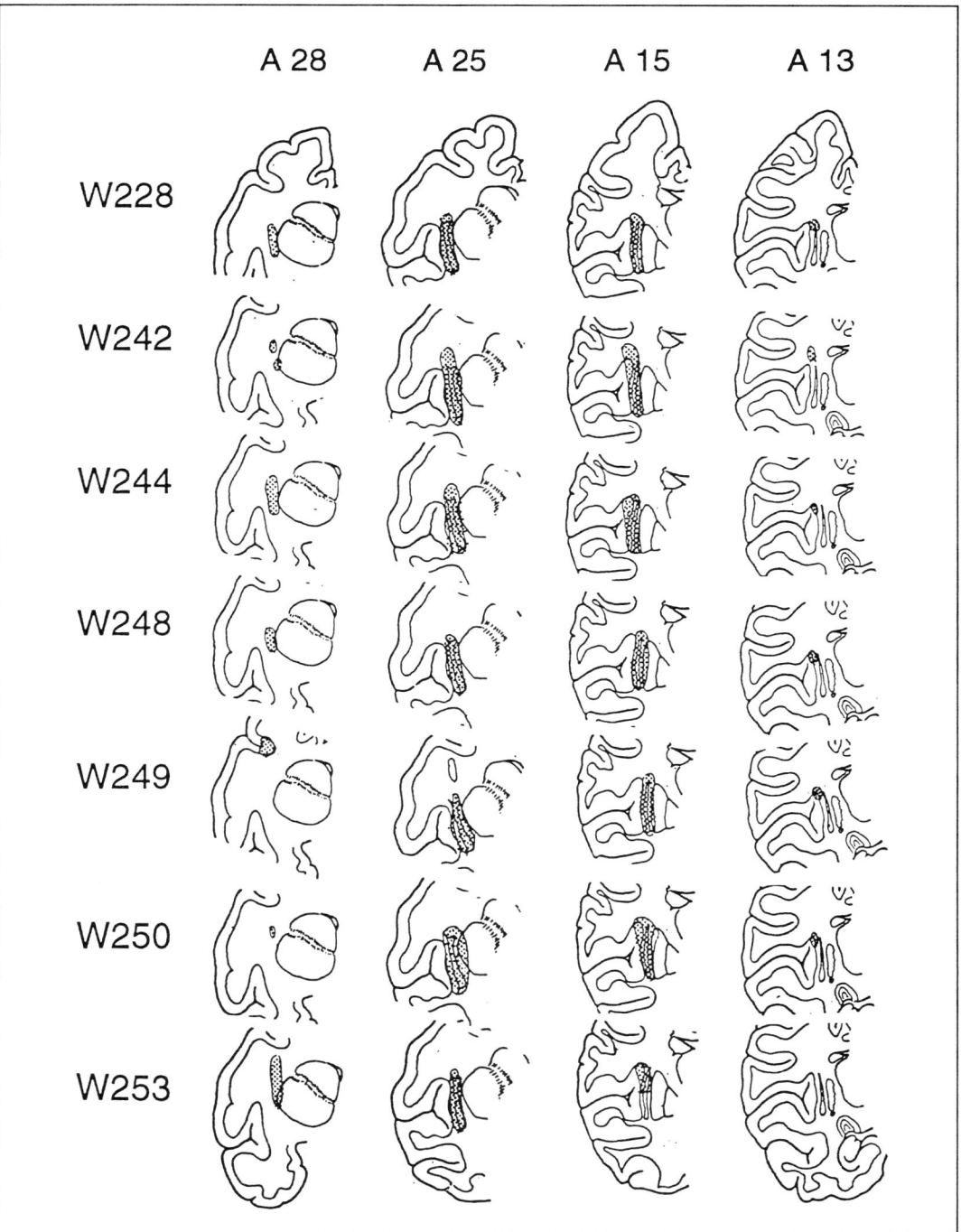

Fig. 9. Extent of claustral lesion.

seizure discharge began in the right frontocentral area, indicating its origin to be within the nonlesioned right hemisphere before becoming secondarily generalized (Fig. 9). Postictal transient left hemiparesis suggested major ictal involvement of the right (nonlesioned) hemisphere. The findings indicate that in primates, the claustrum plays a critical role in transforming visual afferents to a convulsive response following intermittent light stimulation.

Effect of unilateral claustral lesioning on amygdala kindled generalized convulsion

Three male Senegalese baboons, weighing 5.2–7.6 kg, were kindled from the primary site (left) amygdala and underwent secondary site (right) amygdala kindling and primary site retesting. Two animals (W248, W249) attained a stable stage 4 asymmetrical generalized convulsive seizure state and the remaining one animal (W250) attained a stable stage 5 bisymmetrical convulsive seizure state. At the secondary site, one animal (W250) attained a stable stage 5 seizure state, while the remaining two animals remained at a stage 2 nonconvulsive seizure state (W248, W249).

Upon completion of the above, and 2 weeks after the left claustral lesioning, the left primary site amygdala was restimulated. It was found that the after-discharge threshold was elevated from a mean of preoperative 133 µA to a mean of 400 µA postoperatively. However, despite elicitation of after-discharge, kindled convulsion could not be recalled. Instead, nonconvulsive stage 1 (W250) or stage 2 (W48, W49) was observed while the after-discharge duration remained comparable to that of the prelesioning stage 4 or 5 convulsive seizure state (Fig. 10). There was no further clinical seizure development during the subsequent stimulation.

When the stimulation was switched to the right amygdala, contralateral to the claustral lesioning, the presurgically established electroclinical seizure pattern was immediately re-activated with either stage 2 (W248, W249) or stage 5 (W250).

The findings above indicate that in primates the claustrum ipsilateral (but not contralateral) to the amygdala-onset seizure plays an important role in accessing the ipsilateral hemispheric motor mechanism for convulsive seizure development.

Effect of unilateral claustral lesioning on cingulate kindled generalized convulsion

In order to test the hypothesis that the claustrum is the key structure for the evolution of a nonmotor partial seizure originating in an area other than the amygdala to a convulsive one, the effect of claustral lesioning was assessed in baboons kindled from either the anterior (W244) or posterior (W242) cingulate gyrus.

The pattern of cingulate seizure development (Tsuchimochi & Wada, 1991) was essentially the same between anterior and posterior cingulate kindling with stage 1, visual searching; stage 2, repetitive contralateral eye/head deviation followed by oral automatism; stage 3, contralateral hemiconvulsion; and stage 4, asymmetrical generalized convulsion. In both anterior and posterior cingulate kindling, there was a frequent regression of seizure stages between stages 4–2. However, following 120 daily stimulations, a stable stage 4 asymmetrical generalized convulsive seizure state was established. Although the general pattern of both seizure development and developed seizure was similar between anterior and posterior cingulate kindling, there was a significant difference in the latency for convulsive seizure onset between the two areas, i.e. a mean of 20.8 s for the anterior and a mean of 45.6 s for the posterior area, indicating the protracted nature of accessing the hemispheric motor mechanism from the posterior cingulate.

With the contralateral secondary site kindling, W244 developed a stage 4 generalized convulsion identical to that of the primary-site kindled one. This was explained by subsequent histological examination which indicated that the secondary-site electrode was misplaced in the primary site hemisphere near the primary site electrode. On the other hand, contralateral secondary-site posterior cingulate kindling failed to develop convulsive seizure and remained at stage 1 even after 50 daily stimulations. Primary site restimulation readily recalled the kindled stage 4 asymmetrical convulsive seizure in both animals.

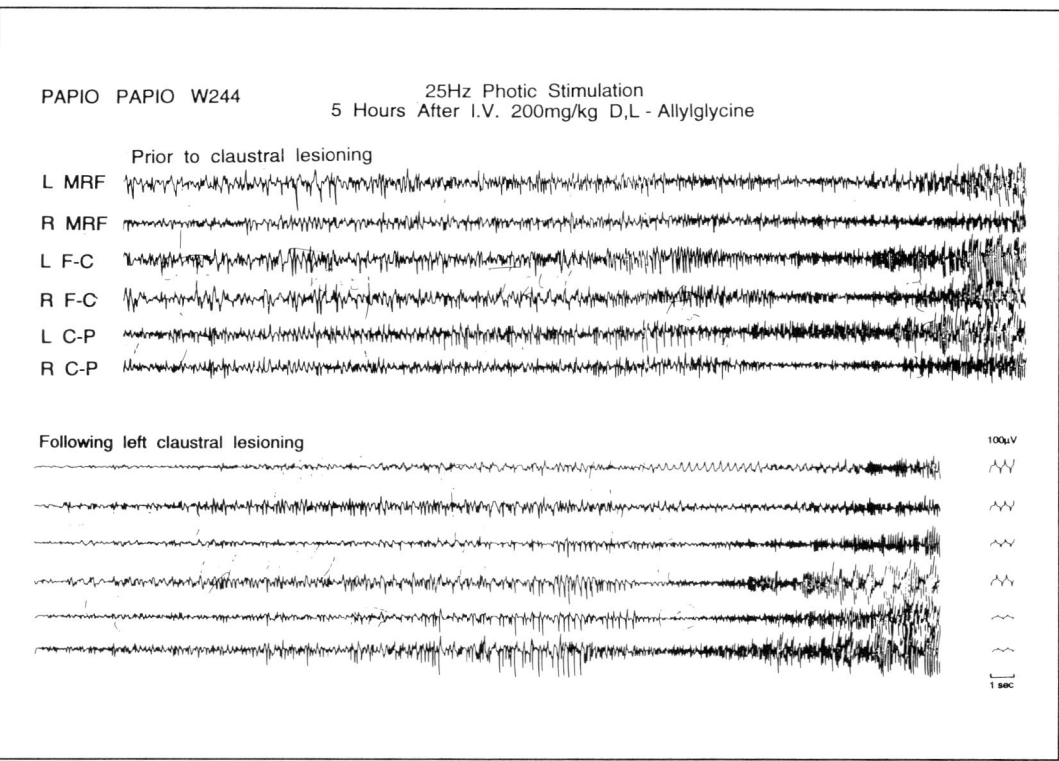

Fig. 10. Effect of left claustral lesioning on photosensitive baboon, Papio papio *W244. Note largely bilateral EEG discharge leading to bisymmetrical convulsion prior to the lesioning (upper trace). Following the lesion, EEG discharge in the non-lesioned right hemisphere predominates with eventual development of adversive left hemiconvulsive seizure which became bilateral.*

When both animals were restimulated at the primary site 2 weeks following ipsilateral claustral lesioning, the kindled convulsive stage was replaced by a nonconvulsive stage 1 seizure in both animals. However, in the anterior cingulate kindled animal, W244, two convulsive seizures were elicited on the fourth and fifth day of stimulation, only to regress again to a nonconvulsive seizure state subsequently. The onset of these convulsive responses had a latency of over 46 s following development of after-discharge, in contrast to a mean of 16 s prior to the lesioning. Furthermore, the ictal electroclinical pattern was a complete mirror-image of the kindled one and was associated with the earlier EEG seizure onset in the contralateral hemisphere (Fig. 11), indicating that the stimulation activated the contralateral, but not the ipsilateral, hemispheric motor mechanism. There was no further seizure development during subsequent daily stimulation.

At the secondary site, there was no change from the previously established stage 1 response in the posterior-kindled animal. However, in the anterior-kindled animal, the previously established stage 4 convulsive seizure could not be activated and was replaced by a stage 1 seizure. As indicated previously, this animal had its secondary site electrode misplaced in the left primary site, i.e. the claustrum lesioned hemisphere. The findings suggested that in primates the claustrum ipsilateral to the cingulate onset seizure plays an important role for convulsive seizure development.

Summary

After unilateral claustral lesioning:

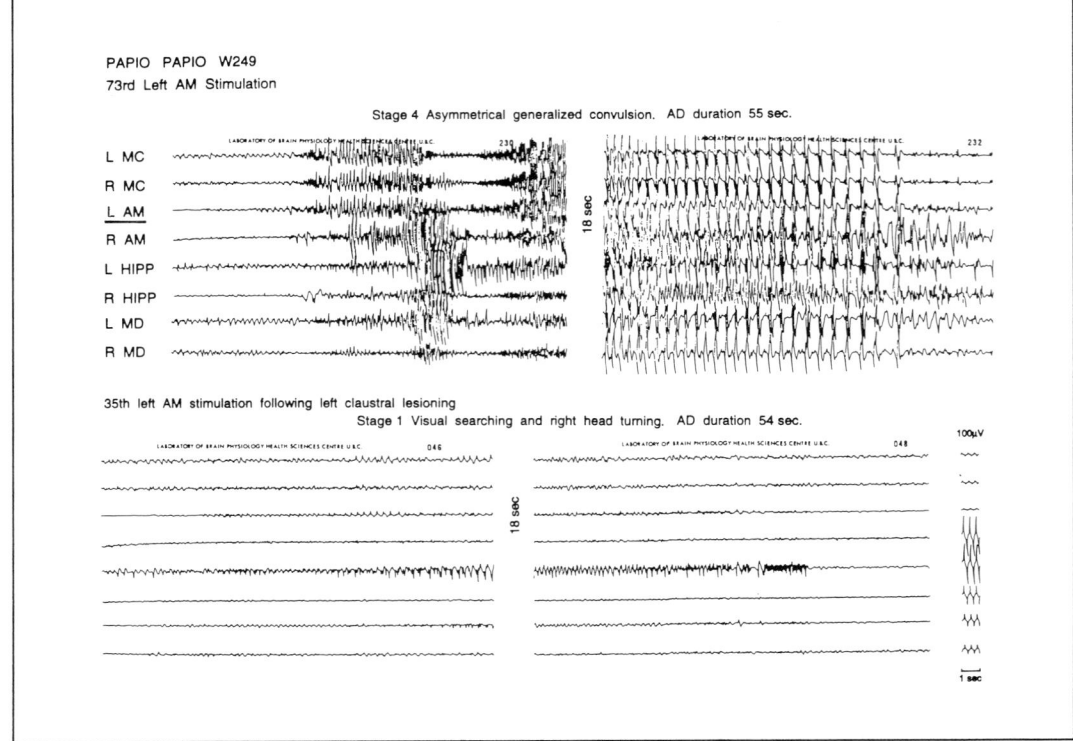

Fig. 11. Effect of left claustral lesioning on left amygdaloid kindled Papio papio W249. Generalized convulsion prior to the lesioning (upper trace). Following the lesion, prolonged limbic seizure is produced but no convulsive seizure development (lower trace).

(i) ILS-induced generalized bisymmetrical convulsion was transformed into a secondarily generalized one originating in the nonlesioned hemisphere.

(ii) Both amygdala- and cingulate-kindled generalized convulsion were replaced by nonconvulsive partial seizure when the ipsilateral kindling site is re-stimulated.

(iii) When the convulsive seizure emerged, it was an exact mirror-image of the kindled one suggesting availability of a transhemispheric pathway to access the contralateral hemisphere motor mechanism.

The findings suggest that the claustrum is essential for transformation of both visual afferents (ILS) and amygdala/cingulate onset partial nonmotor seizure to convulsive seizure. However, it is not involved in the mechanism of secondary generalization.

General discussion

Traditionally, considerable insight into the anatomical substratum of partial epilepsy has been gained through time-honoured and astute clinical observation. This was significantly assisted by the development of the EEG and the availability of surgical intervention, particularly in partial epilepsy, allowing direct stimulation of and recording from the exposed brain. The more recent development of invasive diagnostic approaches has further accelerated this process. This was paralleled by the availability of a number of animal models, both acute and chronic, of partial epilepsy. In contrast, clinical opportunities for the observation of generalized epileptic seizure have been limited mainly to patients with nonconvulsive seizures. Indeed, the now historical notion of a centrencephalic mechanism in idiopathic generalized epilepsy was largely based on the electroclinical observation of petit mal absence. A postulated central midline subcortical mechanism capable of activating widespread cortical areas, explaining both the lapses of awareness and bisymmetrical spike-and-wave discharges, was also presumed to be responsible for primarily generalized convulsive seizures. Unlike partial epilepsy, however, the lack of a justifiable therapeutic surgical opportunity in generalized epilepsy limited exploration of this condition. This was in part alleviated by the development of anterior callosal bisection as a therapeutic modality for intractable generalized seizures (Wada, 1979). Similarly, the experimental problem of a lack of appropriate animal models with recurrent generalized convulsive seizure was considerably ameliorated by the almost concurrent discovery of two chronic animal models, i.e. the photosensitive baboon *Papio papio*, considered to be a model of epilepsy with primarily generalized convulsion, and *kindling* which is considered to be a model of partial epilepsy with secondarily generalized convulsion. Although noninvasive neuro-imaging approaches are becoming available for further study of generalized epilepsy, our understanding of the anatomical substratum of generalized convulsive seizure remains limited. Therefore, exploration through appropriate animal models is highly desirable, though more than one animal model is necessary for the diverse human problem of generalized epilepsies and considerable perspicacity will be required for interpretation of animal data.

In our study, we not only examined the anatomy of ILS-induced generalized convulsions in *Papio papio* but also made comparative observations in different species of primates subjected to kindling. Our findings suggested that intrinsic and genetically dictated factors unique to each species contribute to the ultimate pattern of kindling seizure development. Thus, only *Papio papio* and *Papio cynocephalus* reached stage 5 bisymmetrical and bisynchronous generalized convulsive seizure state while the rhesus monkey and *Papio hamadryas* failed to progress beyond a stage 4 asymmetrical generalized convulsive seizure state. Similarly, the speed of development of both partial convulsive seizures and a convulsive generalization was extremely rapid in both *Papio papio* and *Papio cynocephalus*, while it was extremely slow in the rhesus monkey with *Papio hamadryas* falling in between. Therefore, among the four primate species studied, *Papio papio* and rhesus monkeys are both at extreme ends of the spectrum regarding the speed of limbic seizure migrating out of the temporal lobe and the speed of convulsive seizure bilateralization and generalization. Therefore, two interrelated questions were posed:

(i) What anatomical structure is involved in the transformation of a nonconvulsive limbic seizure to a convulsive one?

(ii) What is the anatomical substratum of seizure bilateralization and generalization?

The same question can be posed regarding ILS-induced generalized convulsion in *Papio papio*, i.e., what structures are responsible for the transformation of visual afferents to convulsive seizures and how do such convulsive seizures become bilateral and generalized. To answer these questions, a number of inter-related studies have been done.

Occipital cortex and its subcortical projection

Our initial study on ILS-induced generalized convulsion in *Papio papio* was aimed at identifying the anatomical pathway underlying photosensitive convulsive seizure. With bilateral ablation of the superior colliculus and the frontal, temporal and occipital cortices, only those animals with resection of the primary visual receiving area in the occipital lobe showed lasting loss of photosensitivity. Bilateral coronal anterior–posterior division of the hemisphere at the parietal junction above the sylvian fissures diminished but did not eliminate photosensitivity, suggesting that the occipotofugal projection to an unknown subcortical site is involved in the development of ILS-induced convulsive seizure.

The substantia innominata

In amygdala kindling, our search for the anatomical substratum for the transformation of nonconvulsive seizure to a convulsive one initially identified the substantia innominata as being critical in strengthening the linkage between the amygdala and the hemispheric motor mechanism. We found that GABAergic enhancement of the substantia innominata ipsilateral to the kindled amygdala eliminated the convulsive component and leaves the limbic seizure intact, while the cortically kindled convulsion was also eliminated but after-discharge cannot be induced at the kindled cortical site. The findings clearly indicated that the role of the substantia innominata in convulsive seizure development is through its modulatory influence on excitability of the hemispheric motor mechanism.

The claustrum

Further search for the specific anatomical site which may be responsible for convulsive seizure development in the kindling of nonmotor structures, such as the amygdala, lead us to study the claustrum which has widespread reciprocal connections with both cortical and subcortical motor structures, as well as the sensory and visual cortices and the limbic system. In cats, the results of unilateral claustral lesioning prior to or upon completion of ipsilateral amygdala kindling were the same with a significant delay of convulsive seizure development. When convulsive seizures developed, it was the mirror image of the expected pattern with an initial ictal engagement of the non-lesioned hemisphere. This finding suggested that convulsive seizure development in amygdala kindling and amygdala-kindled convulsion result from the accession of the amygdala onset limbic seizure to the ipsilateral hemispheric motor mechanism through the claustrum. However, an alternative route is available for the amygdala seizure to access the contralateral hemispheric motor mechanism in the absence of the ipsilateral claustrum. On the other hand, claustral lesioning does not have any effect on convulsive seizures originating in the contralateral amygdala, suggesting that the claustrum is not involved in the mechanism of secondary generalization.

Since the claustrum is partially continuous with the amygdala, the question was raised whether the convulsive seizure suppressive effect described above is only applicable to amygdala kindling and kindled seizure. This is most unlikely since, in primates, claustral lesioning had a profound effect on not only the cingulate-kindled convulsion but also on ILS-induced generalized convulsions. Thus, unilateral claustral lesioning eliminated the generalized convulsion resulting from kindling of the ipsilateral cingulate gyrus anteriorly or posteriorly. Similarly, an ILS-induced generalized convulsion was transformed into a partial onset one involving the non-lesioned hemisphere, becoming secondarily generalized. Therefore, the claustrum does not appear to participate in the mechanism of secondary generalization but is involved in activating the ipsilateral hemispheric motor mechanism. It remains to be seen whether the claustrum is the common final pathway for seizures originating from all other non-motor cortical sites to become convulsive.

The massa intermedia

For the second question of how unilateral motor seizures become bilateral and generalized, the potential role of the two structures in the midline, i.e. the massa intermedia and the corpus callosum, was examined. The reason for our interest in examining the massa intermedia was that it is rather large in all subhuman mammalian brains, while small or absent in the human brain. Since we are using animal models for understanding the mechanisms of human epilepsies, the significance of an obvious morphological difference implying a functional difference must be clearly appreciated.

Electrical kindling of the massa intermedia was slow and difficult but once kindled, subsequent kindling at the amygdala was rapidly accomplished. Injection of an excitatory amino acid into the massa intermedia however caused an initial violent behavioural change followed by the development of temporal limbic seizures. Subsequent kindling at both the amygdala and the hippocampus was accelerated. When the animals kindled from the amygdala or the hippocampus had an excita-

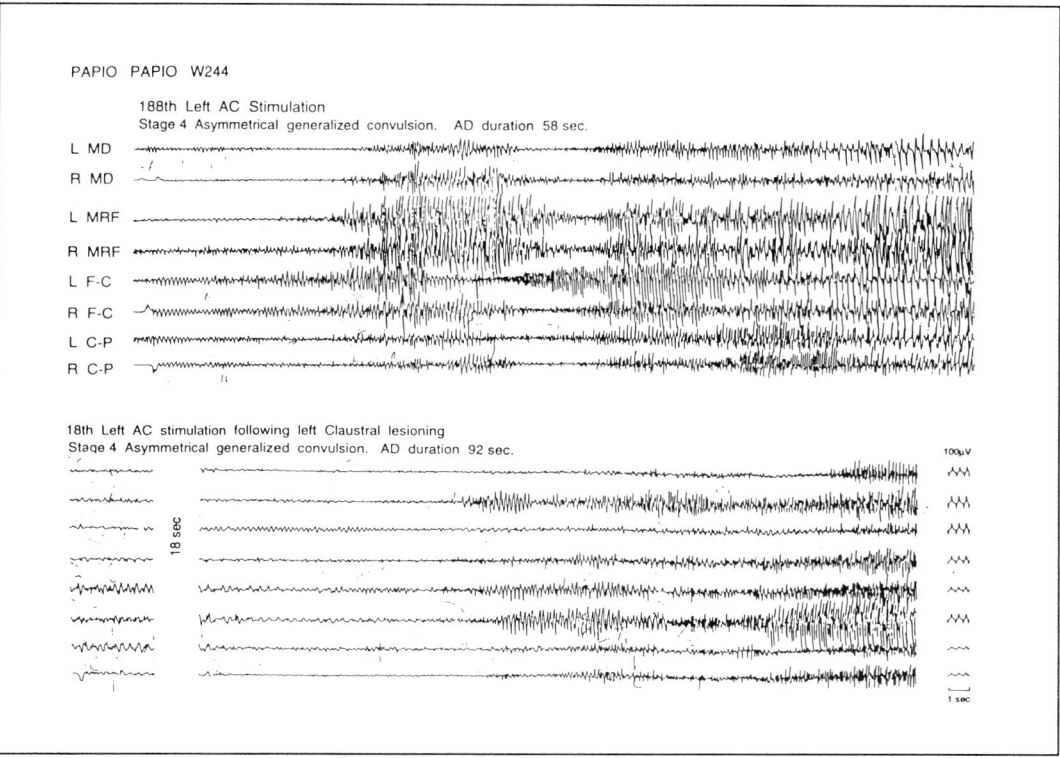

Fig. 12. *Effect of claustral lesioning on left anterior cingulate kindled* Papio papio *W244. Upper trace, before the lesioning. An isolated convulsive seizure induced following the lesioning, latency to convulsive seizure development is markedly increased with predominantly right sided EEG discharge leading to clinical seizure which was the mirror image of stage 4 seizure prior to the lesioning (lower trace).*

tory amino acid injection into the massa intermedia, kindled convulsion was readily precipitated. These findings suggested that the massa intermedia modulates temporal limbic excitability and participates in the generation and expression of generalized convulsion. On the other hand, destruction of the massa intermedia by electrolytic means or ibotenic acid injection had no effects on convulsive seizure development of kindled generalized convulsion. However, the lesioning readily eliminated the positive transfer effect expected from the secondary site amygdala. This does not occur, however, with midline bisection of the massa intermedia suggesting that the perikarya in the massa intermedia plays a role in precipitation of kindled seizure and is an integral part of the kindled network. Since selective midsagittal section of the massa intermedia failed to impact on amygdala kindling or kindled generalized convulsive seizure, the essential kindled network appears to be vertically oriented within the kindled hemisphere. Thus, despite its massiveness in subhuman brains, intrahemispheric networks rather than the transhemispheric connection through the massa intermedia are critical for modulation and expression of generalized convulsive seizure in animals confirming the validity of our animal model findings.

The corpus callosum

Our study on the role of the corpus callosum identified the anterior two-thirds of the corpus callosum to be the major, if not the exclusive, anatomical substratum for convulsive seizure bilateralization and generalization. Despite the fact that both *Papio papio* and rhesus monkeys share the same callosal mechanism in this regard, a significant qualitative difference was found. Thus, callosal bisection caused not only a remarkable acceleration in the speed of seizure development but also intensification of convulsive seizures in the rhesus monkey. This did not occur in *Papio papio*. Therefore, the striking difference of extremely rapid and slow convulsive bilateralization and generalization in *Papio papio* and rhesus monkeys, respectively, suggests a significant difference in the functional capacity of the corpus callosum, and that dysfunction of the callosal neuron may underlie aspects of pathophysiology in the epileptic baboon, *Papio papio*.

Further study on the effect of callosal bisection on ILS-induced generalized convulsion in *Papio papio* showed that each hemisphere has independent seizure susceptibility to intermittent light stimulation and that the anatomical integrity of the corpus callosum is essential for convulsive seizure bilateralization and generalization to occur.

The fact that despite callosal bisection, some aspects of ILS-induced convulsion may be bilateral, and asymmetrical generalized convulsion can occur with prolonged kindling in some bisected baboons, suggests the participation of a subcortical pathway which presumably exists in the brainstem.

Finally, it should be mentioned that the corpus callosum could not be regarded as a mere pathway for transmission of seizure discharge since its bisection can eliminate spontaneous recurrent generalized convulsive seizures in kindled *Papio papio*. This finding suggests that the corpus callosum, i.e. the callosal neuron, also participates in a more dynamic aspect of convulsive seizure initiation and generation.

Conclusion

Until recently, information on the anatomical mechanisms of generalized convulsive seizure was limited due to the lack of a justifiable invasive diagnostic or therapeutic opportunity. Under such circumstances, the availability of an animal model would have been helpful but this was not the case. However, a new era of exploration began with callosal bisection becoming a therapeutic modality for some generalized seizure patients and with the discovery of two animal models of chronic generalized convulsive seizure. The photosensitive baboon, *Papio papio*, was used as a model of idiopathic generalized epilepsy. This is particularly significant for the understanding of generalized convulsive seizure since some members of this species spontaneously show generalized bisymmetrical convulsive seizures. The other animal model is the kindling one which is regarded as a model of partial epilepsy with secondarily generalized convulsion. This development afforded an opportunity for us to gain information on the anatomy of those cerebral structures involved for convulsive seizure development and its generalization.

Evaluation of the striking morphological difference of the massa intermedia between human and subhuman mammalian brains has led to the conclusion that intrahemispheric vertically oriented networks involving its perikarya rather than its transthalamic connection important for the mechanism of precipitation and expression of generalized convulsive seizure.

Results of our studies on *Papio papio* and other primate species in combination with kindling over the past 25 years are selectively reviewed. Results suggest the following:

(i) In the mechanism of generalized convulsive seizures

– The substantia innominata participates through its capacity to modulate excitability of the hemispheric motor mechanism including the fronto-rolandic cortex,

– The perikarya of the mesial thalamus modulates limbic excitability and participates in the process of precipitation and expression of generalized convulsive seizures of limbic origin.

(ii) Convulsive seizure development following intermittent light stimulation or kindling of nonmotor structures such as the amygdala or the cingulate cortex requires accession to the hemispheric motor mechanism through the ipsilateral claustrum. Whether the claustrum is the exclusive pathway for all partial onset nonmotor seizures to become hemiconvulsive ones remains to be clarified.

(iii) Bilateralization and generalization of partial motor or unilateral convulsive seizures requires the availability of the anterior two-thirds of the corpus callosum. However, a high threshold route is also available in the brain-stem. The identity of such a pathway and the specific circumstances under which it becomes available remain the subject of future research.

Acknowledgement

This work was supported by grants from the Medical Research Council of Canada.

References

Andersen, D.L. (1968): Some striatal connections to the claustrum. *Exp. Neurol.* **20**, 261.

Baba, H. & Wada, J.A. (1987): Reciprocal inhibition between seizure induced by intermittent light stimulation and premotor cortical stimulation in Senegalese baboons, *Papio papio. Epilepsia* **28**, 645–650.

Berman, A.L. & Jones, E.G. (1982): The thalamus and basal telencephalon of the cat. A cytoarchitectonic atlas with stereotaxic coordinates. Wisconson: University of Wisconsin Press.

Corcoran, M.E., Cain, P. & Wada, J.A. (1984): Amygdaloid kindling in *Papio cynocephalus* and subsequent recurrent spontaneous seizures. *Folia Psychiatr. Neurol. Jpn* **38**, 151–158.

Druga, R. (1984): Reciprocal connections between the claustrum and the gyrus sigmoideus posterior in the cat. *Anat. Anz.* **156**, 109–118.

Ehara, Y. & Wada, J.A. (1990): Midline thalamus and amygdaloid kindling. In: *Kindling 4*, ed. J.A. Wada, pp. 409–422. New York: Plenum Press.

Ehara, Y. & Wada, J.A. (1989): NMDA injection into the massa intermedia precipitates limbic seizure. *Epilepsia* **30** (5), 701.

Erickson, T.C. (1940): Spread of the epileptic discharge. *Arch. Neurol. Psychiatry* **32**, 429–452.

Fukuda, H., Valin, A., Bryere, P., Riche, D., Wada, J.A. & Naquet, R. (1988): Role of forebrain commissure and hemispheric independence in photosensitive response of epileptic baboon *Papio papio. Electroencephalogr. Clin. Neurophysiol.* **69**, 363–370.

Fukuda, H., Valin, A., Menini, C., Boscher, C., De La Sayette, V., Riche, D., Kunimoto, M., Wada, J.A. & Naquet, R. (1989): Effect of macular and peripheral retina coagulation on photosensitive epilepsy, in the forebrain bisected baboon *Papio papio. Epilepsia* **30**, 623–630.

Gloor, P. (1969): Neurophysiological basis of generalized seizures termed centrencephalic. In: *The physiopathogenesis of the epilepsies*, eds. H. Gastaut, H.H. Jasper, J. Bancaud & A. Waltregny, pp. 209–236. Springfield, IL: C.C. Thomas.

Gloor, P. (1978): Evolution of the concept of the mechanism of generalized epilepsy with bilateral spike-and-wave discharge. In: *Modern perspectives in epilepsy*, ed. J.A. Wada, pp. 99–137. Montreal: Eden Press.

Goddard, G.V. (1967): Development of epileptic seizures through brain stimulation at low intensity. *Nature* **214**, 1020–1021.

Goddard, G.V., McIntyre, D.C. & Leech, C.K. (1969): A permanent in brain function resulting from daily electrical stimulation. *Exp. Neurol.* **25**, 295–330.

Hirayasu, Y. & Wada, J.A. (1992): Convulsive seizure in rats induced by *N*-methyl-D-aspartate injection into the massa intermedia. *Brain Res.* **577**, 36–40.

Hirayasu, Y. & Wada, J.A. (1993): *N*-methyl-D-aspartate injection into the massa intermedia facilitates development of limbic kindling in rats. *Epilepsia* **33**, 965–970.

Hiyoshi, T. & Wada, J.A. (1988a): Midline thalamic lesion and feline amygdaloid kindling. I. Effect of lesion placement prior to kindling. *Electroencephalogr. Clin. Neurophysiol.* **70**, 339–349.

Hiyoshi, T. & Wada, J.A. (1988b): Midline thalamic lesion and feline amygdaloid kindling. II. Effect of lesion placement upon completion of primary site kindling. *Electroencephalogr. Clin. Neurophysiol.* **70,** 339–349.

Ishibashi, M. & Wada, J.A. (1990): Division of massa intermedia has no effect in feline amygdaloid kindling. *Epilepsia* **31 (5),** 632.

Ishikawa, I., Kawamura, S. & Tanaka, O. (1969): An experimental study on the effect of connections of the amygdaloid complex in the cat. *Acta Med. Okayama* **23,** 519.

Kaneko, Y., Kimura, H. & Wada, J.A. (1981): Is the amygdaloid neuron necessary for amygdaloid kindling? In: *Kindling 2,* ed. J.A. Wada, pp. 249–264. New York: Raven Press.

Killam, K.F., Killiam, E.K. & Naquet, R. (1967): An animal model of light sensitive epilepsy. *Electroencephalogr. Clin. Neurophysiol.* **22,** 497–513.

Kimura, H., Kaneko, Y. & Wada, J.A. (1981): Catecholamine and cholinergic systems and amygdaloid kindling. In: *Kindling 2,* ed. J.A. Wada. pp. 265–287. New York: Raven Press.

Krettek, E. & Price, J.L. (1978): A description of the amygdaloid complex in the rat and cat with observations on intra-amygdaloid axonal connections. *J. Comp. Neur.* **178,** 255.

Kudo, T. & Wada, J.A. (1990): Claustrum and amygdaloid kindling. In: *Kindling 4,* ed. J.A. Wada, pp. 397–407. New York: Plenum Press.

Kuenzle, (1976): Thalamic projections from the precentral motor cortex in *Macada fascicularis*. *Brain Res.* **105,** 253–267.

Kusske, J.A. & Rush, J.L. (1978): Corpus callosum and propagation of afterdischarge to contralateral cortex and thalamus. *Neurology* **28,** 905–912.

Macchi, G., Bentivoglio, M., Minciacchi, D. & Molinari, M. (1981): The organization of the claustroneocortical projections in the cat studied by means of the HRP retrograde axonal transport. *J. Comp. Neurol.* **195,** 681.

Marcus, E.M. (1985): Generalized seizure models and the corpus callosum. In: *Epilepsy and the corpus callosum,* ed. A.G. Reeves, pp. 131–206. New York: Plenum Press.

Markowitsch, H.J. Irele, E., Bang-Olsen, R. & Flindt-Egebak, P. (1984): Claustral efferents to the cat's limbic cortex studied with retrograde and anterograde tracing techniques. *Neuroscience* **12,** 409.

Meldrum, B.S., Menini, C., Naquet, R., Laurent, H. & Stutzmann, J.M. (1979): Preconvulsant, convulsant and other actions of the d- and l-stereoisomers of allylglycine in the photosensitive baboon, *Papio papio*. *Electroencephalogr. Clin. Neurophysiol.* **47,** 383–395.

Mori, N. & Wada, J.A. (1989): Suppression of amygdaloid kindled convulsion following unilateral injection of 2-amino-7-phosphonoheptanoic acid (2-APH) into the substantia innominata of rats. *Brain Res.* **486,** 141–146.

Mori, N. & Wada, J.A. (1992): Kindling of the massa intermedia in rats. *Brain Res.* **575,** 148–150.

Mori, N., Wada, J.A., Yokoyama, N., Ariga, K. & Kumashiro, H. (1993): Ipsilateral hemiconvulsive seizure after unilateral injection of procaine into the substantia innominata of amygdaloid-kindled rats. *Brain Res.* **610,** 354–357.

Morita, K., Okamoto, M., Seki, K. & Wada, J.A. (1985): Suppression of amygdala-kindled seizure in cats by enhanced GABAergic transmission in substantia innominata. *Exp. Neurol.* **89,** 225–236.

Naquet, R. & Meldrum, B.S. (1972): Photogenic seizures in baboon, In: *Experimental models of epilepsy: a manual for the laboratory worker,* ed. D.D. Purpura, J.K. Penry, D.B. Tower, D.M. Woodbury & R.D. Walter, pp. 376–406. New York: Raven Press.

Naquet, R. & Wada, J. (1992): Role of the corpus callosum in photosensitive epileptic baboon, *Papio papio*, *Adv. Neurol.* **57,** 579–587.

Okamoto, M., Morita, K., Sato, M. & Wada, J.A. (1986): The role of substantia innominata in the expression of somatomotor manifestations of temporal lobe seizures. In: *Kindling 3,* ed. J.A. Wada, pp. 107–121. New York: Raven Press.

Okamoto, M. & Wada, J.A. (1984): Reversible suppression of amygdaloid-kindled convulsion following unilateral gabaculline injection into the substantia innominata. *Brain Res.* **305,** 389–392.

Ono, K., Mori, K., Baba, H., Seki, K. & Wada, J.A. (1986): A new chronic model of partial onset generalized seizure induced by low frequency cortical stimulation: its relationsip to kindling phenomenon. In: *Kindling 3,* ed. J.A. Wada, pp. 139–156. New York: Raven Press.

Pinel, J.P. (1981): Spontaneous kindled motor seizures in rats. In: *Kindling 2,* ed. J.A. Wada, pp. 179–187. New York: Raven Press.

Riche, D. & Lanoir, I. (1978): Some claustro-cortical connections in the cat and baboon as studied by retrograde horseradish perioxidase transport. *J. Comp. Neurol.* **177,** 435–444.

Sakai, S. & Wada, J.A. (1987): Reversible suppression of amygdaloid and cortically kindled seizures in Senegalese baboon, *Papio papio*, by unilateral injection of gabaculine in the substantia innominata. *Epilepsia* **28** (5), 618.

Sloniewski, P. & Pilgrim, Ch. (1984): Clautro-neocortical connections in the rat as demonstrated by retrograde tracing with lucifer yellow. *Neurosci. Lett.* **49,** 29–32.

Sutula, T., Cascino, G., Cavazos, J., Parada, I. & Ramirez, L. (1988): Mossy fiber synaptic reorganization in the epileptic human temporal lobe. *Ann. Neurol.* **26,** 321–330.

Tsuchimochi, H. & Wada, J.A. (1991): Cingulate kindling in Senegalese baboons, *Papio papio*. *Epilepsia* **32** (3), 36.

Uemura, S. & Wada, J.A. (1981): Seizure predisposition and species. *Epilepsia* **22,** 228.

Wada, J.A. (1971): Longitudinal observation of Senegalese baboon, *Papio papio. EEG Clin. Neurophysiol.* **31,** 296.

Wada, J.A. (1979): Epilepsy: surgery may help patients when medication is ineffective. *Brit. Columbia Med. J.* **6** (2), 129–131.

Wada, J.A. (1980): New surgical treatment through experimental models, In: *Advances in epileptology: Xth Epilepsy International Symposium*, eds. J.A. Wada & J.K. Penry, pp. 195–204. New York: Raven Press.

Wada, J.A. (1987): Anterior 2/3 callosal bisection: comparative observations in animals and man. In: *Fundamental mechanisms of human brain function*, ed. J. Engel, Jr., G.A. Ojemann, H.O. Lueders & P.D. Williamson, pp. 259–266. New York: Raven Press.

Wada, J.A. & Komai, S. (1985): Effect of anterior 2/3 callosal bisection upon bisymmetrical and bisynchronous convulsions kindled from amygdala in epileptic baboon, *Papio papio*. In: *Epilepsy and the corpus callosum*, ed. A.G. Reeves, pp. 75–98. New York: Plenum Press.

Wada, J.A. & Mizoguchi, T. (1984): Effect of forebrain bisection upon amygdaloid kindling in epileptic baboon, *Papio papio. Epilepsia* **25,** 278–387.

Wada, J.A., Mizoguchi, T. & Komai, S. (1981): Cortical motor activation in amygdaloid kindling: observations in non-epileptogenesis rhesus monkeys with anterior 2/3 callosal bisection, In: *Kindling 2* ed. J.A. Wada, pp. 235–248. New York: Raven Press.

Wada, J.A., Mizoguchi, T. & Osawa, T. (1978): Secondarily generalized convulsive seizure induced by daily amygdaloid stimulation in rhesus monkeys. *Neurology* **28,** 1026–1036.

Wada, J.A. & Moyes, P.D. (1982): Anterior callosal bisection in medically refractory generalized seizure patients. *Epilepsia* **24,** 262.

Wada, J.A. & Naquet, R. (1972): Examination of neural mechanisms involved in photogenic seizure susceptibility in epileptic Senegalese baboon, *Papio papio. Epilepsia* **13,** 344.

Wada, J.A., Naquet, R., Catier, J., Charmasson, G. & Menini, C. (1973): Further examination of neural mechanisms underlying photosensitivity in the epileptic Senegalese baboon, *Papio papio. EEG Clin. Neurophysiol.* **35,** 786.

Wada, Y., Okuda, H., Yamaguchi, N. & Yoshida, K. (1986): Effect of allylglycine on photosensitivity in the lateral geniculate-kindled cats. *Exp. Neurol.* **94,** 228– 236.

Wada, J.A. & Osawa, T. (1976): Spontaneous recurrent generalized seizures induced by daily amygdaloid stimulation in Senegalese baboons, *Papio papio. Neurology* **26,** 273–286.

Wada, J.A., Osawa, T. & Mizoguchi, T. (1975): Recurrent spontaneous seizure state induced by prefrontal kindling in the Senegalese baboons, *Papio papio. Can. J. Neurol. Sci.* **2,** 447–492.

Wada, J.A. & Sato, M. (1973): Photosensitivity in deep cerebral structures in epileptic Senegalese baboons, *Papio papio. EEG Clin. Neurophysiol.* **35,** 786.

Wada, J.A. & Sato, M. (1974): Generalized convulsive seizure induced by daily electrical stimulation of the amygdala in cats: correlative electrographic and behavioural features. *Neurology* **24,** 565–574.

Wada, J.A., Sato, M. & Corcoran, M.E. (1974): Persistent seizure susceptibility and recurrent spontaneous seizures in kindled cats. *Epilepsia* **15,** 464–478.

Wada, J.A., Terao, A. & Booker, H.E. (1972): Longitudinal correlative analysis of photosensitive baboons, *Papio papio. Neurology* **22,** 1272–1285.

Wada, J.A., Terao, B. & Jung, B. (1970): Inferior colliculus lesion and audiogenic seizure susceptibility. *Exp. Neurol.* **28**, 326–332.

Wada, J.A. & Tsuchimochi, H. (1992): Claustral activation of hemispheric motor mechanism in partial seizure. *Epilepsia* **33** (3), 37.

Witter, M.P., Groenewegen, H.J. & Lohman, A.H.H. (1983): Reciprocal connections of the insular and piriform claustrum with limbic cortex: an anatomical study in the cat. *Neuroscience* **24**, 519.

Chapter 31

Genetic epilepsy in chickens: new approaches and concepts

N. Guy*†, M.A. Teillet†, G. Le Gal La Salle‡, N. Fadlallah*, N.M. Le Douarin†, R. Naquet‡ and C. Batini*

*Laboratoire de Physiologie de la Motricité, CNRS-URA 14 et Université Pierre et Marie Curie, Paris, France; †Institut d'Embryologie Cellulaire et Moléculaire, CNRS-UMR 9924 et Collège de France, Nogent-sur-Marne, France; ‡Institut Alfred Fessard, CNRS-UPR 2212, Gif-sur-Yvette, France

Starting with a group of five chickens discovered to be 'epileptic' in a colony of Fayoumi chickens, Crawford (1970) built a 'synthetic' strain of epileptic chickens (Crawford, 1983, 1990). These animals are affected by a recessive autosomal gene mutation with complete penetrance. All males and females homozygous for the Epi gene (FEpi) develop convulsions starting at hatching, while heterozygotes (FHtz) are normal in behaviour. Epileptic seizures of the FEpi chickens are either spontaneous or induced by a variety of stimuli including excessive physical exercise, elevated body temperature, and auditory and visual stimulations. However, they are consistently induced by intermittent light stimulations (ILS) at a frequency of 14 flashes per s (Crichlow & Crawford, 1974). Characteristic ILS-induced seizures have been divided into three phases: (i) increased alertness, vocalization and neck extension; (ii) backward movements and loss of standing; (iii) violent thrashing movements due to rapid extensions and flexions of legs and wings. This last period corresponds to the generalized tonic–clonic convulsions and is followed by a brief period of lethargy and unresponsiveness (Johnson & Tuchek, 1987). According to Crichlow & Crawford (1974), the electroencephalogram (EEG) reveals paroxysmal abnormalities characterized by continuous high voltage, slow waves and spikes and waves during interictal periods, while during ILS-induced seizures the EEG would be characterized by repetitive slow potentials at the intermittent light stimulation frequency evolving into high voltage spikes. These behavioural and EEG patterns of epilepsy led Crawford and co-workers to consider FEpi as a model of primary generalized convulsive epilepsy of humans. Moreover, FEpi seizures respond to the antiepileptic drugs commonly used to treat 'grand mal seizures'. Among these drugs, phenobarbital, sodium valproate, diazepam and clonazepam are the most efficient. Phenytoin and trimethadione block the seizures only for doses inducing toxicity. Ethosuximide is not active (Crawford, 1983; Johnson & Davis, 1983; Johnson & Tuchek, 1987).

Brains of FEpi look normal and, except for a megalencephaly recently described by George et al. (1990), present no specific anatomical abnormality (Johnson & Davis, 1983). From the biochemical point of view, in interictal periods FEpi show a weaker concentration of serotonin and dopamine, and a more elevated concentration of norepinephrine (but weaker turnover) than in non-epileptic

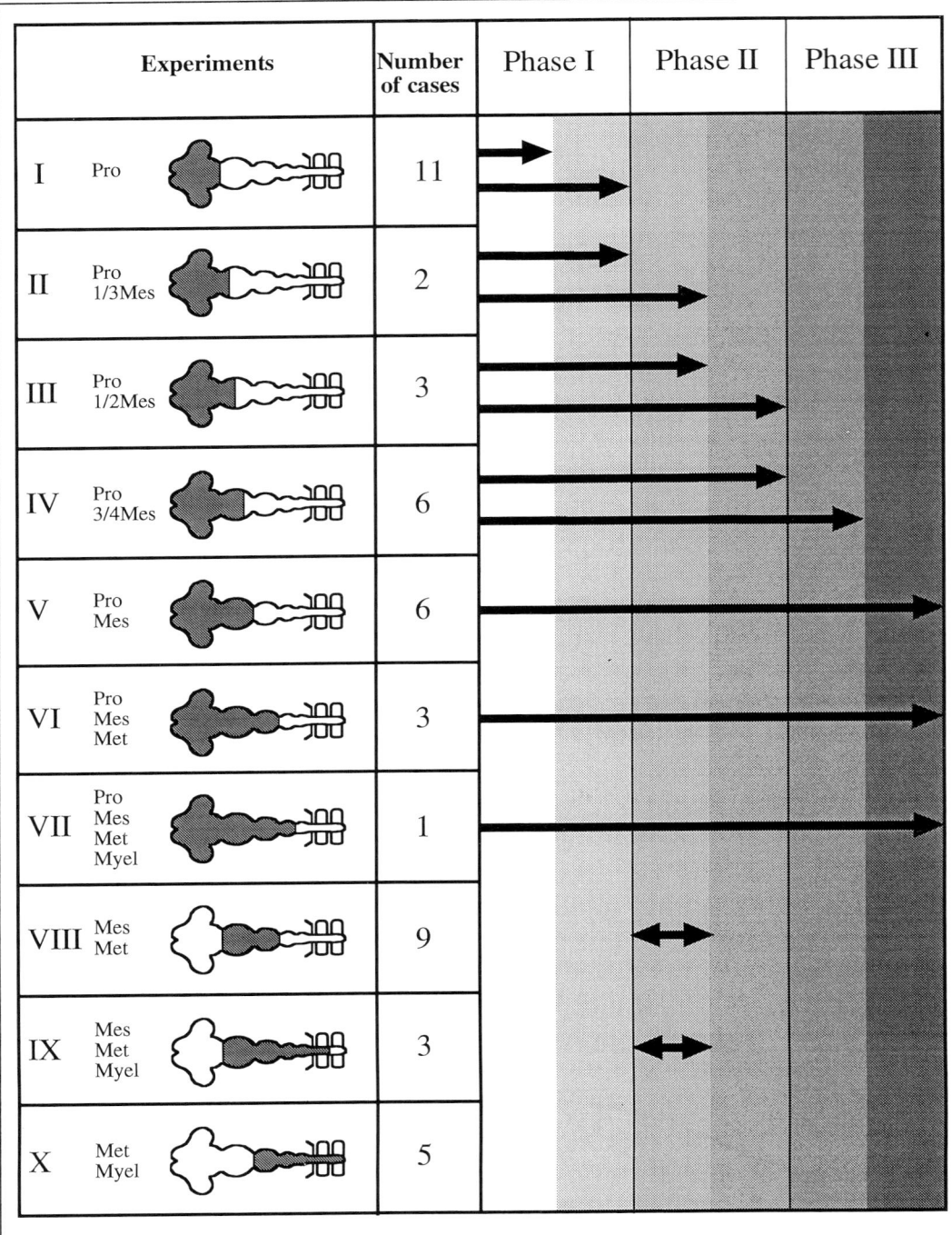

Fig. 1. Different types of transplantation of FEpi brain territories. The grafted encephalic vesicles are represented as grey shaded areas on E2 (2 days of incubation) brain schemes. Extention of arrows indicates the severity of the ILS-induced seizure for each type of chimera.

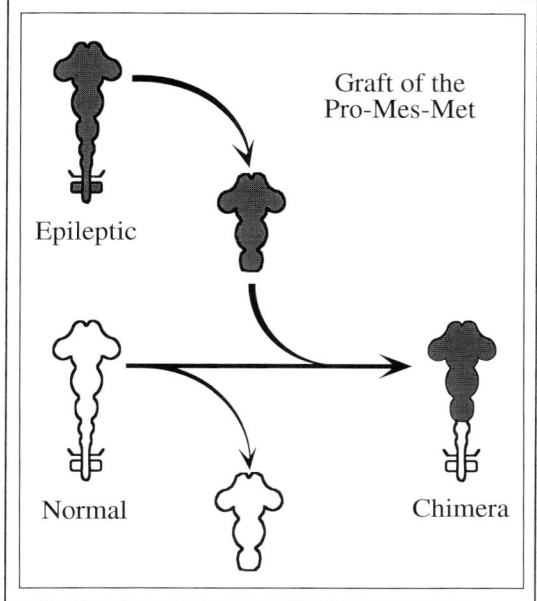

Fig. 2. Schematic representation of the brain transplantation experiment. The constrictions separating the different encephalic vesicles are used as landmarks for microsurgery. Here, the prosencephalic, mesencephalic and metencephalic vesicles are removed from the FEpi embryo at 12-somite stage and grafted onto the place of the same structures in a normal chick embryo of the same stage.

chickens. Treatments to compensate for these biochemical abnormalities are ineffective. Concentrations of aspartate, glutamate, and taurine are analogous between FEpi and normal chickens. The level of GABA is higher in adults FEpi than in other animals. Based on these data of Crawford's group considered that for monoamines, as for amino acids, differences in concentration seem to be secondary to the epileptic seizures rather than at their origin (Johnson & Tuchek, 1987).

Previous work carried out in one of our laboratories (Le Douarin, 1993) led to the production of brain chimeras by microsurgical manipulations in ovo (see Le Douarin, 1993, for a review). Brain chimeras were first made by exchanging specific brain areas between two bird embryos of different species, quail and chick (Balaban et al., 1988; Hallonet et al., 1990). Grafts of quail neuro-epithelium into chicken embryos were performed at 2 days of incubation (E2) before the onset of vascularization of the neural tube. Chimeras with quail brain grafts hatched. These experiments showed that neural transplantation *per se* never induces epileptic manifestations. We therefore decided to apply this method to analyse some aspects of avian epilepsy. In fact this method was appropriate to answer several kinds of questions: is it possible to transfer the epileptic phenotype by grafting an epileptic brain? What part of the brain is necessary or sufficient to transfer epilepsy? Different territories of the brain anlage were replaced in normal chicken embryos by their counterpart from the FEpi strain at E2 (Figs. 1, 2). The chimeras obtained were compared to FEpi, FHtz and normal chickens for the behavioural and electrophysiological observations. We consider here only ILS-induced seizures. Sound-induced seizures are at present under study.

Brain chimeras: transfer of epilepsy

The hatching rate of brain chimeras is about 11 per cent (89 out of 830 operated embryos). Animals with anatomical malformations or behavioural abnormalities were discarded. Fifty chimeras were retained for the present study. Their growth rate is similar to that of the recipient but the feathers have the pigmentation of the donor Fayoumi strain at the level of the graft (Fig. 3), white or variegated, in both cases contrasting with the yellow colour of the JA recipient. The different types of brain substitution and the resulting ILS-induced seizure level transferred in each chimera, are depicted in Fig. 2. In contrast to quail–chick chimeras, chick–chick chimeras usually show no immunological rejection, so they can survive in perfect health to adulthood (Okhi et al., 1987).

The transfer of the epileptic phenotype from FEpi to normal chickens was first obtained by substitution of almost the entire brain anlage. But it was possible to demonstrate that partial substitution may be sufficient to transfer the full pattern of the seizure induced by intermittent light stimulation. Grafting the primordia of both prosencephalon and mesencephalon (Pro-Mes) of FEpi was necessary and sufficient to reproduce the epileptic phenotype in normal chickens (phases I and

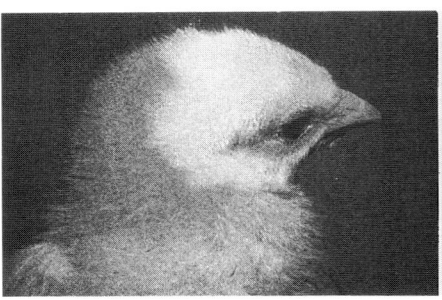 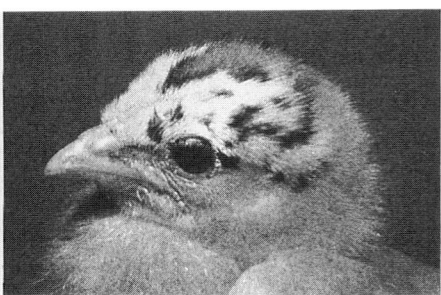

Fig. 3. Ten-days-old epileptic chimeras, made by transplanting prosencephalic, mesencephalic and metencephalic vesicles from FEpi to normal chick embryos at 2 days of incubation. The white pigmentation (left view) or variegated pigmentation (right view) at the level of the graft is due to melanoblasts of neural crest origin transplanted along with the neural anlage. Both of these pigmentations are found in the FEpi strain (see also colour plates).

II and self-sustained phase III after cessation of ILS). Chimeras with only the prosencephalon grafted showed incomplete ILS-induced behavioural manifestations with only phases I and II present. Chimeras having FEpi mesencephalon and rhombencephalon never displayed convulsions under intermittent light stimulation. However, in these animals it was possible to perceive myoclonia of the neck muscles following the frequency of the intermittent light stimulation which are characteristic of the beginning of the phase II of FEpi seizure (Fig. 1).

These results suggest that cooperation of forebrain and midbrain is required to produce the full epileptic phenotype under intermittent light stimulation. (Teillet et al., 1991).

The EEG and the EMG of ILS-induced seizures in FEpi and chimeras

FEpi and chimeras were studied either freely moving (telemetry) or partially restrained or paralysed with flaxedil. EEG and EMG of the neck muscles were recorded.

In the FEpi, the previously described EEG interictal activities composed of paroxysmal slow waves, slow spikes, and spikes and waves (Crichlow & Crawford, 1974; Crichlow, 1983) were confirmed (Figs. 4 & 5). But, in our hands, EEG during ILS-induced seizures was characterized by a 'desynchronization' (D) of the trace usually followed by a 'flattening' (F) (Guy et al., 1992). DF observed in both paralysed and non-paralysed FEpi chickens was never seen in FHtz or normal ones (Fig. 5). This DF may persist after the cessation of intermittent light stimulation and then corresponds to the self-sustained part of the seizure and to the postictal phase. Its duration is longer in freely moving or partially restrained animals than in paralysed ones. Only occasionally, potentials at the intermittent light stimulation frequency were recorded early during stimulation, and bursts of paroxysms were recorded at the end of DF. Moreover, in the non-paralysed FEpi animals, the EMG revealed myoclonus of the neck muscles at the frequency of the intermittent light stimulation. The myoclonus gradually increased in amplitude, invading the body muscles, until generalized convulsions were reached.

Pro-Mes-grafted chimeras and chimeras having only the prosencephalon grafted showed interictal EEG similar to the FEpi (Figs. 4 & 5). During the ictal phase (phases I and II) D and sometimes DF exist. They do not continue after cessation of intermittent light stimulation in prosencephalon-grafted chimeras in contrast to the FEpi chickens and Pro-Mes-grafted chimeras (Fig. 5). Chimeras having the graft of the FEpi mesencephalon without the prosencephalon present a normal interictal EEG; however, during intermittent light stimulation, the EMG showed bursts of potentials at the

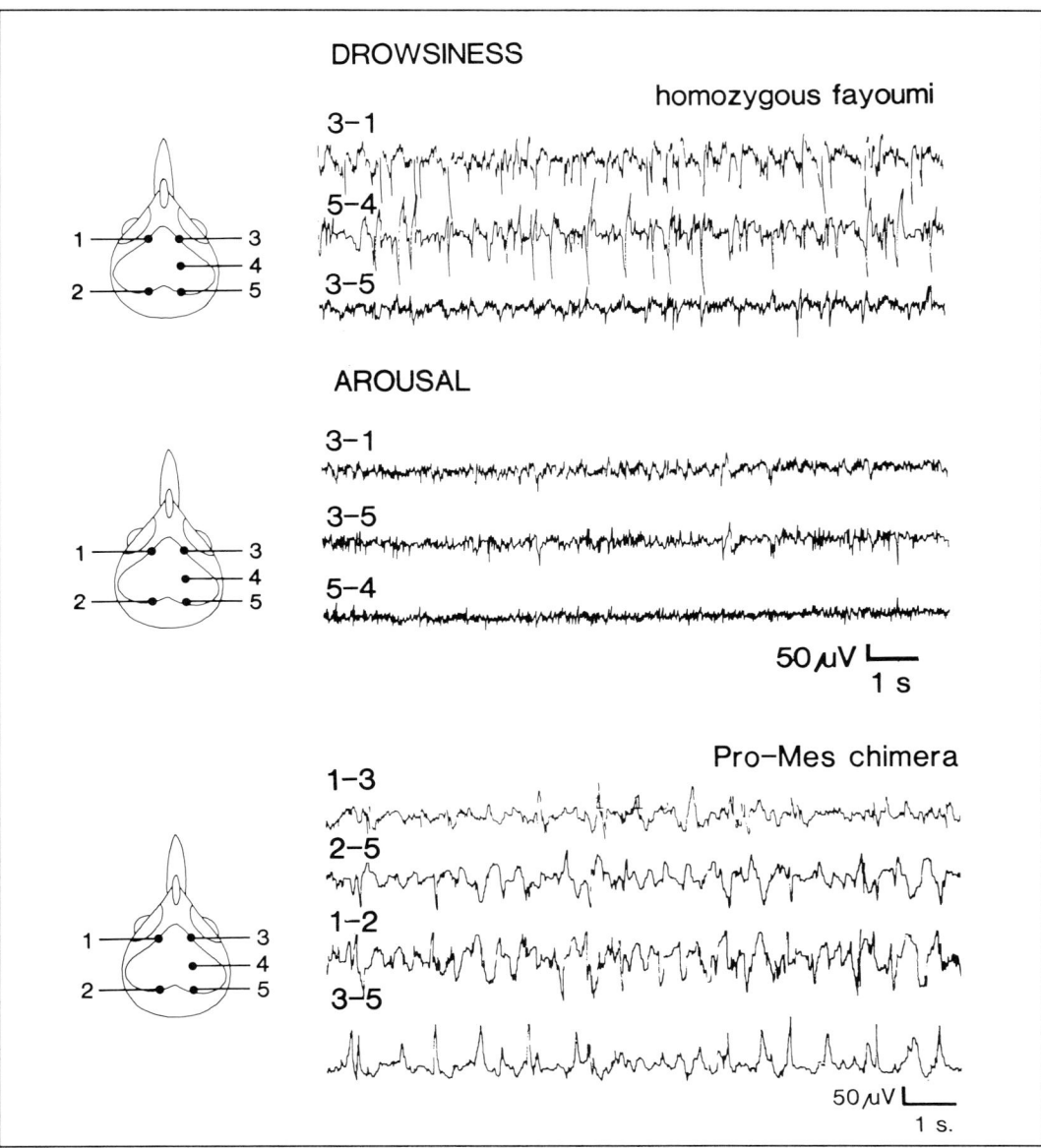

Fig. 4. Examples of EEG during drowsiness and arousal of a Fayoumi homozygous chicken, and during drowsiness of a Pro-Mes chimera (the prosencephalon and mesencephalon coming from an embryo of a homozygous Fayoumi chicken were grafted on a normal chicken embryo). Note the similar continuous high-amplitude spikes, polyspikes and slow waves discharges recorded during drowsiness in homozygous Fayoumi and Pro-Mes chimeras.

intermittent light stimulation frequency which correspond to the myoclonia of the neck muscles. The myoclonus remained localized at these muscles and did not continue after the end of intermittent light stimulation. Metrazol injected intravenously, into all types of paralysed chickens (FHtz, FEpi, chimeras, normal chickens) evoked the EEG ictal paroxysms as described in other species

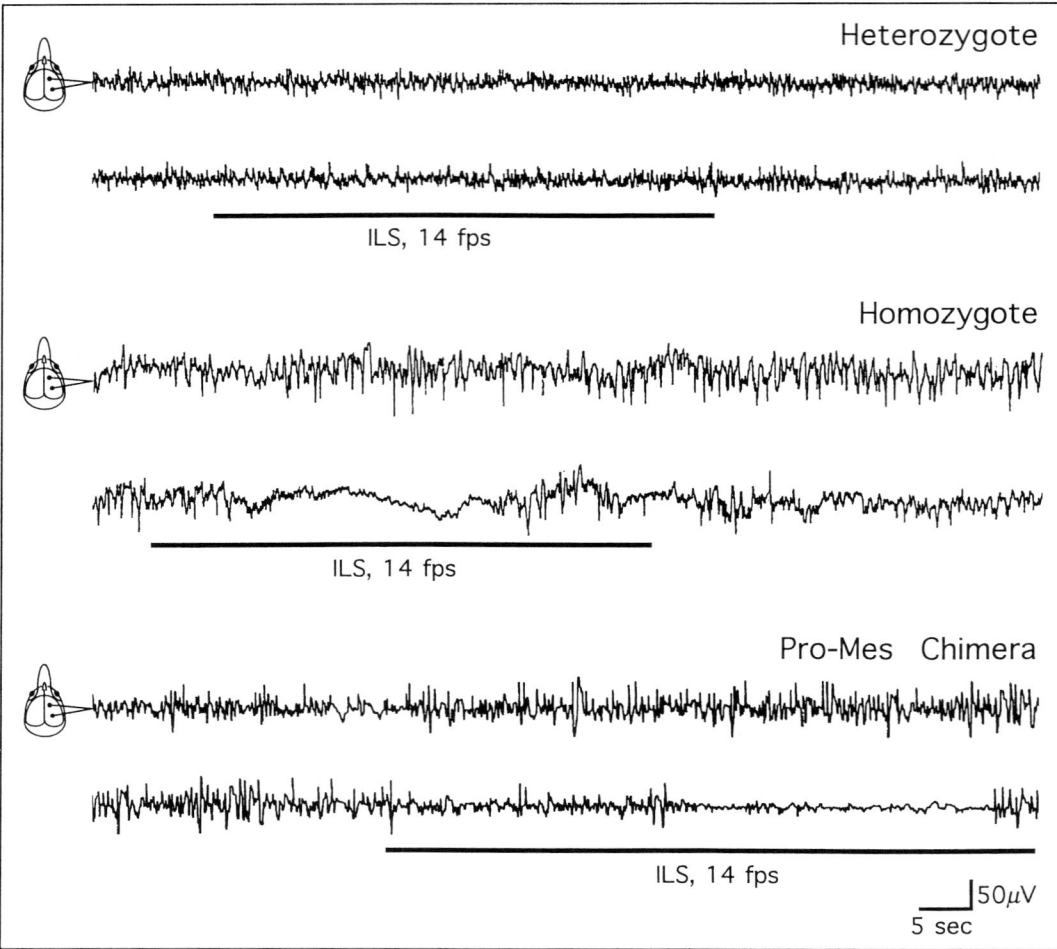

Fig. 5. Three examples of EEG taken at a speed different from the one in Fig. 4. EEG recordings without (first line of each example) and with (second line) intermittent light stimulation (ILS). In heterozygote chick the resting EEG is normal and ILS does not provoke any significant modification. In homozygote FEpi, as in Pro-Mes chimera, the resting interictal EEG is made of paroxysmal slow waves, slow spikes and spikes and waves. In the two last examples, ILS induces a desynchronization followed by a flattening.

(Killam et al., 1967; Vergnes et al., 1990). In FEpi and Pro-Mes chimeras, the threshold to induce a seizure was lower than in FHtz and normal chickens. Mes-Met chimeras presented an intermediate sensitivity (unpublished personal results).

These results show that ILS-induced seizures in FEpi are not expressed as EEG paroxysmal discharges (Guy et al., 1992), although spike or spike-and-wave discharges can be induced in chickens by Metrazol. After embryonic manipulations leading to different types of chimeras between FEpi and non-epileptic chickens, it is possible to transfer the ILS-induced behavioural and EEG patterns of FEpi to normal controls. Moreover EEG data tend to support the idea that large brain areas, presumably the entire prosencephalon and mesencephalon, underlie the genetic dysfunction of FEpi responsible for the predisposition to seizures. Under intermittent light stimulation, each part of the brain responds specifically, by an arousal reaction as confirmed by EEG desynchronization in prosencephalic chimeras, or by myoclonus in Mes-Met chimeras. In the partially grafted chimeras these reactions are not sufficient to permit the full expression of the concomitant self-sustained seizure with its particular EEG.

Unit recordings in the prosencephalon and mesencephalon of FEpi and Pro-Mes chimeras

Unit recordings until now have been carried out only in normal chickens, FHtz, FEpi and Pro-Mes chimeras. Extracellular units were recorded in some visual structures of the prosencephalon (Wulst), and of the mesencephalon (optic tectum) of paralysed animals (Guy *et al.*, 1993). Units recorded in the prosencephalon of FEpi and chimeras showed abnormal interictal bursting activity, distinctly different from the activity of non-epileptic FHtz and normal chickens. Bursting was synchronized with the EEG spike activity. During ILS-induced DF, bursting stopped and units began to fire at random in an irregular, continuous pattern of discharges.

The interictal pattern of the mesencephalic units of FEpi and chimeras was regular and analogous to that of normal chickens. During ILS-induced DF these units showed two types of abnormal activity which were distinct from that of non-epileptic chickens: type I neurons displayed an early high sensitivity to intermittent light stimulation followed by a prolonged suppression of activity; type II neurons displayed an early and prolonged suppression of activity.

Recordings of unitary discharges made in the Wulst of FEpi confirm that even in the absence of sensory stimulation, electrical activity in the brain hemispheres is abnormal. This part of the nervous system obviously has a role in the predisposition of the FEpi chickens to develop epileptic seizures. However, the seizure generator under intermittent light stimulation would lie in the mesencephalon where the optic tectum differentiates. This visual structure receiving afferences from the retina shows signs of hyperexcitability marked by acceleration of unitary discharges under intermittent light stimulation. From this point of view, if one admits that the generator of seizures in the FEpi is in the mesencephalon, this model would be analogous to the audiogenic epilepsy of rodents (Niaussat & Laget, 1963) where seizures originate in the brain-stem (see Marescaux *et al.*, 1987; Le Gal La Salle & Naquet, 1990). However, in contrast to the rodent audiogenic model, the FEpi model responds to different modalities of sensory stimulations. Moreover different parts of the brain are implicated: brain hemispheres and the brain-stem are necessary for ILS-induced seizures to occur in FEpi while the brain-stem alone allows audiogenic seizures to occur in rodents (Fadlallah *et al.*, in preparation).

Conclusions

Experiments combining techniques of embryology and electrophysiology, applied to the study of the mechanisms underlying the avian FEpi reflex epilepsy, have demonstrated the following points.

It is possible to transfer a genetic pathological trait affecting the nervous system in birds through embryonic *in situ* transplantation of neural epithelium. In the present case, the photosensitive epilepsy of the fowl was transferred either totally or partially depending on the part of the brain which had been substituted.

To transfer the full spectrum of the ILS-induced seizure of the FEpi, it is necessary to graft both the prosencephalon and the mesencephalon, each one being responsible for some particular aspects of the epileptic pattern. The graft of an 'epileptic' rhombencephalon is not necessary to permit the full expression of this reflex epilepsy induced by intermittent light stimulation. On the contrary recent experiments (Fadlallah *et al.*, in preparation) show that 'epileptic' mesencephalon is necessary and sufficient for the genesis of audiogenic seizures.

FEpi, which presents similarities and differences with reflex epilepsies in other species, is an interesting model. The intermittent light stimulation frequency required is the same in chickens and in man, while different in baboons. Tonic–clonic seizures and their concomitant EEG paroxysms found in man and baboon under intermittent light stimulation are not observed in reflex seizures in chicken. On the contrary, the EEG expression of seizures in chickens is close to the audiogenic seizures of rodents, although the beginning of the behavioural seizure is not similar (Fadlallah et al., in preparation).

It is also important to note that the behavioural and EEG signs of ILS-induced seizures differ from those induced by convulsants such as metrazol acting preferentially in the anterior part of the brain.

With the present behavioural and electrophysiological data, one can only hypothesize that the mechanism of the motor manifestations of the complete seizure of FEpi is the result of a direct hyper-reactivity of the brain-stem to intermittent light stimulation or from a suppression of the control exerted by the prosencephalon over the brain-stem during such stimuli.

Acknowledgements

We are grateful to R.D. Crawford who provided us with embryonated eggs of his mutant strain allowing us to undertake our own breeding, and P. Mérat, F. Minvielle and G. Coquerelle (INRA, Jouy-en-Josas) who helped us in this enterprise. We also thank D.D. Johnson and R. Gonda who sent us recently epileptic embryonated eggs for our experiments. We thank B. Schuler for excellent technical assistance, and B. Henri, Y. Rantier and T. Guérot who managed the video recordings and photographs. This work was supported by CNRS, INSERM, Fondation pour la Recherche Médicale, Fondation de France and Association pour la Recherche contre le Cancer. N.T.M. Guy was a recipient of a fellowship from Fondation Française pour la Recherche sur l'Epilepsie.

References

Balaban, E., Teillet, M.A. & Le Douarin, N.M. (1988): Application of the quail–chick chimera system to the study of brain development and behaviour. *Science* **241**, 1339–1342.

Crawford, R.D. (1970): Epileptiform seizures in domestic fowl. *J. Hered.* **61**, 185–188.

Crawford, R.D. (1983): Genetics and behavior of the epi mutant chicken. In: *The brain and behavior of the fowl*, ed. T. Ookawa, pp. 259–269. Tokyo: Japan Scientific Society Press.

Crawford, R.D. (1990): Mutations and major variants of the nervous system in chickens. In: *Poultry breeding and genetics*, ed. R.D. Crawford, pp. 257–272. New York: Elsevier.

Crichlow, E.C. (1983): Electroencephalogram and brain biochemistry of the Epi mutant chicken. In: *The brain and behavior of the fowl*, ed. T. Ookawa, pp. 271–280. Tokyo: Japan Scientific Society Press.

Crichlow, E.C. & Crawford, R.D. (1974): Epileptiform seizures in domestic fowl. II. Intermittent light stimulation and the electroencephalogram. *Can. J. Physiol. Pharmacol.* **52**, 424–429.

George, D.H., Munoz, D.G., McConnell, T. & Crawford, R.D. (1990): Megalencephaly in the epileptic chicken: a morphometric study of the adult brain. *Neuroscience* **39**, 471–477.

Guy, N., Teillet, M.A., Schuler, B., Le Gal La Salle, G., Le Douarin, N.M., Naquet, R. & Batini, C. (1992): Pattern of electroencephalographic activity during light induced seizures in genetic epileptic chickens and brain chimeras. *Neurosci. Lett.* **145**, 55–58.

Guy, N.T.M., Teillet, M.A., Naquet, R. & Batini, C. (1993): Avian photogenic epilepsy and embryonic brain chimeras: neural activity of the adult prosencephalon and mesencephalon. *Exp. Brain Res.* **93**, 196–204.

Hallonet, M.E.R., Teillet, M.A. & Le Douarin, N.M. (1990): A new approach to the development of the cerebellum provided by the quail–chick marker system. *Development* **108**, 19–31.

Johnson, D.D. & Davis H.L. (1983): Drug responses and brain biochemistry of the Epi mutant chicken. In: *The brain and behavior of the fowl*, ed. T. Ookawa, pp. 281–296. Tokyo: Japan Scientific Society Press.

Johnson, D.D. & Tuchek, J.M. (1987): The epileptic chickens. In: *Neurotransmitters and epilepsy*, eds. P.C. Jobe & H.E. Laird II, pp. 95–115. Clifton: Humana Press.

Killam, K.F., Killam, E.K. & Naquet, R. (1967): An animal model of light sensitive epilepsy. *Electroencephalogr. Clin. Neurophysiol.* **22**, 497–513.

Le Douarin, N.M. (1993): Embryonic neural chimeras in the study of brain development. *Trends Neurosci.* **16**, 64–72.

Le Gal La Salle, G. & Naquet, R. (1990): Audiogenic seizures evoked in DBA/2 mice induce c-fos oncogene expression into subcortical auditory nuclei. *Brain Res.* **518**, 308–312.

Marescaux, C, Vergnes, M., Kiesmann, M., Depaulis, A., Micheletti, G. & Warter J.M. (1987): Kindling of audiogenic seizures in Wistar rats: an EEG study. *Exp. Neurol.* **97,** 160–168.

Niaussat, M.M. & Laget, P. (1963): Psychophysiologie, neuropharmacologie et biochimie de la crise audiogène. In: *Colloque CNRS 112*, ed. CNRS, pp. 181–197. Paris: Editions du CNRS.

Ohki, H., Martin, C., Corbel, C., Coltey, M. & Le Douarin, N.M. (1987): Tolerance induced by thymic epithelial grafts in bird. *Science* **238,** 1032-1035.

Teillet, M.A., Naquet, R., Le Gal La Salle, G., Merat, P., Schuler, B. & Le Douarin, N.M. (1991): Transfer of genetic epilepsy by embryonic brain grafts in the chicken. *Proc. Natl. Acad. Sci. (USA)* **88,** 6966–6970.

Vergnes, M., Marescaux, C, Depaulis, A., Micheletti, G. & Warter, J.M. (1990): Spontaneous spike-and-wave discharges in Wistar rats: a model of genetic generalized convulsive epilepsy. In: *Generalized epilepsy*, eds. M. Avoli, P. Gloor, G. Kostopoulos & R. Naquet, pp. 238–253. Boston: Birkhaüser.

Chapter 32

The GEPR model of the epilepsies

Phillip C. Jobe[*], Pravin K. Mishra[*], Leah E. Adams-Curtis[*], Kwang Ho Ko[†]
and John W. Dailey[*]

[*]*Department of Basic Sciences, University of Illinois College of Medicine at Peoria, Box 1649, Peoria Il 61656 USA*, [†]*Department of Pharmacy, College of Pharmacy, Seoul National University, Center for Biofunctional Molecules, Postech, Korea*

Introduction

The genetically epilepsy-prone rat (GEPR) is a useful tool in the understanding of seizure predisposition and mechanisms of seizure initiation, propogation and termination. The GEPR model has been derived from Sprague–Dawley stock through selective breeding for audiogenic susceptibility characteristics. In response to acoustical stimulation, these two independently derived strains exhibit either generalized clonus (GEPR-3s) or a complete tonic extensor convulsion (GEPR-9s). In addition to sound, GEPRs are susceptible to other stimuli that are not convulsant in normal animals. Moreover, these animals demonstrate a lower threshold and/or increased responsiveness to modalities that are seizure provoking in normal animals. These seizure predisposition characteristics make GEPRs an advantageous model for the study of the characteristics of the underlying pathophysiology of epilepsy. Additionally, all known antiepileptic drugs that have been tested in GEPRs are effective against seizures in these animals. In contrast, tests in GEPRs do not appear to detect false positives. This makes the GEPRs useful models for screening potential antiepileptic drugs. Moreover, the GEPR, and other genetic models of epilepsy, can play a unique role in the development of drugs for abnormalities which underly seizure predisposition as well as seizure initiation and spread.

Brief description of the GEPR

As shown in Fig. 1, the genetically epilepsy-prone rat (GEPR) stems from Sprague–Dawley stock. Two independently derived GEPR strains have been developed: the moderate seizure GEPR-3s and severe seizure GEPR-9s (Jobe *et al.*, 1991, 1992b). An extensive description of the derivation of the two strains has been reported (Dailey *et al.*, 1989). In response to audiogenic stimulation, each strain exhibits its own characteristic convulsive pattern. GEPR-3s exhibit generalized clonus (a class 3 brain-stem seizure as measured by the severity scale developed by Jobe *et al.* (1973) and further modified by Dailey *et al.* (1985)), (Fig. 2). GEPR-9s exhibit tonic extensor convulsions (a class 9 seizure on the severity scale). These class 3 and class 9 responses are the basis for the acronyms GEPR-3 and GEPR-9 since these two types of GEPRs exhibit audiogenic response scores of 3 and 9 respectively (Fig. 2). On first exposure to the acoustical stimulus, currently over 90 per

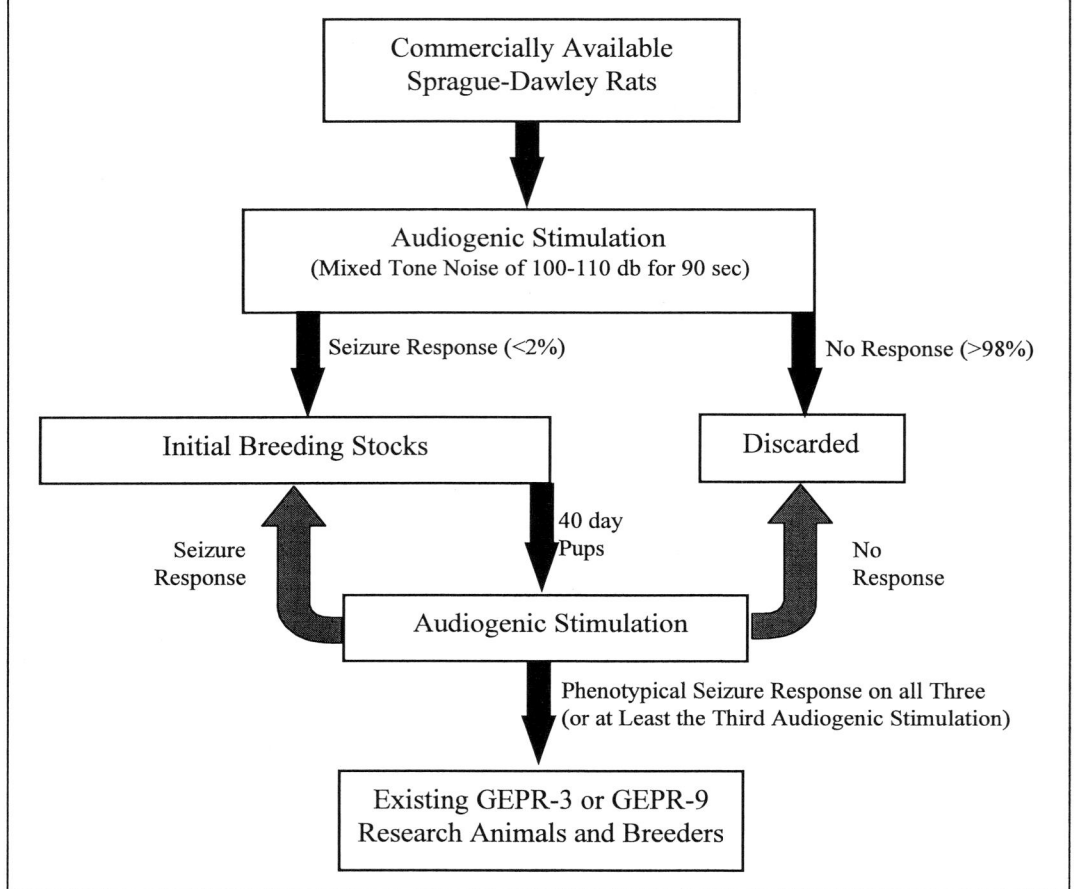

Fig. 1. Development of the two GEPR strains (GEPR-3s and GEPR-9s) and protocol for their breeding.

cent of GEPR-3s and GEPR-9s display their phenotypical seizures. By the third exposure to the sound stimulus, over 98 per cent of the GEPRs display the characteristic seizure (Mishra et al., 1993a). A consistent phenotypical seizure pattern as well as uniform latency to its onset upon audiogenic stimulation persist throughout life (Thompson et al., 1991). The breeding protocol used in the maintainance of the GEPR strains is shown in Fig. 1.

Seizure predisposition in GEPR-3s and GEPR-9s

Seizure predisposition in both GEPR models encompasses spontaneous seizures; exaggerated seizure responsiveness to stimuli which also provoke seizures in normal animals; and susceptibility to seizures induced by stimuli that do not cause seizures in normal rats (Table 1). The incidence of spontaneous seizures has been noted to be approximately two per 600 GEPR-9s per month and less frequently in GEPR-3s (Dailey et al., 1989). The exaggerated seizure responsiveness in the GEPR, as compared to non-epileptic rats, is characterized by a more intense response to an equivalent amount of a seizure-producing stimulus, and/or a lower threshold for an equivalent seizure response to the stimulus (Jobe et al., 1991). For example, an equivalent electroshock current produces a seizure response of a greater severity in the GEPR than in non-epileptic animals. Further, in the

ARS Score	RESPONSE TO SOUND STIMULATION	Characteristic Convulsive Posture
0	No response	no convulsion
1	Running only	
2	two running phases; ⎤ -clonic convulsion	
3	one running phase; ⎦	
4	two running phases; ⎤ tonus of neck, trunk and	
5	one running phase; ⎦ forelimb; hindlimb clonus	
6	two running phases; ⎤ nearly complete tonic	
7	one running phase; ⎦ extension except hindfeet	
8	two running phases; ⎤ -complete tonic extension	
9	one running phase; ⎦	

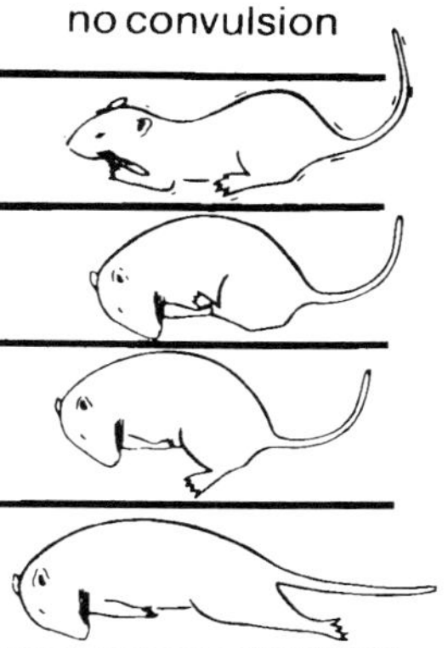

Fig. 2. The severity scale for rating the audiogenic seizures in GEPRS developed by Jobe et al. *(1973) and further modified by Dailey et al. (1985): (reproduced with permission).*

GEPR fewer kindling stimuli and smaller doses of chemoconvulsants are required to produce seizure responses equivalent to those observed in normal animals. The susceptibility of GEPRs to stimuli which fail to produce seizures in normal rats includes: (1) brain-stem audiogenic seizures; (2) seizure-induced exacerbation of brain-stem audiogenic seizures; (3) forebrain seizures secondary to brain-stem seizures; (4) hyperthermic brain-stem seizures; and (5) handling-induced seizures (Jobe *et al.*, 1991).

Approaches to the study of seizure susceptibility and expression

The brains of normal rats and other normal mammals, including humans, can exhibit seizures upon stimulation with a convulsant drug or an electrical stimulus. Thus, seizure mechanisms can be studied experimentally in normal brain. Brains of genetic models of epilepsy also exhibit seizures in response to these stimuli. Models of epilepsy developed in normal brain are useful in part because they include traits of seizure mechanisms that normal brains share with epileptic mammals, including those of the GEPRs. Because of these shared traits, both normal and epileptic mammals are useful in the study of seizure initiation and expression. Since both types of mammals are susceptible to forebrain and brain-stem seizures, they can be employed for investigations of seizure mechanisms operative in either the rostral or caudal circuitry (Jobe *et al.*, 1991, 1992b). Accordingly, either type can be used for ontogenetic studies of seizure susceptibility and expression. When used for these purposes, experimentation with GEPRs is comparable to that with non-epileptic mammals.

The GEPR as a model of innate seizure predisposition

At least some humans with epilepsy and the mammalian models of genetic epilepsy exhibit seizure predisposition: they exhibit seizures in response to stimuli that do not cause such episodes in normal people or other normal mammals (Jobe *et al.*, 1991). Because of this trait, epileptic mammals including the GEPR are useful for distinguishing the underlying mechanisms of epileptic dysfunction from seizure mechanisms of normal brain. Moreover, a predisposition to seizures in GEPRs exists in the seizure naive state (Jobe *et al.*, 1991). These animals provide a means for establishing

Table 1. Comparison of GEPRs with non-epileptic animals

Seizure triggering/ causing modality	Manifestation of seizures in		
	Non-epileptic animals	GEPR-3s	GEPR-9s
Idiopathic	No spontaneous seizures	Less frequent spontaneous seizures than GEPR-9s (Dailey et al., 1989)	2 seizures per 600 with or without continuing status epilepticus (Dailey et al., 1989)
Sound	No seizure	Class-3 brain-stem seizure[1] (Mishra et al., 1989). EEG field potential spiking occurs in the brain-stem in response to the first sound stimulation (Wang et al., 1993). Prominent cortical spiking with repeated stimulations (Naritoku et al., 1992)	Class-9 brain-stem seizure[2] (Mishra et al., 1988b). EEG field potential spiking occurs in the brain-stem in response to the first sound stimulation (Wang et al., 1993). Prominent cortical spiking with repeated stimulations (Naritoku et al., 1992).
Hyperthermia	No convulsion in adult non-epileptic rats (Jobe et al., 1982)	Not studied	Class-9 brain-stem seizure[2] (Jobe et al., 1982)
Hyperbaria	Tremor and convulsions	Not studied	Abnormally low threshold (Millan et al., 1991)
Pentylenetetrazole	FFC[3] with rearing followed in some cases by class-5 brain-stem seizure[4] with doses between 35 & 50 mg/kg i.p. (Browning et al., 1990)	Occasional GEPR-3 exhibits FFC in response to doses between 35 & 50 mg/kg i.p. (Browning et al., 1990). Progression to class-5 brain-stem convulsion with prodromal running component. Mean seizure severity more intense than for control rats. Latency to onset of initial myoclonic jerk equal to control value. Another study: convulsant dose fifty lower than in control rats (Dailey et al., 1988)	No FFC with rearing with i.p. doses 35 & 50 mg/kg i.p. (Browning et al., 1990). Rapid progression to class-9 brainstem convulsions without running component with 50 mg/kg i.p. Mean seizure severity more intense than for GEPR-3. Latency to onset of initial myoclonic jerk equal to control value. Another study: convulsant dose fifty lower than for control but equal to GEPR-3 (Dailey et al., 1988)
Corneal electroshock low current range	FFC	Abnormally low threshold for FFC (Mishra et al., 1991; Browning et al., 1990)	Threshold for FFC lower than in GEPR-3; threshold for FFC higher than threshold for brain-stem-type seizures. Nevertheless, currents sufficient to produce FFC usually do not do so. These forebrain seizure-induced behaviours are typically masked by the dominant influence of the brain-stem-driven seizure (Browning et al., 1990)
Earclip electroshock intermediate current range	Class-3 and class-9 brain-stem convulstions at lower and higher end of range, respectively. An appreciable fraction of control rats fail to exhibit convulsions above class 5 (Browning, 1992)	Abnormally low thresholds for class-3 and class-9 brain-stem convulsions (Browning et al., 1990). Major fraction of GEPR-3s exhibit class-9 convulsions with higher currents	Both thresholds lower than for GEPR-3s (Browning et al., 1990). Essentially all GEPR-9s exhibit class 9 convulsions with higher current
Earclip electroshock supramaximal current	Lowest incidence of Class-9 brain-stem seizures (unpublished observations) and lowest pelvic limb extension/flexion ratios (Jobe et al., 1992a)	Higher incidence of class-9 brain-stem seizures and higher pelvic limb extension/ flexion ratios (Jobe et al., 1992a)	Highest incidence of class-9 brain-stem seizures and highest pelvic limb extension/ flexion ratios (Jobe et al., 1992a)
Limbic kindling	An average of 24 stimulations are required to reach a class-5 kindled stage (Savage et al., 1986	An average of 19 stimulations are required to get a class-5 kindled stage (Savage et al., 1986)	An average of 12 stimulations are required to get a class-5 kindled stage (Savage et al., 1986)

[1] A class-3 brain-stem seizure is a running episode followed by generalized clonus with loss of righting; [2] A class-9 brainstem seizure is a complete tonic extensor convulsion with or without a preceding wild running episode; [3] FFC denotes facial and forelimb clonus stemming from a forebrain seizure; [4] A class-5 brain-stem seizure is a tonic extensor convulsion with a running episode.

Chapter 32 The GEPR model of the epilepsies

Manifestation of seizures in

Seizure triggering/causing modality	Non-epileptic animals	GEPR-3s	GEPR-9s
Corneal kindling	Small reduction in facial and forelimb clonus threshold with increasing number of electroshocks (unpublished observations)	Accelerated and more pronounced reduction in facial and forelimb clonus threshold as compared to non-epileptic controls (Mishra et al., 1990; unpublished observations)	Not studied
Three repetitions of audiogenic seizures	No seizure	Reduction in latency to onset of class-3 seizure from first to third weekly stimulation; of littermates exhibiting less than a Class-3 response, most progress to a class-3 seizure (Mishra et al., 1989)	Reduction in latency to onset of class-9 seizure from first to third weekly stimulation. Of animals exhibiting less than a Class-9 response, most progress to a class-9 seizure (Mishra et al., 1988)
Repeated audiogenic seizures, > 20 daily stimulations	Increase in grooming behaviour (Garcia-Cairasco et al., unpublished observations)	Increase in seizure duration. Appearance of FFC after termination of class-3 brain-stem seizure (Narioku et al., 1992); EEG field potential spiking occurs in the brain-stem in response to the first sound stimulation (Wang et al., 1993). Prominent cortical spiking with repeated stimulations (Narioku et al., 1992)	Increase in seizure duration. A clonic phase appears upon termination of class-9 brain-stem convulsion (Narioku et al., 1992). EEG field potential spiking occurs in the brainstem in response to the first sound stimulation (Wang et al., 1993). Prominent cortical spiking with repeated stimulations (Narioku et al., 1992)
ICV morphine	Dose-dependent (5–120 μg) progression from wetdog shakes, bilateral forelimb clonus with rearing, class-3 brain-stem clonus to class-9 brain-stem tonic extensor convulsions (Reigel et al., 1988)	Less sensitive than control rats to wetdog shakes and forelimb clonus with rearing. Equally sensitive to class-3 brain-stem clonus. No class-9 brain-stem seizures at any dose (Reigel et al., 1988)	More sensitive than controls or GEPR-3s to wetdog shakes and forelimb clonus with rearing, class-3 brain-stem clonus and class-9 brain-stem seizures (Reigel et al., 1988)
Aminophylline	Mostly clonic, occasionally tonic seizure (De Sarro & De Sarro, 1991).	Not studied	Rapid progression into tonic seizure with lower proconvulsant dose (De Sarro & De Sarro, 1991)
Bicuculine	Intravenous administration produces both electrographic seizures and convulsions (Faingold, 1987)	Greater threshold than controls for electrographic seizures following intravenous administration (Reigel et al., 1984). Extinct GEPR-2 colony showed reduced threshold compared to controls when injected into the inferior colliculus (Duplisse, 1976). Effect of injection into inferior colliculus not studied in extant GEPR-3s.	Greater threshold than controls for electrographic seizures following intravenous administration (Reigel et al., 1984).

[1] A class-3 brain-stem seizure is a running episode followed by generalized clonus with loss of righting; [2] A class-9 brainstem seizure is a complete tonic extensor convulsion with or without a preceding wild running episode; [3] FFC denotes facial and forelimb clonus stemming from a forebrain seizure; [4] A class-5 brain-stem seizure is a tonic extensor convulsion with a running episode

the 'pristine mechanisms of seizure predisposition in brain unadulterated by seizure-induced seizure propensity' (Jobe et al., 1994). Conversely, the GEPR model also allows evaluation of the consequences of seizures as opposed to the biological factors that underly predisposition. This is an important experimental control in the evaluation of the GEPR.

Evidence that seizure predisposition in the GEPR resides in forebrain circuitry stems partially from investigations showing that angular bundle kindling is accelerated markedly in GEPR-9s and moderately in GEPR-3s. Also, studies with corneal electroshock show that forebrain seizure thresholds are abnormally low both in GEPR-3s and GEPR-9s, with the lowest threshold in GEPR-9s (Jobe et al., 1992b).

Quantitative documentation of brain-stem seizure predisposition stems from several types of observations including those with audiogenic, hyperthermic, and electroshock seizures (Jobe et al., 1992b). The fraction of current GEPR-3 and GEPR-9 strains which exhibit brain-stem driven audiogenic seizures upon first exposure to the acoustical stimulus exceeds 90 per cent (Mishra et al., 1988a,b, 1993a). The expression of such seizures in commercially available Sprague–Dawley control rats is infrequent. Susceptibility to hyperthermic convulsions, apparently driven by brain-stem circuitry, is high in GEPRs, but seemingly not in adult members of a non-epileptic control colony (Jobe et al., 1982). Corneal electroshock studies have shown that the threshold for brain-stem convulsions is rank ordered: highest in non-epileptic control rats, intermediate in GEPR-3s and lowest in GEPR-9s. Moreover, in GEPR-9s the ratio of brain-stem to forebrain convulsions threshold is less than 1, whereas in GEPR-3s and non-epileptic control rats it is more than 1 (Browning et al. 1990).

The GEPR as a model of innately determined, age-dependent epileptogenesis

Seizure predisposition in GEPRs becomes evident early in postnatal life (Jobe et al., 1980; Hjeresen et al., 1987; Ribak et al., 1988b; Franck et al., 1989; Reigel et al., 1989; Thompson et al. 1991). Although many aspects of innately determined epileptogenesis remain undetermined, evidence shows that audiogenic seizures upon initial exposure to the acoustic stimulus develop similarly in GEPR-3s and GEPR-9s until divergence appears in the fourth postnatal week. At this last age of equivalence, the audiogenic seizure severity of GEPR-3s has exceeded its adult phenotype. In contrast, severity in the GEPR-9 has not yet escalated to the adult level. Soon after, GEPR-3s exhibit a decline in severity, achieving the adult phenotype by 45 days of age. But ontogenetic epileptogenesis in GEPR-9s is characterized by a final period of progressively increasing severity. The maximal severity equivalent to that of adulthood is achieved around postnatal day 45 (Reigel et al., 1989).

The GEPR also has potential as a model of ontogenetically determined epileptogenesis involving interactions between forebrain and brain-stem seizure circuitry (Jobe et al., 1991). Moreover, the characteristic seizure development pattern may be informative of normal excitatory and inhibitory neural pathways. Studies which examine the relative roles of these systems in the severity of seizure expression can indicate whether this is the case. Audiogenic forebrain seizures appear to occur within a narrow window of time in developing GEPR-3s (Reigel et al., 1989). At 15 days of age, in half of the GEPR-3s exhibiting the running–bouncing clonus of brain-stem seizures (upon initial exposure to the sound stimulus), the seizures subside into a period of quiescence followed by the forelimb clonus and rearing typical of forebrain seizures. At 21 days of age, all GEPR-3 pups exhibit both the clonus and the secondary forebrain seizures. However, brain-stem seizure-induced forebrain seizures are no longer evident by day 45 in GEPR-3s which have had received no prior exposure to the acoustical stimulus. Further investigations in the ontogeny of seizures, and the corresponding changes in neurophysiology will enable us to determine how much the GEPR can contribute to the understanding of ontogeny of the nervous system in general, and the ontogeny of the seizure disorders in specific.

A model of stimulus-exacerbated genetically determined seizure predisposition

Seizure-induced aggravation of epileptogenesis has been documented in adult GEPRs. This phenomenon appears to occur both in forebrain and brain-stem seizure circuitry. With regard to brain-stem seizures, GEPRs experience increasing severity of audiogenic convulsions between their first and third sound-induced seizure (Jobe *et al.*, 1992b). One aspect of this increasing severity may be related to the rostral extension of brain-stem seizure spiking into the forebrain that occurs with repeated audiogenic seizures. Accordingly, forebrain-like behaviours with facial and forelimb clonus occur in response to repetitive audiogenic seizures (Naritoku *et al.*, 1992).

A model for studies of the aetiology of seizure predisposition

The significant pathophysiology of GEPR predisposition to seizure entails several features (Faingold & Naritoku, 1992; Jobe *et al.*, 1993a,b). For example, noradrenergic (Jobe *et al.*, 1973, 1984a; Ko *et al.*, 1982, 1984; Dailey & Jobe, 1986; Mishra *et al.*, 1988a, 1993b, 1994; Browning *et al.*, 1989b; Lauterborn & Ribak, 1989; Dailey *et al.*, 1991; Yan *et al.* 1993a,b; Yourick *et al.*, 1991; Razani Boroujerdi *et al.*, 1993), serotonergic (Dailey *et al.*, 1992a,b, 1993; Yan *et al.*, 1992, 1994), GABAergic (Roberts *et al.*, 1985; Booker *et al.*, 1986; Faingold *et al.*, 1986a,b,c; Roberts & Ribak, 1986,1988; Ribak *et al.*, 1988a, 1989, 1993; Browning *et al.*, 1989a; Evans *et al.*, 1991; Faingold & Anderson, 1991; Lasley, 1991; Doretto *et al.*, 1994) opioidergic (Reigel *et al.*, 1988; Savage *et al.*, 1988;) and glutamatergic and aspartatergic (Faingold *et al.*, 1988, 1989; Millan *et al.*, 1988; Meyerhoff *et al.*, 1992a,b) abnormalities appear to participate as contributing factors. The possibility of aetiologically significant abnormalities in the GEPR 'wiring diagram' or circuitry has been reported (Roberts *et al.*, 1985; Roberts & Ribak, 1986; Ribak *et al.*, 1988b, 1989, 1993; Lauterborn & Ribak, 1989). Both noradrenergic and GABAergic systems are characterized by deficient presynaptic and post-synaptic function and the contributions of these systems to seizure predisposition appear to derive from these defects (Jobe *et al.* 1993a,b). The specific roles of these abnormalities in all aspects of seizure predisposition in GEPRs have not been investigated. But useful hypotheses are emerging. Neuroanatomical evidence supports the concept that GABAergic deficits in the inferior colliculus function as one element in the audiogenic triggering mechanism responsible for the appearance of seizure spiking first in the brain-stem reticular formation and then in the inferior colliculus (Wang *et al.*, 1993). Recent observations in our laboratory suggest that experimentally induced noradrenergic increments outside of the inferior colliculus can prevent spiking within this structure (Browning *et al.*, 1989a; Wang *et al.*, 1993).

A model for studies of anticonvulsants and development of antiepileptic drugs

Since the discovery of antiepileptic properties of phenytoin (Merrit & Putnam, 1938), investigations in epileptology have been dominated by two informative experimental approaches. In the first, investigators have evaluated seizure mechanisms and anticonvulsant processes in the normal brain. In the second, they have studied kindling mechanisms and the resulting stimulus-induced seizure propensity in normal brain. The current drugs used for the clinical management of the epilepsies were largely developed through the preclinical evaluation of anticonvulsant processes in normal mammalian brain. Moreover, most of what we know today about anticonvulsant drug therapy has been learned from study of animal models of epilepsy (Fisher, 1989, 1991).

There are several advantages in using the GEPR for anticonvulsant-drug screening protocols. Both GEPR-3 and GEPR-9 have a reproducible and more consistent seizure intensity than those observed in the maximal electroshock rat model. The incidence of undesired seizures (such as novelty-induced seizures in mongolian gerbils) is insignificant in the GEPR. Unlike the kindling model, seizure-induction processes in the GEPR do not require extensive preparation. An audiogenic seizure is easier to administer than electroshock, pentylenetetrazole or other drug-induction or threshold paradigms. Moreover, the two levels of seizure predisposition in the GEPR-3 and GEPR-9 offer advantages in interpretation of the drug-screening data that are unmatched by any other model system for routine screening of potential anticonvulsant drugs.

While all antiepileptic drugs that have been tested in GEPRs are effective in these animals, the two strains of GEPRs do respond differently to these drugs. Accordingly, the ratio of anticonvulsant effective doses in GEPR-3s and GEPR-9s predicts the effectiveness of a particular drug against various types of seizures (Dailey & Jobe, 1985). Drugs with a ratio of the GEPR-3 CC_{50}/GEPR-9 CC_{50} of more than 1, such as phenytoin and carbamazepine, are effective in generalized tonic–clonic and complex partial seizures. Drugs with a ratio of 1, such as phenobarbital and ethosuximide are effective in convulsive and/or absence seizures. Drugs with a ratio of less than 1 such as valproic acid and loreclozole are broad-spectrum drugs for generalized convulsive and absence seizures (Dailey & Jobe, 1985; Reigel et al., 1986).

GEPRs also have additional advantages. Firstly, false positives are avoided in the anticonvulsant drug evaluation protocols. Accordingly, GEPRs distinguish drugs that have been found anticonvulsant in other models but are not effective in humans. For example, we have observed that chlorpromazine, haloperidol and baclofen do not produce anticonvulsant effects in GEPRs, even when given in doses (10 mg/kg for chlorpromazine and baclofen; 1 mg/kg for haloperidol) that block spontaneous motor activity. These observations are in contrast to those reported for other models. For example, chlorpromazine blocks tonic hindlimb extension in non-paralytic doses in non-epileptic rats (Raines et al., 1976) and is anticonvulsant against audiogenic seizures in DBA/1 mice (Plotnikoff, 1963). Neither haloperidol nor baclofen are recognized as anticonvulsant in humans, and baclofen blocks ictal epileptiform events induced by removal of extracellular magnesium in slices of entorhinal cortex (Jones, 1989). Secondly, the GEPR is a superior model for assessing toxicity profiles of anticonvulsant drugs as it distinguishes the toxicity on a wider scale than do other models (Dailey & Jobe, 1985).

A model for studies of the proconvulsant and anticonvulsant potential of psychoactive drugs

Since psychotropic drugs are shown to have anticonvulsant effects in GEPRs and human responses to these agents are sometimes convulsions, it may be argued that the GEPR does not accurately mimic such effects in humans. Based on this belief, the value of the GEPR is sometimes questioned. However, a careful evaluaton of the published literature proves that the response of GEPRs to these drugs closely parallels that of the human and other species. Documentation of these analogous effects is summarized below.

Prior to the recognition that anticonvulsant effects were produced by antidepressant drugs in humans, clinical attention was largely focused on these drugs as causes of convulsions (Legg & Swash, 1974; Pineda & Russell, 1974; Trimble, 1978, 1980a,b, 1984; Callaham, 1979; Itil & Soldatos, 1980; Edwards et al., 1986; Rickels & Schweizer, 1990; Nierenberg & Cole, 1991; Preskorn & Fast, 1992; Skowron & Stimmel, 1992). Other mammalian species – including GEPRs (Dailey & Jobe, 1985; Jobe et al., 1984b), epileptic mice, epileptic baboons (Meldrum et al., 1982), non-epileptic rats (Jobe et al., 1984b; Dailey & Jobe, 1985), cats (Polc et al., 1979) and rhesus monkeys (Yanagita et al., 1980) – mimic humans by exhibiting seizures in response to antidepressant drugs. However, anticonvulsant effects of the antidepressants in humans and other animals are less well known than the convulsant effects. Nevertheless, the body of evidence clearly supports the concept that anticonvulsant properties are part of the antidepressant pharmacological repertory broadly shared across species (Vernier, 1961; Piette et al., 1963; Stille & Sayers, 1964; Baker & Kratky, 1967; Lehmann, 1967; Chen et al., 1968; Lange et al., 1976; Babington, 1977; McIntyre et al., 1979; Meldrum et al., 1982; Leander, 1992). In humans, these anticonvulsant properties have been documented in retrospective and prospective investigations including case reports, open studies and double-blind crossover studies (Millichap, 1965; Fromm *et al.*, 1971, 1972, 1978; Buge *et al.*, 1974; Pineda & Russell, 1974; Ojemann *et al.*, 1983)

The anticonvulsant effects of the antidepressants in GEPRs are also extensively documented. The anticonvulsant effects of imipramine were reported by Jobe *et al.* (1973). Since that time, the anticonvulsant effects of many other antidepressants have been documented in GEPRs (Jobe *et al.*, 1984b; Dailey & Jobe, 1985; Reigel *et al.*, 1986; Dailey *et al.*, 1992b; Wang *et al.* 1993; Yan *et al.*, 1993b, 1994).

In summary, neither the anticonvulsant nor the convulsant effects of the antidepressant drugs are unique to GEPRs. Rather, they are characteristic of mammalian responses in mice, rats, cats, subhuman primates and in people. Dosage appears to be a prominent factor in determining whether antidepressant drugs produce anticonvulsant or convulsant effects. The convulsant dose$_{50}$s of antidepressants are approximately two to nine times the anticonvulsant dose$_{50}$s in GEPRs (Dailey & Jobe, 1985; Jobe *et al.*, 1984b), genetically epileptic baboons, and in non-epileptic cats and mice (Lange *et al.*, 1976; Dailey & Jobe, 1985; Reigel *et al.*, 1986). In humans, dosage also appears to play the same prominent role in determining whether antidepressant drugs produce anticonvulsant or convulsant effects (Fromm *et al.*, 1972; Legg & Swash, 1974). Some of the clinical literature fostered the idea that doses of the antidepressants used therapeutically in psychiatry sometimes caused convulsions in patients. Now, however, this concept seems less tenable. A recent study (Preskorn & Fast, 1992) shows that seizures occurred only in those patients who had excessive plasma antidepressant drug levels despite the ingestion of 'therapeutic doses' of several different antidepressants. As a specific example, the patient with 1200 ng/ml of desipramine was on a therapeutic regimen of 200 mg/day. This plasma level contrasts markedly with the estimates of the therapeutic range of 40 to 160 ng/ml (Benet & Williams, 1990). According to Preskorn & Fast (1992) there are no reports in the literature of tricyclic-induced seizures at therapeutic concentrations of the antidepressants.

The role of the GEPR in the development of novel drugs

The GEPR model has the potential to contribute to the development of novel drugs that can selectively ameliorate innately determined seizure-predisposing abnormalities (Jobe *et al.*, 1991). Present antiepileptic drugs suppress symptoms. Future agents developed through an understanding of the genetically determined epileptic states and their interactions with environmental factors may increase the likelihood for the development of preventions and cures.

References

Babington, R.G. (1977): The pharmacology of kindling. In: *Animal models in psychiatry and neurology*, eds. I. Hanin & E. Usdin, pp. 141–149. New York: Pergamon Press.

Baker, W.W. & Kratky, M. (1967): Acute effects of chlorpromazine and imipramine on hippicampal foci. *Arch. Int. Pharmacodyn. Ther.* **162**, 265–275.

Benet, L.Z. & Williams, R.L. (1990): Appendix II. Design and optimizatiion of dosage regimens; pharmacokinetic data. In: *Goodman and Gilman's the pharmacological basis of therapeutics*, 8th edn. eds. A.G. Gilman, T.W. Rall, A.S Nies & P. Taylor, pp. 1650–1735. New York: Pergamon Press.

Booker, J.G., Dailey, J.W., Jobe, P.C. & Lane, J.D. (1986): Cerebral cortical GABA and benzodiazepine binding sites in genetically seizure prone rats. *Life Sci.* **39**, 799–806.

Browning, R.A., Lanker, M.L. & Faingold, C.L. (1989a): Injections of noradrenergic and GABAergic agonists into the inferior colliculus: effects on audiogenic seizures in genetically epilepsy-prone rats. *Epilepsy Res.* **4**, 119–125.

Browning, R.A., Wade, D.R., Marcinczyk, M., Long, G.L. & Jobe, P.C. (1989b): Regional brain abnormalities in norepinephrine uptake and dopamine beta-hydroxylase activity in the genetically epilepsy-prone rat. *J. Pharmacol. Exp. Ther.* **249**, 229–235.

Browning, R.A., Wang, C., Lanker, M.L. & Jobe, P.C. (1990): Electroshock- and pentylenetetrazol-induced seizures in genetically epilepsy-prone rats (GEPRs): differences in threshold and pattern. *Epilepsy Res.* **6**, 1–11.

Buge, A., Poisson, M., Rancurel, G., Bestel, B. & Cross, P. (1974): An intractable case of petit mal. Effects of clomipramine. *Nouv. Presse Med.* **3**, 373–375.

Callaham, M. (1979): Tricyclic antidepressant overdose. *J. Am. Coll. Exp. Pharmacol.* **8**, 413–425.

Chen, G., Ensor, C.R. & Bohner, B. (1968): Studies of drug effects on electrically induced extensor seizures and clinical implications. *Arch. Int. Pharmacodyn. Ther.* **172**, 183–218.

Dailey, J.W., Reigel, C.E., Woods, T.W., Penney, J.E. & Jobe, P.C. (1985): Types of seizure predisposition in the genetically epilepsy-rone rats (GEPRs). *Fed. Proc.* **44**, 1107(Abstract).

Dailey, J.W., Lasley, S.M., Bettendorf, A.F., Burger, A.F., Mishra, P.K. & Jobe, P.C. (1988): Aspartame does not facilitate pentylenetetrazol-induced seizures in genetically epilepsy-prone rats. *Epilepsia* **29**, 651 (Abstract).

Dailey, J.W., Reigel, C.E., Mishra, P.K. & Jobe, P.C. (1989): Neurobiology of seizure predisposition in the genetically epilepsy-prone rat. *Epilepsy Res.* **3**, 3–17.

Dailey, J.W., Mishra, P.K., Ko, K.H., Penny, J.E. & Jobe, P.C. (1991): Noradrenergic abnormalities in the central nervous system of seizure-naive genetically epilepsy-prone rats. *Epilepsia* **32**, 168–173.

Dailey, J.W., Mishra, P.K., Ko, K.H., Penny, J.E. & Jobe, P.C. (1992a): Serotonergic abnormalities in the central nervous system of seizure-naive genetically epilepsy-prone rats. *Life Sci.* **50**, 319–326.

Dailey, J.W., Yan, Q., Mishra, P.K., Burger, R.L. & Jobe, P.C. (1992b): Effects of fluoxetine on convulsions and on brain serotonin as detected by microdialysis in genetically epilepsy-prone rats. *J. Pharmacol. Exp. Ther.* **260**, 533–540.

Dailey, J.W., Yan, Q., Ko, K.H. & Jobe, P.C. (1993): The anticonvulsant effect of the broad spectrum anticonvulsant loreclezole may be mediated in part by serotonin: a microdialysis study. *Epilepsia* **34**, 78–79 (Abstract).

Dailey, J.W. & Jobe, P.C. (1985): Anticonvulsant drugs and the genetically epilepsy-prone rat. *Fed. Proc.* **44**, 2640–2644.

Dailey, J.W. & Jobe, P.C. (1986): Indices of noradrenergic function in the central nervous system of seizure-naive genetically epilepsy-prone rats. *Epilepsia* **27**, 665–670.

De Sarro, A. & De Sarro, G.B. (1991): Responsiveness of genetically epilepsy-prone rats to aminophylline-induced seizures and interactions with quinolone. *Neuropharmacology* **30**, 169–176.

Doretto, M.C., Burger, R.L., Mishra, P.K., Garcia-Cairasco, N., Dailey, J.W. & Jobe, P.C. (1994): A microdialysis study of amino acid concentrations in the extracellular fluid of the substantia nigra of freely behaving GEPR-9s: relationship to seizure predisposition. *Epilepsy Res.* in press.

Duplisse, B.R. (1976): *Mechanism of susceptibility of rats to audiogenic seizure.* University of Arizona: Xerox University Microfilms.

Edwards, J.G., Long, S.K., Sedgwick, E.M. & Wheal, H.V. (1986): Antidepressants and convulsive seizures: clinical, electroencephalographic, and pharmacological aspects. *Clin. Neuropharmacol.* **9(4)**, 329–360.

Evans, M.S., McCabe, K.E., Caspary, D.M., Faingold, C.L., Kalita, S. & Pencek, T.L. (1991): Paired pulse facilitation is increased in genetically epilepsy-prone rat (GEPR) hippocampus. *Neurology* **41**, 404.

Faingold, C.L., Gehlbach, G. & Caspary, D.M. (1986a): Decreased effectiveness of GABA-mediated inhibition in the inferior colliculus of the genetically epilepsy-prone rat. *Exp. Neurol.* **93**, 145–159.

Faingold, C.L., Gehlbach, G., Travis, M.A. & Caspary, D.M. (1986b): Inferior colliculus neuronal response abnormalities in genetically epilepsy-prone rats: evidence for a deficit of inhibition. *Life Sci.* **39**, 869–878.

Faingold, C.L., Travis, M.A., Gehlbach, G., Hoffmann, W.E., Jobe, P.C., Laird, H.E. & Caspary, D.M. (1986c): Neuronal response abnormalities in the inferior colliculus of the genetically epilepsy-prone rat. *Electroencephalogr. Clin. Neurophysiol.* **63**, 296–305.

Faingold, C.L., Millan, M.H., Boersma, C.A. & Meldrum, B.S. (1988): Excitant amino acids and audiogenic seizures in the genetically epilepsy-prone rat. I. Afferent seizure initiation pathway. *Exp. Neurol.* **99**, 678–686.

Faingold, C.L., Millan, M.H., Boersma Anderson, C.A. & Meldrum, B.S. (1989): Induction of audiogenic seizures in normal and genetically epilepsy-prone rats following focal microinjection of an excitant amino acid into reticular formation and auditory nuclei. *Epilepsy Res.* **3**, 199–205.

Faingold, C.L. & Anderson, C.A. (1991): Loss of intensity-induced inhibition in inferior colliculus neurons leads to audiogenic seizure susceptibility in behaving genetically epilepsy-prone rats. *Exp. Neurol.* **113**, 354–363.

Faingold, C.L. & Naritoku, D.K. (1992): The genetically epilepsy-prone rat: neuronal networks and actions of amino acid neurotransmitters. In: *Drugs for the control of epilepsy: actions on neuronal networks involved in seizure disorder*, eds. C.L. Faingold & G.H. Fromm, pp. 277–308. Boca Raton, LA: CRC Press.

Fisher, R.S. (1989): Animal models of the epilepsies. *Brain Res. Brain Res. Rev.* **14**, 245–278.

Fisher, R.S. (1991): Animal models of the epilepsies. In: *Neurotransmitters and epilepsy*, eds. R.S. Fisher & J.T. Coyle, pp. 61–76. New York: Wiley-Liss, Inc..

Franck, J.E., Ginter, K.L. & Schwartzkroin, P.A. (1989): Developing genetically epilepsy-prone rats have an abnormal seizure response to flurothyl. *Epilepsia* **30**, 1–6.

Fromm, G.H., Rosen, J.A. & Amores, C.Y. (1971): A clinical and experimental investigation of the effect of imipramine on epilepsy. *Epilepsia* **12**, 282–283 (Abstract).

Fromm, G.H., Amores, C.Y. & Thies, W. (1972): Imipramine in epilepsy. *Arch. Neurol.* **27**, 198–204.

Fromm, G.H., Wessel, H.B., Glass, J.D., Alvin, J.D. & VanHorn, G. (1978): Imipramine in absence and myoclonic–astatic seizures. *Neurology* **28**, 953–957.

Hjeresen, D.L., Franck, J.E. & Amend, D.L. (1987): Ontogeny of seizure incidence, latency, and severity in genetically epilepsy prone rats. *Dev. Psychobiol.* **20**, 355–363.

Itil, T.M. & Soldatos, C. (1980): Epileptogenic side effects of psychotropic drugs. *J.A.M.A.* **244**, 1460–1463.

Jobe, P.C., Picchioni, A.L. & Chin, L. (1973): Role of brain norepinephrine in audiogenic seizure in the rat. *J. Pharmacol. Exp. Ther.* **184**, 1–10.

Jobe, P.C., Brown, R.D., Dailey, J.W., Ray, T.B., Woods, T.W., Mims, M.E. & Bairnsfather, S. (1980): Effects of multiple exposures to intense acoustic stimulation on audiogenic seizure (AGS) susceptibility (S) and intensity (I) in rats. I. A developmental study in progency from a genetically susceptible colony. *Soc. Neurosci. Abstr.* **6**, 824(Abstract).

Jobe, P.C., Woods, T.W., McNatt, L.E., Kearns, G.L., Wilson, J.T. & Dailey, J.W. (1982): Genetically epilepsy-prone rats (GEPR) a model for febrile seizures?. *Fed. Proc.* **41**, 1560 (Abstract).

Jobe, P.C., Ko, K.H. & Dailey, J.W. (1984a): Abnormalities in norepinephrine turnover rate in the central nervous system of the genetically epilepsy-prone rat. *Brain Res.* **290**, 357–360.

Jobe, P.C., Woods, T.W. & Dailey, J.W. (1984b): Proconvulsant and anticonvulsant effects of tricyclic antidepressants in genetically epilepsy-prone rats. In: *Advances in epileptology: XVth epilepsy international symposium*, ed. R.J. Porter, pp. 187–191. New York: Raven Press.

Jobe, P.C., Mishra, P.K., Ludvig, N. & Dailey, J.W. (1991): Scope and contribution of genetic models to an understanding of the epilepsies. *CRC Crit. Rev. Neurobiol.* **6**, 183–220.

Jobe, P.C., Lasley, S.M., Burger, R.L., Bettendorf, A.F., Mishra, P.K. & Dailey, J.W. (1992a): Absence of an effect of aspartame on seizures induced by electroshock in epileptic and non-epileptic rats. *Amino Acids* **3**, 155–172.

Jobe, P.C., Mishra, P.K. & Dailey, J.W. (1992b): Genetically epilepsy-prone rats: actions of antiepileptic drugs and monoaminergic neurotransmitters. In: *Drugs for the control of epilepsy: actions on neuronal networks involved in seizure disorders*, eds. C.L. Faingold & G.H. Fromm, pp. 253–275. Boca Raton, FL: CRC Press.

Jobe, P.C., Mishra, P.K., Ludvig, N. & Dailey, J.W. (1993a): Genetic models of the epilepsies. In: *Concepts and models in epilepsy research*, ed. P.A. Schwartzkroin, pp. 94–140. Cambridge: Cambridge University Press.

Jobe, P.C., Mishra, P.K., Ludvig, N. & Dailey, J.W. (1993b): Genetic models of the epilepsies. In: *Concepts and models in epilepsy research*, ed. P.A. Schwartzkroin, pp. 494–499. Cambridge: Cambridge University Press.

Jobe, P.C., Mishra, P.K., Browning, R.A., Wang, C.D., Adams-Curtis, L. & Dailey, J.W. (1994): Noradrenergic abnormalities in the genetically epilepsy-prone rat. *Brain Res. Bull.* Invited review, in press .

Jones, R.S.G. (1989): Ictal epileptiform events induced by removal of extracellular magnesium slices of entorhinal cortex are blocked by baclofen. *Exp. Neurol.* **104**, 155–161.

Ko, K.H., Dailey, J.W. & Jobe, P.C. (1982): Effect of increments in norepinephrine concentrations on seizure intensity in the genetically epilepsy-prone rat. *J. Pharmacol. Exp. Ther.* **222**, 662–669.

Ko, K.H., Dailey, J.W. & Jobe, P.C. (1984): Evaluation of monoaminergic receptors in the genetically epilepsy prone rat. *Experientia* **40**, 70–73.

Lange, S.C., Julien, R.M. & Fowler, G.W. (1976): Biphasic effects of imipramine in experimental models of epilepsy. *Epilepsia* **17**, 183–196.

Lasley, S.M. (1991): Roles of neurotransmitter amino acids in seizure severity and experience in the genetically epilepsy-prone rat. *Brain Res.* **560**, 63–70.

Lauterborn, J.C. & Ribak, C.E. (1989): Differences in dopamine beta-hydroxylase immunoreactivity between the brains of genetically epilepsy-prone and Sprague–Dawley rats. *Epilepsy Res.* **4**, 161–176.

Leander, J.D. (1992): Fluoxetine, a selective serotonin-uptake inhibitor, enhances the anticonvulsant effects of phenytoin, carbamazepine, and ameltolide (LY201116). *Epilepsia* **33**, 573–576.

Legg, N.J. & Swash, M. (1974): Clinical note: seizures and EEG activation after trimipramine. *Epilepsia* **15**, 131–135.

Lehmann, A. (1967): Audiogenic seizures data in mice supporting new theories of biogenic amines mechanisms in the central nervous system. *Life Sci.* **6**, 1423–1431.

McIntyre, D.C., Saari, M. & Pappas, B.A. (1979): Potentiation of amygdala kindling in adult or infant rats by injections of 6-hydroxydopamine. *Exp. Neurol.* **63**, 527–544.

Meldrum, B.S., Anlezark, G.M., Adam, H.K. & Greenwood, D.T. (1982): Anticonvulsant and proconvulsant properties of viloxazine hydrochloride: pharmacological and pharmacokinetic studies in rodents and the epileptic baboon. *Psychopharmacology* **76**, 212–217.

Meritt, H.H. & Putnam, T.J. (1938): A new series of anticonvulsant drugs tested by experiments on animals. *Arch. Neurol. Psychiatry* **39**, 1003–1015.

Meyerhoff, J.L., Carter, R.E., Yourick, D.L., Slusher, B.S. & Coyle, J.T. (1992a): Activity of a NAAG-hydrolyzing enzyme in brain may affect seizure susceptibility in genetically epilepsy-prone rats. *Mol. Neurobiol. Epilepsy (Epilepsy Research Supp. 9)* 163–172.

Meyerhoff, J.L., Carter, R.E., Yourick, D.L., Slusher, B.S. & Coyle, J.T. (1992b): Genetically epilepsy-prone rats have increased brain regional activity of an enzyme which liberates glutamate from N-acetyl-aspartyl-glutamate. *Brain Res.* **593**, 140–143.

Millan, M.H., Meldrum, B.S., Boersma, C.A. & Faingold, C.L. (1988): Excitant amino acids and audiogenic seizures in the genetically epilepsy-prone rat. II. Efferent seizure propagating pathway. *Exp. Neurol.* **99**, 687–698.

Millan, M.H., Wardley Smith, B., Durmuller, N. & Meldrum, B.S. (1991): The high pressure neurological syndrome in genetically epilepsy prone rats: protective effect of 2-amino-7-phosphono heptanoate. *Exp. Neurol.* **112**, 317–320.

Millichap, J.G. (1965): Anticonvulsant drugs. In: *Physiological pharmacology: a comprehensive treatise*, eds. W.S. Root & F.G. Hofmann, pp. 97–173. New York: Academic Press.

Mishra, P.K., Dailey, J.W., Reigel, C.E. & Jobe, P.C. (1988a): Brain norepinephrine and convulsions in the genetically epilepsy-prone rat: sex-dependent responses to Ro 4-1284 treatment. *Life Sci.* **42**, 1131–1137.

Mishra, P.K., Dailey, J.W., Reigel, C.E., Tomsic, M.L. & Jobe, P.C. (1988b): Sex-specific distinctions in audiogenic convulsions exhibited by severe seizure genetically epilepsy-prone rats (GEPR-9s). *Epilepsy Res.* **2**, 309–316.

Mishra, P.K., Dailey, J.W., Reigel, C.E. & Jobe, P.C. (1989): Audiogenic convulsions in moderate seizure genetically epilepsy-prone rats (GEPR-3s). *Epilepsy Res.* **3**, 191–198.

Mishra, P.K., Dailey, J.W., Wang, C., Browning, R.A. & Jobe, P.C. (1990): Effects of 6-hydroxydopamine injected into the locus ceruleus on indices of forebrain and brain-stem seizures in genetically epilepsy-prone rats. *Epilepsia* **31**, 633–634 (Abstract).

Mishra, P.K., Bettendorf, A.F., Burger, R.L., Dailey, J.W., Eldadah, M.K., Wang, C., Browning, R.A. & Jobe, P.C. (1991): Noradrenergic regulation of forebrain and brain-stem seizures in non-epileptic and genetically epilepsy-prone rats (GEPRs). *Soc. Neurosci. Abstr.* **17**, 172 (Abstract).

Mishra, P.K., Dailey, J.W. & Jobe, P.C. (1993a): Selective inbreeding for seizure traits has further refined convulsive characteristics of the two genetically epilepsy-prone rat strains. *Soc. Neurosci. Abstr.* **19**, (Abstract).

Mishra, P.K., Kahle, E.H., Bettendorf, A.F., Dailey, J.W. & Jobe, P.C. (1993b): Anticonvulsant effects of intracerebroventricularly administered norepinephrine are potentiated in the presence of monoamine oxidase inhibition in severe seizure genetically epilepsy-prone rats (GEPR-9s). *Life Sci.* **52**, 1435–1441.

Mishra, P.K., Burger, R.L., Bettendorf, A.F., Browning, R.A. & Jobe, P.C. (1994): Role of norepinephrine in forebrain and brain-stem seizures: chemical lesioning of locus ceruleus with DSP4.. *Exp. Neurol.* in press.

Naritoku, D.K., Mecozzi, L.B., Aiello, M.T. & Faingold, C.L. (1992): Repetition of audiogenic seizures in genetically epilepsy-prone rats induces cortical epileptiform activity and additional seizure behaviors. *Exp. Neurol.* **115**, 317–324.

Nierenberg, A.A. & Cole, J.O. (1991): Antidepressant adverse drug reactions. *J. Clin. Psychiatry* **52**, 40–47.

Ojemann, L.M., Friel, P.N., Trejo, W.J. & Dudley, D.L. (1983): Effect of doxepin on seizure frequency in depressed epileptic patients. *Neurology* **33**, 646–648.

Piette, Y., Delaunois, A.L., De Shaepdryver, A.F. & Heymans, C. (1963): Imipramine and electroshock threshold. *Arch. Int. Pharmacodyn. Ther.* **144**, 293–297.

Pineda, M.R. & Russell, S.C. (1974): The use of a tricyclic antidepressant in epilepsy. *Dis. Nerv. Syst.* **35**, 322–323.

Plotnikoff, N. (1963): A neuropharmacological study of escape from audiogenic seizures. In: *Psychophysiologie, Neuropharmacologie et Biochimie de la Crise Audiogene, Colloques Internationaux du Centre National de la Recherche Scientifique*, ed. Anonymous, pp. 429–443. Paris: CNRS.

Polc, P., Schneeberger, J. & Haefely, W. (1979): Effects of several centrally active drugs on the sleep-wakefulness cycle of cats. *Neuropharmacology* **18**, 259–267.

Preskorn, S.H. & Fast, G.A. (1992): Tricyclic antidepressant-induced seizures and plasma drug concentration. *J. Clin. Psychiatry* **53**, 160–162.

Raines, A., Helke, C.J., Iadarola, M.J., Britton, L.W. & Anderson, R.J. (1976): Blockade of the tonic hindlimb extensor component of maximal electroshock and pentylenetetrazol-induced seizures by drugs acting on muscle and muscle spindle systems: a perspective on method. *Epilepsia* **17**, 395–402.

Razani Boroujerdi, S., Tso Olivas, D.Y., Hoffman, T.J., Weiss, G.K. & Savage, D.D. (1993): Decrease in locus coeruleus ^{3}H-β-idazoxan binding site density in genetically epilepsy-prone (GEPR) rats. *Brain Res.* **600**, 181–186.

Reigel, C.E., Jobe, P.C., Woods, T.W. & Dailey, J.W. (1984): A GABA-ergic convulsant profile in the genetically epilepsy-prone rat. *Soc. Neurosci. Abstr.* **10**, 408 (Abstract).

Reigel, C.E., Dailey, J.W. & Jobe, P.C. (1986): The genetically epilepsy-prone rat: an overview of seizure-prone characteristics and responsiveness to anticonvulsant drugs. *Life Sci.* **39**, 763–774.

Reigel, C.E., Jobe, P.C., Dailey, J.W. & Stewart, J.J. (1988): Responsiveness of genetically epilepsy-prone rats to intracerebroventricular morphine-induced convulsions. *Life Sci.* **42**, 1743–1749.

Reigel, C.E., Jobe, P.C., Dailey, J.W. & Savage, D.D. (1989): Ontogeny of sound-induced seizures in the genetically epilepsy-prone rat. *Epilepsy Res.* **4**, 63–71.

Ribak, C.E., Byun, M.Y., Ruiz, G.T. & Reiffenstein, R.J. (1988a): Increased levels of amino acid neurotransmitters in the inferior colliculus of the genetically epilepsy-prone rat. *Epilepsy Res.* **2**, 9–13.

Ribak, C.E., Roberts, R.C., Byun, M.Y. & Kim, H.L. (1988b): Anatomical and behavioral analyses of the inheritance of audiogenic seizures in the progeny of genetically epilepsy-prone and Sprague–Dawley rats (a published erratum appears in *Epilepsy Res.* 1989 **3**, 262.) *Epilepsy Res.* **2**, 345–355.

Ribak, C.E., Ghaderi, L. & Byun, M.Y. (1989): Seizure severity correlates with an increase in the number of small GABAergic neurons in the moderate seizure line of genetically epilepsy-prone rat. *Epilepsia* **30**, 698.

Ribak, C.E., Lauterborn, J.C., Navetta, M.S. & Gall, C.M. (1993): The inferior colliculus of GEPRs contains greater numbers of cells that express glutamate decarboxylase (GAD67) mRNA. *Epilepsy Res.* **14**, 105–113.

Rickels, K. & Schweizer, E. (1990): Clinical overview of serotonin reuptake inhibitors. *J. Clin. Psychiatry* **51**, 9–12.

Roberts, R.C., Kim, H.L. & Ribak, C.E. (1985): Increased numbers of neurons occur in the inferior colliculus of the young genetically epilepsy-prone rat. *Brain Res.* **355**, 277–281.

Roberts, R.C. & Ribak, C.E. (1986): Anatomical changes of the GABAergic system in the inferior colliculus of the genetically epilepsy-prone rat. *Life Sci.* **39**, 789–798.

Roberts, R.C. & Ribak, C.E. (1988): The ultrastructure of the central nucleus of the inferior colliculus of the genetically epilepsy-prone rat. *Epilepsy Res.* **2**, 196–214.

Savage, D.D., Reigel, C.E. & Jobe, P.C. (1986): Angular bundle kindling is accelerated in rats with a genetic predisposition to acoustic stimulus-induced seizures. *Brain Res.* **376**, 412–415.

Savage, D.D., Mills, S.A., Jobe, P.C. & Reigel, C.E. (1988): Elevation of naloxone-sensitive ^{3}H-dihydromorphine binding in hippocampal formation of genetically epilepsy-prone rats. *Life Sci.* **43**, 239–246.

Skowron, D.M. and Stimmel, G.L. (1992): Antidepressants and the risk of seizures. *Pharmacotherapy* **12**, 18–22.

Stille, G. & Sayers, A. (1964): The effect of antidepresssant drugs on the convulsive excitability of brain structures. *Int. J. Neuropharmacol.* **3**, 605–609.

Thompson, J.L., Carl, F.G. & Holmes, G.L. (1991): Effect of age on seizure susceptibility in genetically epilepsy-prone rats (GEPR-9s). *Epilepsia* **32**, 161–167.

Trimble, M. (1978): Non-monoamine oxidase inhibitor antidepressants and epilepsy: a review. *Epilepsia* **19**, 241–250.

Trimble, M.R. (1980a): New antidepressant drugs and the seizure threshold. *Neuropharmacology* **19**, 1227–1228.

Trimble, M.R. (1980b): Antidepressant drugs and convulsions. *Lancet* **1**, 307.

Trimble, M.R. (1984): Epilepsy, antidepressants, and the role of nomifensine. *J. Clin. Psychiatry* **45**, 39–42.

Vernier, V.G. (1961): The pharmacology of antidepressant agents. *Dis. Nerv. Syst.* **22**, 7–13.

Wang, C., Mishra, P.K., Yan, Q., Dailey, J.W., Browning, R.A. & Jobe, P.C. (1993): Electrographic activity in the inferior colliculus or medullary reticular formation during audiogenic seizures in severe seizure genetically epilepsy-prone rats (GEPR-9s). *Soc. Neurosci. Abstr.* **19**, 602 (Abstract).

Yan, Q., Mishra, P.K., Burger, R.L., Bettendorf, A.F., Jobe, P.C. & Dailey, J.W. (1992): Evidence that carbamazepine and antiepilepsirine may produce a component of their anticonvulsant effects by activating serotonergic neurons in genetically epilepsy-prone rats. *J. Pharmacol. Exp. Ther.* **261**, 652–659.

Yan, Q., Jobe, P.C. & Dailey, J.W. (1993a): Thalamic deficiency in norepinephrine release detected via intracerebral microdialysis: a synaptic determinant of seizure predisposition in the genetically epilepsy-prone rat. *Epilepsy Res.* **14**, 229–236.

Yan, Q., Jobe, P.C. & Dailey, J.W. (1993b): Noradrenergic mechanisms for the anticonvulsant effects of desipramine and yohimbine in genetically epilepsy-prone rats: studies with microdialysis. *Brain Res.* **610**, 24–31.

Yan, Q., Jobe, P.C. & Dailey, J.W. (1994): Evidence that serotonergic mechanism is involved in the anticonvulsant effect of fluoxetine in genetically epilepsy-prone rats. *Eur. J. Pharmacol.* **252**, 105–112.

Yanagita, T., Wakasa, Y. & Kiyohara, H. (1980): Drug-dependence potential of viloxazine hydrochloride tested in rhesus monkeys. *Pharmacol. Biochem. Behav.* **12**, 155–161.

Yourick, D.L., LaPlaca, M.C. & Meyerhoff, J.L. (1991): Norepinephrine-stimulated phosphatidylinositol metabolism in genetically epilepsy-prone and kindled rats. *Brain Res.* **551**, 315–318.

Chapter 33

Anatomy of generalized convulsive seizures

Ronald A. Browning

Departments of Physiology and Pharmacology, Southern Illinois University School of Medicine, Carbondale, Illinois 62901, USA

Historical aspects

The concept that the motor concomitants of seizures (i.e. convulsions) are a consequence of and are directly correlated with paroxysmal discharge in a discrete region of the brain was first advanced by J.H. Jackson (see Meldrum, 1988). Today the correlation between localized cerebral epileptiform discharge and specific clinical signs is well established for cortical focal and other partial seizures. However, the correlation between motor events during generalized seizures and paroxysmal activity in discrete circuits is less well accepted. Nevertheless, the view that the motor concomitants of generalized seizures have distinct neural substrates has a long history. According to Gastaut & Fischer-Williams (1959) the hypothesis that tonic and clonic convulsions have different sites of origin was essentially elevated into law by Bechterew in 1897. However, this view was strongly challenged by Horsley and others who believed that tonic and clonic seizures could be produced by stimulating any motor centre (Gastaut & Fischer-Williams, 1959). Examination of the literature reveals that several investigators in the early to mid-twentieth century used surgical manipulations (e.g. transections or lesions) to determine the origin of clonic and tonic convulsions in animals undergoing pentylenetetrazol-induced seizures. However, these investigators failed to distinguish between the different types of clonus and often concluded that brain-stem transections failed to alter the seizure (Asuad, 1940; Gutiérrez-Noriega, 1944; Schoen, 1926). Other investigators examined the effect of brain-stem transections on tonic convulsions produced by maximal electroshock and found that tonic seizures still occur after transections at the ponto-medullary border indicating that tonic seizures can originate in the brain-stem (Tanaka & Mishima, 1953). Studies carried out since then have provided more direct evidence for the hypothesis that tonic and some types of clonic seizures have separate anatomical substrates and these are considered in some detail in the subsequent sections.

The concept of forebrain and brain-stem separation of seizure substrates (networks)

Having worked with several different seizure models in the 1980s our laboratory became intrigued with the observation that convulsive behaviour (i.e. motor seizures) in rodents consisted of three predominant motor patterns: (1) facial and forelimb (F&F) clonus with or without rearing similar

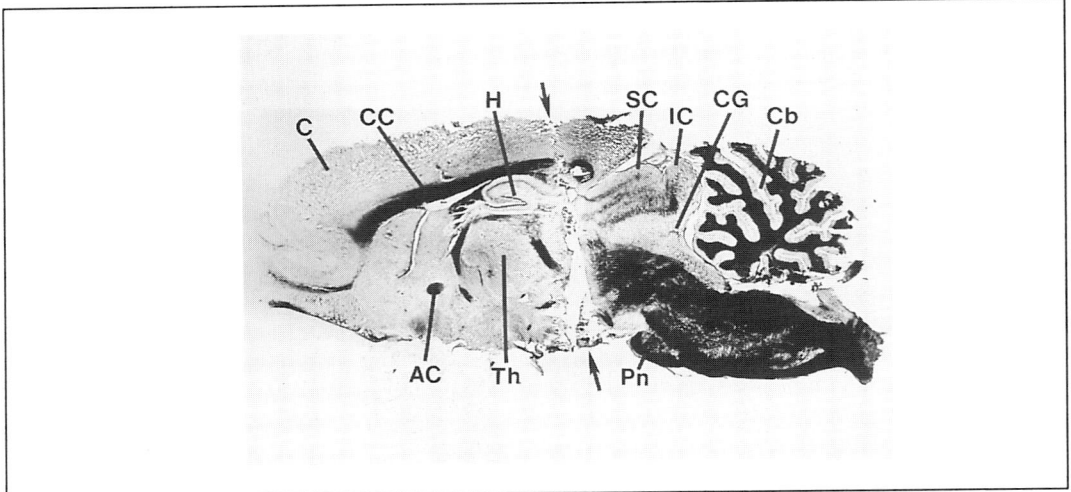

Fig. 1. Sagittal section of rat brain transected at the precollicular level. The transection separated the diencephalon from the mesencephalon, sparing the colliculi and most of the midbrain. Some damage to the ventral aspects of the rostral mesencephalon occurred. Arrows indicate the plane of transection. AC=anterior commissure; C = cortex; Cb = cerebellum; CC = corpus callosum; CG = central grey; H = hippocampus; IC = inferior colliculus; Pn = pontine nuclei; SC = superior colliculus, Th = thalamus. Reproduced from Browning & Nelson (1986).

to the pattern described by the Racine (1972) kindling scale, (2) running followed by clonus in all four limbs (sometimes involving bouncing or jumping), which we described as running–bouncing (R/B) clonus, and (3) tonic convulsions characterized by tonic forelimb extension (forelimbs extended caudally and pressed down against the chest), with or without hindlimb extension (hindlimbs extended caudally), as seen in maximal electroshock seizures. Behaviours (2) and (3) are also seen in genetically epilepsy-prone rats (GEPRs) undergoing audiogenic seizures and can be quantified by the behavioural rating scale of Jobe et al. (1973a). Some convulsive stimuli can elicit one of these behaviours independently of the others, while other stimuli (e.g. i.v. infusion of chemoconvulsant drugs) cause a sequential progression from facial and forelimb clonus to tonic convulsions. In general, it has long been known that low doses of chemoconvulsant drugs such as pentylenetetrazol (PTZ) and low currents of electroshock produce facial and forelimb clonus, while high doses of chemoconvulsants and high-intensity electrical stimulation produce tonic convulsions. Thus, past dogma held that these behaviours represent a continuum of increasing seizure severity (Woodbury & Esplin, 1959; Piredda et al., 1985). Implicit in this notion was the concept that the progression from facial and forelimb clonus to tonus involved the recruitment of larger and larger numbers of neurons into a common paroxysmal discharge until the whole brain is involved, resulting in tonic convulsions.

About 12 years ago my laboratory began to make observations which suggested the above concept was not entirely correct. These findings suggested that specific motor components of a generalized seizure may have distinct anatomical substrates. A key observation that provided support for this concept was made while comparing two forms of electroshock seizures. Surprisingly, we found that the site of stimulation rather than the intensity of the stimulus determined the type of convulsion observed. For example, it was found that stimulation of rats through transcorneal electrodes resulted in facial and forelimb clonus with rearing at current intensities just exceeding threshold (Table 1). However, when transauricular electrodes were used to deliver the electroshock, the first response observed (when threshold was reached) was running–bouncing (R/B) clonus and further increases in current intensity resulted in a tonic convulsion (Table 1). Indeed, facial and forelimb clonus could

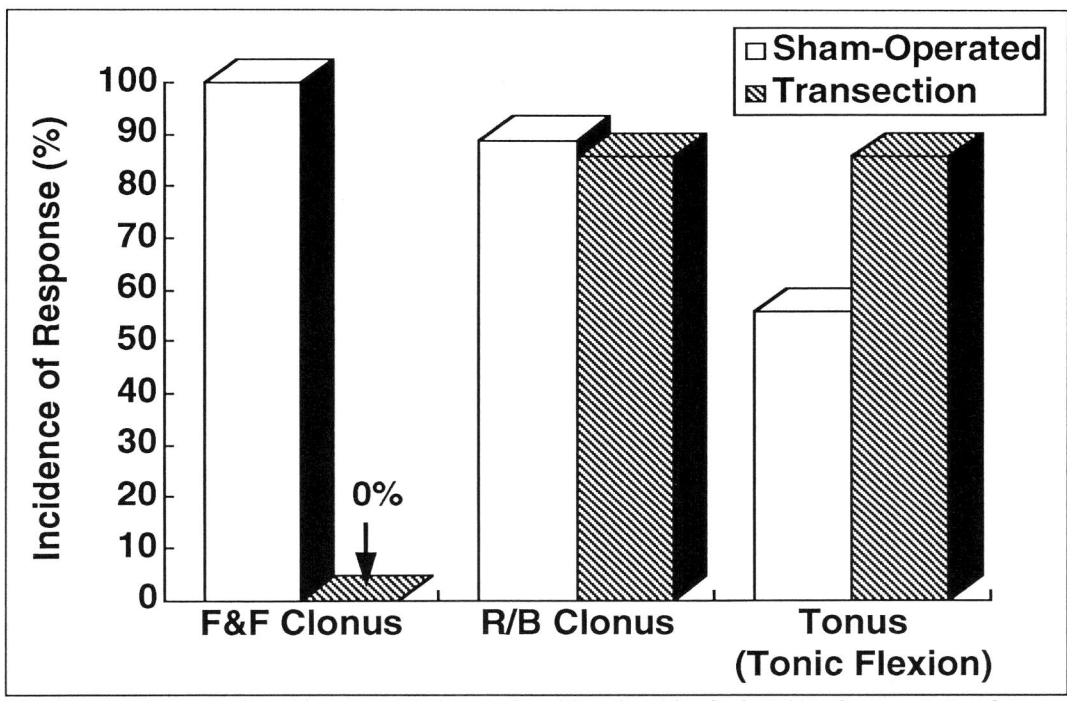

Fig. 2. The incidence of pentylenetetrazol (PTZ)-induced facial and forelimb (F&F) clonus, running–bouncing (R/B) clonus, and tonus following a precollicular transection or sham-surgery is shown. Rats received PTZ (50 mg/kg, i.p.) 3 h after the transection. There were seven to nine rats per group. Note that transected rats failed to display F&F clonus. Reproduced from Browning & Nelson (1986).

not be produced using transauricular electrodes irrespective of the current intensity. Our interpretation of this unexpected finding was that after transcorneal stimulation the highest density of current passed through the forebrain, while the predominant path of current spread after transauricular stimulation was through the brain-stem (Browning & Nelson, 1985). These observations led to the following hypothesis: there are two separate anatomical systems in the brain that are responsible for the expression of generalized convulsions: (1) a system in the forebrain responsible for the expression of facial and forelimb clonus which is observed with kindled seizures and low current corneal electroshock; and (2) a system in the brain-stem responsible for the expression of running–bouncing clonus and tonic convulsions, which are observed in audiogenic and maximal electroshock seizures.

Table 1. Influence of electrode placement on electroshock-induced clonus

Stimulation	n	Incidence of clonus		Threshold
		F&F	R/B	mA
Transcorneal	9	100%	0%	20.06 ± 0.6
Transauricular	10	0%	100%	25.40 ± 0.4*

*$P < 0.01$ compared to transcorneal stimulation using t-test. F&F = facial and forelimb clonus; R/B = running–bouncing clonus. Data taken from Browning & Nelson (1985).

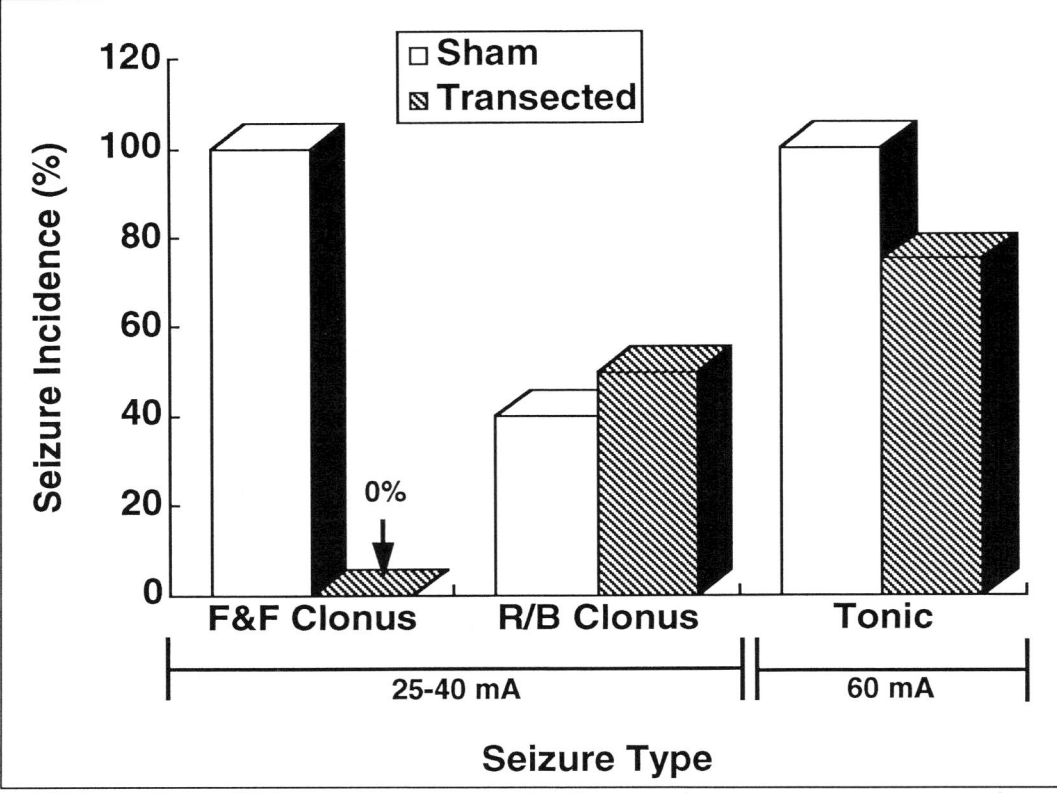

Fig. 3. The incidence of transcorneal electroshock-induced facial and forelimb (F&F) clonus, running-bouncing (R/B) clonus, and tonus following a precollicular transection or sham-surgery. Note the absence of F&F clonus in transected rats. Data summarized from Browning & Nelson (1986).

Testing of the hypothesis

The hypothesis that there are separate anatomical substrates (circuits, networks) for clonic and tonic generalized convulsions was tested by examining the effect of a precollicular brain transection (separating midbrain from diencephalon) on generalized convulsions produced by pentylenetetrazol or electroshock (Browning & Nelson, 1986). In rats that had received a precollicular transection separating forebrain from brain-stem (Fig. 1) 3 h earlier under ether anaesthesia, pentylenetetrazol (50 mg/kg, i.p.) produced running–bouncing clonus which progressed to tonic forelimb extension; but facial and forelimb clonus, which occurred in rats with sham-transections, was never observed in the transected animals (Fig. 2). Similarly, when rats were transected and subjected to transcorneal electroshock using currents ranging from threshold to suprathreshold (25–60 mA) the responses consisted of running–bouncing clonus and tonic convulsions, while facial and forelimb clonus was never observed (Fig. 3). However, all sham-transected rats displayed facial and forelimb clonus at low intensity and tonic convulsions at high-intensity electroshock stimulation (Fig. 3).

As indicated above, genetically epilepsy-prone rats (GEPRs) display R/B clonus or tonus in response to sound stimulation depending on the substrain (GEPR-3s or GEPR-9s) involved as described in Ch. 32 by Jobe. According to the above hypothesis these behaviours are manifestations of brain-stem driven convulsions and a precollicular transection should not alter the response of GEPRs to sound stimulation. Recent studies (Browning et al., 1991) showed that the majority of

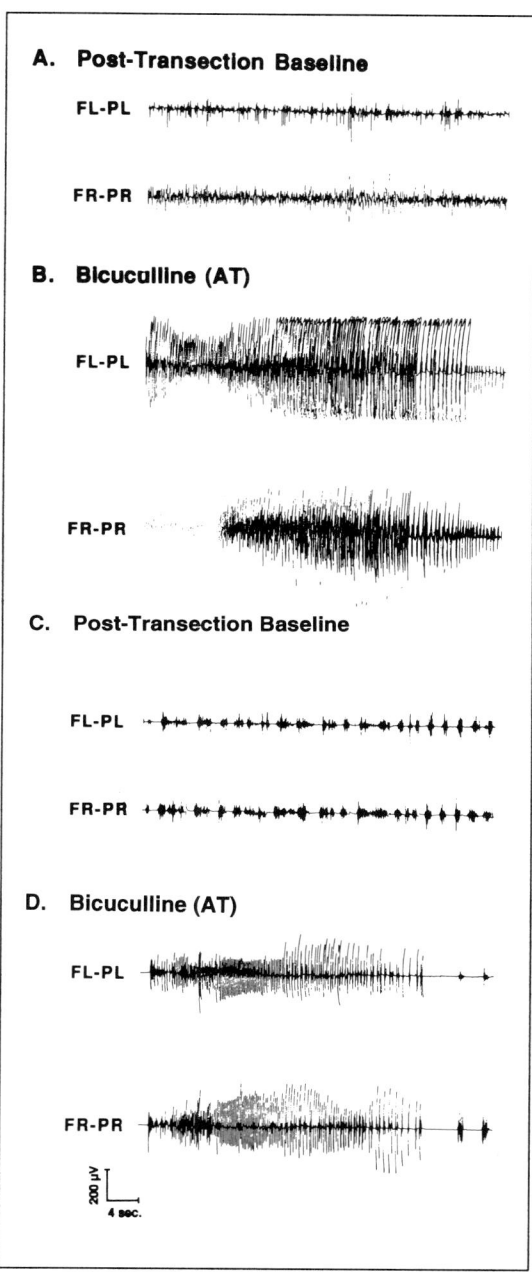

Fig. 4. Effect of midcollicular and precollicular transection on seizures initiated from area tempestas (deep prepiriform cortex). A: Baseline EEG in a rat 3 h after a midcollicular transection. B: EEG record after bicuculline (118 pmol) infusion into area tempestas (AT) of same rat shown in A. C: Baseline EEG in a rat after a precollicular transection. D: EEG record after bicuculline (118 pmol) infusion into AT of same rat shown in C. FL–PL = frontal left–parietal left; FR–PR = frontal right–parietal right.
Reproduced from Browning et al. (1993).

GEPR-9s display a tonic convulsion in response to sound stimulation following a precollicular transection, but only a minority of the GEPR-3s (which display running–bouncing clonus in response to sound) are susceptible to sound-induced seizures after this transection. However, all GEPRs with a precollicular transection displayed a seizure in response to the sound if they were pretreated with a subconvulsant dose of pentylenetetrazol 5 min before sound stimulation (Browning et al., 1991). These findings indicate that the brain-stem contains all the circuitry necessary to sustain an audiogenic seizure but that the transection somehow elevates the threshold for such a seizure. The mechanism by which the transection elevates the audiogenic seizure threshold is currently unknown.

In more recent studies it has been found that forebrain-evoked seizures can occur in the absence of connections with the brain-stem (Browning et al., 1993). In these studies forebrain seizures were evoked by microinfusion of bicuculline (118 pmoles) into the deep prepiriform cortex (area tempestas) and seizures were monitored electrographically using epidural EEG recording electrodes after a brain-stem transection separating forebrain from brain-stem. As can be seen in Fig. 4, bilateral forebrain electrographic seizures occurred in the complete absence of connections between forebrain and brain-stem showing that the brain-stem is not required for forebrain evoked seizures.

Other lines of evidence provide further support for the separation of forebrain and brain-stem seizure networks. Autoradiograpic metabolic mapping studies using ^{14}C-2-deoxyglucose (2DG) in rats showed activation of limbic forebrain structures in animals displaying facial and forelimb clonic status epilepticus with no activation of brain-stem structures except for the substantia nigra (Lothman & Collins, 1981; Handforth & Ackerman, 1988a; McIntyre et al., 1991). Moreover, mapping the expression of immediate early genes (IEG), such as c-fos (a putative index of neuronal excitation) during F&F clonic seizures has revealed a similar pattern of limbic system activation (Popovici et al., 1990; Maggio et al., 1993), with essentially no brain-stem involvement. However, brain-stem-evoked seizures produced by chemical stimulation of the inferior colliculus was associated with little or no expression of c-fos in the limbic system (Maggio et al., 1993). In agreement, the inferior colliculus and other brain-stem auditory structures showed an increase in c-fos-like immunoreactivity, while limbic structures showed little change in fos immunoreactivity following audiogenic seizures in DBA/2 mice (Le Gal La Salle & Naquet, 1990).

Forebrain structures responsible for facial and forelimb clonus

Despite the fact that electrophysiological recording may provide a more sensitive technique (Lothman & Collins, 1981), the most complete picture concerning the anatomical structures involved in generalized limbic (forebrain) seizures has been obtained by mapping 2DG uptake and/or IEG expression (see above). However, limitations associated with 2DG autoradiographic mapping such as the period required for radionuclide equilibration between blood and brain and the requirement for sustained seizure activity has restricted observations to models that display prolonged seizures. For this reason several investigators have examined 2DG uptake in rats undergoing status epilepticus induced by prolonged electrical stimulation of limbic nuclei or olfactory cortex (Lothman & Collins, 1981; Handforth & Ackerman, 1988a; McIntyre et al., 1991). These studies have revealed at least three behavioural states of status epilepticus, each of which is associated with a distinct anatomical map of ^{14}C-2DG uptake. In viewing these findings, one is struck by the remarkable agreement among different labs (irrespective of the technique employed) showing widespread involvement of the limbic and olfactory systems in animals undergoing generalized facial and forelimb clonus. These types of convulsions have, therefore, become known as limbic motor seizures (Lothman & Collins, 1981; Turski et al., 1984; Handforth & Ackerman, 1988b; Patel, 1988; Gale, 1992).

It appears that in all models of limbic motor seizures the paroxysmal discharge quickly spreads from a site of origin within limbic or olfactory areas to other limbic structures which eventually include

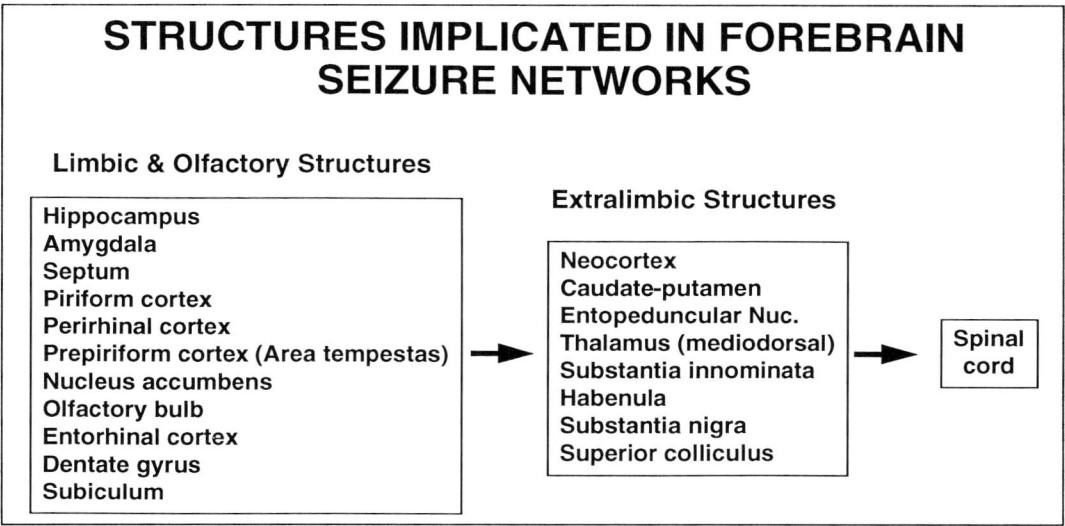

Fig. 5. *Proposed sequence for the involvement of brain structures in the seizure discharge leading to limbic motor seizures (based on assessment of the literature).*

the amygdala, hippocampal formation, subiculum, septum, entorhinal cortex, piriform cortex, perirhinal cortex, insular cortex, and olfactory bulbs (Lothman & Collins, 1981; Collins et al., 1983; Handforth & Ackerman, 1988a; McIntyre et al., 1991; Gale, 1992). However, the onset of the clonic motor convulsion (facial and forelimb clonus) is accompanied by the activation of additional structures outside the limbic–olfactory system, such as the neocortex, thalamus, and basal ganglia (Handforth & Ackerman, 1988b). Except for the substantia nigra, limbic motor seizures do not appear to increase 2DG uptake in the brain-stem (Handforth & Ackerman, 1988b).

Recent work by White & Price (1993a) has extended the metabolic mapping studies by comparing 2-DG activation with *c*-fos immunoreactivity in rats undergoing different stages of limbic status epilepticus. These investigators were able to correlate EEG, *c*-fos and 2DG mapping with the behavioural concomitants of the seizure. Such studies suggest that the amygdalohippocampal area and the basal nucleus of the amygdala serve as the foci for the various types of limbic status. Moreover, with the exception of three areas (parataenial and mediodorsal nuclei of thalamus and the substantia nigra) there was remarkable agreement between the 2DG and *c*-fos mapping techniques (White & Price, 1993a). The importance of the basal amygdaloid nucleus in generalized limbic status epilepticus was confirmed by showing that inactivation of this area by lidocaine prevented the behavioural, electrographic and metabolic concomitants of the seizure (White & Price, 1993b)

Because of the extensive interconnectivity and redundancy of pathways among limbic and olfactory structures in the forebrain and the nature of 2DG metabolic mapping, it is difficult to identify sequential pathways of seizure propagation. Nevertheless, several authors have proposed pathways of seizure spread during limbic motor seizures. The major differences among them appear to be due to the different sites of initiation prior to generalization. A general scheme for the sequential involvement of specific structures in forebrain seizures is depicted in Fig. 5. A more detailed discussion of the various forebrain seizure networks involved in limbic motor seizures can be found in several reviews (Handforth & Ackerman, 1988b; Patel, 1988; Faingold & Riaz, 1992; Gale, 1992).

Although it is beyond the scope of this review, it should be pointed out that an additional seizure network has been identified in the forebrain. The latter network appears to be responsible for *non-convulsive seizures* (i.e. absence seizures) and has been shown to involve a thalamocortical circuitry (Avoli, 1988; Avanzini *et al.*, 1992; Marescaux *et al.*, 1992; Vergnes & Marescaux, 1992). Other chapters in this book describe the neuronal networks of absence seizures.

Brain-stem structures responsible for R/B clonic and tonic convulsions

Our knowledge of the structures involved in brain-stem mediated convulsions, albeit incomplete, comes from studies that have employed electrical stimulation, lesions or microinjections of drugs. Such studies have led to the identification of several brain-stem structures that appear to play an important role in regulation of brain-stem-driven convulsions. These include the areas of the brain-stem reticular core (such as the nucleus reticularis pontis oralis (RPO) and reticularis pontis caudalis (RPC), the superior cerebellar peduncle (cerebellum), the substantia nigra, the superior colliculus and the inferior colliculus).

Areas of the reticular core

Electrical stimulation of widespread areas of the brain-stem reticular core from the medulla to the midbrain of cats and rats was found to produce convulsive attacks which were described as tonic in nature (Kreindler *et al.*, 1958). Subsequent studies by other laboratories (Bergmann *et al.*, 1963; Burnham *et al.*, 1981) confirmed and extended these findings. Considering that such attacks could be evoked after precollicular transections separating forebrain from brain-stem, these studies provided some of the first evidence for independent brain-stem seizures (Kreindler *et al.*, 1958; Bergmann *et al.*, 1963). An examination of the different sites from which brain-stem seizures could be triggered suggested that the midbrain reticular formation (MRF) has the lowest threshold, but showed that these seizures can be evoked independently from every level of the reticular core (Burnham, 1987). Indeed, a comparison of stimulation parameters, anatomical sites of stimulation, and convulsive behaviours used by different labs to produce electrically evoked brain-stem seizures can be found in an excellent review by Burnham (1987).

Large bilateral mechanical lesions of the pontine reticular formation in the areas stimulated by Kreindler *et al.* (1958) were found to attenuate the tonic components of seizures induced by maximal electroshock (MES), maximal pentylenetetrazol (PTZ) and audiogenic stimulation while having no effect on facial and forelimb clonus induced by minimal electroshock (corneal stimulation), pentylenetetrazol, flurothyl (Browning *et al.*, 1981b, 1985) or amygdala kindling (Applegate *et al.*, 1991). Further attempts to identify the sites responsible for the lesion-induced attenuation of tonic seizures showed that damage to the reticularis pontis oralis and reticularis pontis caudalis nuclei of the pons could produce these effects (Browning, 1981a; Browning *et al.*, 1985). However, damage to the midbrain reticular formation failed to have an effect despite the fact that this area had the lowest threshold for electrically-evoked brain-stem seizures (Burnham, 1987).

Further evidence for involvement of the pontine reticular formation in brain-stem seizures was provided by studies showing that microinjections of the excitant amino acid antagonist, 2-amino-phosphonoheptanoate (2-APH), into the RPC inhibits sound-induced tonic and running–bouncing clonic convulsions in GEPRs (Millan *et al.*, 1988)

Cerebellum

Bilateral lesions of the superior cerebellar peduncles, a major efferent pathway of the cerebellum, were found to inhibit electroshock-induced tonic convulsions (Browning *et al.*, 1981a). Such findings are in agreement with studies showing that cerebellectomy markedly attenuates tonic extensor convulsions induced by maximal electroshock (Raines & Anderson, 1976). However, it appears that lesions of the cerebellum facilitate neocortical focal epileptiform discharge (Dow, 1965; Dow *et al.*, 1962). Moreover, cerebellectomized cats were shown to display an exacerbation of clonic seizures kindled from the amygdala (Paz *et al.*, 1985). Recently, Miller *et al.* (1993) have found that microinjection of GABA agonists into the fastigial nucleus of the cerebellum inhibits seizures induced by systemic administration of bicuculline. Thus, the cerebellum has been shown to regulate seizures in several animal models. While there is evidence that reducing cerebellar efferent activity inhibits tonic seizures and facilitates forebrain (clonic) seizures, more work is needed before a full understanding of the role of the cerebellum in seizures can be realized.

Inferior colliculus (IC)

Electrical or chemical stimulation of the IC has been shown to produce running and running–bouncing clonic convulsions in rats (McCown et al., 1984, 1991; Bagri et al., 1992). Moreover, infusion of NMDA (10 nmoles/side) into the inferior colliculus renders normal rats susceptible to audiogenic seizures which consist of running–bouncing clonic convulsions. Considerable evidence now supports the concept that audiogenic seizures are initiated from the inferior colliculus (Faingold & Naritoku, 1992). However, the inferior colliculus does not appear to be necessary for tonic convulsions induced by maximal electroshock in normal rats (R.A. Browning, unpublished observation). Such findings show that the inferior colliculus is not a crucial part of the MES brain-stem seizure network.

Substantia nigra

A substantial body of evidence indicates that the efferent activity of the neurons in the pars reticulata of the substantia nigra exert control over both forebrain and brain-stem driven generalized seizures. Treatments that inhibit nigral efferent activity (such as microinjections of $GABA_A$ agonists or nigral lesions) consistently exert antiepileptic effects (Gale, 1985; Gale & Browning, 1988). These studies have suggested that inhibition of nigral output elevates seizure threshold and suppresses both motor and electrographic seizures (McNamara et al., 1983; Garant & Gale, 1986). The substantia nigra has been shown to regulate seizures in essentially all forebrain (limbic motor and absence) seizure models examined (DePaulis, Ch. 42). However, the only type of brain-stem seizure that has been consistently shown to be suppressed by inhibiting nigral efferent activity is the maximal electroshock-induced seizure. Indeed, the role of the substantia nigra in audiogenic seizures remains equivocal (DePaulis, Ch. 42). Gale (1990, 1993) has concluded that the substantia nigra is neither a site of seizure initiation nor of propagation since its integrity is not required for seizures to occur. Rather, the substantia nigra appears to be one of the remote endogenous systems that is capable of providing control over generalized seizures (see below), an effect that appears to be mediated through disinhibition of neurons in the superior colliculus. The reader is referred Ch. 42 by Depaulis for a detailed discussion of this system.

Superior colliculus

The superior colliculus receives efferent projections from the substantia nigra (pars reticulata), and is believed to be part of the nigral system involved in the control of seizures (see Depaulis et al., 1994; Depaulis, Ch. 42). Lesions of the superior colliculus have been shown to prevent the anticonvulsant effects of GABAergic agonists microinjected into the substantia nigra (Garant & Gale, 1987). Similarly, disinhibition at the level of the superior colliculus (e.g. microinfusion of bicuculline) has been shown to suppress forebrain (Gale, 1993) as well as MES-induced seizures (Garant & Gale, 1987; Dean & Gale, 1989; Redgrave et al., 1991a,b). While the superior colliculus appears to be part of the remote nigral control system as indicated by Depaulis (Ch. 42), it may be an integral part of the audiogenic seizure network. For example, large bilateral lesions of the superior colliculus were shown to suppress audiogenic seizures in DBA mice (Willot & Lu, 1980) and knife cuts between the inferior and superior colliculus were reported to attenuate audiogenic seizures in a susceptible strain of Wistar rats (Tsutsui et al., 1993). More recent evidence suggests that the superior colliculus is a site where norepinephrine exerts its anticonvulsant effect on audiogenic seizures in the GEPR (Jobe et al., 1992). Whether the latter findings are unique to the audiogenic seizure circuitry or whether the superior colliculus is also an essential component of the brain-stem seizure network remains to be determined.

Pathways of propagation

Although the above-mentioned structures have been implicated in brain-stem-driven convulsions, it is not yet possible to make detailed circuit diagrams of the brain-stem seizure network. In the case of the audiogenic seizure where more information is available and the afferent pathway leading to seizure initiation is known, it is possible to make more accurate predictions about pathways (Faingold et al., 1988; Garcia-Cairasco et al., 1993). There is evidence that the audiogenic seizure is initiated in the inferior colliculus and then propagates to brain-stem reticular formation either directly or via the superior colliculus (Faingold & Naritoku, 1992). Considerable evidence now suggests that the audiogenic seizure is actually initiated in the dorsal cortex or external nuclei of the inferior colliculus rather than the central nucleus. The central nucleus is, however, essential for relaying the auditory stimulus to the dorsal cortex (see Garcia-Cairasco et al., 1993, for review). An hypothesized pathway for the initiation and propagation of the audiogenic seizures has been provided by Faingold & Naritoku (1992).

Remote systems that exert regulatory control over forebrain and brain-stem seizures networks

It now appears that there are a number of endogenous systems (that are not themselves part of the seizure-propagating network) which exert control over the forebrain and brain-stem seizure networks. The most widely studied of these systems is the substantia nigra and its connections with the striatum and the tectum. The role of this system in various types of experimental seizures has been extensively reviewed by Depaulis (Ch. 42; and Depaulis et al., 1994) and the reader is referred to these accounts for more detail.

There are a variety of neurotransmitter systems whose cell bodies are located in the brain-stem and whose terminals are located in widespread areas of brain. Many of these, such as the noradrenergic, cholinergic, and serotonergic systems have been shown to influence states of sleep and rhythmic oscillations of the brain (Steriade et al., 1993). These neurotransmitter systems are known to alter seizures in a wide variety of experimental models (Jobe & Laird, 1987). The noradrenergic system has been shown to exert anticonvulsant effects in essentially every experimental seizure model except genetic absence seizures in the tottering mouse (Noebels, 1984; also see Noebels, Ch. 20). Serotonin also appears to exert anticonvulsant activity in both brain-stem (Jobe et al., 1973b; Browning, 1985) and forebrain seizure models (Pasani et al., 1992; Wada et al., 1992). The cholinergic pathways projecting from the laterodorsal tegmental and pedunculopontine tegmental nuclei have been shown to exert important influences on PTZ-induced seizures (see Miller, 1992, for review). At least part of the influence of cholinergic projections on pentylenetetrazol seizures appears to be mediated via cells in the central medial intralaminar nucleus of thalamus which also apparently receive GABAergic innervation (Miller & Ferrendelli, 1990a,b). Some of the remote seizure regulatory systems, such as the noradrenergic pathways, can exert rather powerful influences in that they can determine whether or not a seizure occurs. These systems should be examine in more detail as targets for drugs directed at the control of epilepsy.

Interactions between forebrain and brain-stem seizure networks

From the above discussion, it is clear that the forebrain and brain-stem seizure networks can operate independently of one another. However, it has also become clear that under certain conditions, these networks interact. For example, as can be seen in Table 2, several laboratories have now demonstrated that daily repetition of brain-stem seizures produced by audiogenic stimulation in genetically susceptible rats can trigger a secondary forebrain seizure together with its electrographic and motor concomitants (Marescaux et al., 1987; Hirsch et al., 1993; Naritoku et al., 1992). Moreover, repeated audiogenic-like seizures triggered by electrical stimulation of the cortical nuclei of the IC have been shown to produce myoclonic forebrain-like seizures together with limbic seizure discharge (McCown et al., 1987; Maton et al., 1992; Hirsch et al., 1993). The neuroanatomical pathways through which these interactions occur have not been widely studied but, in the case of the audiogenic seizure, appear to involve the medial geniculate and the amygdala (Naritoku et al., 1989). It should be kept in mind that first trial audiogenic or electrically evoked audiogenic-like seizures do not trigger secondary forebrain seizures and therefore this phenomenon has been referred to as audiogenic kindling of limbic motor seizures (Naritoku et al., 1992; Hirsch et al., 1993).

Table 2. Ability of brain-stem seizures to trigger forebrain seizures

Initiating stimuli	Rat strain	Secondarily triggered forebrain seizure		References
		EEG	Behavioural	
Sound (AGS)				
First trial	Wistar	0	0	Marescaux et al., 1987
	GEPR	0	0	Naritoku et al., 1992
	GEPR-3 pup	ND	+	Reigel et al., 1989
Seizure repetition (kindling)	Wistar	+	+	Marescaux et al., 1987
	GEPR	+	+	Naritoku et al., 1992
IC electrical stimulation				
First trial	Sprague–Dawley	0	0	McCown et al., 1987
Seizure repetition	Sprague–Dawley	+	+	McCown et al., 1987
Dorsal tegmental kindling				
First trial	Wistar	0	0	Maton et al., 1992
Seizure repetition	Wistar	+	+	Maton et al., 1992

AGS = audiogenic seizure; IC = inferior colliculus; ND = not determined; 0 = no response to stimulus; + = seizure occurred in response to stimulus.

Can forebrain seizures trigger secondary brain-stem seizures? This would appear to be the normal progression of seizure development in secondarily generalized tonic–clonic seizures in humans. Yet, the incidence of this in experimental models of limbic motor seizures is remarkably low. This may result because the threshold of the brain-stem is normally much higher than that of the forebrain or that forebrain seizures actually inhibit brain-stem seizure discharge. There is, however, some evidence that repeated forebrain seizures can facilitate brain-stem seizures. For example, amygdala kindling has been shown to increase the incidence of hindlimb extension in male Sprague–Dawley rats undergoing maximal electroshock (Applegate et al., 1991). Moreover, seizures evoked by the systemic administration of kainic acid in GEPR-9s begin as limbic motor convulsions but quickly trigger tonic convulsions with full hindlimb extension typical of a brain-stem seizure (Jobe, personal communication). Thus, it appears that forebrain seizures, like brain-stem seizures, do not normally activate other seizure networks. However, under conditions of seizure repetition or when one seizure substrate has an abnormally low threshold (as does the brain-stem of the GEPR), secondary generalization to the other seizure network occurs.

Another feature of the relationship between forebrain and brain-stem seizure networks is that if both systems are activated simultaneously, the brain-stem network has dominance in terms of motor expression (i.e. has control over seizure behaviour). This was illustrated in a study showing that GEPR-9s never display facial and forelimb clonus when stimulated with transcorneal electroshock (Browning et al., 1990) because the brain-stem threshold of GEPR-9s is lower than that of the forebrain, and it is not possible to activate the forebrain system without also having brain-stem activation. This was also illustrated by the inability of transauricular electroshock to evoke facial and forelimb clonus, despite the fact that transcorneal electroshock evokes facial and forelimb clonus at low currents (when forebrain network is activated exclusively) and tonic seizures at high currents (when both systems are activated simultaneously) (Browning & Nelson, 1985; discussed above).

In conclusion, a substantial body of evidence now supports the hypothesis that facial and forelimb clonic convulsions seen in rodents are a manifestation of seizure discharge occurring in the limbic forebrain, while running–bouncing clonic and tonic convulsions are manifestations of a seizure discharge in the brain-stem. The available evidence also indicates that seizures in the forebrain and brain-stem can occur independently of one another. However, under certain conditions (e.g. seizure repetition or brain pathology) the forebrain and brain-stem seizure networks can interact and seizures in one network can affect the susceptibility and/or the severity of seizures in the other network. Finally, it appears that there are a wide variety of remote endogenous systems in the brain that are not themselves part of a seizure network, but which exert control over the seizure networks. It would appear that, while the task is far from complete, we are well on our way to identifying the anatomical substrates for the various subtypes of generalized seizures.

Acknowledgements

Thanks are due to Drs Phillip Jobe and Michael Statnick for their comments on the manuscript.

References

Applegate, C.D., Samoriski, G.M. & Burchfiel, J.L. (1991): Evidence for the interaction of brain-stem systems mediating seizure expression in kindling and electroconvulsive shock seizure models. *Epilepsy Res.* **10**, 142–147.

Asuad, J. (1940): Contribution à l'étude de l'épilepsie expérimentale chez les animaux décérébrés, mésencéphaliques, protubérantiels, bulbaires et spinaux. *Pr. Méd.* **48**, 1043–1047.

Avanzini, G., de Curtis, M., Marescaux, C., Panzica, F., Spreafico, R. & Vergnes, M. (1992): Role of the thalamic reticular nucleus in the generation of rhythmic thalamocortical activities subserving spike and wave. *J. Neural. Trans.* **35**, 85–95.

Avoli, M. (1988): Primary generalized seizures with spike and wave. In: *Mechanisms of epileptogenesis: transition to seizure*, ed. M.A. Dichter, pp. 73–83. New York: Plenum Press.

Bagri, A., Di Scala, G. & Sandner, G. (1992): Wild running elicited by microinjections of bicuculline or morphine into the inferior colliculus of rats: lack of effect of periaqueductal gray lesions. *Pharmacol. Biochem. Behav.* **41**, 727–732.

Bergmann, F., Costin, A. & Gutman, J. (1963): A low threshold convulsive area in the rabbit mesencephalon. *Electroencephalogr. Clin. Neurophysiol.* **15**, 683–690.

Browning, R.A., Turner, F.J., Simonton, R.L. & Bundman, M.C. (1981a): Effect of midbrain and pontine tegmental lesions on the maximal electroshock seizure pattern in rats. *Epilepsia* **22**, 583–594.

Browning, R.A., Simonton, R.L. & Turner, F.J. (1981b): Antagonism of experimentally-induced tonic seizures following a lesion of the midbrain tegmentum. *Epilepsia* **22**, 595–601.

Browning, R.A. (1985): Role of the brain-stem reticular formation in tonic–clonic seizures: lesion and pharmacological studies. *Fed. Proc.* **44**, 2425–2431.

Browning, R.A. & Nelson, D.K. (1985): Variation in threshold and pattern of electroshock-induced seizures in rats depending on site of stimulation. *Life Sci.* **37**, 2205–2211.

Browning, R.A., Nelson, D.K., Mogharreban, N., Jobe, P.C. & Laird, H.E. (1985): Effect of midbrain and pontine tegmental lesions on audiogenic seizures in genetically epilepsy-prone rats. *Epilepsia* **26**, 175–183.

Browning, R.A. & Nelson, D.K. (1986): Modification of electroshock and pentylenetetrazol seizure patterns in rats after precollicular transections. *Exp. Neurol.* **93**, 546–556.

Browning, R.A., Wang, C., Lanker, M.L. & Jobe, P.C. (1990): Electroshock- and pentylenetetrazol-induced seizures in genetically epilepsy-prone rats (GEPRs): differences in threshold and pattern: *Epilepsy Res.* **6**, 1–11.

Browning, R.A., Wang, C. & Jobe, P.C. (1991): Effect of precollicular transection on audiogenic seizures in genetically epilepsy-prone rats (GEPRs). *Soc. Neurosci. Abst.* **17**, 172.

Browning, R.A., Maggio, R., Sahibzada, N. & Gale, K. (1993): Role of brain-stem structures in seizures initiated from the deep prepiriform cortex of rats. *Epilepsia* **34**, 393–407.

Burnham, W.M., Albright, P., Schneiderman, J., Chiu, P. & Ninchoji, T. (1981): 'Centrencephalic' mechanisms in the kindling model. In: *Kindling 2*, ed. J. Wada, pp. 161–178. New York: Raven Press.

Burnham, W.M. (1987): Electrical stimulation studies: generalized convulsions triggered from the brain-stem. In: *Epilepsy and the reticular formation: the role of the reticular core in convulsive seizures*, eds. G.H. Fromm, C.L. Faingold, R.A. Browning & W.M. Burnham, pp. 25–38. New York: Alan R. Liss.

Collins, R.C., Tearse, R.G. & Lothman, E.W. (1983): Functional anatomy of limbic seizures: focal discharges from medial entorhinal cortex in rats. *Brain Res.* **280**, 25–40.

Dean, P. & Gale, K. (1989): Anticonvulsant action of GABA receptor blockade in the nigro-collicular target region. *Brain Res.* **477**, 391–395.

Depaulis, A., Vergnes, M. & Marescaux, C. (1994): Endogenous control of epilepsy: the nigral inhibitory system. *Prog. Neurobiol.* **42**, 33–56.

Dow, R.S. (1965): Extrinsic regulatory mechanisms of seizure activity. *Epilepsia* **6**, 122–140.

Dow, R.S., Fernandez-Guariola, A. & Manni, E. (1962): The influence of the cerebellum on experimental epilepsy. *Electroencephalogr. Clin. Neurophysiol.* **14**, 383–398.

Faingold, C.L. & Naritoku, D.K. (1992): The genetically epilepsy-prone rat: neuronal networks and actions of amino acid neurotransmitters. In: *Drugs for the control of epilepsy*, eds. C.L. Faingold & G.H. Fromm, pp. 277–308. Boca Raton: CRC Press.

Faingold, C.L. & Riaz, A. (1992): Neuronal networks in convulsant drug-induced seizures. In: *Drugs for control of epilepsy: actions on neuronal networks involved in seizure disorders*, eds. C.L. Faingold & G.H. Fromm, pp. 213–251. Boca Raton: CRC Press.

Faingold, C.L., Millan, M.H., Boersma, C.A. & Meldrum, B.S. (1988): Excitant amino acid and audiogenic seizures in the genetically epilepsy-prone rat. I. Afferent seizure initiation pathway. *Exp. Neurol.* **99**, 678–686.

Gale, K. (1985): Mechanisms of seizure control mediated by γ-aminobutyric acid: role of the substantia nigra. *Fed. Proc.* **44**, 2414–2424.

Gale, K. (1990): Animal models of generalized convulsive seizures: some neuroanatomical differentiation of seizure types. In: *Generalized epilepsy: cellular, molecular and pharmacological approaches*, eds. M. Avoli, P. Gloor, G. Kospopoulos & R. Naquet, pp. 329–343. Boston: Birkhauser.

Gale, K. (1992): Subcortical structures and pathways involved in convulsive seizure generation. *J. Clin. Neurophysiol.* **9**, 264–277.

Gale, K. (1993): Focal trigger zones and pathways of propagation in seizure generation. In: *Epilepsy: models, mechanisms, and concepts*, ed. P.A. Schwartzkroin, pp. 48–93. Cambridge: Cambridge University Press.

Gale, K. & Browning, R.A. (1988): Anatomical and neurochemical substrates of clonic and tonic seizures. In: *Mechanisms of epileptogenesis: transition to seizures*, ed. M.A. Dichter, pp. 111–152. New York: Plenum Press.

Garant, D.S. & Gale, K. (1986): Intranigral muscimol attenuates electrographic signs of seizure activity induced by intravenous bicuculline. *Eur. J. Pharmacol.* **124**, 365–369.

Garant, D.S. & Gale, K. (1987): Substantia nigra-mediated anticonvulsant actions: role of nigral output pathways. *Exp. Neurol.* **97**, 143–159.

Garcia-Cairasco, N., Terra, V.C. & Doretto, M.C. (1993): Midbrain substrates of audiogenic seizures in rats. *Behav. Brain Res.* **58**, 57–67.

Gastaut, H. & Fischer-Williams, M. (1959): The physiopathology of epileptic seizures. In: *Handbook of physiology*, Section I, Neurophysiology, eds. J. Field, H.W. Magoun & V.E. Hall, pp. 329–363. Washington DC: American Physiology Society.

Gutiérrez-Noriega, C. (1944): Interpretacion fisiologica de la action del cardiazol. *Rev. Neuro-psiquiat.* **7**, 14–38.

Handforth, A. & Ackermann, R.F. (1988a): Functional [^{14}C]-2-deoxyglucose mapping of progressive states of status epilepticus induced by amygdala stimulation in rat. *Brain Res.* **460**, 94–102.

Handforth, A. & Ackermann, R.F. (1988b): Electrically induced limbic status and kindled seizures. In: *Anatomy of epileptogenesis*, eds. B.S. Meldrum, J.A. Ferrendelli & H.G. Wieser, pp. 71–87. London: John Libbey.

Hirsch, E., Maton, B., Vergnes, M., Depaulis, A. & Marescaux, C. (1993): Reciprocal positive transfer between kindling of audiogenic seizures and electrical kindling of inferior colliculus. *Epilepsy Res.* **15,** 133–139.

Jobe, P.C. & Laird II, H.E. (1987): *Neurotransmitters and epilepsy.* Clifton, NJ: The Humana Press.

Jobe, P.C., Picchioni, A.L. & Chin, L. (1973a): Role of brain norepinephrine in audiogenic seizure in the rat. *J. Pharmacol. Exp. Ther.* **184,** 1–10.

Jobe, P.C., Picchioni, A.L. & Chin, L. (1973b): Role of brain 5-hydroxytryptamine in audiogenic seizure in the rat. *Life Sci.* **13,** 1–13.

Jobe, P.C., Burger, R.L., Dailey, J.W., Wang, C., Browning, R.A., & Mishra, P.K. (1992): Is the noradrenergic site for brain-stem seizure regulation located within the midbrain? Studies with desipramine infused via microdialysis in the GEPR. *Epilepsia* **33,** 35.

Kreindler, A., Zuckermann, E., Steriade, M. & Chimion, J. (1958): Electroclinical features of convulsions induced by stimulation of brain-stem. *J. Neurophysiol.* **21,** 430–436.

LeGal La Salle, G. & Naquet, R. (1990): Audiogenic seizures evoked in DBA/2 mice induce c-fos oncogene expression into subcortical auditory nuclei. *Brain Res.* **518,** 308–312.

Lothman, E.W. & Collins, R.C. (1981): Kainic acid induced limbic seizures: metabolic, behavioral, electroencephalographic, and neuropathological correlates. *Brain Res.* **218,** 299–318.

Maggio, R., Lanaud, P., Grayson, D.R. & Gale, K. (1993): Expression of c-fos mRNA following seizures evoked from an epileptogenic site in the deep prepiriform cortex: regional distribution in brain as shown by *in situ* hybridization. *Exp. Neurol.* **119,** 11–19.

Marescaux, C., Vergnes, M., Kiesmann, M., Depaulis, A., Micheletti, G. & Warter, J.M. (1987): Kindling of audiogenic seizures in Wistar rats: an EEG study. *Exp. Neurol.* **97,** 160–168.

Marescaux, C., Vergnes, M. & Depaulis, A. (1992): Genetic absence epilepsy in rats from Strasbourg – a review. *J. Neural Trans. (Suppl.)* **35,** 37–69.

Maton, B., Hirsch, E., Vergnes, M., Depaulis, A. & Marescaux, C. (1992): Dorsal tegmentum kindling in rats. *Neurosci. Lett.* **134,** 284–287.

McCown, T.J., Greenwood, R.S., Frye, G.D. & Breese, G.R. (1984): Electrically elicited seizures from the inferior colliculus: a potential site for the genesis of epilepsy. *Exp. Neurol.* **86,** 527–542.

McCown, T.J., Greenwood, R.S., Frye, G.D. & Breese, G.R. (1987): Inferior colliculus interactions with limbic seizure activity. *Epilepsia* **28,** 234–241.

McCown, T.J., Duncan, G.E. & Breese, G.R. (1991): Neuroanatomical characterization of inferior collicular seizure genesis: 2-deoxyglucose and stimulation mapping. *Brain Res.* **567,** 25–32.

McIntyre, D.C., Don, J.C. & Edson, N. (1991): Distribution of [^{14}C]-deoxyglucose after various forms and durations of status epilepticus induced by stimulation of a kindled amygdala focus in rats. *Epilepsy Res.* **10,** 119–133.

McNamara, J-O, Rigsbee, L.C. & Galloway, M.T. (1983): Evidence that substantia nigra is crucial to neural network of kindled seizure. *Eur. J. Pharmacol.* **86,** 485–486.

Meldrum, B.S. (1988): Historical introduction. In: *Anatomy of epileptogenesis,* eds. B.S. Meldrum, J.A. Ferrendelli & H.G. Wieser, pp. 1–11. London: John Libbey.

Millan, M.H., Meldrum, B.S., Boersma, C.A. & Faingold, C.L. (1988): Excitant amino acids and audiogenic seizures in the genetically epilepsy-prone rat. II. Efferent seizure propagating pathway. *Exp. Neurol.* **99,** 687–698.

Miller, J.W. (1992): The role of mesencephalic and thalamic arousal systems in experimental seizures. *Prog. Neurobiol.* **39,** 155–178.

Miller, J.W. & Ferrendelli, J.A. (1990a): The central medial nucleus: thalamic site of seizure regulation. *Brain Res.* **508,** 297–300.

Miller, J.W. & Ferrendelli, J.A. (1990b): Characterization of GABAergic seizure regulation in the midline thalamus. *Neuropharmacology* **29,** 649–655.

Miller, J.W., Gray, B.C. & Turner, G.M. (1993): Role of the fastigial nucleus in generalized seizures as demonstrated by GABA agonist microinjections. *Epilepsia* **34,** 973–978.

Naritoku, D.K., Mecozzi, L.B., Randall, M.E. & Faingold, C.L. (1989): Infusions of GABA agonists or 2-APH into the amygdala (AMY) or medial geniculate (MGB) reversibly reduce seizure duration and clonus after repeated audiogenic seizures (AGS) in the genetically epilepsy-prone rat (GEPR-9) *Soc. Neurosci. Abst.* **15,** 46.

Naritoku, D.K., Mecozzi, L.B., Aiello, M.T. & Faingold, C.L. (1992): Repetition of audiogenic seizures in genetically epilepsy-prone rats induces cortical epileptiform activity and additional seizure behaviors. *Exp. Neurol.* **115**, 317–324.

Noebels, J.L. (1984): A single gene error of noradrenergic axon growth synchronizes central neurons. *Nature* **310**, 409–411.

Pasini, A., Tortorella, A. & Gale, K. (1992): Anticonvulsant effect of intranigral fluoxetine. *Brain Res.* **593**, 287–290.

Patel, S. (1988): Chemically induced limbic seizures in rodents. In: *Anatomy of epileptogenesis*, eds. B.S. Meldrum, J.A. Ferrendelli & H.G. Wieser, pp. 89–106. London: John Libbey.

Paz, C., Reygadas, E. & Fernandez-Guardiola, A. (1985): Amygdala kindling in totally cerebellectomized cats. *Exp. Neurol.* **88**, 418–424.

Piredda, S.G., Woodhead, J.H. & Swinyard, E.A. (1985): Effect of stimulus intensity on the profile of anticonvulsant activity of phenytoin, ethosuximide and valproate. *J. Pharmacol. Exp. Ther.* **232**, 741–745.

Popovici, T., Represa, A., Crepel, V., Barbin, G., Beaudoin, M. & Ben-Ari, Y. (1990): Effect of kainic acid-induced seizures and ischaemia on c-fos-like proteins in rat brain. *Brain Res.* **536**, 183–194.

Racine, R.J. (1972): Modification of seizure activity by electrical stimulation II. Motor seizures. *Electroencephalogr. Clin. Neurophysiol.* **32**, 281–294.

Raines, A. & Anderson, R.J. (1976): Effects of acute cerebellectomy on maximal electroshock seizures and anticonvulsant efficacy of diazepam in the rat. *Epilepsia* **17**, 177–182.

Redgrave, P., Simkins, M., Overton, P. & Dean, P. (1991a): Anticonvulsant role of nigrotectal projection in the maximal electroshock model of epilepsy. I. Mapping of dorsal midbrain with bicuculline. *Neuroscience* **46**, 379–390.

Redgrave, P., Marrow, L.P. & Dean, P. (1991b): Anticonvulsant role of nigrotectal projection in the maximal electroshock model of epilepsy-II. Pathways from substantia nigra pars lateralis and adjacent peripeduncular area to dorsal midbrain. *Neuroscience* **46**, 391–406.

Reigel, C.E., Jobe, P.C., Dailey, J.W. & Savage, D.D. (1989): Ontogeny of sound-induced seizures in the genetically epilepsy-prone rat. *Epilepsy Res.* **4**, 64–71.

Schoen, R. (1926): Beiträge zur Pharmakologie der Körperstellung und der Labyrinthreflexe 22. *Mitteilung: Hexeton und Cardiazol Arch. exp. Path. Pharmak.* **113**, 257–274.

Steriade, M., McCormick, D.A. & Sejnowsk, T.J. (1993): Thalamic oscillations in the sleep and aroused brain. *Science* **262**, 679–685.

Tanaka, K. & Mishima, O. (1953): The localization of the center dealing with the tonic extensor seizure of electroshock. *Jpn. J. Pharmacol.* **3**, 6–9.

Tsusui, J., Terra, V.C., Oliveira, J.A.C. & Garcia-Cairasco, N. (1992): Neuroethological evaluation of audiogenic seizures and audiogenic-like seizures induced by microinjection of bicuculline into the inferior colliculus. I. Effects of midcollicular knife cuts. *Behav. Brain Res.* **52**, 7–17.

Turski, W.A., Cavalheiro, E.A., Bortolotto, Z.A., Mello, L.M., Schwartz, M. & Turski, L. (1984): Seizures produced by pilocarpine in mice: a behavioral, electroencephalographic and morphological analysis. *Brain Res.* **321**, 237–253.

Vergnes, M. & Marescaux, C. (1992): Cortical and thalamic lesions in rats with genetic absence epilepsy. *J. Neural. Trans. (Suppl.)* **35**, 71–83.

Wada, Y., Nakamura, M., Hasegawa, H. & Yamaguchi, N. (1992): Role of serotonin receptor subtype in seizures kindled from the feline hippocampus. *Neurosci. Lett.* **141**, 21–24.

White, L.E. & Price, J.L. (1993a): The functional anatomy of limbic status epilepticus in the rat. I. Patterns of ^{14}C-2-deoxyglucose uptake and fos immunocytochemistry. *J. Neurosci.* **13**, 4787–4809.

White, L.E. & Price, J.L. (1993b): The functional anatomy of limbic status epilepticus in the rat. II. The effect of focal deactivation. *J. Neurosci.* **13**, 4810–4830.

Willott, J.F. & Lu, S.M. (1980): Midbrain pathways of audiogenic seizures in DBA/2 mice. *Exp. Neurol.* **70**, 288–299.

Woodbury, D.M. & Esplin, D.W. (1959): Neuropharmacology and neurochemistry of anticonvulsant drugs. *Res. Publ. Assoc. Nerv. Ment. Dis.* **37**, 24–56.

Chapter 34

Propagation of generalized seizures from brain-stem to forebrain networks

E. Hirsch*[†], M. Vergnes*, S. Simler*, B. Maton[‡], A. Nehlig* and C. Marescaux*[†]

*INSERM U 398, Centre de Neurochimie du CNRS, 5 rue Blaise Pascal, 67084 Strasbourg Cedex, France; [†]Unité d'Explorations Fonctionnelles des Epilepsies, Hôpitaux Universitaires, 1 place de l'Hôpital, 67091 Strasbourg Cedex, France; [‡]Division de Neurophysiologie Clinique, Hôpital Cantonal Universitaire, rue Micheli du Crest 24, 1211 Genève 14, Switzerland

Audiogenic seizures in rodents are one of the most common animal models of generalized convulsive epilepsy (Jobe et al., Ch. 32). A strain of Wistar rats (Wistar AS) was inbred in our laboratory for its susceptibility to sound. In contrast to GEPR stemming from a Sprague–Dawley strain, Wistar AS do not appear to have lower seizure thresholds for any epileptogenic stimulus other than their susceptibility to sound (Hirsch et al., 1992, 1993; Jobe et al., Ch. 32). In Wistar AS, an intense acoustic stimulus induces an epileptic seizure characterized by one or two fits of wild running followed by a tonic phase with dorsal hyperextension, the head up, the forelimbs stretched out forward, the hind limbs most often flexed. In contrast, GEPR-9s exhibit a flexion of the neck with a complete tonic extension of the limbs (Jobe et al., Ch. 32). No high amplitude spikes are detectable on the cortical EEG during any of these phases. The tonic phase is associated with a short cortical flattening, followed by a regular low-voltage 10–12 c/s rhythm for 20 to 30 s, due to simultaneous recording through the cortex of a high amplitude hippocampal theta rhythm. This hippocampal theta activity is related to the intense activation of brain-stem structures, without any characteristics of an epileptic discharge. Similar 10–12 c/s hippocampal theta waves are recorded under physiological conditions during REM sleep, in 'cerveau isolé' preparations and following a non-convulsant electrical stimulation of the nucleus reticularis pontis oralis (Hirsch et al., 1992).

The absence of cortical discharges is explained by the fact that audiogenic seizures, in Wistar AS as in other rodent strains, originate in the brain-stem and do not involve forebrain structures (Browning, Ch. 33). In order to examine the possibility of inducing a process of kindling, we have studied the effects of repeated auditory stimulation in Wistar AS. When sound-susceptible Wistar rats are submitted to 10–40 daily sound stimulations, the tonic phase progressively evolves into myoclonic seizure characterized by facial and forelimb clonus, rearing and falling or into tonic–clonic seizures. These myoclonic or tonic–clonic seizures are accompanied by paroxysmal cortical spike and spike-wave discharges for 40–120 s. These behavioural and EEG modifications, which can be elicited by a renewed acoustic stimulation several months after discontinuation of daily acoustic stimulations, evoke a phenomenon similar to kindling (Marescaux et al., 1987; Vergnes et al., 1987). Identical observations were made in GEPR (Naritoku et al., 1992). Similar behavioral and EEG concomitants are observed during daily electrical stimulation of the inferior colliculus (Maton et al., 1992). Moreover, an immediate reciprocal positive transfer between electrical kindling of inferior colliculus and kindling of audiogenic seizures was obtained (Hirsch et al., 1993).

Several lines of evidence demonstrate that usually forebrain and brain-stem seizure networks operate independently (Browning, Ch. 33). However, the above data suggest that under certain circumstances, these two networks can interact. In order to define the neuroanatomical pathways through which these interactions occur, different experiments were performed comparing control rats, naïve Wistar AS and kindled Wistar AS submitted to repeated auditory stimulus.

Male Wistar rats were chosen from the two strains inbred in our laboratory for 18–20 generations: the non epileptic control strain (NE) insensitive to acoustic stimulation, and the Wistar AS strain. Animals were submitted to a suprathreshold sound stimulus (10 000–20 000 Hz, 120 dB, 90 s) at 2 months of age. Only Wistar AS displaying a full audiogenic seizure and controls failing to show any behavioural response were included in the different groups. All rats were then housed in individual cages on a standard 12 h/12 h light–dark cycle with free access to food and water, until the age of 4 months, when the experimental procedure took place. From 2 to 4 months of age, the rats were either left free of sound stimulation (group control NE and group AS) or submitted to repeated sound stimulations (group KAS).

Table 1. Behavioural development of (A) hippocampal, (B) amygdalar kindling in NE (non-epileptic control), AS (single audiogenic seizure) and KAS (kindled audiogenic seizure)

Stage		(A) Hippocampal kindling		
		NE n = 7	AS n = 8	KAS n = 8
3–4	number of rats	6/7	6/8	8/8
	number of stimuli			
	median	22.5	22	4**
	range	19–39	10–37	1–16
5–6	number of rats	5/7	5/8	8/8
	number of stimuli			
	median	30	22	4**
	range	22–36	10–32	1–16
Stage		(B) Amygdalar kindling		
		NE n = 7	AS n = 8	KAS n = 8
3–4	number of rats	7/7	7/7	7/7
	number of stimuli			
	median	6.5	5	1**
	range	5–11	3–14	1–3
5–6	number of rats	7/7	7/7	7/7
	number of stimuli			
	median	10	11	1**
	range	6–14	6–16	1–5

Number of rats reaching at least one stage 3–4 and 5–6 (Racine's scale modified by Pinel) and number of stimuli necessary to reach these stages for the first time. **$P < 0.01$, statistically significant differences from NE control.

Experiment I: Positive transfer of audiogenic kindling to electrical hippocampal and amygdalar kindling in Wistar AS

Following kindling of a primary brain site, the number of electrical stimuli necessary to induce kindled seizures at a secondary site may be reduced. This positive transfer results from the spread of after-discharges from the primary site to the secondary one during the kindling process (Goddard et al., 1969). To confirm that repeated audiogenic stimulations cause a propagation of the epileptic activity towards the forebrain, we examined a possible positive transfer of audiogenic kindling to electrical kindling of limbic structures.

The behavioural and EEG development of electrical hippocampal kindling were compared in controls, naïve AS and kindled KAS rats. Under pentobarbital anesthesia, the three groups were implanted with frontal and parietal single contact cortical electrodes, and with a bipolar electrode placed in the right dorsal hippocampus. Ten days later, the threshold for elicitation of local after-discharges was defined and a stimulus (2 s, 50 Hz) twice as high as threshold was delivered daily, for a total of 40 stimulations. For each electrical stimulus, motor seizures were scored using Racine's scale modified by Pinel (Racine et al., 1972; Pinel & Rovner, 1978). In each group, the number of animals demonstrating at least one seizure of stage 3–4 and/or 5–6, and the mean number of stimuli necessary to reach each of these stages for the first time were noted. The total duration of the after-discharge was measured. Statistical analyses were performed using Mann–Whitney and χ^2 tests.

Results are summarized in Table 1 (A). Hippocampal kindling was similar in the AS and the control rats. In the KAS rats, the hippocampal kindling was clearly facilitated, as compared to controls and AS rats. Behavioural stage 5 was reached in a median of four stimulations in KAS vs 30 and 22 stimulations respectively in controls and AS rats.

The same procedure was applied to three groups of rats implanted in the right amygdala. Results (Table 1 (B), Fig. 1) were similar. Amygdalar kindling was not accelerated in the AS group when compared to the control group. However, in the KAS group, an immediate transfer between kindling of audiogenic seizure and electrical kindling of amygdala was observed: behavioural stage 5 was observed after the first stimulation in KAS, whereas this stage was reached only after 10 and 11 stimulations respectively in controls and AS rats.

These positive transfer phenomena suggest that during kindling of audiogenic seizures, epileptic discharges spread from the brain-stem to the forebrain and progressively involve the amygdala and the hippocampus. This hypothesis was confirmed in the same studies by the recordings of hippocampal and amygdalar paroxysmal high-amplitude spike-wave discharges during kindled audiogenic seizures (Hirsch et al., 1992).

Experiment II: Effects of audiogenic seizures on c-fos expression in naïve and kindled Wistar AS

As expression of the nuclear proto-oncogene c-fos can rapidly and transiently be induced in the central nervous system in response to a wide variety of epileptic seizures (Dragunow & Faull, 1989; Morgan & Curran, 1991; Represa et al., Ch. 36), regional elevation of c-fos protein expression was used to map the pathways involved in single and kindled audiogenic seizures.

Control (NE), AS and KAS rats were submitted to a suprathreshold acoustic stimulation, killed 2 h later, and their brains were processed for c-fos protein immunochemistry. The method was slightly modified from that reported by Dragunow & Faull (1989). Coronal sections were incubated for 36 h with a polyclonal, affinity-purified sheep antibody against the c-fos family of antigens. Sections were stained by the avitin–biotin method.

Results are summarized in Table 2 and Fig. 2. The density and intensity of labelled cells within anatomically defined regions of the brain were subjectively rated on a four-point scale (0, absence

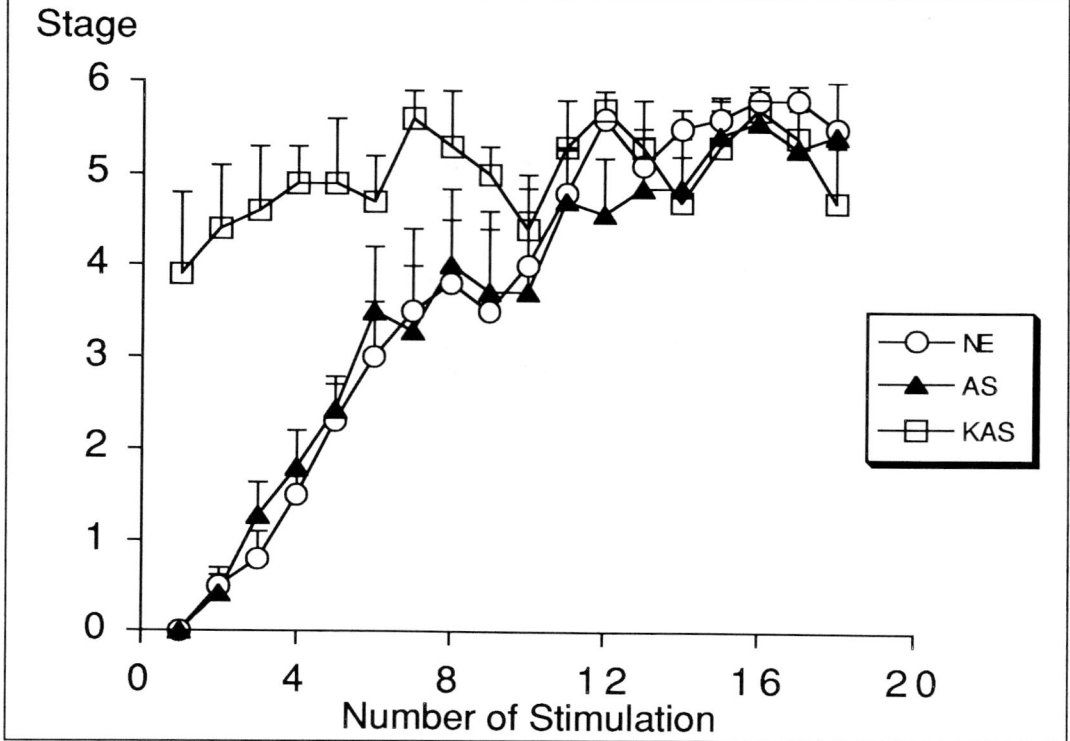

Fig. 1. *Behavioural response during amygdalar kindling in non-epileptic controls (NE, open circles), naïve Wistar AS (AS, black triangles) and kindled Wistar AS (KAS, open squares). Stages, defined according to Racine, are represented as mean ± SEM.*

of labelling; 1, low labelling; 2, moderate labelling; 3, intense labelling). The observers were blind to the experimental procedures.

The experimental white noise did not induce any *c*-fos expression in NE control rats. In Wistar AS rats, a single typical audiogenic seizure induced the expression of *c*-fos in specific subsets of neurons which belong with only minor exception to the subcortical auditory nuclei (inferior colliculus, dorsal nucleus of the lateral lemniscus and medial geniculate nucleus) and the reticular formation. The hippocampus, which is commonly associated with seizures in a large number of epilepsy models, was completely devoid of any labelling. A few scattered cells were labelled in the amygdala and the piriform cortex. The induction of *c*-fos in the inferior colliculus and in the related auditory nuclei of Wistar AS after single audiogenic seizures, agrees with previous data obtained in the genetically susceptible DBA/2 mice (Le Gal La Salle & Naquet, 1990) and in rats normally resistant to audiogenic seizures, but made susceptible by exposing them to a loud noise on postnatal day 14 (Snyder-Keller & Pierson, 1992).

Kindling did not significantly change audiogenic seizure-induced *c*-fos expression in the brainstem. In contrast, it strongly increased *c*-fos expression in forebrain areas. Intense additional staining was induced in the amygdala and the piriform cortex. The hypothalamus and the neocortex which are occasionally and slightly positive after a single audiogenic seizure, are clearly positive. Moreover, the hippocampus which was not labelled at all after a single audiogenic seizure, displayed an intense labelling after a kindled audiogenic seizure. Preliminary data obtained after 5 to 15 acoustic stimulations when kindling is in progress, suggested that the amygdala is involved

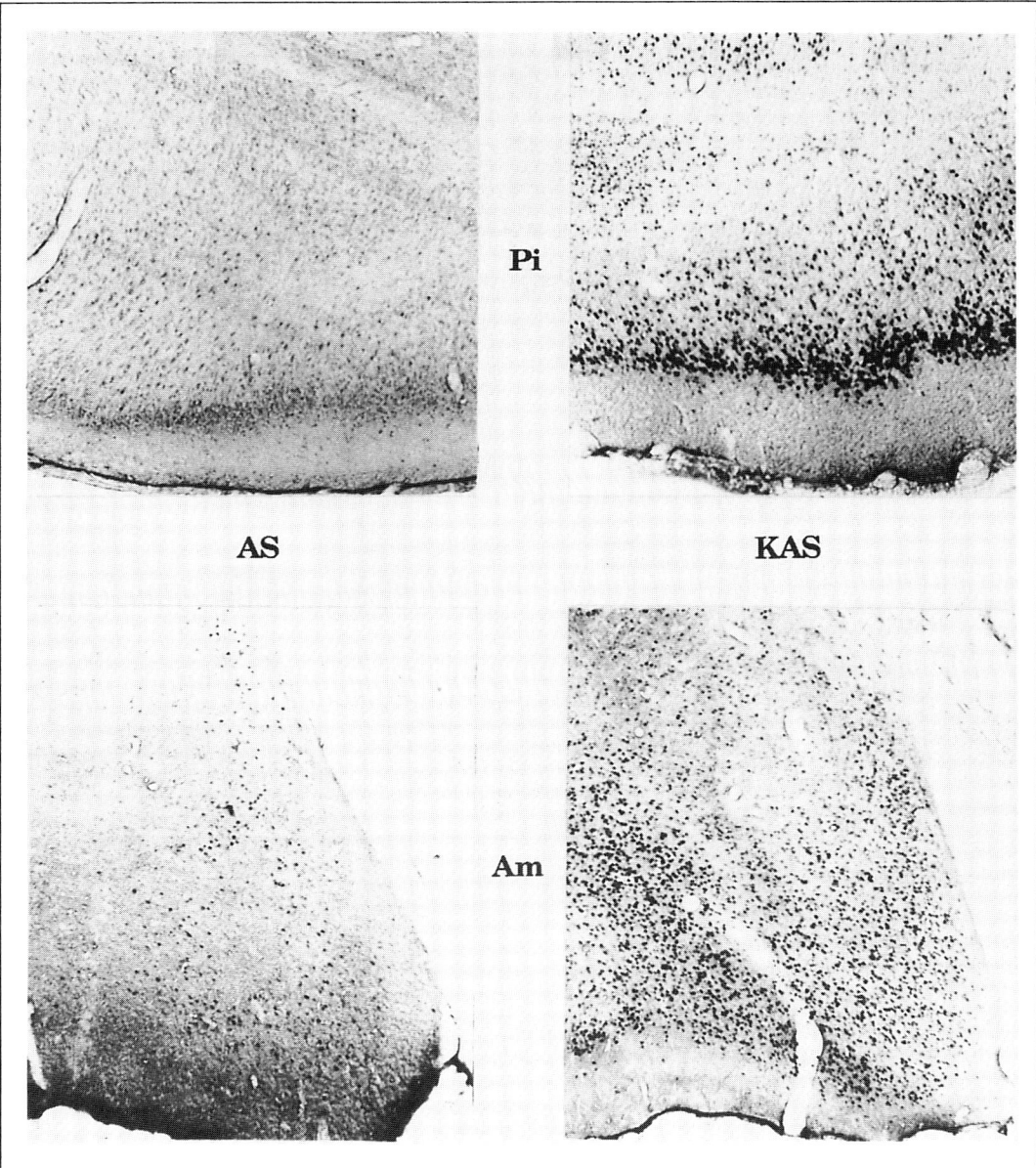

Fig. 2. C-fos expression in amygdala (Am) and piriform cortex (Pi) in naïve (AS) and kindled (KAS) Wistar AS rats 2 h after an audiogenic seizure.

before the piriform cortex and hippocampus. This pattern of c-fos protein accumulation is very similar to those seen after experimental seizures involving the forebrain, induced by convulsant drugs (pentylenetetrazol, kainic acid, pilocarpine), maximum electroshock and amygdalar or hippocampal electrical kindling (Morgan & Curran, 1991).

Thus, our results show that audiogenic seizure-induced expression of c-fos protein, which is limited

Table 2. Sound or seizure-induced local c-fos expression in NE (non-epileptic control), AS (single audiogenic seizure) and KAS (kindled audiogenic seizure)

Structures	Groups		
	NE n = 3	AS n = 6	KAS N = 5
Auditory pathways			
Inferior colliculus			
Central nucleus	0 (3/3)	0 (6/6)	3 (1/5); 2 (4/5)
External cortex	0 (3/3)	2 (6/6)	3 (5/5)
Medial geniculate nucleus	0 (3/3)	2 (6/6)	3 (2/5); 2 (3/5)
Temporal cortex	1 (1/3); 0 (2/3)	1 (2/6); 0 (4/6)	2 (3/5); 1 (2/5)
Brain-stem structures			
Pontine reticular nucleus	0 (3/3)	1 (6/6)	2 (3/5); 1 (2/5)
Giganto-cellular nucleus	0 (3/3)	1 (6/6)	1 (5/5)
Forebrain structures			
Amygdala	0 (3/3)	1 (6/6)	3 (5/5)
Piriform cortex	0 (3/3)	1 (2/6); 0 (4/6)	3 (5/5)
Hippocampus			
CA_1	0 (3/3)	0 (6/6)	2 (5/5)
CA_2	0 (3/3)	0 (6/6)	2 (5/5)
CA_3	0 (3/3)	0 (6/6)	1 (2/5); 0 (3/5)
Dentate gyrus	0 (3/3)	0 (6/6)	3 (4/5); 2 (1/5)

The density of labelled cells is rated from 0 to 3 (see text). In parentheses: number of rats displaying a given score/total number of animals in the group.

to brain-stem nuclei after a single seizure, spreads to limbic and cortical structures after completion of kindling. The extent of c-fos induction reflects the extent of propagation of EEG discharges. C-fos expression in forebrain areas may indicate long-term neuronal changes associated with kindling of brain-stem seizures.

Experiment III: Effects of audiogenic seizures on cerebral blood flow in naïve and kindled Wistar AS

Mapping of cerebral blood flow has been performed during the course of audiogenic seizures in naïve and kindled Wistar AS by means of the quantitative autoradiographic [^{14}C]iodoantipyrine technique of Sakurada et al., (1978). This technique allows the mapping of local rates of cerebral blood flow during very short periods ranging from 20–90 s and could therefore be used for the quantitative approach of cerebral functional activity over an event as short as an audiogenic seizure. Control (NE) rats submitted to the same auditory stimulus serve as controls.

Both NE, AS and KAS were exposed to the same suprathreshold sound stimulus. Iodoantipyrine infusion was initiated after the beginning of the first running phase in Wistar AS, and after approximately the same period of exposure to sound (about 20 s) in controls. As shown in Table 3 summarizing the data for four representative brain structures, cerebral blood flow was significantly increased over control values during audiogenic seizures in both naïve and kindled rats. In naïve Wistar AS, rates of cerebral blood flow massively increased (200–300 per cent) in the two posterior areas, inferior colliculus and the reticular gigantocellularis nucleus, both known to be involved in the expression of audiogenic seizures (Browning, Ch. 33). In these AS rats, rates of cerebral blood flow increased much less (62–79 per cent) in forebrain areas such as amygdala and cerebral cortex that are not involved in the expression of single audiogenic seizures (Browning, Ch. 33).

In kindled KAS rats, rates of cerebral blood flow were significantly lower during audiogenic seizures than in naïve AS in the two brain-stem structures. In the cerebral cortex, cerebral blood flow was similar in both kindled KAS and naïve AS while, in amygdala, the rate of cerebral blood flow was higher in KAS than in AS.

Table 3. *Effects of sound or audiogenic seizures on cerebral blood flow in representative structures of naïve (AS) and kindled (KAS) Wistar AS rats and of non-epileptic controls (NE)*

Structures	NE n = 8	AS n = 9	Variation from control (%)	KAS n = 7	Variation from control (%)
Inferior colliculus	143.0 ± 21.2	426.3 ± 47.9**	+198	239 ± 21.0*††	+ 67
Gigantocellularis nucleus	58.2 ± 6.3	228.2 ± 24.0**	+292	143.8 ± 11.1**††	+147
Basolateral amygdala	71.2 ± 6.8	127.7 ± 7.8**	+ 79	158.4 ± 9.0**†	+122
Frontal cortex	133.0 ± 15.1	215.0 ± 18.2*	+ 62	182.6 ± 13.5	+ 37

Values expressed as ml/10 g/min, are means ± SEM of the number of animals in parentheses. $^*P < 0.05$, $^{**}P < 0.01$, statistically significant differences from control; $^†P < 0.05$, $^{††}P < 0.01$, statistically significant differences from naïve Wistar AS rats.

These data show that the extension of seizures from brain-stem to forebrain during kindling occurs via mechanisms that do not translate into increases in rates of cerebral blood flow rates in forebrain structures, but that they rather induce a decrease in cerebral blood flow rates in posterior areas as compared to those during single audiogenic seizures. A similar pattern has been previously described for energy metabolism and blood flow after repeated electroconvulsive seizures (Orzi *et al.*, 1987; Barkai *et al.*, 1991).

Conclusion

In conclusion, the positive and immediate transfer of audiogenic seizure kindling to amygdalar kindling, the early and massive expression of amygdalar *c*-fos during audiogenic seizure kindling and finally, the selective increase of cerebral blood flow in the amygdala by kindled audiogenic seizures, indicate the primacy of the amygdala in the propagation of audiogenic seizures.

These data are in accordance with recent results obtained in our laboratory. Selective deactivation of the amygdala by microinfusion of lidocaine, a local anaesthetic, in kindled Wistar AS rats suppressed myoclonic components and cortical spike-wave discharges during sound-induced seizures, restoring EEG and behavioural patterns similar to the prekindled ones. Comparable results were obtained by Naritoku *et al.* (1989) after amygdalar injections of GABA agonists or NMDA antagonists in kindled GEPRs.

The relationship between the brain-stem and cortical structures in generalized seizures is still a subject of interest and controversy (Jobe *et al.*, 1991; Jasper, 1991; Browning, Ch. 33; Guy *et al.*, Ch. 31; Menini *et al.*, Ch. 29; Wada, Ch. 30). Taken together, the results of our experiments reveal the amygdala as a crucial relay in the neuroanatomical pathways through which audiogenic seizures spread from the brain-stem towards the forebrain during seizure repetition. This propagation secondarily involves other forebrain structures such as the hippocampus and the cortex. Implications of similar processes during the development of tonic and tonic–clonic seizures in humans should be clarified.

References

Barkai, A.I., Prohovnik, I., Young, W.L., Durkin, M. & Nelson, H.D. (1991): Alterations of local cerebral blood flow and glucose uptake by electroconvulsive shock in rats. *Biol. Psychiatr.* **30**, 269–282.

Dragunow, M. & Faull, R. (1989): The use of c-fos as a metabolic marker in neuronal pathway tracing. *J. Neurosci. Methods* **29**, 261–265.

Goddard, G.V., McIntyre, C. & Leech, C.K. (1969): A permanent change in brain function resulting from daily electrical stimulation. *Exp. Neurol.* **25**, 295–330.

Hirsch, E., Maton, B., Vergnes, M., Depaulis, A. & Marescaux, C. (1992): Positive transfer of audiogenic kindling to electrical hippocampal kindling in rats. *Epilepsy Res.* **11**, 159–166.

Hirsch, E., Maton, B., Vergnes, M., Depaulis, A. & Marescaux, C. (1993): Reciprocal positive transfer between kindling of audiogenic seizures and electrical kindling of inferior colliculus. *Epilepsy Res.* **15**, 133–139.

Jasper, H.H. (1991): Current evaluation of the concepts of centrencephalic and cortico-reticular seizure. *Electroencephalogr. Clin. Neurophysiol.* **78**, 2–11.

Jobe, P.C., Mishra, P.K., Ludvig, N. & Dailey, J.W. (1991): Scope and contribution of genetic models to an understanding of the epilepsies. *Crit. Rev. Neurobiol.* **6**, 183–220.

Le Gal La Salle, G. & Naquet, R. (1990): Audiogenic seizures evoked in DBA/2 mice induce c-fos oncogene expression into subcortical auditory nuclei. *Brain Res.* **518**, 308–312.

Marescaux, C., Vergnes, M., Kiesmann, M., Depaulis, A., Micheletti, G. & Warter, J.M. (1987): Kindling of audiogenic seizures in Wistar rats: an EEG study. *Exp. Neurol.* **97**, 160–168.

Maton, B., Hirsch, E., Vergnes, M., Depaulis, A. & Marescaux, C. (1992): Dorsal tegmentum kindling in rats. *Neurosci. Lett.* **134**, 284–287.

Morgan, J.I. & Curran, T. (1991): Proto-oncogene transcription factors and epilepsy. *Trends Pharmacol. Sci.* **12**, 343–349.

Naritoku, D.K., Mecozzi, L.B., Randall, M.E. & Faingold, C.L. (1989): Infusions of GABA agonists or 2-APH into the amygdala (AMY) or medial geniculate (MGB) reversibly reduce seizure duration and clonus after repeated audiogenic seizures (AGS) in the genetically epilepsy-prone rat (GEPR-9). *Soc. Neurosci. Abst.* **15**, 46.

Naritoku, D.K., Mecozzi, L.B., Aiello, M.T. & Faingold, C.L. (1992): Repetition of audiogenic seizures in genetically epilepsy-prone rats induces cortical epileptiform activity and additional seizure behaviors. *Exp. Neurol.* **115**, 317–324.

Orzi, F., Passarelli, F., Diana, G. & Fieschi, C. (1987): Effects of single and repeated ECS on local cerebral glucose utilization in conscious rats. *Brain Res.* **423**, 144–148.

Pinel, J.P. & Rovner, L.I. (1978): Experimental epileptogenesis: kindling-induced epilepsy in rats. *Exp. Neurol.* **58**, 190–202.

Racine, R., Okujava, V. & Chipasvili, S. (1972): Modification of seizure activity by electrical stimulation. *Electroencephalogr. Clin. Neurophysiol.* **32**, 269–299.

Sakurada, O., Kennnedy, C., Jehle, J., Brown, J.D., Carbin, G.L. & Sokoloff, L. (1978): Measurement of local cerebral blood flow with [^{14}C]iodoantipyrine. *Am. J. Physiol.* **234**, H59–H66.

Snyder-Keller, A.M. & Pierson, M.G. (1992): Audiogenic seizures induce c-fos in a model of developmental epilepsy. *Neurosci. Lett.* **135**, 108–112.

Vergnes, M., Kiesmann, M., Marescaux, C., Depaulis, A., Micheletti, G. & Warter, J.M. (1987): Kindling of audiogenic seizures on the rat. *Int. J. Neurosci.* **36**, 167–176.

Part VII
Fundamental and therapeutic aspects

Introductory remarks

Dominique Broglin and Raymond Bernasconi

In the therapeutic field, progress necessarily results both from developments in basic research and the more pragmatic experience gained by clinicians while treating the patients themselves. The final part of this book provides a review of the principal areas in which progress has already been achieved, or can reasonably be envisaged for the treatment of idiopathic generalized epilepsies (IGEs).

How much is known about the role of conventional antiepileptic drugs in the treatment of these disorders? This question is not paradoxical and is worth asking. These drugs are certainly highly effective in controlling seizures in these idiopathic epilepsies and syndromes, and, if chosen appropriately according to the type of seizure, result in disappearance of seizures in approximately three-quarters, or more, of patients. Their true long-term impact remains much more difficult to evaluate. Does appropriate and early treatment change the natural course of IGEs, does it decrease the duration and/or severity of their course? Some clinical data seem to provide a positive answer to these questions for certain IGE syndromes, but they remain open to criticism from a methodological viewpoint. Therefore, larger clinical trials which are both methodologically coherent and ethically irreproachable are necessary before these partial and insufficient data can be confirmed, corrected or invalidated.

Of course, Gower's concept, according to which 'seizures beget seizures', is not unrelated to these questions. Besides the clinical findings, this assumption is now supported by a great deal of experimental data showing that epileptic discharges induce genic, molecular, functional and morphological cellular – neuronal as well as glial – alterations which are obviously likely to favour the process of epileptogenesis and the auto-perpetuation of recurrent spontaneous discharges. Most of these data, it is true, concern experimental models of focal seizures, but a few do involve induced convulsive generalized seizures. However, the clinical significance of such experimental observations remains unclear in the specific context of idiopathic generalized epilepsies, particularly with respect to some of their essential characteristics: age-dependence, predisposition or indeed pre-existing genetic cause.

The hypotheses concerning the mechanisms of action of antiepileptic drugs remain mainly deductive in nature. More specifically, a link can be presumed between the clinical efficacy of a drug in a given type of seizure on the one hand, and one of the neurobiological and pharmacological effects – which is considered essential – of this drug on the other. But the exact relationship between this essential effect and the action of the drug on the specific physiopathological mechanisms of epileptic discharges themselves still needs to be more clearly defined.

One of the most important new acquisitions concerning the mechanisms of action of antiepileptic drugs is undoubtedly the demonstration of the reduction in low-threshold T calcium currents in thalamic neurons by the specifically anti-absence molecules ethosuximide and dimethadione, whose mechanism of action has until now remained unknown. But other question still need to be answered, for example: on what mechanism(s) is the anti-absence action of benzodiazepines based? What are the probably multiple mechanisms of action of valproate? Does an antiepileptic drug which is effective in various types of seizure have several different mechanisms of action or a single, but polyvalent, mechanism? Why are drugs with apparently different mechanisms of action nonetheless active in a same type of seizure?

What about new antiepileptic drugs for the treatment of IGEs? For obvious ethical and methodological reasons, there are relatively little data on these types of epilepsies in comparison with the information collected in patients who suffer from pharmaco-resistant epilepsy, mainly symptomatic or cryptogenic, whether localization-related or generalized. Several of these new drugs are effective in convulsive generalized seizures, particularly tonic–clonic attacks. But data from a different approach, that is involving patients suffering from a particular IGE syndrome, remain preliminary, particularly in single drug therapy and in untreated patients.

What are the prospects for the future? In the coming years, significant therapeutic progress in certain types of seizures which occur in IGEs – notably primary generalized tonic–clonic seizures, absences – could emerge from improved understanding of the pathophysiological mechanisms of the genesis and/or propagation of the discharges which characterize these seizures. Such progress involves several domains and lines of research, in particular:

* the role of $GABA_B$ receptors. The long-lasting hyperpolarizing currents induced by the activation of these receptors probably play an important role in the deinactivation of the low-threshold T calcium currents in thalamic neurons and, consequently, in the genesis of spike-and-wave discharges. Antagonist substances in these receptors could thus be valuable anti-absence drugs. The experimental data acquired to date on several animal models of absence seizures support this theory.

* the endogenous systems and circuits presumed to play a role in limiting the onset and/or propagation of epileptic discharges. In convulsive and non-convulsive primary generalized seizures, an essential role is attributed, at a sub-cortical level, to the GABAergic neurons of the pars reticulata of the substantia nigra, and to their afferent and efferent neurons. GABAergic mechanisms involving several phases result in the deinhibition of certain neurons which are the target of the GABAergic neurons of the substantia nigra, and it is this deinhibition which is responsible for the protective effect against seizure discharges. The identification of suitable targets within these circuits, open to appropriate pharmacological action, could lead to significant progress in the treatment of such types of seizures.

* the excitatory neurotransmission mediated by the excitatory amino acids, mainly glutamate. The ability to modulate or decrease this synaptic excitation, by competitive and non-competitive antagonists at various levels – NMDA, AMPA/kaïnate and metabotropic glutamate receptors, ionic channel itself or modulatory sites – remains a very important line of research. However, clinical results are lacking in IGEs and not very encouraging to date in partial seizures. Nevertheless, several new drugs do appear to have an effect on the neurotransmission process mediated by the excitatory amino acids.

* the role of second messengers, such as nitric oxide, even if data relating to the role of this molecule in epilepsies – and eventual therapeutic implications – are still at a very primary stage and remain somewhat contradictory.

Thus, thanks to progress in both the pathophysiology of IGEs and molecular biology and pharmacology, a mechanistic approach to the treatment of such conditions is no longer utopian. Rather than basing the approach on systematic screening of the anti-convulsant efficacy of compounds against convulsive seizures induced in non-epileptic animals, which remains the predominant approach, the idea would be to 'design' – and not discover in a more or less empirical fashion – molecules or therapeutic strategies capable of modifying a given pathophysiological mechanism, and then validate these molecules or strategies on animal models of epilepsy, appropriately selected in the specific context of IGEs.

It will, or should soon, be possible to act in a known anatomical and functional system and/or at the level of given receptors on a sub-type and a clearly identified site of these receptors. In this case, it can be envisaged that our therapeutic battery would include the following:

* either molecules, effective in the treatment of epileptic seizures such as our current antiepileptic drugs, but with a significantly better efficacy/side effects ratio.

* or molecules capable of curing, or even preventing, the epileptogenic process itself underlying the seizures. Such molecules might or might not also have an anti-seizure effect and might or might not have to be administered on a long-term basis.

However, in the specific case of IGEs, genic therapy could be a more fruitful approach for effective action on the epileptogenic process itself. Genic therapy in the central nervous system is not just a dream. Most of the basic experimental techniques have been mastered, thanks chiefly to the viruses which carry modified genes. Nevertheless, numerous important ethical and scientific questions remain: the innocuity of the methods, the transfer of the modified gene to the necessary and sufficient area of the brain and its subsequent long-term expression, *a fortiori* the 'replacement' of a causative pathological gene by a 'normalized' gene.

Chapter 35

Influence of drugs on the outcome of idiopathic generalized epilepsies

Pierre Loiseau

Department of Neurology, Bordeaux University Hospital, France

The classification of epilepsies *per se* is beyond the scope of this chapter, yet at the same time fundamental to the subject. Some epileptologists ('the splitters') insist on the existence of distinct epileptic syndromes (Commission, 1989), others ('the lumpers') view the epilepsies as a broad neurobiological continuum (Berkovic *et al.*, 1987; Holmes *et al.*, 1987) and would almost certainly dismiss any attempt to evaluate the influence of drugs on the outcome of idiopathic generalized epilepsies (IGEs) as futile. In fact, however, the two approaches are not irreconcilable; there is much to be said in favour of each.

Splitting is a more clinical way of thinking. IGEs undoubtedly encompass several syndromes for which different therapies are indicated and different outcomes can be expected (e.g. childhood absence epilepsy and juvenile myoclonic epilepsy). With regard to therapy, the type of seizures determines the choice of medication. 'A further rationale for classification into seizures types and epilepsy syndromes is the use of the most appropriate therapeutic regimen, the judicious withholding of treatment, and the prediction of prognosis on which may be predicated the decision about whether and when to attempt the termination of treatment' (Dreifuss, 1989). Note that, by itself, the type of seizure does not predict the result of treatment.

Lumping is a more scientific attitude. The pathophysiological basis of the present classification is debatable (Aicardi, 1988). Disorders with a known genetic basis may have highly variable phenotypes. Even single-gene disorders can cause heterogeneous phenotypes. Complex genetic factors associated with acquired factors may lead to various clinical pictures. Furthermore, the manifestations may change with the passage of time, from one category to another (e.g. absence seizures in childhood, and generalized tonic–clonic seizures and myoclonic jerks in adolescence). An overlapping of the idiopathic generalized epileptic syndromes is quite frequent (Panayiotopoulos *et al.*, 1992). All the foregoing factors have to be taken into account when choosing a medication.

As regards the influence of drugs on the outcome of IGEs, a distinction has to be made between the short-term outcome and the long-term outcome.

Short-term outcome

On the whole, medication improves the short-term prognosis of IGEs more than that of other epilepsies. Complete control of seizures is achieved in about 75 to 80 per cent of patients, whatever the syndrome may be. The type of seizures is the main clue for the choice of medication.

Generalized tonic–clonic seizures

Most of the published data are inconclusive, because true IGEs have been mixed with other epilepsies presenting either with generalized tonic–clonic seizures (GTCS) but without characteristic EEG abnormalities, or with secondarily generalized seizures. Gastaut *et al.* (1973) considered a rather large group of patients (517 in all) presenting with generalized tonic–clonic seizures and bilateral spike and waves. After a 2 year follow-up period, 68 per cent of patients with an onset after 15 years of age and 61 per cent with an onset before 15 years of age were seizure free. Twenty-two per cent and 27 per cent, respectively, experienced a more than 50 per cent reduction in seizure rate. So the short-term outcome of generalized tonic–clonic seizures may be considered very favourable, since only 10 to 12 per cent of patients were found to be drug-resistant. Most of Gastaut's patients were on polytherapy. However, the efficacy of single drug-treatment has been documented.

* Phenobarbitone (PB) is the oldest drug still in use. Its efficacy is beyond doubt, even if, to our knowledge, no placebo-controlled trial has ever been undertaken. In a small prospective study, phenobarbitone was used to treat nine patients presenting with generalized tonic–clonic seizures alone. Eight were seizure-free over a period of 15 months (Feely *et al.*, 1980). Phenobarbitone still has a place in the modern treatment of epilepsy, especially in developing countries. Only 9 per cent of patients with primary generalized seizures are not helped by it (Watts, 1992). However, sedation and behavioural side-effects have led to a gradual shift away from phenobarbitone towards the use of other medications.

* Primidone (PRM): the evidence remains unclear as to whether primidone is more effective than phenobarbitone, but it may prove effective in some patients when other medications have failed (Smith, 1989).

* Phenytoin (PHT) is obviously effective in the control of patients with generalized tonic–clonic seizures (Reynolds *et al.*, 1981; Callaghan *et al.*, 1985), with 73 to 80 per cent of previously untreated patients becoming seizure free. However, in these two studies, as in others, the diagnosis of IGE is not certain.

* Several comparisons of phenytoin and valproate (VPA) as sole therapy in untreated patients with only primary generalized tonic–clonic seizures demonstrated a similar efficacy (Wilder *et al.*, 1983). No statistically significant difference between the two drugs was noted. However, some studies showed a trend towards a better efficacy of valproate. For instance, a 2 year remission rate was achieved in 73 per cent of patients on valproate and 56 per cent on phenytoin (Turnbull *et al.*, 1985), and a 6 month remission rate was reported in 64 per cent of patients on valproate and 53 per cent on phenytoin (Ramsay *et al.*, 1992). In the last study, the trend was magnified in the patient subpopulation with spike and wave abnormalities: 58 per cent and 37 per cent, respectively.

* The efficacy of carbamazepine against generalized tonic–clonic seizures has been documented in adults as well as in children (Parsonage *et al.*, 1980; Dulac *et al.*, 1983; Jeavons, 1983). However, it is probably less effective than phenytoin and valproate: 39 per cent of excellent control *vs.* 73 per cent and 59 per cent, respectively (Callaghan *et al.*, 1985).

* Soon after its first clinical use in France, valproate was recognized as a highly effective drug in idiopathic epilepsies (Pinder *et al.*, 1977). Pivotal studies demonstrated its efficacy as a sole drug in idiopathic generalized tonic–clonic seizures, giving a complete control of seizures in 73 per cent (Covanis *et al.*, 1982), 75 per cent (Feuerstein *et al.*, 1983) and 85 per cent (Bourgeois *et al.*, 1987) of patients. It was documented in children also (Dulac *et al.*, 1986). Valproate is at present the drug of first choice in idiopathic grand mal.

*   Investigational drugs: patients suffering from generalized tonic–clonic seizures are not usually admitted to clinical trials, for two reasons: (1) a seizure rate incompatible with classical designs, and (2) fear of occurrence of status epilepticus.

Absence seizures

*   Neither phenobarbitone, nor phenytoin, nor, later, carbamazepine proves effective against absence seizures.
*   Trimethadione, discovered in 1945, was the first anti-absence drug. However, trimethadione and paradione are both toxic.
*   In the 1960s, they were supplanted by ethosuximide (ESM). Comprehensive prospective studies demonstrated its efficacy in controlling absence seizures (Sherwin, 1989).
*   Absence seizures were the first indication for valproate. Double-blind studies in which ethosuximide was compared with valproate indicated that the two drugs were equally effective in controlling absence seizures (Sato et al., 1982). Valproate was even considered to be superior (Covanis et al., 1982). In a summary of five studies comparing the two, it is reported that complete control was achieved in 58 per cent of patients on ethosuximide and 65 per cent of those on valproate (Fromm & Crumrine, 1986). In current practice, valproate appears to be more effective. Complete control of absence seizures was achieved in 87 per cent (Feuerstein et al., 1983), 92 per cent (Dulac et al., 1986), and 95 per cent (Bourgeois et al., 1987) of patients.

    In the United States, however, ethosuximide remains the drug of first choice for absence seizures (Browne & Mirsky, 1983; Sherwin, 1989), on the principle that: 'If absence seizures are the sole seizure pattern, ethosuximide provides a relatively safe and effective form of monotherapy. If tonic–clonic seizures occur, ethosuximide can be readily combined with carbamazepine, phenytoin or others agents. Ethosuximide remains the contemporary drug of choice for children with typical absence seizures, in whom the potential hepatotoxicity of valproate is an important consideration' (Sherwin, 1989); and: 'The administration of prophylactic tonic–clonic antiepileptic drugs is of questionable value' (Browne & Mirsky, 1983). Conversely, we in Europe, consider that valproate as a sole drug is not hepatotoxic in the age range of absence seizures and is the drug of choice in this form of idiopathic generalized epilepsy. In clinical practice, individual patients may respond to one or the other drug in monotherapy. Other patients benefit from combined therapy (Rowan et al., 1983).

*   Benzodiazepines, including clonazepam, clobazam and others are also active in the control of absence seizures (Pinder et al., 1976; Gastaut & Low, 1979), but development of tolerance and frequent adverse effects relegate these agents to second place.
*   Fifteen to 20 per cent of patients with absence seizures are waiting for novel drugs. The place of lamotrigine has not yet been firmly established. It may become an important anti-absence drug, alone or in combination with valproate.

Myoclonic seizures

The assessment of the efficacy of drugs in myoclonic epilepsies is made difficult by a somewhat loose classification.

*   Valproate is the drug of first choice in benign myoclonic epilepsy in infants (Dulac et al., 1986; Dravet et al., 1992).
*   Phenobarbitone and primidone have been more effective than phenytoin in the treatment of juvenile myoclonic epilepsy: 67 per cent of patients on phenobarbitone, 82 per cent of patients on primidone, and 32 per cent on phenytoin became seizure free (Janz & Christe, 1992). Valproate is now the drug of first choice 'because it controls all the primary generalized seizure types characteristic of juvenile myoclonic epilepsy and has minimal

adverse effects' (Penry *et al.*, 1989). Complete control was achieved in 80 to 95 per cent of patients (Feuerstein *et al.*, 1983; Delgado-Escueta & Enrile-Bacsal, 1984; Janz & Christe, 1992). Clonazepam may be a useful concomitant drug when patients are not controlled by valproate alone (Obeid & Panayiatopoulos, 1989).

Photosensitive epilepsies

In these conditions valproate is the drug of choice (Bruni *et al.*, 1980; Jeavons *et al.*, 1986).

Long-term outcome

The question arises whether modern therapy changes the long-term outcome of IGEs. In other words, in suppressing seizures does the treatment improves the long-term prognosis? A century ago, Gowers suggested that seizures might be self-provoking, each one predisposing to the next. More recently, Reynolds and the King's College Group (Reynolds *et al.*, 1983) supported this hypothesis, stressing a contrast between the easy control of newly diagnosed epilepsies and the poor progonosis of chronic epilepsy.

Some epileptic syndromes, such as childhood absence epilepsy, tend to disappear with advancing age, regardless of whether or not medications are used. 'The tendency for petit mal to cease is present at all ages and not just at puberty. In about a quarter of patients, the attacks cease before the age of 15 years and, by the age of 30, petit mal has ceased in about three quarters of the patients . . . It was noted that the attacks became shorter and less frequent as the patient became older. . . the attacks faded away rather than stopped abruptly' (Gibberd, 1966). It is impossible to tell whether a favourable long-term outcome of treated childhood absence epilepsy reflects the natural history of the disorder, or whether early control affects the long-term prognosis. Absence seizures are thus probably not an appropriate example.

However, later in life, many patients with childhood absence epilepsy develop generalized tonic–clonic seizures. If the proportion of patients developing generalized tonic–clonic seizures were lower after a correct treatment than without it, one might assume that this treatment modified the natural course of the syndrome. In 1965, two studies gave an affirmative answer:

Livingston *et al.* (1965) published the results of a prolonged follow-up study of 100 patients with petit mal epilepsy, most of them with childhood absence epilepsy. The duration of follow-up ranged from 5 to 28 years. Tonic–clonic seizures developed in 21 of the 59 patients (35.6 per cent) who were treated with a major anticonvulsant drug in addition to anti-absence drugs, as against 33 of the 41 patients (80.5 per cent) treated with an anti-absence drug alone who developed tonic–clonic seizures. Bergamini *et al.* (1965) followed up 78 patients presenting with 'pure petit mal', i.e. childhood absence epilepsy, over periods ranging from 5 to 14 years. They considered that 46 patients had received an early and correct therapy, whereas 32 had received a late or incorrect therapy, or both. Only 14 (30 per cent) in the first group developed tonic–clonic seizures, *vs* 22 (68 per cent) in the second group.

In 1985, Dietrich *et al.* set out to determine whether modern therapy with ethosuximide and/or valproate, with or without other drugs, improves the long-term prognosis of absence epilepsies compared to former treatments. They concluded that an early and appropriate therapy improved the ultimate prognosis. However, the authors themselves emphasize the important methodological shortcomings of this retrospective study.

Hence, some indications favour the proposition that drugs might modify the outcome of childhood absence epilepsy; but to what extent is not clear. Are the patients better controlled with medication, or really cured without need of medication?

A different problem arises with juvenile myoclonic epilepsy. Recurrence of seizures remains a lifelong possibility. Even early control does not prevent relapses, when therapy is stopped, after many seizure-free years (Delgado-Escueta & Enrile-Bacsal, 1984; Janz & Christe, 1992). But we do not know the influence of drugs on the severity of the disorder, i.e. on the seizure rate.

Idiopathic generalized epilepsies are now so easily controlled that they no longer worry the specialist. However, intractable cases exist. One may ask if they are due to the disorder itself, or to late therapy. Large prospective studies would be of great help in assessing the influence of drugs on the long-term outcome. One might compare patients with childhood absence epilepsy treated early, with published data on the pre-valproate period. Another longitudinal study of patients with juvenile myoclonic epilepsy would be useful in assessing their outcome according to the moment of the beginning of the correct treatment, i.e. early, after the first generalized tonic–clonic seizures or even earlier, when only myoclonic jerks are present, or later, after numerous seizures.

Future prospects

Most currently available anti-epileptic drugs (AEDs) were discovered by testing new compounds in animal models of seizures; that is to say they were discovered almost by serendipity. A better understanding of the cellular and molecular mechanisms that underlie normal central nervous system function and seizure phenomena is now used in a mechanistic approach to drug discovery. Much new drug development is targeted at modulating the excitatory and inhibitory events playing a role in the onset and spread of epileptic discharges. For instance, the importance of intrinsic, voltage-dependent currents, and especially of calcium currents, in the pathophysiology of epileptic processes is well documented.

However, the outcome of epilepsies will not be very much affected by the availability of the drugs at present under investigation, either undergoing clinical testing, or awaiting final approval. No dramatic change can be expected.

An interesting approach would be to develop drugs acting at the beginning of the pathophysiological process, i.e. truly preventing the epilepsy. That appears to be possible in focal epilepsies. These epilepsies develop in areas of cortex that are damaged, either developmentally or by trauma or ischaemia. Restorative processes, axon sprouting, new synaptic formation and circuit reorganization occur. But they also are likely to produce local circuits that will be epileptogenic. Drugs interrupting these noxious processes would be real anti-epileptic drugs. However, idiopathic generalized epilepsies are different: they originate not from an acquired lesion, but from an inherited metabolic abnormality, for instance, insufficient $GABA_A$-ergic inhibition, excessive sodium current and/or T-calcium current, either in the cortical layers or in thalamic neurons, or noradrenergic hyperinnervation in the cortex. Multiple isoforms of sodium, calcium channels, of NMDA receptors and $GABA_A$-receptor channels, that have unique pharmacological and/or biophysical properties have been identified. The receptor and channel isoforms have discrete regions of distribution and various patterns of expression in the central nervous system. It has been shown that $GABA_A$-receptors with different combinations of subunits have distinct pharmacological properties. These findings suggest that anti-epileptic drugs that target specific receptors or channels may have more selective actions and, therefore, be less toxic. They explain why, due to their lack of specificity, the currently available calcium blockers are poor anti-epileptic drugs. Such very specific drugs, capable of modifying a specific function, will be difficult to find.

References

Aicardi, J. (1988): Epileptic syndromes in childhood. *Epilepsia* **29** (Suppl. 3), S1–S5.

Bergamini, L., Bram, S., Broglia, S. & Alessandro, R. (1965): L'insorgenza tardiva di crisi Grande Male nel Piccolo Male puro. Studio catamnestico di 78 casi. *Arch. Suisses. Neurol. Neurochir. Psychiatr.* **96**, 306–317.

Berkovic, S.F., Andermann, F., Andermann, E. & Gloor, P. (1987): Concepts of absence epilepsies: discrete syndromes or biological continuum? *Neurology* **37**, 993–1000.

Bourgeois, B., Beaumanoir, A., Blajev, B. *et al.* (1987): Monotherapy with valproate in primary generalized epilepsies. *Epilepsia* **28** (Suppl. 2), S8–S11.

Browne, T.R. & Mirsky, A.F. (1983): Absence (petit mal) seizures. In: *Epilepsy, diagnosis and management*, eds. T.R. Brown & R.G. Feldman, pp. 61–74. Boston: Little, Brown.

Bruni, J., Wilder, B.J., Bauman, A.W. & Willmore, L.J. (1980): Clinical efficacy and long-term effects of valproic acid therapy on spike and wave discharges. *Neurology* **30**, 42–46.

Callaghan, N., Kenny, R.A. & O'Neill, B. *et al.* (1985): A prospective study between carbamazepine, phenytoin and sodium valproate as monotherapy in previously untreated and recently diagnosed patients with epilepsy. *J. Neurol. Neurosurg. Psychiatry* **48**, 639–644.

Commission on Classification and Terminology of the International League Against Epilepsy (1989): Proposal for revised classification of epilepsies and epileptic syndromes. *Epilepsia* **30**, 389–399.

Covanis, A., Gupta, A.K. & Jeavons, P.M. (1982): Sodium valproate: monotherapy and polytherapy. *Epilepsia* **23**, 693–720.

Delgado-Escueta, A.V. & Enrile-Bacsal, F. (1984): Juvenile myoclonic epilepsy of Janz. *Neurology* **34**, 285–294.

Dietrich, E., Baier, W.K., Doose, H., Tuxhorn, I. & Fichsel, H. (1985): Long-term follow-up of childhood epilepsy with absences. I. Epilepsies with absences at onset. *Neuropediatrics*, **16**, 149–154.

Dravet, C., Bureau, M. & Roger, J. (1992): Benign myoclonic epilepsy in infants. In: *Epileptic syndromes in infancy, childhood and adolescence*, 2nd edn, eds. J. Roger, M. Bureau, Ch. Dravet, F.E. Dreifuss, A. Perret & P. Wolf, pp. 67–74. London: John Libbey.

Dreifuss, F.E. (1989): Classification of epileptic seizures and the epilepsies. *Pediatr. Clin. North Am.* **36**, 265–279.

Dulac, O., Bouguerra, L., Rey, E., de Lauture, D. & Arthuis, M. (1983): Monothérapie par la carbamazépine dans les épilepsies de l'enfant. *Arch. Fr. Pediatr.* **40**, 415–419.

Dulac, O., Steru, D., Rey, E., Perret, A. & Arthuis, M. (1986): Sodium valproate monotherapy in childhood epilepsy. *Brain Dev.* **8**, 47–52.

Feely, M., O'Callagan, M., Duggan, B. & Callaghan, N. (1980): Phenobarbitone in previously untreated epilepsy. *J. Neurol. Neurosurg. Psychiatry* **43**, 365–368.

Feuerstein, J., Revol, M., Roger, J., Sallou, C., Truelle, J.L. Vercelletto, P. & Weber, M. (1983): La monothérapie par le valproate de sodium dans les épilepsies généralisées primaires. *Sem. Hop. Paris* **59**, 1263–1274.

Fromm, G.H. & Crumrine, P. (1986): Ethosuximide: an update. In: *Recent advances in epilepsy 3*, eds. T.A. Pedley & B.S. Meldrum, pp. 279–294. Edinburgh: Churchill Livingstone.

Gastaut, H., Gastaut, J.A. & Gastaut, J.L. (1973): Epilepsie généralisée primaire grand mal. In: *Evolution and prognosis of epilepsies*, eds. E. Lugaresi, P. Pazzaglia & C.A. Tassinari, pp. 24–41. Milano: Aulo Gaggi.

Gastaut, H. & Low, M.D. (1979): Antiepileptic properties of clobazam, a 1–5 benzodiazepine in man. *Epilepsia* **20**, 437–446.

Gibberd, F.B. (1966): The prognosis of petit mal. *Brain* **89**, 531–538.

Holmes, G.L., Mc Keever, M. & Adamson, M. (1987): Absence seizures in children: clinical and electroencephalographic features. *Ann. Neurol.* **21**, 268–273.

Janz, D. & Christe, W. (1992): Generalized epilepsies. In: *The medical treatment of epilepsy*, eds. S.R. Resor & H. Kutt, pp. 145–162. New York: Marcel Dekker.

Jeavons, P.M. (1983) Monotherapy with sodium valproate and carbamazepine. In: *Research progress in epilepsy*, ed. F. Rose Clifford, pp. 406–412. Bath: Pitman.

Jeavons, P.M., Bishop, A. & Harding, G.F.A. (1986): The prognosis of photosensitivity. *Epilepsia* **27**, 569–575.

Livingston, S., Torres, I., Pauli, L.L. & Rider, R.V. (1965): Petit mal epilepsy. Results of a prolonged follow-up of 117 patients. *J.A.M.A.* **194**, 113–118.

Obeid, T. & Panayiotopoulos, C.P. (1989): Clonazepam in juvenile myoclonic epilepsy. *Epilepsia* **30**, 603–606.

Panayiotopoulos, C.P., Chroni, E., Daskalopoulos, Baker A., Rowlinson, S. & Walsh, P. (1992): Typical absence seizures in adults: clinical, EEG, video-EEG findings and diagnostic/syndromic considerations. *J. Neurol. Neurosurg. Psychiatry* **55**, 1002–1008.

Parsonage, M.J., Yeung, R. & Laljee, H.C.K. (1980): Clinical experience with carbamazepine in the treatment of grand mal epilepsy. In: *Epilepsy updated: causes and treatment*, ed. P. Robb, pp. 213–228. Chicago: Year Book.

Penry, J.K., Dean, J.C. & Riela, A.K. (1989): Juvenile myclonic epilepsy: long term response to therapy. *Epilepsia* **30** (Suppl. 4), S19–S23.

Pinder, R.M., Brogden, R.N., Speight, T.M. & Avery, G.S. (1976): Clonazepam: a review of its pharmacological properties and therapeutic efficacy in epilepsy. *Drugs* **12**, 321–361.

Pinder, R.M., Brogden, R.N., Speight, T.M. & Avery, G.S. (1977): Sodium valproate. A review of its pharmacological properties and therapeutic efficacy in epilepsy. *Drugs* **13**, 81–123.

Ramsay, R.E., Wilder, B.J., Murphy, J.V. *et al.* (1992): Efficacy and safety of valproic acid *vs* phenytoin as sole therapy for newly diagnosed primary generalized tonic–clonic seizures. *J. Epilepsy* **5**, 55–60.

Reynolds, E.H., Elwes, R.D.C. & Shorvon, S.D. (1983): Why does epilepsy become intractable? *Lancet* **ii**, 952–954.

Reynolds, E.H., Shorvon, S.D., Galbraith, A.W., Chadwick, D., Dellaportas, C.I. & Vydelingum, L. (1981): Phenytoin monotherapy for epilepsy: a long term prospective study, assisted by serum level monitoring, in previously untreated patients. *Epilepsia* **27**, 475–488.

Rowan, A.J., Meijer, J.W., De Beer-Pawlikowski, N., Van Der Greest, P. & Meinardi, H. (1983): Valproate-ethosuximide combination therapy for refractory absence seizures. *Arch. Neurol.* **40**, 797–802.

Sato, S., White, B.G., Penry, J.K., Dreifuss, F.E., Sackellares, J.C. & Kupferberg, H.J. (1982): Valproic acid *vs* ethosuximide in the treatment of absence seizures. *Neurology* **32**, 157–163.

Sherwin, A.L. (1989): Ethosuximide. Clinical use. In: *Antiepileptic drugs*, 3rd edn, eds. R. Levy *et al.* pp. 689–698. New York: Raven Press.

Smith, D.B. (1989): Primidone. Clinical use. In: *Antiepileptic drugs*, 3rd edn, eds. R. Levy *et al.*, pp. 423–438. New York: Raven Press.

Turnbull, D.M., Howel, D., Rawlins, M.D. & Chadwick, D.W. (1985): Which drug for the adult epileptic patient: phenytoin or valproate? *Br. Med. J.* **290**, 815–819.

Watts, A.E. (1992): The natural history of untreated epilepsy in a rural community in Africa. *Epilepsia* **33**, 464–468.

Wilder, B.J., Ramsay, R.E., Murphy, J.V., Karas, B.J., Marquardt, K. & Hammond, E.S. (1983): Comparison of valproic acid and phenytoin in newly diagnosed tonic–clonic seizures. *Neurology* **33**, 1474–1476.

Chapter 36

Seizures induce molecular and morphological changes in rat brains

Alfonso Represa, Jérôme Niquet, Hélène Pollard, Joëlle Moreau, Michel Khrestchatisky and Yehezkel Ben-Ari

INSERM U29, 123 Boulevard Port Royal, 75014 Paris, France

Introduction

Epilepsy may be considered as an ongoing process in which repeated seizures may have an important impact on brain and subsequently account for the evolution of this pathology. Thus, different reports demonstrated that seizures set in motion a cascade of complex molecular and genomic changes, including modification of receptor expression, that may contribute to the abnormally increased neuronal excitability and be responsible for the development of seizure-induced neuronal lesions. Furthermore, seizures may induce a glial reaction and synaptic remodelling which, by generating recurrent excitatory neuronal networks, may also increase the neuronal activity and contribute to the maintenance of the epilepsy. Such processes have been particularly well analysed in models of focal, secondarily generalized epilepsy, such as those induced by the administration of convulsant agents (e.g. kainic acid (KA)) or by electric stimulation of limbic pathways (kindling, electrolytic shocks), but have also been studied in models of generalized tonic–clonic seizures induced by the administration of pentrylenetetrazole or bicuculline.

Seizure-induced changes may be rapid and transient (i.e. increased expression of transcription factors, trophic factors, neurotransmitter receptors), or may be delayed and long lasting (i.e. neuronal lesion, glial reaction and neosynaptogenesis), so that they may be separated into two major phases: an induction phase and a reinforcement or maintenance phase (Fig. 1). *During the induction phase*, the expression of some genes occurs rapidly and often transiently. It is assumed that the effects of these alterations are reversible, provided that stimulations are kept within a range close to normal. If not, repeated and/or powerful stimulations of a given neuronal circuit may set into motion a cascade of molecular events which may induce irreversible and eventually deleterious modifications in neurons. The *maintenance phase* is characterized by the consolidation of the epileptic process and the recurrence of seizures. The study of such processes is of interest in order to better understand the mechanisms underlying focal epilepsy, and is in addition of general interest to better understand the consequences of seizures in brain.

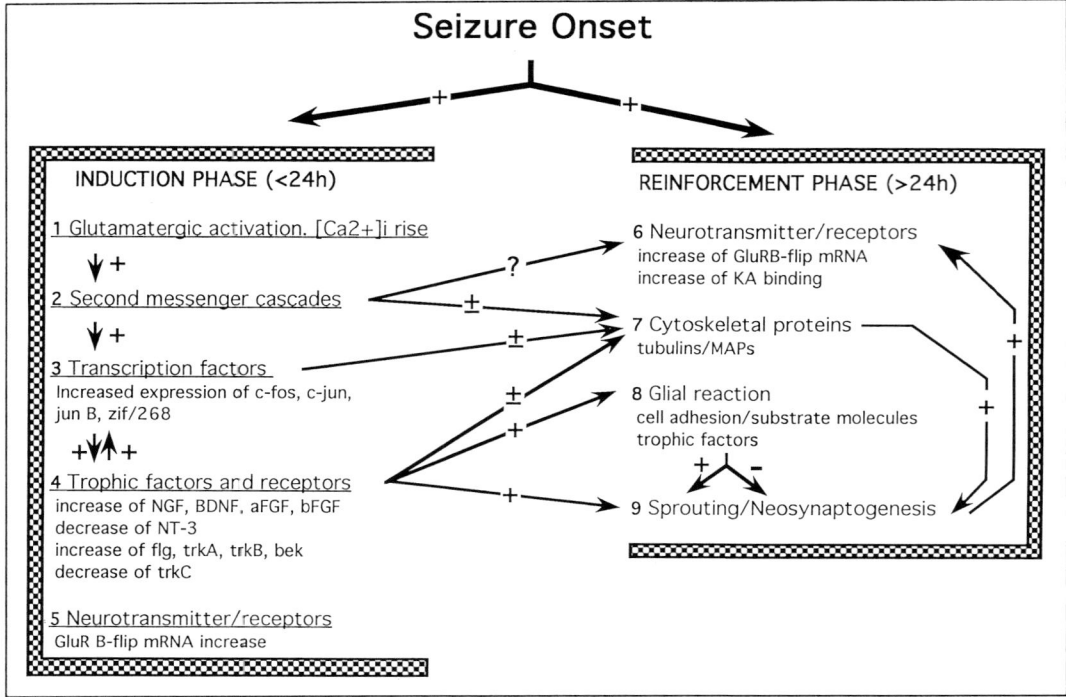

Fig. 1. Seizures set in motion molecular and morphological changes, which may be early and transient (induction phase) or delayed and long-lasting (reinforcement phase). Some of these changes are likely to be connected (arrows) and may constitute different links in the process which lead from seizures to glial and synaptic remodelling.

Early changes induced by seizures (induction phase)

Excitatory neurotransmitter glutamate is involved in bursting activity

Different procedures or chemicals generate synchronized bursts in hippocampus. They include train stimulus (Anderson et al., 1987), repetitive electrical stimulation (kindling; Slater et al. (1985)) or the application of various convulsive agents including high K$^+$ solution (Korn et al., 1987; Ben-Ari & Gho, 1988), mast cell degranulating peptide (Cherubini et al., 1988), reduced Mg^{2+} concentrations (Walther et al., 1986), α-tubocurarine (Johnston & Brown, 1984) and GABA$_A$ receptor channel blockers (Fischer & Alger, 1984). These bursts are driven by giant post-synaptic excitatory potentials (i.e. are not endogenous pacemaker events), as demonstrated on hippocampal slices maintained *in vitro*. They are blocked by glutamate receptor antagonists of amino-hydroxy-methyl-isoxazolepropionic acid (AMPA) type (Traub & Wong, 1982; Miles & Wong, 1986; Ben-Ari & Gho, 1988), receptors that mediate fast synaptic neurotransmission (Mayer & Westbrook, 1987).

Interestingly, in CA3, a brief epileptiform episode produces a long-lasting enhancement of synaptic responses (Ben-Ari & Gho, 1988) which is reminiscent of long-term potentiation (LTP). Thus, after a short application of a convulsant (e.g. 3–5 min of kainic acid) a further stimulation of hippocampal inputs will generate, instead of the usual single excitatory post-synaptic potential (EPSP) followed by an inhibitory one, an EPsp followed by a burst (Ben-Ari & Gho, 1988). This evoked response persists for several hours after removal of the drug. Furthermore, in this process, as in long-term potentiation, there is no persistent change in intrinsic cell properties or in inhibition mediated through GABA$_A$ receptors. Also, as in long-term potentiation, the long-lasting change induced by the convulsants, involves the activation of glutamatergic receptors of NMDA (N-methyl-D-aspartate) type. Thus, application of NMDA receptor antagonists simultaneously with the convulsant results in spontaneous synchronized bursts, but prevents the long-lasting change. NMDA receptors are characterized by slow rise time in synaptic transmission, voltage-dependent block by Mg^{2+} and high Ca^{2+} permeability. Because their channels carry Ca^{2+}, NMDA receptors may be actively involved in the calcium-mediated activation of molecular cascades, including increased gene expression (see below).

To summarize, the initial phases of the seizures is most likely to result from an accumulation of glutamate in the extracellular space of neurons. The enhanced release and/or reduced uptake of glutamate leads to increased activation of glutamatergic receptors. While the induction of this process requires the activation of NMDA receptors, it is largely mediated by an increase of the post-synaptic AMPA receptor responses (Müller et al., 1988; Staubli et al., 1992). This observation may also suggest that quantitative and/or qualitative modifications of glutamate receptors may contribute towards increasing the neuronal excitability as described below.

Seizures induce a rapid activation of transcription and trophic factors

Increased intracellular Ca^{2+} levels generated by glutamatergic-receptor activation and voltage-dependent calcium channels, stimulate transduction mechanisms involving second messenger cascades – including phosphorylation – and lead to the activation of existing but quiescent transcription factors (Greenberg et al., 1986). This results in a rapid and often massive increase in the expression of genes encoding other transcription factors like c-fos, c-jun, jun B and zif/268. The expression of such immediate early genes was indeed strongly increased after limbic or generalized seizures (see Kiessling & Gass (1993) for a review). Some of these factors as well as many others, yet to be identified, may interact in a daunting number of transcription complexes which will determine positive or negative regulation of the promoter sequences of numerous effector genes. Remarkably, the transcription of genes enconding nerve growth factor (NGF) and brain-derived neurotropic factor (BNDF) (Gall & Isackson, 1989; Zafra et al., 1990; Ernfors et al., 1991) is also rapidly induced) while the expression of neurotrophin-3 (NT-3) is decreased. Changes in neurotrophin receptors (trkA and trkB, which are membrane-associated tyrosine kinases) have also been reported. Even very brief seizure episodes (a few seconds) are sufficient to induce these transcriptional modifications. It has been shown that these mRNA increases result in increased protein levels. More recently, we have shown (Bugra et al., 1994) that the mRNA levels for basic and acidic fibroblast growth factors (bFGF and aFGF) and one of their receptors, flg, are also increased following KA-induced seizures. Importantly, we have shown that these inductions are seizure dependent, since anticonvulsant treatment prior to administration of kainic acid prevents alterations of the mRNA levels. Interestingly, the most rapid induction of bFGF mRNA levels occurs in area CA1, where pyramidal neurons are not prone to cell death in epileptic rats, at least in kindled rats or in rats injected with KA in the amygdala. Various data suggest that aFGF and bFGF may actively participate in hippocampal cell survival as well as in sprouting and neosynaptogenesis: (i) in the adult brain, FGF concentration is four times that of nerve growth factor; (ii) aFGF and one of its receptors, flg are abundantly expressed in pyramidal and granular layers of the hippocampus (Wanaka et al., 1990; Wilcox & Unnerstall, 1991); (iii) during development, aFGF expression coincides with the formation of granular and pyramidal cell connections; (iv) in vitro, fibroblast growth factors are active in enhancing the survival and neurite outgrowth of hippocampal primary cultures (Walicke et al., 1986).

Although these increases are globally described as rapid, time courses vary between factors (anywhere from 30 min to 24 h) as well as between the neuronal types and brain regions examined. This suggests that signal transduction mechanisms may differ in neurons of distinct networks, but also that the combined effects of these factors may vary spatially and temporally, eliciting a wide variety of responses spanning from survival and sprouting to cell death. Indeed, it is unlikely that a single

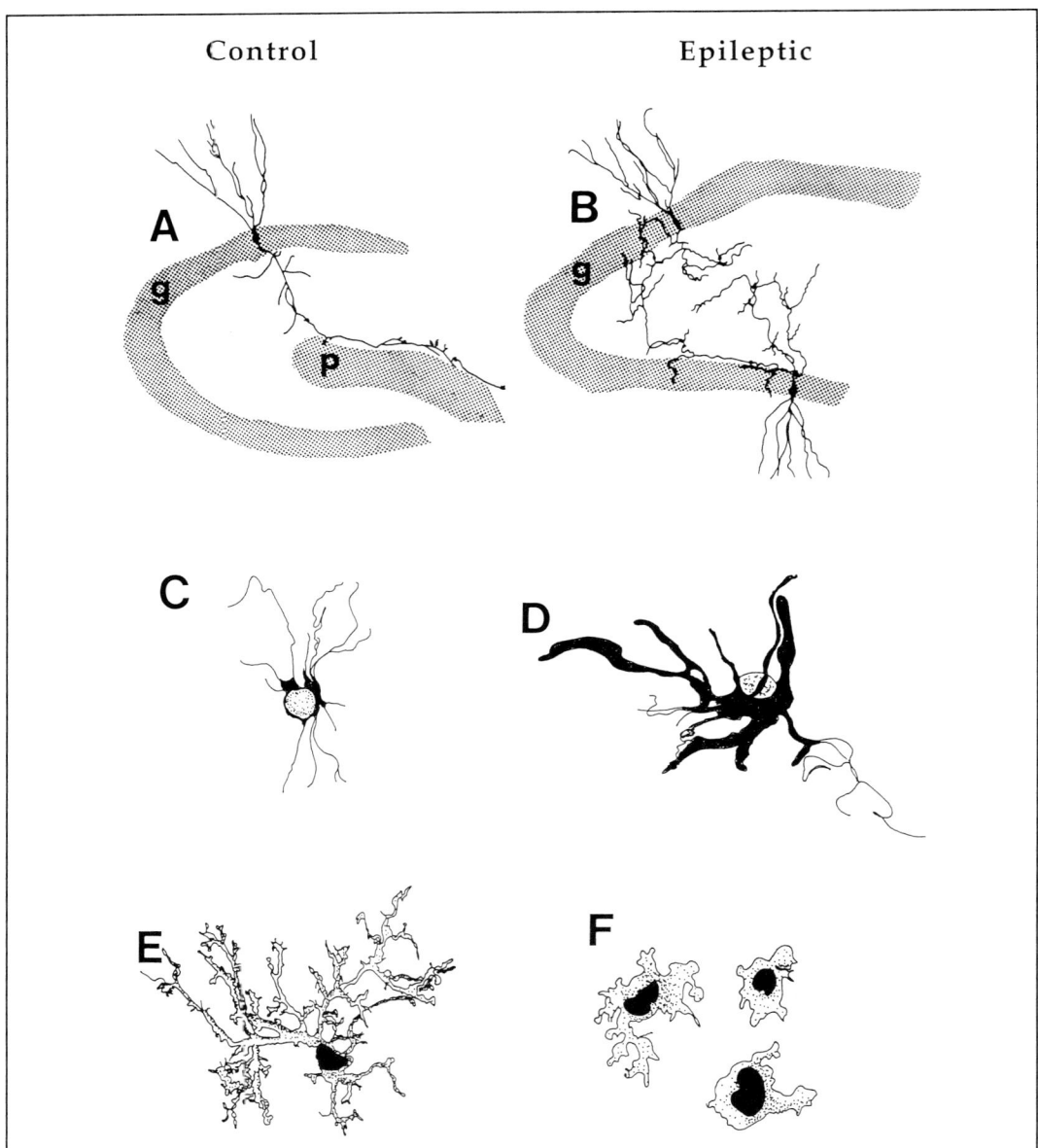

Fig. 2. KA-induced seizures generate morphological changes in rat hippocampus. The present camera lucida reconstruction demonstrates: A,B: a collateral sprouting of mossy fibres (Golgi impregnation of control (A) or epileptic (B) dentate gyrus. Dotted lines represent the granule cell layer (g) or the pyramidal cell layer (p); the latter was destroyed after seizures. C,D: An astroglial hypertrophy. Astrocytes were stained with GFAP antibodies. As compared with control astrocytes (C) hippocampal astrocytes developed larger and more intensely immunostained extensions after seizures. These astrocytes were also A2B5 immunoreactive, suggesting that in epileptic rats hippocampal astrocytes acquire the phenotypic features of type 2-astrocytes. E,F: An activation of microglial cells. These cells were stained with MRC OX-42 antibody. In control rats (E) stained cells have the ramified configuration of resting microglial cells. After treatment with the convulsant agent kainate (F) immunoreactive cells acquire the amoeboid configuration of activated macrophages.

factor will promote survival or that the absence – or over-expression – of another will induce cell death. A detailed study of the expression kinetics and spatial distributions of the trophic factors following seizures may yield precious information on which combinations bring about these responses.

It is known that the promoter of the NGF gene carries regulatory elements for the c-fos/c-jun dimer (Hengerer et al., 1990). In addition, recent data obtained in our laboratory (Ferhat et al., 1993) indicate that in pyramidal neurons, bFGF very rapidly (15–30 min) modulates the expression of genes encoding transcription factors. The aforementioned use-dependent up-regulation of NGF, BDNF, aFGF and bFGF expression as well as that of some of the receptors for these growth factors, linked to their crucial role in neuronal development and survival and in modulating gene expression, strongly suggests that in the initial phases of neuronal stimulation, an interplay of transcription and growth factors may be critical in initiating the subsequent events leading to sustained hyperactivity and eventually to axonal sprouting and synaptic remodelling (see below).

Delayed changes induced by seizures (maintenance phase)

Seizures generate neuronal cell loss and glial reaction

Intracerebral injection of kainic acid, which is a powerful convulsant analogue of glutamate, induces neuronal cell loss associated with glial reaction at the site of the injection (Ben-Ari, 1985; Anderson et al., 1991; Dusart et al., 1991; Marty et al., 1991; Finsen et al., 1993; Jorgensen et al., 1993). This is characterized by a clear hypertrophy of astrocytes and microglia-macrophages and an apparent increase in the number of stained cells. These changes may result from both an extravasation of peripheral blood marrow cells and an eventual glial cell proliferation *in situ*, within the injured field.

In addition to the local effects of the neurotoxin, neuronal degeneration and glial changes occur in brain structures located at a distance from the injection of kainic acid. Thus, when kainic acid is injected into the amygdala, a pathological alteration develops in the hippocampus (Ben-Ari et al., 1979; Ben-Ari et al., 1980; Okazaki & Nadler, 1988). This lesion is characterized by the loss of CA3-CA4 pyramidal cells and hilar interneurons. This cell loss starts as early as 12 h after the injection of the convulsants and develops within the first 3 days. Seizure-induced neuronal cell loss may have necrotic features (cell picnosis, vacuolization and membrane leaking), but may also have some apoptotic features (i.e. laddering pattern of DNA segmentation (Pollard et al. (1994a)). It is interesting to note that fos expression is abnormally persistent in cells suffering programmed cell death after ischaemia (Smeyne et al., 1993), and that in epilepsy, vulnerable pyramidal cells also show a more delayed expression of this oncogene.

In conclusion, the presently described observations suggest that different mechanisms of cell death may be responsible for the seizure-induced damage. Neuronal cell death after seizures is associated with astroglial hypertrophy measured with glial fibrillary acid protein (GFAP) antibodies (Represa et al., 1993b) (Fig. 2d) and astroglial proliferation demonstrated with proliferation cell markers such as ^{3}H-thymidine incorporation (unpublished results). Besides astrocytes, there is also an important change in microglial–macrophagic cells. Thus, microglial cells proliferate *in situ*, at the level of cell loss, and acquire the typical ameboid morphology of activated macrophages (Fig. 2F). In contrast, oligodendrocytes do not proliferate in the hippocampus of these animals. In agreement with previous observations (Ben-Ari, 1985), this hippocampal damage is seizure related and not induced by diffusion of the drug. Thus, hippocampal lesion is avoided when animals are pre-treated with anticonvulsant drugs (i.e. diazepam, Ben-Ari et al. (1979)) or when propagation of the abnormal activity to the hippocampus is prevented by cutting off various inputs to this structure (i.e. mossy fibres (Okazaki & Nadler, (1988)).

In a previous report (Represa et al., 1993b) we demonstrated that reactive astrocytes in the hippocampus of kainic-acid-treated rats acquire new properties, such as the expression of immunoreactivity to A2B5 (antibodies that *in vitro* labelled the 0–2A lineage: precursor cells; type-2 astrocytes and oligodendrocytes (Raff *et al.*, 1983). These results may suggest that resident astrocytes in the hippocampus are transformed to type 2-like astrocytes after convulsions. Nevertheless, one can suggest that a new cell lineage from resident precursor cells or adult astrocytes develop after kainic acid treatment; the newly developing cells then express immunoreactivity to antibodies which are usually expressed, at least *in vitro*, by immature cells. In agreement with this hypothesis is the fact that hippocampal reactive astrocytes also express immunoreactivity against embryonic neural cell adhesion molecules (Le Gal La Salle *et al.*, 1992). Nevertheless A2B5 immunoreactivity is observed not only in proliferating astrocytes but in resident reactive astrocytes also (unpublished results) and we have never observed the presence of precursor 0–2A cells in the hippocampus of epileptic animals (Represa *et al.*, 1993b).

Similar hippocampal cell loss has been evoked by repeated electric stimulation of hippocampal afferences (Cavazos & Sutula, 1990) and seems to be a common event after severe seizures in rats. Previous reports also demonstrated a similar loss of CA4-hilar neurons in hippocampal tissue from patients with temporal lobe epilepsy (Falconer *et al.*, 1964; Margerison & Corsellis, 1966; Mouritzen Dam, 1980). Unfortunately the glial cell reaction has not yet been well analysed in other models of epilepsy or in human epileptic tissue, and we do not know if these glial changes constitute a common change induced by seizures in brain. Whatever it may be, it should be of interest to determine if reactive astrocytes acquire new and different functional properties. They may regulate the extracellular ionic equilibrium and glutamate uptake and metabolism in a different way than normal resting astrocytes. Gliosis, which may be a common event in epilepsy, would therefore play a much more important role in paroxymal discharges than that so far suspected.

Seizures increase the expression of cytoskeletal proteins and induce reactive sprouting of hippocampal mossy fibres

Microtubule protein expression changes after seizures

In the days following seizures, we have also observed alterations of the genes encoding cytoskeletal proteins (Represa *et al.*, 1993c) known to be active components of microtubule formation and neurite extension. The levels of mRNAs encoding tubulin increase in the dentate granule cell bodies after 3 days of kainic acid treatment and peak on day 12. These changes correlate with an enhancement of α-tubulin immunoreactivity in both granule cell dendrites and mossy fibres (MF), already noticeable 4 days after kainic acid.

In addition we recently observed that 6–12 days after kainic acid the mRNA encoding for the microtubule-associated protein MAP2 as well as MAP2 immunoreactivity are also selectively enhanced in the dendrites of granule cells. The mRNA encoding for the microtubule-associated protein TAU is increased in granule cells, whereas TAU immunoreactivity is increased in mossy fibres and granule cells and granule cell bodies within the same time (Pollard *et al.*, 1994b). The levels of mRNA and protein immunoreactivity return to control values by 20 and 30 days after kainic acid treatment, respectively.

Seizures induce collateral and terminal sprouting of mossy fibres

In the fascia dentata of both kindled and KA-treated rats we observed a collateral sprouting of mossy fibres (Represa *et al.* 1993a). In fact, numerous branches originating from mossy fibres in the hilus distribute within the polymorph cells layer or pass through the granule cell layer to reach the inner third of the molecular layer (Represa *et al.*, 1993a) (Fig. 2B). Similar sprouting has been demonstrated after generalized tonic–clonic seizures (Golarai *et al.*, 1992).

The granule cells of epileptic rats show a normal dendritic arborization. Some impregnated neurons (about 10 per cent of impregnated cells) display clusters of giant excrescences in their primary and/or secondary dendrites. In some impregnated granule cells from KA-treated rats, clear giant thorny excrescences have been observed (Represa et al., 1993a).

In the fascia dentata of epileptic animals (in both kindled and KA-treated rats), giant synaptic boutons develop in the inner third of the molecular layer. These boutons have all the characteristic features of mossy boutons, giant size, complex shape, multiple synaptic contacts with complex dendritic spines, high density of synaptic vesicles, desmosome-like contacts with dendritic shafts or other mossy fibre boutons, and post-synaptic spines embedded in the bouton (Represa et al., 1993a). This strongly suggests that sprouted collateral mossy fibres do establish synaptic contacts with granule cell dendrites.

We now have evidence that experimental epilepsy is associated with sprouting of MF not only in the fascia dentata (Tauck & Nadler, 1985; Represa et al., 1987; Sutula et al., 1988; Represa et al., 1989; Sutula et al., 1989; Represa et al., 1993a) but also in the infrapyramidal band of CA3 (Represa & Ben-Ari, 1992). This terminal sprouting only develops in epileptic rats which do not have CA3 degeneration (i.e. kindled rats). This sprouting is also associated with the formation of ectopic, axo-spinous mossy fibre synapses with basilar dendrites of CA3 pyramidal neurons. The difference between control and kindled is significant ($P < 0.01$) and may represent 7.2 additional asymmetric synaptic contacts for each neuron (since each mossy fibre bouton made 3.82 ± 2.7 synaptic contacts with 3.4 ± 1.7 spines, Represa & Ben-Ari (1992)).

The first manifestations of mossy fibre sprouting have been observed in rats 10–12 days after the initial treatment. Thus, in rats killed 3 or 7 days after injection of kainic acid, no signs of collateral sprouting were detected either with Timm staining or with Golgi impregnations. The maximum degree of mossy fibre sprouting seems to be reached 2 weeks later (around 30 days after the treatment), so that this sprouting develops between the second and fourth week after seizure onset. This point is of interest since the changes observed in microtubule proteins (see above) precede the initiation of branching and sprouting and are maintained during the period of greater axonal outgrowth. Therefore we suggest that the production and stabilization of tubulin polymers with TAU contribute to both the initiation of the sprouting and to the axonal growth and side-branching of mossy fibres. The dendritic increase of tubulin and MAP2, which also develops during the period of synapse formation, may be related to a local synthesis involved in the formation of post-synaptic specializations during neosynaptogenesis.

Synaptogenesis in adult brain is reminiscent of developmental synaptogenesis

Tubulin heterogeneity is mainly generated at the level of transcription and differentially regulated during development. Thus, $T\alpha_1$-tubulin mRNA is expressed at high levels in the developing nervous system and decreases significantly by adulthood (Lewis et al., 1986; Miller et al., 1987). This expression correlates with the process of neurite outgrowth (Miller et al., 1987). In contrast, T26 tubulin mRNA is expressed in neurons at a level and time consistent with the maintenance of the microtubule framework (Miller et al., 1987). In our recent report (Pollard et al., 1994b), we depicted an increased expression of the 'immature' tubulin isoform in epileptic animals. This result agrees with previous reports (Hoffman & Cleveland, 1988; Miller et al., 1989; Tetzlaff et al., 1991) showing a rapid induction of $T\alpha_1$-tubulin mRNA in rat motoneurons or sensory neurons after nerve crush. Taken together, these results support the notion that synaptic remodelling in adulthood depends on re-expression of developmental programmes (also see Hoffman & Cleveland, 1988). Further analysis would clarify this point.

Consequences of MF sprouting and synaptogenesis

Several lines of evidence strongly support a major role for mossy fibres in the induction and propagation of epileptic discharges and underlying pathological changes (Ben-Ari, 1985; Okazaki & Nadler, 1988). In fact, limbic motor seizures and the subsequent sclerosis of Ammon's horn do not develop before the maturation of mossy fibres has taken place (Nitecka et al., 1984). The destruction of mossy fibres (by γ-ray irradiation or colchicine injection) also has a protective effect on adult animals, since status epilepticus fails to be produced and pyramidal cells do not degenerate in such animals (Okazaki & Nadler, 1988).

It is therefore likely that an aberrant and enhanced mossy fibre synaptogenesis may impair hippocampal function and contribute to the maintenance of the epilepsy (Tauck & Nadler, 1985). The increased number of mossy fibres synapses represents at least an amplification of the excitatory signal impinging on CA3 neurons or on granule cells. Since each mossy fibre will innervate a greater number of target cells in epileptic patients, mossy fibres sprouting would facilitate their synchronization.

Though not compelling, previous data indeed suggested that sprouting and development of recurrent excitatory circuits increase granule cell excitability. Thus, in hippocampal slices from epileptic rats, antidromic stimulation of mossy fibres elicits multiple population spikes in granule cells, in contrast to the single population spikes obtained in control slices (Tauck & Nadler, 1985). A positive correlation between the intensity of mossy fibre sprouting analysed by Timm staining and the frequency of spontaneous epileptic seizures in KA-treated rats has been described (Cronin & Dudek, 1988). In kindled rats density of sprouting was also found to be correlated with the amplitude of evoked after-discharges (Sutula et al., 1992). In conclusion, these data strongly support the hypothesis that seizure-induced synaptic remodelling increases the hippocampal excitability and contributes to the development of new seizure episodes.

Glutamatergic receptor changes after seizures

It is interesting to note that KA-induced seizures dramatically alter the expression of genes encoding subunits of the glutamate receptor of the AMPA type, designated $GluR_{A\ to\ D}$ (or $GluR_{1\ to\ 4}$) (Boulter et al., 1990; Keinänen et al., 1990). For each subunit, alternative splicing of the mRNA yields variants named flip and flop, with distinct expression patterns during development as well as in the adult brain (Sommer et al., 1990; Monyer et al., 1991). *In vitro* expression studies show that the flip and flop modules different pharmacological and kinetic properties on currents generated by glutamate and AMPA, the flip versions allowing more current entry into cells. Homomeric or heteromeric receptors composed of $GluR_1$ and $GluR_3$ ($GluR_A$ and $_C$ respectively) display inward calcium currents while those composed of $GluR_2$ ($GluR_B$) show no such Ca^{2+} permeability (Hollmann et al., 1991). We have found that the levels and the alternative splicing of the $GluR_B$ mRNA are differentially altered in distinct areas of the hippocampus. KA-induced epilepsy provokes a rapid (3 h) but transient increase of $GluR_B$ flip mRNA levels in CA1, CA3 and dentate gyrus (Fig. 3). This early phase is followed by a second one characterized by (i) a persistent $GluR_B$ flip increase in regions in which neurons are known to be seizure-resistant (i.e. CA1 and dentate gyrus) and (ii) a large decrease in the vulnerable CA3 area (Fig. 3). In keeping with the properties of GluR flip variants, our results suggest that altered AMPA receptor subunit stoichiometry may lead to a rapid and long-lasting enhanced efficiency of fast synaptic transmission in the epileptic hippocampus. Since AMPA receptors deprived of $GluR_B$ are Ca^{2+} permeable, our results also suggest increased Ca^{2+} permeability in the pyramidal neurons of CA3, which are known to be vulnerable in the epileptic hippocampus, but not in CA1 or dentate gyrus. Similar observations have been reported in kindled rats (Kamphuis et al., 1992).

Hence, while the short, transient increase in $GluR_B$ flip mRNA may participate in the induction process, the second increase observed 24 h after the onset of seizures is likely to be sustained for days or even weeks, subserving enhanced fast synaptic transmission which perpetuates the events described above.

In regard to the repercussion of mossy fibre sprouting it is interesting to note that in epileptic rats it is associated with a selective increased binding of ^3H-kainate. In fact, kainic acid binding sites are significantly increased in the molecular layer of both kindled and KA-treated rats (up to 30 per cent as compared to control rats (Represa et al., 1987, 1989). Furthermore, in the stratum oriens of

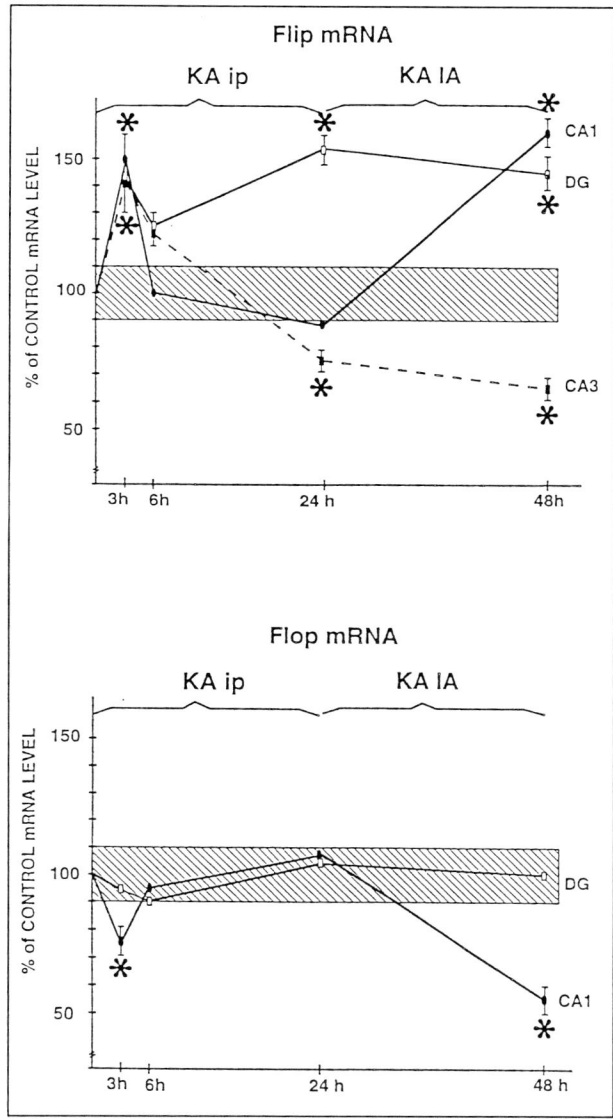

Fig. 3. Modifications of GluR-B flip and flop mRNA levels in hippocampal subfields as a function of time following KA induced seizures. In each panel, values are plotted as per cent (± SEM) of optical densities measured from saline-treated rats (by intraperitoneal (ip) or intra-amygdaloid (IA) route) on autoradiograms. A general transient increase in the GluR-B flip variant is observed in the hippocampus, 3 hours after KA-ip. Significant increases in GluR-B flip expression in the granule cell layer of the dentate gyrus (DG) and a concomitant decrease in the pyramidal cell layer of the CA3 subfield are observed later (24 and 48 h after the KA treatments). In the same areas, flop expression is either unchanged (DG) or decreased (CA1).
*$P < 0.05$ (Student's t-test) as compared to control values.

CA3, kainic acid binding dramatically increases after kindling and forms an ectopic band of labelling (Represa et al., 1989). These changes in binding are without effect on the affinity constant and are likely to reflect an increase in the mean number of kainic acid receptors. The increased density of kainic acid receptors will promote further excitability of the hippocampal circuitry.

To conclude, though the stoichiometry of glutamate receptors is not yet well understood, it seems clear that the different subunits cloned up to now may confer different functional properties on the receptors, mainly in calcium permeability. These changes may develop in the absence of other histopathological alterations and may be induced by the paroxysmal activity. A better understanding of such changes would help the search for new antiepileptic drugs.

Conclusions

In conclusion, seizures set in motion a complex number of molecular and morphological changes in vulnerable structures such as the hippocampal complex. A number of these changes are responsible for the lesion and scanning of brain tissue. Others will permanently disturb certain neuronal networks so that they may contribute to the maintenance of the epileptic process and in addition account for the clinical evolution of the pathology. Though most of these observations mainly apply to focal – secondarily generalized or not – forms of epilepsy, the presently described modifications may also be the consequence of generalized seizures.

Although the molecular and cellular changes described here have been characterized in experimental animals, preliminary studies of resected hippocampi from human temporal lobe epilepsy have found similar changes. The morphological analysis of such material with *in situ* hybridization and immunohistochemistry, combined with stereo-electroencephalography and clinical studies, will provide interesting information on the functional consequences of degenerative and regenerative processes which occur after seizures.

References

Anderson, P.-B., Perry, V.H. & Gordon, S. (1991): The kinetics and morphological characteristics of the macrophage–microglial response to kainic acid-induced neuronal degeneration. *Neuroscience* 42, 201–214.

Anderson, W.W., Swartzwelder, H.S. & Wilson, W.A. (1987): The NMDA receptor antagonist 2-amino-phosphonovalerate blocks stimulus train-induced epileptogenesis but not epileptiform bursting in the rat hippocampal slice. *J. Neurophysiol.* 57, 1–21.

Ben-Ari, Y. (1985): Limbic seizures and brain damage produced by kainic acid: mechanisms and relevance to human temporal lobe epilepsy. *Neuroscience* 14, 375–403.

Ben-Ari, Y. & Gho, M. (1988): Long-lasting modification of the synaptic properties of rat CA3 hippocampal neurones induced by kainic acid. *J. Physiol.* 404, 365–384.

Ben-Ari, Y., Tremblay, E. & Ottersen, O.P. (1980): Injection of kainic acid into the amygdaloid complex of the rat: an electrographic, clinical and histological study in relation to the pathology of the epilepsy. *Neuroscience* 5, 515–528.

Ben-Ari, Y., Tremblay, E., Ottersen, O.P. & Naquet, R. (1979): Evidence suggesting secondary epileptogenic lesion after kainic acid: pretreatment with diazepam reduces distant but not local brain damage. *Brain Res.* 165, 362–365.

Boulter, J., Hollmann, M., O'Shea-Greenfield, A., Hartley, M., Deneris, E., Maron, C. & Heinemann, S. (1990): Molecular cloning and functional expression of glutamate receptor subunit genes. *Science* 249, 1033–1037.

Bugra, K., Pollard, H., Charton, G., Moreau, J., Ben-Ari, Y. & Khrestchatisky, M. (1994): $_a$FGF, $_b$FGF and flgm RNAs show distinct patterns of induction in the hippocampus following kainate-induced seizures. *Eur. J. Neurosci.* 6, 58–66.

Cavazos, J.E. & Sutula, T.P. (1990): Progressive neuronal loss induced by kindling: a possible mechanism for mossy fiber synaptic reorganization and hippocampal sclerosis. *Brain Res.* 527, 1–6.

Cherubini, E., Neuman, R.S., Roviara, C. & Ben-Ari, Y. (1988): Epileptogenic properties of the mast cell degranulating peptide in CA3 hippocampal neurons. *Brain Res.* 445, 91–100.

Cronin, J. & Dudek, F.E. (1988): Chronic seizures and collateral sprouting of dentate mossy fibers after kainic acid treatment in rats. *Brain Res.* 474, 181–184.

Dusart, I., Marty, S. & Peschanski, M. (1991): Glial changes following an excitotoxic lesion in the CNS. II: astrocytes. *Neuroscience* **45**, 541–549.

Ernfors, P., Bengzon, J., Kokaia, Z., Persson, H. & Lindvall, O. (1991): Increased levels of messenger RNAs for neurotrophic factors in the brain during kindling epileptogenesis. *Neuron* **7**, 165–176.

Falconer, M.A., Serafetinides, E.A. & Corsellis, J.A. (1964): Etiology and pathogenesis of temporal lobe epilepsy. *Arch. Neurol.* **19**, 233–248.

Ferhat, L., Krestchatisky, M., Roisin, M.P. & Barbin, G. (1993): Basic Fibroblast growth factor-induced increase in zif/268 and c-fos mRNA levels is Ca^{2+}-dependent in primary cultures of hippocampal neurons. *J. Neurochem.* **61**, 1105–1112.

Finsen, B.R., Jorgensen, M.B., Diemer, N.H. & Zimmer, J. (1993): Microglial MHC expression after ischemic and kainic acid lesions of the adult rat hippocampus. *Glia* **7**, 41–49.

Fischer, R.S. & Alger, B.E. (1984): Electrophysiological mechanisms of kainic acid induced epileptiform activity in the rat hippocampal slice. *J. Neurosci.* **4**, 1312–1323.

Gall, C.M. & Isackson, P.J. (1989): Limbic seizures increase neuronal production of messenger RNA for nerve growth factor. *Science* **245**, 758–761.

Greenberg, M.E., Ziff, E.B. & Greene, L.A. (1986): Stimulation of neuronal acetylcholine receptors induces rapid gene transcription. *Science* **234**, 80–83.

Golarai, G., Cavazos, J.E. & Sutula, T.P. (1992) Activation of the dentate gyrus by pentylenetetrazol evoked seizures induces mossy fiber synaptic reorganization. *Brain Res.* **593**, 257–264.

Hengerer, B., Lindholm, D., Heumann, R., Ruther, U., Wagner, E.F. & Thoenen, H. (1990): Lesion-induced increase in nerve growth factor mRNA is mediated by cfos. *Proc. Natl. Acad. Sci. USA* **87**, 3899–3903.

Hoffman, P.N. & Cleveland, D.W. (1988): Neurofilament and tubulin expression recapitulates the developmental program during axonal regeneration: induction of a specific β-tubulin isotype. *Proc. Natl. Acad. Sci. USA* **85**, 4530–4533.

Hollmann, M., Hartley, M. & Heinemann, S. (1991): Ca^{2+} permeability of KAAMPA-gated glutamate receptor channels depends on subunit composition. *Science* **252**, 851–853.

Johnston, D. & Brown, T.H. (1984): Mechanisms of neuronal burst generation. In: *Electrophysiology of epilepsy*, pp. 227–301. New York: Academic press.

Jorgensen, M.B., Finsen, B.R., Jensen, M.B., Castellano, B., Diemer, N.H. & Zimmer, J. (1993): Microglial and astroglial reactions to ischemic and kainic acid-induced lesions of the adult rat hippocampus. *Exp. Neurol.* **120**, 70–88.

Kamphuis, W., Monyer, H., De Rijk, T.C. & Lopes da Silva, F.H. (1992): Hippocampal kindling increases the expression of glutamate receptor–A Flip and B-Flip mRNA in dentate granule cells. *Neurosci. Lett.* **148**, 51–54.

Keinänen, K., Wisden, W., Sommer, B., Werner, P., Herb, A., Verdoorn, T.A., Sakmann, B. & Seeburg, P.H. (1990): A family of AMPA-selective glutamate receptors. *Science* **249**, 556–560.

Kiessling, M. & Gass, P. (1993): Immediate early gene expression in experimental epilepsy. *Brain Pathol.* **3**, 381–393.

Korn, S.J., Giacchino, J.L., Chamberlin, N.L. & Dingledine, R. (1987): Epileptiform burst activity induced by potassium in the hippocampus and its regulation by GABA-mediated inhibition. *J. Neurophysiol.* **57**, 325–340.

Le Gal La Salle, G., Rougon, G. & Valin, A. (1992): The embryonic form of neural cell surface molecule (E-NCAM) in the rat hippocampus and its reexpression on glial cells following kainic acid-induced status epilepticus. *J. Neurosci.* **12**, 872–882.

Lewis, S.A., Villasante. A., Sherline, P. & Cowan, N. (1986): Brain specific expression of MAP2 detected using cloned cDNA probe. *J. Cell Biol.* **102**, 2098–2105.

Margerison, J.H. & Corsellis, J.A.N. (1966): Epilepsy and the temporal lobes: a clinical, electroencephalographic and neuropathological study of the brain in epilepsy, with particular reference to the temporal lobes. *Brain* **89**, 499–530.

Marty, S., Dusart, I. & Peschanski, M. (1991): Glial changes following an excitotoxic lesion in the CNS-I. Microglia/macrophages. *Neuroscience* **45**, 529–539.

Mouritzen Dam, A. (1980): Epilepsy and neuron loss in the hippocampus. *Epilepsia* **21**, 617–629.

Mayer, M.L. & Westbrook, G.L. (1987): The physiology of excitatory amino acids in the vertebrate central nervous system. *Prog. Neurobiol.* **28**, 197–276.

Miles, R. & Wong, R.K.S. (1986): Excitatory synaptic interactions between CA3 neurons in the guinea-pig hippocampus. *J. Physiol.* **373**, 371–373.

Miller, F.D., Naus, C.C.G., Durant, M., Bloom, F.E. & Milner, R.J. (1987): Isotypes of α-tubulin are differentially regulated during neuronal maturation. *J. Cell. Biol.* **105**, 3065–3073.

Miller, F.D., Tezlaff, W., Bisby, M.A., Fawcett, J.W. & Milner, R.J. (1989): Rapid induction of the major embryonic α-tubulin mRNA, Tα1, during nerve regeneration in adult rats. *J. Neurosci.* **9**, 1452–1463.

Monyer, H., Seeburg, P.H. & Wisden, W. (1991): Glutamate- operated channels: developmentally early and mature forms arise by alternative splicing. *Neuron* **6**, 799–810.

Müller, D., Joly, M. & Lynch, G. (1988): Contributions of quisqualate and NMDA receptors to the induction and expression of LTP. *Science* **242**, 1694–1697.

Nitecka, L., Tremblay, E., Charton, G., Bouillot, J.P., Berger, M.L. & Ben-Ari, Y. (1984): Maturation of kainic acid seizure-brain damage syndrome in the rat. II Histopathological sequelae. *Neuroscience* **13**, 1073–1094.

Okazaki, M.M & Nadler, J.V. (1988): Protective effects of mossy fiber lesions against kainic acid-induced seizures and neuronal degeneration. *Neuroscience* **26**, 763–781.

Pollard, H., Cantagrel, S., Charriaut-Marlangue, C., Moreau, J. & Ben-Ari, Y. (1994a): Apoptosis associated DNA fragmentation in epileptic brain damage. *Neuro. Report* **5**, 1053–1055.

Pollard, H., Khrestchatisky, M., Moreau, J., Ghilini, G., Ben-Ari, Y. & Represa, A. (1994b): Correlation between reactive sprouting and microtubule protein expression in epileptic hippocampus. *Neuroscience* **61**, 773–784.

Raff, M.C., Miller, R.H. & Noble, M. (1983): A glial progenitor cell that develops *in vitro* into an astrocyte or an oligodendrocyte depending on culture medium. *Nature* **303**, 390–396.

Represa, A. & Ben-Ari, Y. (1992): Kindling is associated with the formation of novel mossy fiber synapses in the CA3 region. *Exp. Brain Res.* **92**, 69–78.

Represa, A., Jorquera, I., Le Gal La Salle, G. & Ben-Ari, Y. (1993a): Epilepsy induced collateral sprouting of hippocampal mossy fibers: does it induce the development of ectopic synapses with granule cell dendrites? *Hippocampus* **3**, 257–268.

Represa, A., Le Gall La Salle, G. & Ben-Ari, Y. (1989): Hippocampal plasticity in the kindling model of epilepsy in rats. *Neurosci. Lett.* **99**, 345–350.

Represa, A., Niquet, J., Charriaut-Marlangue, C. & Ben-Ari, Y. (1993b): Reactive astrocytes in the KA-damaged hippocampus have the phenotypic features of type-2 astrocytes. *J. Neurocytol.* **22**, 299–310.

Represa, A., Pollard, H., Moreau, J., Ghilini, G., Krestchatisky, M. & Ben-Ari, Y. (1993c): Mossy fiber sprouting in epileptic rats is associated with a transient increased expression of α-tubulin. *Neurosci. Lett.* **156**, 149–152.

Represa, A., Tremblay, E. & Ben-Ari, Y. (1987): Kainate binding sites in the hippocampal mossy fibers: Localization and plasticity. *Neuroscience* **20**, 739–748.

Slater, N.T., Stelzer, A. & Galvan, M. (1985): Kindling-like stimulus patterns induce epileptiform discharges in the guinea pig *in vitro* hippocampus. *Neurosci. Lett.* **60**, 25–31.

Smeyne, R.S., Vendrell, M., Hayward, M., Baker, S.J., Miao, G.G., Schilling, K., Robertson, L.M., Curran, T. & Morgan, J.I. (1993): Continuous c-fos expression precedes programmed cell death *in vivo*. *Nature* **363**, 166–169.

Sommer, B., Keinänen, K., Verdoorn, T.A., Wisden, W., Burnashev, N., Herb, A., Köhler, M., Takagi, T., Sakmann, B. & Seeburg, P.H. (1990): Flip and flop: a cell-specific functional switch in glutamate-operated channels of the CNS. *Science* **249**, 1580–1585.

Staubli, U., Ambros-Ingerson, J. & Lynch, G. (1992): Receptor changes and LTP: an analysis using aniracetam, a drug that reversibly modifies glutamate (AMPA) receptors. *Hippocampus* **2**, 49–58.

Sutula, T., Cascino, G., Cavazos, J., Parada, I. & Ramirez, L. (1989): Mossy fiber synaptic reorganization in the epileptic human temporal lobe. *Ann. Neurol.* **26**, 321–330.

Sutula, T.P., Golarai, G. & Cavazos, J. (1992): Assessing the functional significance of mossy fiber sprouting. *Epilepsy Res.* **Suppl. 7**, 251–257.

Sutula, T., Xiao-Xian, H., Cavazos, J. & Scott, G. (1988): Synaptic reorganization in the hippocampus induced by abnormal functional activity. *Science* **239**, 1147–1150.

Tauck & Nadler, J.V. (1985) Evidence for functional mossy fiber sprouting in hippocampal formation of kainic acid treated rats. *J. Neurosci.* **5**, 1016–1022.

Tetzlaff, W., Alexander, S.W., Miller, F.D. & Bisby, M.A. (1991): Response of facial and rubrospinal neurons to axotomy: changes in mRNA expression for cytoskeletal proteins and GAP-43. *J. Neurosci.* **11,** 2528–2544.

Traub, R.D & Wong, R. (1982): Cellular mechanism of neuronal synchronization in epilepsy. *Science* **216,** 745–747.

Walicke, P.A., Cowan, W.M., Ueno, N., Baird, A. & Guillemin, R. (1986): Fibroblast growth factor promotes survival of dissociated hippocampal neurons and enhances neurite extension. *Proc. Natl. Acad. Sci. USA* **83,** 3012–3016.

Walther, H., Lambert, J.D.C., Jones, R.S.G., Heinemann, U. & Hamon, B. (1986): Epileptiform activity in combined slices of the hippocampus, subiculum and entorhinal cortex during perfusion with low magnesium medium. *Neurosci. Lett.* **69,** 156–161.

Wanaka, A., Jonson, E.M. & Milbrandt, J. (1990): Localization of FGF receptor mRNA in the adult central nervous system by *in situ* hybridization. *Neuron* **5,** 267–281.

Wilcox, B.J. & Unnerstall, J.R. (1991): Expression of acidic fibroblast growth factor mRNA in the developing and adult rat brain. *Neuron* **6,** 397–409.

Zafra, F., Hengerer, B., Leibrock, J., Thoenen, H. & Lindholm, D. (1990): Activity dependent regulation of BDNF and NGF mRNAs in the rat hippocampus is mediated by non-NMDA glutamate receptors. *EMBO J.* **9,** 3545–3550.

Chapter 37

Possible mechanisms of action of first choice drugs for the treatment of idiopathic generalized epilepsies

P.E. Keane[*] & D. Broglin[†]

[*]*Sanofi Recherche, 195 Route d'Espagne, 31036 Toulouse Cedex, France;* [†]*Clinique Paul Castaigne, Groupe Hospitalier Pitié-Salpêtrière, 47–83 Blvd de l'Hôpital, 75651 Paris Cedex 13, France and Sanofi Winthrop, 9 Rue du Président Allende, 94258 Gentilly Cedex, France*

Generalized idiopathic epilepsies consist of a variety of diverse syndromes characterised by different types of generalized seizures (convulsive: myoclonic or tonic–clonic, or non-convulsive: absences), ages of onset, and EEG features. In the absence of a precise aetiological understanding of any of the human seizure disorders, drug therapy has been directed at the control of the symptoms, i.e. the suppression of seizures. Both clinical observations and experimental studies have nevertheless shown clear differences in the profiles of the first choice drugs for the treatment of generalized idiopathic epilepsies (Table 1; see also Macdonald (1989), and Rogawski & Porter (1990)). Thus, phenytoin, carbamazepine and valproate appear as the drugs of choice in generalized tonic–clonic (as well as partial) seizures, whereas ethosuximide and trimethadione are without effect. Although not drugs of first choice, phenobarbital and benzodiazepines are also used for treatment of generalized tonic–clonic seizures. Valproate, clonazepam and, to a lesser extent, phenobarbital are effective against myoclonic seizures, whereas phenytoin, carbamazepine, ethosuximide and trimethadione are not. Finally, generalized absence seizures are improved by ethosuximide, trimethadione, valproate and clonazepam, but not by phenytoin or carbamazepine.

A large number of hypotheses have been proposed to explain the antiepileptic efficacy of these compounds, and it is difficult to determine which effects may be serious contenders for mechanisms of action, and which are only epiphenomena. The object of the present review is to look separately at the antiepileptics used for the treatment of idiopathic generalized epilepsies, and to determine to what extent they may share pharmacological effects which could be the basis of a common mechanism of action against the seizures observed in these types of epilepsy.

Generalized tonic–clonic seizures

In studying this class of seizures, we should determine whether there exist any pharmacological effects that are shared by phenytoin, carbamazepine and valproate, but not by ethosuximide or trimethadione. Phenytoin exerts a wide variety of pharmacological actions on neurons, many of which are possible mechanisms of anticonvulsant activity. The most widely studied of these actions in recent years, however, has been the interaction of phenytoin with the voltage-dependent inward Na^+ currents that are responsible for the action potential upstroke. Phenytoin modifies this system in a highly specific voltage- and frequency-dependent manner.

Table 1. *Efficacy of classical antiepileptic drugs on different types of seizures of idiopathic generalized epilepsies*

Antiepileptic drug	Generalized tonic–clonic	Myoclonic	Generalized absence
Phenytoin	++	–	–
Carbamazepine	++	–	–
Valproate	++	++	++
Phenobarbital	++	+	–
Clonazepam	+	++	+
Ethosuximide	–	–	++
Trimethadione	–	–	++

Toman (1949) was the first to show that phenytoin could block high-frequency repetitive firing of the frog sciatic nerve, without, however, modifying the first action potential of the series. More recent studies have confirmed that phenytoin inhibits high-frequency repetitive firing of mammalian central neurons in culture at clinically relevant concentrations (McLean & Macdonald, 1983). This effect of phenytoin was shared by both carbamazepine and valproate, also at therapeutically relevant concentrations (McLean & Macdonald, 1986). All three antiepileptics shared several important properties. The block of repetitive firing was voltage-dependent, as it could be reversed by sustained membrane hyperpolarization. The block was also use-dependent, the first action potential being unaltered, while the second and successive action potentials were progressively reduced in amplitude, or suppressed. Finally, the effect was time-dependent. In contrast to these three antiepileptics that were effective against generalized tonic–clonic seizures, ethosuximide did not modify high-frequency repetitive firing (McLean & Macdonald, 1986).

Differences do, however, occur between the effect of valproate and those of phenytoin and carbamazepine. Phenytoin and carbamazepine can block batrachotoxin-induced influx of $^{22}Na^+$ into synaptosomes (Willow et al., 1984), and displace [^{3}H]batrachotoxin binding to Na^+ channels on synaptosomes (Willow & Catterall, 1982). Their mechanism of action is at present considered to be by binding to the inactivated form of the Na^+ channels, and reducing the rate of recovery of the channel from the inactivated to the resting, activable state. In contrast, valproate does not share these effects on [^{3}H]batrachotoxin binding and $^{22}Na^+$ influx (Willow & Catterall, 1982; Willow et al., 1984), and therefore may act at a different site. Another hypothesis for the mechanism of action of valproate in generalized tonic–clonic seizures remains possible in view of the activity of phenobarbital and the benzodiazepines against this type of seizure, as all three potentiate the transmission at $GABA_A$ receptors (see below), a possible anatomical site for this action being the substantia nigra (see e.g. Depaulis et al., 1994).

Generalized myoclonic seizures

The most effective antiepileptics for this seizure category are generally considered to be valproate, clonazepam and, to a lesser extent, phenobarbital, the other major antiepileptics being ineffective. The principal molecular effect of the benzodiazepines is the allosteric potentiation of the effects of the inhibitory neurotransmitter γ-amino-butyric acid (GABA) at the $GABA_A$ receptor. This has been shown by many laboratories both in terms of electrophysiological responses (Choi et al., 1977; Macdonald & Barker, 1978) and of the binding of GABA to this receptor (Skerrit & Johnston, 1983).

Barbiturates also potentiate the interaction of GABA with the $GABA_A$ receptor; but the site of action of this effect differs from that of the benzodiazepines (Olsen & Snowman, 1982). In electrophysiological terms, whereas benzodiazepines increase the frequency of GABA-induced chloride channel openings, barbiturates do not modify this parameter, but prolong the duration of each channel opening, so that there is a greater chloride passage per burst (Study & Barker, 1981).

The outcome of the potentiation of the post-synaptic effects of GABA at $GABA_A$ receptors is an increased inhibition of the post-synaptic neurone. Valproate has also been shown to potentiate the inhibitory effects of GABA and the $GABA_A$ receptor agonist muscimol, both *in vitro* (Macdonald & Bergey, 1979; Harrison & Simmonds, 1982) and *in vivo* (Schmutz *et al.*, 1979; Gent & Phillips, 1980; Kerwin *et al.*, 1980), although some studies have not found this result (McLean & Macdonald, 1986). At first, this effect of valproate was discounted as a possible antiepileptic mechanism, as Harrison & Simmonds (1982) found it was necessary to use very high concentrations of valproate (≥ 1 mM) to potentiate the effects of GABA in rat cuneate nucleus slices, whereas the generally accepted range of therapeutic free valproate concentrations is much lower (~ 20–200 μM). More recently, however, Olpe *et al.* (1988) have found that valproate could potentiate the post-synaptic effects of GABA and muscimol in locus coeruleus slices *in vitro* at therapeutically relevant concentrations (50 μM and above). Nevertheless, the significance of this effect of valproate will remain dubious until it is demonstrated that valproate can potentiate endogenous, i.e. synaptically evoked, inhibitory responses (Capek & Esplin, 1990)

The molecular mechanism by which valproate potentiates the effects of GABA is not known, but differs from that of the benzodiazepines and barbiturates in that valproate does not modify the binding characteristics of GABA or muscimol to the $GABA_A$ receptor, nor interfere with associated binding sites at concentrations below 500 μM (see Chapman *et al.*, 1982a). In our present state of knowledge, it is only possible to speculate on the mechanisms underlying this effect of valproate. In contrast to the barbiturates, benzodiazepines and valproate, the other first choice antiepileptics have not been shown to potentiate the effects of GABA (Macdonald, 1989). This may explain their inefficacy against myoclonic seizures.

Generalized absence seizures

Effective treatment of generalizd absence seizures can be obtained using valproate, ethosuximide, or, more rarely, trimethadione, whereas phenytoin, carbamazepine and phenobarbital are unable to improve this seizure type. No single pharmacological effect is known today to be shared by the anti-absence drugs, so the possibility remains that multiple mechanisms of action are responsible for anti-absence activity.

The most likely mechanism of action of ethosuximide is its ability to reduce the low-threshold, T-type calcium current. This effect has been observed both in primary afferent neurons, and in thalamic neurons (Coulter *et al.*, 1989a). The latter site of action may well be involved in the antiepileptic effect of ethosuximide, in view of the importance of thalamocortical circuitry in the production of the EEG abnormalities of absence seizures. The active metabolite of trimethadione, dimethadione, also reduces T-type calcium currents, while succinimide and other non-antiepileptic analogues of ethosuximide do not (Coulter *et al.*, 1989b). Initial studies showed that valproate could not modify the T-type calcium current of thalamic neurons (Coulter *et al.*, 1989b), but more recently, Kelly *et al.* (1990) have found that valproate is able to reduce T-type calcium currents in the nodose ganglion. The effect of valproate was small, however (a maximum of about 15 per cent inhibition), and occurred at concentrations above the therapeutic range (≥ 250 μM), so that its relevance for anti-absence mechanisms remains unclear (Macdonald & Kelly, 1993).

Another possible anti-absence mechanism may involve γ-hydroxybutyrate (GHB). This compound has long been known to produce absence-like spike-and-wave discharges when administered to rats, an effect which was aggravated by phenytoin and carbamazepine, but reduced by ethosuximide, trimethadione and valproate (Snead, 1988). Interest in a possible role of γ-hydroxybutyric acid in the pathological processes underlying absence seizures has increased with the appearance of publications suggesting a possible physiological role of γ-hydroxybutyric acid as a neuromodulator.

γ-Hydroxybutyric acid has been found to be an endogenous substance in the brain (Roth & Giarman, 1970), and heterogeneously distributed binding sites for this compound have also been described in the brain (Benavides et al., 1982; Snead & Liu, 1984). Furthermore, uptake (Hechler et al., 1985) and release of γ-hydroxybutyric acid have been described in rat brain slices (Maitre et al., 1983).

Both ethosuximide and valproate have been found to reduce the release of [^{3}H]GHB from rat hippocampal slices, albeit at concentrations somewhat above the therapeutic range (Vayer et al., 1987a). γ-Hydroxybutyric acid has also been described to produce post-synaptic effects, such as an increase in cGMP in the rat hippocampus (Vayer et al., 1987b), and a decrease in the cerebellum and thalamus (Bernasconi et al., 1992). This effect of γ-hydroxybutyric acid can also be antagonized by valproate (Vayer et al., 1987b) and ethosuximide (Vayer et al., 1988). The ability to reduce the post-synaptic effects of γ-hydroxybutyric acid could constitute a possible mechanism of anti-absence activity, if it is considered that a hyperactivity of endogenous GHB-mediated neuromodulation contributes to the pathological processes underlying the occurrence of absence seizures (Vayer et al., 1988). Unfortunately, no data have yet been published concerning the effects of dimethadione on the release or post-synaptic effects of γ-hydroxybutyric acid. Such studies might help to reinforce (or undermine) the γ-hydroxybutyric acid hypothesis.

GABAergic processes have also been implicated in the effects of anti-absence compounds, albeit in a complex manner. In animal models of absence seizures, the direct stimulation of $GABA_A$ receptors (by administering receptor agonists, or GABA transaminase (GABA-T) inhibitors) aggravates absence seizures (Vergnes et al., 1984). Similarly, clinical studies show that the GABA-T inhibitor vigabatrin also aggravates the occurrence of absence seizures (Grant & Heel, 1991). Conversely, allosteric potentiation of $GABA_A$-receptor activity (e.g. by benzodiazepines) actually reduces them (Marescaux et al., 1984). Further studies are clearly necessary to resolve this apparent paradox. The only action of ethosuximide that has been described on GABA processes is the ability to reduce GABA receptor mediated effects at therapeutic concentrations (Barnes & Dichter, 1984). The ability of valproate to potentiate post-synaptic $GABA_A$ receptor stimulation, mentioned above, is not the only effect of this drug on GABA processes. Many studies have shown that valproate increases whole brain and synaptosomal GABA levels (see Chapman et al., 1982a). These effects were initially attributed to the inhibition of the enzymes GABA-T or succinic-semialdehyde-dehydrogenase (SSA-DH), which are responsible for the degradation of GABA. However, subsequent studies have suggested that the situation is more complex. A number of studies have shown that the rate of synthesis of GABA is reduced in brain tissue after the administration of valproate (Bernasconi, 1982; Chapman et al., 1982b), although an increased synthesis rate has been described in the substantia nigra (Löscher, 1989).

More recently, two independent studies have found that valproate reduces GABA release into the extracellular space, at doses that are pharmacologically active in animal models of anti-absence activity (up to 200 mg/kg i.p., see e.g. Marescaux et al., 1992a), and at concentrations in the therapeutic anti-absence range. Biggs et al. (1992) showed that 100 mg/kg i.p. valproate significantly reduced extracellular GABA in the rat hippocampus, using a dialysis method, and Wolf and colleagues found that therapeutic concentrations of valproate, perfused locally via a push–pull cannula into the pre-optic area (Wolf et al., 1988), and the substantia nigra (Wolf & Tscherne, 1994), also significantly reduced extracellular GABA concentrations. Based upon the known ability of valproate to enhance the effects of GABA on post-synaptic $GABA_A$ receptors (see above), Wolf & Tscherne (1994) suggested that valproate reduced GABA release by potentiating the negative feedback effect of the transmitter on presynaptic $GABA_A$ autoreceptors. The overall consequence of this would be that, while valproate increases the effects of GABA at the post-synaptic $GABA_A$ receptor, it would concomitantly reduce GABAergic neurotransmission at post-synaptic $GABA_B$ receptors. This phenomenon could be relevant to the antiabsence effect of valproate, as a role for the activation of $GABA_B$ receptors has recently been postulated in the generation of the spike-and-wave EEG discharges characteristic of absence seizures. The $GABA_B$ agonist baclofen increases EEG spike-and-wave discharges in spontaneously epileptic rats, and induced this EEG abnormality in non-epileptic rats (Marescaux et al., 1992a). Furthermore, the $GABA_B$ receptor antagonist CGP 35348 suppressed the spike-and-wave EEG discharges (Marescaux et al., 1992b). It is thus possible that valproate might reduce absence seizures by indirectly reducing GABAergic transmission at the level of $GABA_B$ receptors. There is indeed evidence that valproate treatment can lead to a reduced neurotransmission at $GABA_B$ receptors. When a receptor's stimulation is reduced over a long period, a frequent occurrence is the upregulation of the receptor, and chronic valproate treatment has been shown to upregulate $GABA_B$ receptors (Lloyd et al., 1985; Motohashi, 1992)

Discussion

The object of the present review has been to determine to what extent there may be common mechanisms of action of the antiepileptic drugs that are active against each of the three major categories of seizures which characterize idiopathic generalized epilepsies. It should be pointed out that although this approach may lead to a clearer view of what is happening in the various epileptic processes, it nevertheless relies heavily on mechanisms of action which are as yet still unproven. The tentative conclusions of this review are summarized in Table 2.

Table 2. Possible mechanisms of action of antiepileptics for the treatment of different types of seizures of idiopathic generalized epilepsies

Tonic–clonic seizures	(a) $\downarrow Na^+$ currents (PHT, CBZ, VPA)
	(b) Allosteric $\uparrow$ GABA transmission (BZ, VPA, PhB)
Myoclonic seizures	Allosteric $\uparrow$ GABA transmission (BZ, VPA, PhB)
Absence seizures	(a) $\downarrow$ T-type Ca^{2+} currents (ESM, TMD)
	(b) $\downarrow$ γ-hydroxybutyrate transmission (VPA, ESM)
	(c) Effect on GABA transmission
	(i) allosteric modulation of $GABA_A$ transmission (VPA, BZ)
	(ii) $\downarrow$ $GABA_B$ transmission (VPA, $GABA_B$ antagonists)

BZ= benzodiazepines; CBZ = carbamazepine; ESM = ethosuximide; PhB = phenobarbital; PHT = phenytoin; TMD = trimethadione; VPA = valproate.

For both the generalized tonic–clonic, and the generalized myoclonic seizures, it has been possible for researchers to find pharmacological effects which are common to the first choice antiepileptic drugs used in their treatment, and which appear to be able to explain an antiepileptic action. Thus, in the case of tonic–clonic seizures, the first choice drugs phenytoin, carbamazepine and valproate all reduce sustained repetitive firing without modifying single action potentials, while the antiepileptics which are without efficacy against this class of seizure (ethosuximide, trimethadione) do not. First choice drugs for the treatment of myoclonic seizures (valproate, clonazepam, phenobarbital) can all potentiate GABAergic neurotransmission at the $GABA_A$ receptor (and this might also explain the effects of these three drugs on tonic–clonic seizures), whereas the antiepileptics inactive against myoclonia (phenytoin, carbamazepine, ethosuximide, trimethadione) do not.

For the third type of seizure belonging to idiopathic generalized epilepsies, the absence seizure, it has not been possible to find a single phenomenon that is known to be shared by the first choice drugs, although several candidate mechanisms appear interesting. The most likely candidate for the mechanism of action of ethosuximide and trimethadione (via its active metabolite, dimethadione) appears to be the antagonism of the low-threshold T-type calcium currents in thalamic neurons, while valproate may act by indirectly reducing GABAergic transmission at $GABA_B$ receptors. Despite the clear differences between the hypotheses that ethosuximide and trimethadione act via T-type calcium channels, and valproate via reduced $GABA_B$ transmission, there is some evidence that these pharmacological targets could constitute different links in the same circuitry involved in the generation of spike-and-wave discharges, and thus lead to the same final effect (see e.g. Marescaux et al., 1992a). Absence seizures are generally considered to involve the production of rhythmic activities by thalamocortical neuronal circuits (Gloor & Fariello, 1988). Thalamic neurons can generate repeated bursts of action potentials because they create rhythmic low-threshold calcium currents, via the T-type calcium channel (Coulter et al., 1989a). Once opened, T-type channels become inactivated, and require a long-lasting hyperpolarization to reverse their inactivation (Coulter et al., 1989a). The activation of $GABA_B$ receptors in the thalamus produces a long-lasting inhibitory post-synaptic potential which may participate in the reactivation of the T-type calcium channel (Crunelli & Leresche, 1991; Marescaux et al., 1992a). Thus, there is reason to believe that a reduction of neurotransmission via $GABA_B$ receptors by valproate might maintain T-type calcium channel inactivation, and produce, more indirectly, the same ultimate effect as direct T-type channel inhibition by ethosuximide or dimethadione. If this hypothesis were to be confirmed by subsequent studies, it would provide an elegant explanation of how different mechanisms of action could lead to the same antiepileptic effect. An alternative hypothesis is that these compounds may prevent absence seizures via the antagonism of a hyperactive endogenous epileptogenic system mediated by γ-hydroxybutyric acid. The credibility of this concept will largely depend on the validation of the physiological and/or pathological roles of γ-hydroxybutyric acid in the brain.

In conclusion, it may be possible to understand the profiles of activity of the major antiepileptic drugs within the context of a few different but well-defined mechanisms of action. Some of the first-choice antiepileptics may act predominantly on only one type of generalized seizure, due to the specificity of the mechanisms underlying each seizure type. Others may act on more than one type of seizure, either because they have a single mechanism of action which is common to more than one kind of seizure, or alternatively because they have multiple mechanisms of action (on different functional systems, or having different effects on a single system, e.g. by potentiating $GABA_A$ receptor processes while attenuating those related to $GABA_B$ receptors, as may be the case for valproate). Our present concepts are mainly based upon a study of the pharmacological effects of the major antiepileptics, but it remains necessary to demonstrate the exact links between these mechanisms and those responsible for the epileptic phenomena themselves.

References

Barnes, D.M. & Dichter, M.A. (1984): Effects of ethosuximide and tetramethylsuccinimide on cultured cortical neurons. *Neurology*, **34**, 620–65.

Benavides, J., Rumigny, J.F., Bourguignon, J.J., Cash, C., Wermuth, C.G., Mandel, P., Vincendon, G. & Maitre, M. (1982): High affinity binding site for γ-hydroxybutyric acid in rat brain. *Life Sci.* **30**, 953–961.

Bernasconi, R. (1982): The GABA hypothesis of affective illness: influence of clinically effective antimanic drugs on GABA turnover. In: *Basic mechanisms in the action of lithium*, eds. H.M. Emrich, J.B. Aidenhoff & H.D. Lux, pp. 183–192. Oxford: Excerpta Medica.

Bernasconi, R., Lauber, J., Marescaux, C., Vergnes, M., Martin, P., Rubio, V., Leonhardt, T., Reymann, N. & Bittiger, H. (1992): Experimental absence seizures: potential role of γ-hydroxybutyric acid and $GABA_B$ receptors. *J. Neural Transm.* (Suppl.) **35**, 155–177.

Biggs, C.S., Pearce, B.R., Fowler, L.J. & Whitton, P.S. (1992): The effect of sodium valproate on extracellular GABA and other amino acids in the rat ventral hippocampus: an *in vivo* microdialysis study. *Brain Res.* **594**, 138–142.

Capek, R. & Esplin, B. (1990): Mechanisms of anticonvulsant action of valproate: an overview and perspective. In: *Generalised epilepsy: neurobiological approaches*, eds. M. Avoli, P. Gloor, G. Kostopoulos & R. Naquet, pp. 436–459. Boston: Birkhauser.

Chapman, A., Keane, P.E., Meldrum, B.S., Simiand, J. & Vernières, J.C. (1982a). Mechanism of anticonvulsant action of valproate. *Prog. Neurobiol.* **19**, 315–359.

Chapman, A.G., Riley, K., Evans M.C. & Meldrum, B.S. (1982b): Acute effects of sodium valproate and γ-vinyl GABA on regional amino-acid metabolism in the rat brain: incorporation of 2-(^{14}C)-glucose into amino-acids. *Neurochem. Res.* **7,** 1089–1105.

Choi, D.W., Farb, D.H. & Fischbach, G.D. (1977): Chlordiazepoxide selectively augments GABA action in spinal cord cell cultures. *Nature* **269,** 342–344.

Coulter, D.A., Huguenard, J.R. & Prince, D.A. (1989a): Characterisation of ethosuximide reduction of low-threshold calcium current in thalamic neurons. *Ann. Neurol.* **25,** 582–593.

Coulter, D.A., Huguenard, J.R. & Prince, D.A. (1989b): Specific petit mal anticonvulsants reduce calcium currents in thalamic neurons. *Neurosci. Lett.* **98,** 74–78.

Crunelli, V. & Leresche, N. (1991): A role for $GABA_B$ receptors in excitation and inhibition of thalamocortical cells. *TINS* **14,** 16–21.

Depaulis, A., Vergnes, M. & Marescaux, C. (1994): Endogenous control of epilepsy: the nigral inhibitory system. *Prog. Neurobiol.* **42,** 33–52.

Gent, J.P. & Phillips, N.I. (1980): Sodium di-n-propylacetate (valproate) potentiates responses to GABA and muscimol on single central neurones. *Brain Res.* **197,** 275–278.

Gloor, P. & Fariello, R.G. (1988): Generalised epilepsy: some of its cellular mechanisms differ from those of focal epilepsy. *TINS* **11,** 63–68.

Grant, S.M. & Heel R.C. (1991): Vigabatrin. A review of its pharmacodynamic and pharmacokinetic properties, and therapeutic potential in epilepsy and disorders of motor control. *Drugs* **41,** 889–926.

Harrison, N.L. & Simmonds, M.A. (1982): Sodium valproate enhances responses to GABA receptor activation only at high concentrations. *Brain Res.* **250,** 201–204.

Hechler, V., Bourguignon, J.J., Wermuth, C.G., Mandel, P. & Maitre, M. (1985): γ-Hydroxybutyrate uptake by rat brain slices. *Neurochem. Res.* **3,** 387–396.

Kelly, K.M., Gross, R.A. & Macdonald, R.L. (1990): Valproic acid selectively reduces the low-threshold (T) calcium current in rat nodose neurons. *Neurosci. Lett.* **116,** 233–238.

Kerwin, R.W., Olpe, H.R. & Schmutz, M. (1980): The effect of sodium n-dipropylacetate on γ-aminobutyric acid-dependent inhibition in the rat cortex and substantia nigra in relation to its anticonvulsant activity. *Br. J. Pharmacol.* **71,** 545–551.

Lloyd, K.G., Thuret, F. & Pilc, A. (1985): Upregulation of γ-aminobutyric acid (GABA) binding sites in rat frontal cortex: a common action of repeated administration of different classes of antidepressants and electroshock. *J. Pharmacol. Exp. Ther.* **235,** 191–199.

Löscher, W. (1989): Valproate enhances GABA turnover in the substantia nigra. *Brain Res.* **501,** 198–203.

Macdonald, R.L. (1989): Antiepileptic drug actions. *Epilepsia* **30,** (Suppl. 1), S19–S28.

Macdonald, R.L. & Barker, J.L. (1978): Benzodiazepines specifically modulate GABA-mediated postsynaptic inhibition in cultured mammalian neurones. *Nature* **271,** 563–564.

Macdonald, R.L. & Bergey, G.K. (1979): Valproic acid augments GABA-mediated postsynaptic inhibition in cultured mammalian neurons. *Brain Res.* **170,** 558–562.

Macdonald, R.L. & Kelly, K.M. (1993): Antiepileptic drug mechanisms of action. *Epilepsia* **34,** (suppl.5), S1–S8.

Maitre, M., Cash, C., Weissmann-Nanopoulos, D. & Mandel, P. (1983): Depolarisation-evoked release of γ-hydroxybutyrate from rat brain slices. *J. Neurochem.* **41,** 287–290.

Marescaux, C., Micheletti, G., Vergnes, M., Depaulis, A., Rumbach, L. & Warter, J.M. (1984): A model of chronic spontaneous petit mal-like seizures in the rat: comparison with pentylenetetrazol-induced seizures. *Epilepsia* **25,** 326–331.

Marescaux, C., Vergnes, M. & Depaulis, A. (1992a): Genetic absence epilepsy in rats from Strasbourg – a review. *J. Neural Transm.* [suppl] **35,** 37–69.

Marescaux, C., Vergnes, M. & Bernasconi, R. (1992b): $GABA_B$ receptor antagonists: potential new anti-absence drugs. *J. Neural Transm.* (Suppl.) **35,** 179–188.

McLean, M.J. & Macdonald, R.L. (1983): Multiple actions of phenytoin on mouse spinal cord neurons in cell culture. *J. Pharmacol. Exp. Ther.* **227,** 779–789.

McLean, M.J. & Macdonald, R.L. (1986): Sodium valproate, but not ethosuximide, produces use- and voltage-dependent limitation of high frequency repetitive firing of action potentials of mouse central neurons in cell culture. *J. Pharmacol. Exp. Ther.* **237**, 1001–1011.

Motohashi, N. (1992): GABA receptor alterations after chronic lithium administration. Comparison with carbamazepine and sodium valproate. *Prog. Neuropsychopharmacol. Biol. Psychiat.* **16**, 571–579.

Olpe, H.R., Steinmann, M.W., Pozza, M.F., Brugger, F. & Schmutz, M. (1988): Valproate enhances $GABA_A$ mediated inhibition of locus coeruleus neurones *in vitro. Naunyn Schmiedebergs Arch. Pharmacol.* **338**, 655–657.

Olsen, R.W. & Snowman, A.M. (1982): Chloride-dependent barbiturate enhancement of GABA receptor binding. *J. Neurosci.* **2**, 1812–1823.

Rogawski, M.A. & Porter, R.J. (1990): Antiepileptic drugs: pharmacological mechanisms and clinical efficacy with consideration of promising developmental stage compounds. *Pharmacol. Rev.* **42**, 223–285.

Roth, R.H. & Giarman, N.J. (1970): Natural occurrence of γ-hydroxybutyrate in mammalian brain. *Biochem. Pharmacol.* **19**, 1087–1093.

Schmutz, M., Olpe, H.R. & Koella, W.P. (1979): Central actions of valproate sodium. *J. Pharm. Pharmacol.* **31**, 413–414.

Skerritt, J.H. & Johnston, G.A.R. (1983): Enhancement of GABA binding by benzodiazepines and related anxiolytics. *Eur. J. Pharmacol.* **89**, 193–198.

Snead, O.C. (1988): γ-Hydroxybutyrate model of generalised absence seizures: further characterisation and comparison with other absence models. *Epilepsia* **29**, 361–368.

Snead, O.C. & Liu, C.C. (1984): γ-Hydroxybutyric acid binding sites in rat and human brain synaptosomal membranes. *Biochem. Pharmacol.* **33**, 2587–2590.

Study, R.E. & Barker, J.L. (1981): Diazepam and (–)-pentobarbital: fluctuation analysis reveals different mechanisms for potentiation of γ-aminobutyric acid responses in cultured central neurones. *Proc. Natl. Acad. Sci. USA* **78**, 7180–7184.

Toman, J.E.P. (1949): The neuropharmacology of antiepileptics. *EEG Clin. Neurophysiol.* **1**, 33–44.

Vayer, P., Charlier, B., Mandel P. & Maitre, M. (1987a): Effect of anticonvulsant drugs on γ-hydroxybutyrate release from hippocampal slices: inhibition by valproate and ethosuximide. *J. Neurochem.* **49**, 1022–1024.

Vayer, P., Gobaille, S., Mandel, P. & Maitre, M. (1987b): 3'-5' cyclic-guanosine monophosphate increase in rat brain hippocampus after gamma-hydroxybutyrate administration. Prevention by valproate and naloxone. *Life Sci.* **41**, 605–610.

Vayer, P., Cash, C.D. & Maitre, M. (1988): Is the anticonvulsant mechanism of valproate linked to its interaction with the cerebral γ-hydroxybutyrate system? *TIPS* **9**, 127–129.

Vergnes, M., Marescaux, C., Micheletti, G., Depaulis, A., Rumbach, L. & Warter, J.M. (1984): Enhancement of spike and wave discharges by GABAmimetic drugs in rats with spontaneous petit mal-like epilepsy. *Neurosci. Lett.* **44**, 91.

Willow, M. & Catterall, W.A. (1982): Inhibition of binding of [^{3}H]-batrachotoxin A 20-benzoate to sodium channels by the anticonvulsant drugs diphenylhydantoin and carbamazepine. *Mol. Pharmacol.* **22**, 627–635.

Willow, M., Kuenze, E.A. & Catterall, W.A. (1984): Inhibition of voltage-sensitive sodium channels in neuroblastoma cells and synaptosomes by the anticonvulsant drugs diphenylhydantoin and carbamazepine. *Mol. Pharmacol.* **25**, 228–234.

Wolf, R., Tscherne, U. & Emrich, H.M. (1988): Suppression of preoptic GABA release caused by push-pull-perfusion with sodium valproate. *Naunyn Schmiedebergs Arch. Pharmacol.* **338**, 658–663.

Wolf, R. & Tscherne, U. (1994): Valproate effect on γ-aminobutyric acid release in pars reticulata of substantia nigra: combination of push-pull perfusion and fluorescence histochemistry. *Epilepsia* **35**, 226–233.

Chapter 38

New anti-epileptic drugs and idiopathic generalized epilepsies

Mogens Dam

University Clinic of Neurology, Hvidovre Hospital, Copenhagen, Denmark

Since the great majority of the patients recruited for clinical trials of new anti-epileptic drugs are patients suffering from refractory epilepsies, in which partial seizures tend to predominate, experience in idiopathic generalized epilepsies (IGEs) is limited. Although few, if any, of the new anti-epileptics are designed for the treatment of IGE, they generally elicit a better effect on these syndromes than on partial epilepsies. One exception is vigabatrin, which is clearly most effective in the treatment of partial seizures.

Oxcarbazepine

Oxcarbazepine (OXC) is the keto analogue of carbamazepine (CBZ). Photo-myoclonic seizures in monkeys are inhibited by this compound, which may suggest that oxcarbazepine will be effective in the treatment of primary generalized tonic–clonic seizures (Killam & Killam, 1972). Conversely, on the basis of the observation that rats that have undergone amygdala kindling show a prolonged duration of after-discharge when treated with oxcarbazepine, the drug is not supposed to have any effect on absence seizures (Schmutz *et al.*, 1988).

Oxcarbazepine is almost completely absorbed in man. It is a pro-drug for the active metabolite, 10,11-dihydro-10-hydroxycarbamazepine (DH-OH-CBZ). About 50 per cent of the active metabolite is bound to plasma proteins.

The concentrations of the parent compound, oxcarbazepine, and the other metabolite, DH-trans-DOH-CBZ, which is pharmacologically inactive, are both negligible. There are no indications of auto-induction or accumulation (Dickinson & Hooper, 1989). Substituting oxcarbazepine for carbamazepine results in decreased enzyme induction, causing an increase in serum levels of concomitantly administered anti-epileptic drugs.

It has been noted that oxcarbazepine affords significantly better control of tonic and tonic–clonic seizures and atypical absences. It is known to be a very effective anti-epileptic drug in the treatment of simple and complex partial seizures with or without secondary generalized convulsions, and also of primary generalized convulsions (Houtkooper *et al.*, 1987; Sillanpää & Pihlaja, 1989). In cases of refractory seizures, substitution of oxcarbazepine for carbamazepine is associated with reduced seizure frequency in some patients, while others experience improved alertness and cognition. Fewer side-effects are provoked, and it is therefore possible to increase the dose of oxcarbazepine to a level allowing better control of seizures. Allergic skin reactions are rare during therapy with oxcarbazepine, and cross-reactivity is only seen in about 25 per cent of patients hypersensitive to carbamazepine (The Danish Oxcarbazepine Study Group, 1984). Most patients showing allergic skin reactions to carbamazepine can therefore be switched over to oxcarbazepine without any similar signs of hypersensitivity occurring.

The diminished propensity to induce oxidative metabolism is a great advantage, as it is much easier in polytherapy to reach the therapeutically effective levels of other anti-epileptic drugs during treatment with oxcarbazepine than with carbamazepine. This is a particular problem with the combination of carbamazepine and valproate in children, where it may be impossible to attain therapeutic concentrations of valproate. Changing to oxcarbazepine raises the level of valproate, resulting in an improved anti-epileptic effect. Overall, oxcarbazepine has been shown to be as effective as carbamazepine in the treatment of generalized tonic–clonic seizures (Reinikainen et al., 1987; Dam et al., 1989). It is ineffective in the treatment of absence epilepsy.

Lamotrigine

Lamotrigine (LMT) is said to stabilize neuronal membranes and is thought to inhibit excitatory neurotransmitter release, principally of glutamate (Leach et al., 1986). It is active in models of tonic–clonic and partial seizures, displaying effects similar to those of phenytoin and carbamazepine (Miller et al., 1986). It suppresses the visually evoked after-discharge, as does valproate, and it may therefore be speculated as to whether it could be effective against the same spectrum of seizures as valproate. It is effective in reducing electro-encephalographic photosensitivity and interictal epileptiform spike discharges. Lamotrigine is extensively metabolized and excreted predominantly as a glucuronide conjugate. It does not cause enzyme induction with regard to cytochrome P_{450}. Protein binding amounts to 55 per cent, and the metabolism follows linear kinetics. Co-medication with enzyme-inducing drugs such as carbamazepine or phenytoin may reduce the half-life of lamotrigine to 5 h, and concomitant treatment with valproate may prolong its half-life to 90 h.

Lamotrigine reduces the frequency of primary generalized seizures by more than 50 per cent and may be at least as effective against IGE as it is against partial epilepsies. Preliminary results suggest that it is active against generalized absences, myoclonic jerks, and tonic and clonic seizures.

Timmings & Richens (1992a) reviewed their case records of all patients that had taken lamotrigine on an open label. They found that the frequency of seizures had been reduced by more than 50 per cent in 58 per cent of these cases. They further noted that in 79 per cent of patients with primary generalized epilepsy seizure frequencies were reduced by more than 50 per cent. They concluded that lamotrigine may be at least as effective against primary generalized seizures as it is in the treatment of partial epilepsies.

Stewart et al. (1992) found that two of four patients with primary generalized epilepsy treated with lamotrigine remained seizure-free for up to 3 years, while the other two showed an improvement of more than 75 per cent.

We have treated 37 of our patients (21 men and 16 women of ages ranging from 17 to 61 years) with lamotrigine, either in open clinical trials or with special permission from the National Health Board. Seven patients had a generalized epilepsy, and the remaining 30 partial seizures with or without secondary generalization. Most of the patients were suffering from refractory seizures. They were treated for periods of 1 to 22 months (average 9 months) with lamotrigine, alone or concomitantly with one to three other anti-epileptic drugs. The maintenance dose of lamotrigine was 100–600 mg. At present, 30 patients are still receiving lamotrigine; in the other seven cases the drug has been withdrawn because of adverse effects or lack of efficacy. Six patients are currently seizure-free on lamotrigine. One of these patients is allergic to carbamazepine and oxcarbazepine and was not seizure-free on phenytoin, but her partial seizures are now well controlled with lamotrigine in monotherapy. Three of the patients are fresh cases with partial seizures.

Another two patients (one with juvenile myoclonic epilepsy and one with partial seizures) were seizure-free on valproate and vigabatrin, respectively, but suffered from side-effects, which they no longer have.

In eight patients, the therapeutic effect has been good or markedly better than that of their previous treatment (50–99 per cent reduction in seizure frequency), and in another four some effect has been evident (25–49 per cent reduction), whereas 18 patients have had only very little or no benefit from lamotrigine. Again, it should be noted that the majority of these patients had also shown unsatisfactory responses to other available drugs. One fresh patient has been free from generalized seizures since she started on lamotrigine treatment, but it has not been possible to assess the effect on her simple partial seizures.

Since special attention has been paid to the possible effect of lamotrigine on Lennox–Gastaut syndrome (Timmings & Richens, 1992b), it should be mentioned that we have treated two patients suffering from this syndrome with lamotrigine. In one patient with a symptomatic Lennox–Gastaut syndrome the frequency of seizures has been reduced by 33 per cent. In the other patient, in whom the condition is idiopathic, the drug initially had some effect, but the seizure frequency increased again after some time.

It is our impression that lamotrigine represents a major step forward in the treatment of epilepsy. Until now it has mainly been used in the treatment of severe cases and as an adjunctive therapy. We feel that the drug is very effective in the treatment of primary generalized epilepsy and idiopathic partial epilepsy. Lamotrigine may well turn out to be a drug that can be used in many of the same situations as valproate. As lamotrigine seems to provoke fewer side-effects than valproate, and as they are also less severe than the side-effects of valproate, such as hepatotoxicity, weight-gain, and tremor, we foresee that this drug may very soon become the drug of first choice in the treatment of some types of primary generalized epilepsy.

Zonisamide

Zonisamide is a 1,2-benzisoxazole derivative. Results of *in vitro* and *in vivo* studies in which the effects of anti-epileptic drugs on neuronal firing were assessed appear to indicate that a common denominator is the capacity to selectively inhibit paroxysmal firing in the neurons of the central nervous system, enabling them to prevent seizures without significantly affecting normal neuronal activity (Fromm *et al.*, 1987). It is suggested that the mechanism of action of zonisamide could involve a blockade of the spread or propagation of seizure discharges and a suppression of the epileptogenic focus (Seino *et al.*, 1991). Zonisamide has been shown to inhibit brain and blood carbonic anhydrase, although the effect is only slight and considerably less than that of acetazolamide (Hammond *et al.*, 1987; Masuda *et al.*, 1980). It is not suggested that zonisamide exerts its anti-epileptic action through inhibition of carbonic anhydrase.

Peak plasma concentrations of orally administered zonisamide are reached within 2.4 to 3.6 h (Taylor *et al.*, 1986). The drug is highly concentrated in the red blood cells (Ito *et al.*, 1982) and exhibits non-linear pharmacokinetics (Wagner *et al.*, 1984). Zonisamide, gabapentin, and valproate equipotently suppress tonic–clonic and myoclonic seizures in reflex epilepsy in genetically epileptic gerbils (Bartoszyk & Hamer, 1987).

Consistent with these findings, zonisamide is as effective as valproate in paediatric patients with IGE (Oguni *et al.*, 1988). In large groups of patients, efficacy rates of 59 per cent have been recorded among those with generalized tonic–clonic convulsions. Other generalized seizures also respond to therapy with zonisamide. It is effective in the treatment of West's syndrome and Lennox–Gastaut's syndrome (Yagi & Seino, 1992). Clinical experience with zonisamide has thus documented its efficacy in the treatment of IGE.

One drawback may be a high frequency of renal calculi, which was found in the patients taking part in drug trials in the USA (Henry & Sackellares, 1992). All trials in the USA and Europe were consequently stopped. In Japan, however, the drug has been on the market for several years and does not seem to cause a greater incidence of kidney stones than any other drug (Seino et al., 1991). Zonisamide is therefore due to be taken up again for further investigations, in Europe at least.

Gabapentin

Gabapentin is an amino acid related to γ-aminobutyric acid (GABA). It was synthesized as a structural analogue of the inhibitory neurotransmitter GABA, in the expectation that it could mimic the actions of GABA in the brain. Tests *in vitro* showed that it almost doubled the release of ^{3}H-GABA from incubated neostriatal slices. This effect was seen in response to therapeutically relevant concentrations of gabapentin. The apparent involvement of $GABA_A$ receptors may contribute to the anti-epileptic activity of gabapentin (Gotz et al., 1993).

Gabapentin is readily absorbed in man and has an elimination half-life of 5–6 h. It is not bound to plasma proteins and is not metabolized (Vollmer et al., 1986). Its pharmacokinetics are not altered in patients with epilepsy receiving phenytoin, phenobarbitone, valproate, or carbamazepine (Graves et al., 1989b, 1990; Basim et al., 1990; Hooper et al., 1991). With increasing age, the elimination rate and renal clearance decrease, suggesting that the age-related alterations in renal function are responsible for changes in the pharmacokinetics of the drug (Boyd et al., 1990).

Gabapentin prevents seizures induced by a wide variety of convulsant treatments in rodents as well as spontaneous seizures in several genetic models. Its action in these animal models suggests that it may prevent generalized tonic–clonic seizures (Taylor, 1993). Although the drug may thus be effective against IGE, there are no data available to support this assumption, as all the published studies were restricted to partial epilepsies and cases stubbornly refractory to drug therapy.

Felbamate

Felbamate (FBM) is a 2-phenyl-1,3-propanediol dicarbamate. It binds to plasma proteins to the extent of 22 to 36 per cent (Adusumalli et al., 1991) and has a half-life of about 20 h in man (Palmer & McTavish, 1993). Felbamate interacts strongly with other drugs: it reduces the clearance and consequently increases the plasma concentrations of phenytoin. On the other hand, it reduces the steady-state plasma concentration of carbamazepine by about 20 per cent, but increases that of CBZ-epoxide by 46 per cent (Fuerst et al., 1988; Graves et al., 1989a; Albani et al., 1991). It also increases the steady-state plasma concentration of valproate by about 20 per cent (Wagner et al., 1991). Other anti-epileptic drugs likewise affect the pharmacokinetics of felbamate: the steady-state concentration is decreased by phenytoin and carbamazepine, but increased by valproate (Wagner et al., 1990).

Felbamate seems to check the spread of seizures, as it inhibits the induction of hind-limb extension by electroshock. It may therefore be effective against primary generalized seizures (Graves & Leppik, 1991). The activity of felbamate against seizures induced both by maximal electroshock and by some chemical convulsants indicates that it could be clinically effective against generalized tonic–clonic seizures and absences. In a trial in patients with Lennox–Gastaut's syndrome, it has also been shown to be effective in the treatment of myoclonic seizures, atonic seizures, and atypical absences (Felbamate Study Group in Lennox–Gastaut's syndrome, 1993).

Vigabatrin

Vigabatrin is a structural analogue of GABA. It has been demonstrated to exert an anti-epileptic effect in various experimental models of epilepsy. The mechanism of action of vigabatrin is supposed to consist in irreversible inhibition of GABA transaminase (Lippert et al., 1977). This action has also been shown to result in an increase in whole-brain levels of GABA (Schechter *et al.*, 1979). All the available clinical data point towards a better effect against partial than against generalized epilepsies, which is the opposite of the typical effects of most other anti-epileptic drugs. However, in a small group of patients suffering from juvenile myoclonic epilepsy, a 50 per cent reduction in the frequency of seizures was observed (Pedersen *et al.*, 1985), which is consistent with the findings in generalized photosensitive epilepsy (Rimmer *et al.*, 1987).

On the other hand, absences in animals and IGE in man seem to respond adversely to vigabatrin (Mumford & Dam, 1989). Hyperfunction of GABAergic inhibitory pathways has been implicated.

Tiagabine

Tiagabine is an *N*-alkylated nipecotic acid derivative that has been developed along rational lines for a specific anti-epileptic effect. It is a highly potent and specific inhibitor of GABA uptake, raising the levels of GABA (Bræstrup *et al.*, 1990; Nielsen *et al.*, 1991). It has been found to display a potent anti-epileptic effect when administered orally in animal models of epilepsy, including audiogenic and pentylenetetrazol-induced seizures. It affords partial protection against photically induced myoclonic seizures in the photosensitive baboon (Meldrum *et al.*, unpublished data).

As tiagabine is an inhibitor of GABA re-uptake, it may be speculated as to whether it has the same effect as vigabatrin, being more potent in partial epilepsy than in generalized epilepsy. This aspect has not yet been investigated.

Conclusion

Many new anti-epileptic drugs have been developed in the last few years, and more still are on the way. None of them has been designed for the treatment of IGE, but many may have some effect on these epileptic syndromes, and some look promising.

As valproate and ethosuximide, the drugs now typically used for the treatment of IGE, both provoke rather disturbing side-effects such as liver damage, weight-gain or weight-loss, tremor, and gastro-intestinal symptoms, it is hoped that the future will bring new drugs rationally designed for the treatment of IGE and devoid of severe side-effects.

References

Adusumalli, V.E., Yang, J.T., Wong, K.K., Kucharczyk, N. & Sofia, R.D. (1991): Felbamate pharmacokinetics in the rat, rabbit and dog. *Drug Metab. Disp.* **19**, 1116–1125.

Albani, F., Theodore, W.H., Washington, P., Devinsky, O., Bromfield, E., Porter, R.J. & Nice, F.J. (1991): Effect of felbamate on plasma levels of carbamazepine and its metabolites. *Epilepsia* **32**, 130–132.

Bartoszyk, G.D. & Hamer, M. (1987): The genetic animal model of reflex epilepsy in the Mongolian gerbil: differential efficacy of new anticonvulsive drugs and prototype antiepileptics. *Pharmacol. Res. Comm.* **19**, 429–441.

Basim, M., Uthman, E.J., Hammond, E.J. & Wilder, B.J. (1990): Absence of gabapentin and valproate interaction: an evoked potential and pharmacokinetic study, *Epilepsia* **31**, 645.

Boyd, R.A., Bockbrader, H.N., Türck, D., Sedman, A.J., Posvar, E.L. & Chang, T. (1990): Effect of subject age on the single dose pharmacokinetics of orally administered gabapentin (CI-945). *Pharm. Res.* **7** (Suppl. 9), S215.

Braestrup, C., Nielsen, E.B., Sonnewald, U., Knutsen, L.J.S., Andersen, K.E., Jansen, J.A., Frederiksen, K., Andersen, P.H., Mortensen, A. & Suzdak, P.D. (1990): (R)-*N*-(4,4-bis(3-methyl-2-thienyl)but-3-en-1-yl)nipecotic acid binds with high affinity to the brain γ-amino-butyric acid uptake carrier. *J. Neurochem.* **54**, 639–647.

Dam, M., Ekberg, R., Loyning, Y., Waltimo, O. & Jakobsen, K. (1989): A double-blind study comparing oxcarbazepine and carbamazepine in patients with newly diagnosed previously untreated epilepsy. *Epilepsy Res.* **3**, 70–76.

Dickinson, R.G. & Hooper, W.D. (1989): First dose and steady-state pharmacokinetics and oxcarbazepine and its 10-hydroxy-metabolite. *Eur. J. Clin. Pharmacol.* **37**, 69–74.

Felbamate Study Group in Lennox–Gastaut syndrome (1993): Efficacy of felbamate in childhood epileptic encephalopathy (Lennox–Gastaut syndrome). *New Engl. J. Med.* **328**, 29–33.

Fromm, G.H., Shibuya, T. & Terrence, C.F. (1987): Effect of zonisamide (CI-912) on a synaptic system model. *Epilepsia* **28**, 673–679.

Fuerst, R.H., Graves, N.M., Leppik, I.E., Brundage, R.C., Holmes, G.B. & Remmel, R.P. (1988): Felbamate increases phenytoin but decreases carbamazepine concentrations. *Epilepsia* **29**, 488–491.

Gotz, E., Feuerstein, T.J., Lais, A. & Meyer, D.K. (1993): Effects of gabapentin on release of gamma-aminobutyric acid from slices of rat neostriatum. *Arzneimittelforsch./Drug Res.* **43**, 636–638.

Graves, N.M., Holmes, G.B., Fuerst, R.H. & Leppik, I.E. (1989a): Effect of felbamate on phenytoin and carbamazepine serum concentrations. *Epilepsia* **30**, 225–229.

Graves, N.M., Holmes, G.B., Leppik, I.E., Rask, C., Slavin, M., Anhut, H. & Schmidt, B. (1989b): Pharmacokinetics of gabapentin in patients treated with phenytoin. *Pharmacotherapy* **9**, 196.

Graves, N.M., Leppik, I.E., Wagner, M.L., Spencer, M.M. & Erdman, G.R. (1990): Effect of gabapentin on carbamazepine levels. *Epilepsia* **31**, 644.

Graves, N.M. & Leppik, I.E. (1991): Antiepileptic medications in development. *Ann. Pharmacother.* **25**, 978–986.

Hammond, E.J., Perchalski, R.J., Wilder, B.J. & McLean, J.R. (1987): Neuropharmacology of zonisamide, a new antiepileptic drug. *Gen. Pharmacol.* **18**, 303–307.

Henry, T.R. & Sackellares, J.C. (1992): Zonisamide. In: *The medical treatment of epilepsy*, eds. S.R. Resor Jr. & H. Kutt, pp. 423–427. New York: Marcel Dekker.

Hooper, W.D., Kavanagh, M.C., Herkes, G.K. & Eadie, M.J. (1991): Lack of pharmacokinetic interaction between phenobarbital and gabapentin. *Br. J. Clin. Pharmacol.* **31**, 171–174.

Houtkooper, M.A., Lammertsma, A., Meyer, J.W.A., Goedhart, D.M., Meinardi, H., van Oorshot, C.A.E.H., Blom, G.F., Höppener, R.J.E.A. & Hulsman, J.A.R.J. (1987): Oxcarbazepine (GP 47680): a possible alternative to carbamazepine? *Epilepsia* **28**, 693–698.

Ito, T., Yamaguchi, T., Miyazaki, H., Sekine, Y., Shimizu, M., Ishida, S., Yagi, K., Kakegawa, N., Seino, M. & Wada, T. (1982): Pharmacokinetic studies of AD-810, a new antiepileptic compound. *Arzneimittelforsch./Drug Res.* **32**, 1581–1586.

Killam, E.K. & Killam, K.F. (1972): Control of photomyoclonic seizures in the baboon by a carbamazepine analogue. *5th International Congress Pharmacology. July 23–28, San Francisco (Abstr.):* **24**, 743.

Leach, M., Harden, C.M. & Miller, A.A. (1986): Pharmacological studies of lamotrigine, a novel potential antiepileptic drug: II. Neurochemical studies of the mechanism of action. *Epilepsia* **27**, 490–497.

Lippert, B., Metcalf, B.W., Jung, M.J. & Casare, P. (1977): 4-amino-hex-5-enoic acid, a selective catalytic inhibitor of 4-aminobutyric acid in mammalian brain. *Eur. J. Biochem.* **74**, 441–445.

Masuda, Y., Karasawa, T., Shiraishi, Y., Hori, M., Yoshida, K. & Shimizu, M. (1980): 3-Sulphamoylmethyl-1,2-benzisoxazole, a new type of anticonvulsant drug. Pharmacological profile. *Arzneimittelforsch./Drug Res.* **30**, 477–483.

Miller, A.A., Whetley, P.L., Sawyer, D.A., Baxter, M.G. & Roth, B. (1986): Pharmacological studies on lamotrigine, a new potential antiepileptic drug: I. Anticonvulsant profile in mice and rats. *Epilepsia* **27**, 483–489.

Mumford, J.P. & Dam, M. (1989): Meta-analysis of European placebo-controlled studies of vigabatrin in drug resistant epilepsy. *Br. J. Clin. Pharmacol.* **27**, 101S–107S.

Nielsen, E.B., Suzdak, P.D., Andersen, K.E., Knutsen, L.J.S., Sonnewald, U. & Braestrup, C. (1991): Characterization of tiagabine (NO-328), a new potent and selective GABA uptake inhibitor. *Eur. J. Pharmacol.* **196**, 257–266.

Oguni, H., Hayashi, K., Fukuyama, Y., Iinuma, K., Seki, T., Seino, M., Watanabe, K., Mimaki, T., Ohtahara, S., Kurokawa, T. & Kuriya, N. (1988): Phase III study of AD-810 (zonisamide (ZNS)), a new antiepileptic, in the treatment of pediatric epilepsy. *Jap. J. Paediatrics* **41** (Suppl), 439–450 (in Japanese).

Palmer, K.J. & McTavish, D. (1993): Felbamate. A review of its pharmacodynamic and pharmacokinetic properties, and therapeutic efficacy in epilepsy. *Drugs* **45**, 1041–1065.

Pedersen, S.A., Klosterskov, P., Gram, L. & Dam, M. (1985): Long-term study of gamma-vinyl GABA in the treatment of epilepsy. *Acta Neurol. Scand.* **72**, 295–298.

Reinikainen, K.J., Keränen, T., Halonen, T., Komulainen, H. & Riekkinen, P.J. (1987): Comparison of oxcarbazepine and carbamazepine: a double-blind study. *Epilepsy Res.* **1**, 284–289.

Rimmer, E.M., Miligan, N.M. & Richens, A. (1987): A comparison of the acute effect of single doses of vigabatrin and sodium valproate on photosensitivity in epileptic patients. *Epilepsy Res.* **1**, 339–346.

Schechter, P.J., Tranier, Y. & Grove, J. (1979): Attempts to correlate alterations in brain GABA metabolism by $GABA_T$ inhibitors with their anticonvulsant effect. In: *GABA–biochemisrty and brain function*, eds. P. Mandel & F.V. DeFeudis, pp. 43–57. New York: Plenum Press.

Schmutz, M., Klebs, K. & Baltzer, V. (1988): Inhibition or enhancement of kindling evolution by antiepileptics. *J. Neural. Trans.* **72**, 245–257.

Seino, M., Miyazaki, H. & Ito, T. (1991): Zonisamide. In: *New antiepileptic drugs*, (Epilepsy Research Suppl. 3), eds. F. Pisani, E. Perucca, G. Avanzini & A. Richens, pp. 169–174. Amsterdam: Elsevier Science.

Sillanpää, M. & Pihlaja, T. (1989): Oxcarbazepine (GP 47680) in the treatment of intractable seizures. *Acta Paediatr. Hung.* **29**, 359–361.

Stewart, J., Hughes, E. & Reynolds, E.H. (1992): Lamotrigine for generalized epilepsies. *Lancet* **340**, 8829.

Taylor, C.P., McLean, J.R., Brockbrader, H.N., Buchanan, R.A., Karasawa, T., Miyazaki, M., Rock, D.M., Takemoto, Y., Uno, H. & Walker, R. (1986): Zonisamide (AD-810, CI-912). In: *New anticonvulsant drugs*, eds. B. Meldrum & R. Porter, pp. 277–294. London: John Libbey.

Taylor, C.P. (1993): Mechanism of action of new-antiepileptic drugs. In: *New trends in epilepsy management: the role of gabapentin*, ed. D. Chadwick, pp. 13–40. London: Royal Society of Medicine Services.

The Danish Oxcarbazepine Study Group (1984): Oxcarbazepine in patients hypersensitive to carbamazepine (Abstr.). *Acta Neurol. Scand.* **70**, 223.

Timmings, P.L. & Richens, A. (1992a): Lamotrigine in primary generalized epilepsy. *Lancet* **339**, 1300.

Timmings, P.L. & Richens, A. (1992b): Lamotrigine as an add-on drug in the management of Lennox–Gastaut syndrome. *Eur. Neurol.* **32**, 305–307.

Vollmer, K.O., Thomann, P., Most, M., von Hodenberg, A., Meyerson, N. & Schmidt, B. (1986): Pharmacokinetics of the new anticonvulsant gabapentin in man. In: *Golden Jubilee Conference and Northern European Epilepsy Meeting* (Abstract). University of York.

Wagner, J.G., Sackellares, J.C., Donofrio, P.D., Berent, S. & Sakmar, E. (1984): Nonlinear pharmacokinetics of CI-912 in adult epileptic patients. *Ther. Drug Monit.* **6**, 277–293.

Wagner, M.L., Leppik, I.E., Graves, N.M., Remmel, R.P. & Campell, J.I. (1990): Felbamate serum concentrations: effect of valproate, carbamazepine, phenytoin and phenobarbital. Abstract. *Epilepsia* **31**, 642.

Wagner, M.L., Graves, N.M., Leppik, I.E., Remmel, R.P., Ward, D.L. & Shumaker, R.V. (1991): The effect of felbamate on valproate disposition. Abstract. *Epilepsia* **32** (Suppl. 3), 15.

Yagi, K. & Seino, M (1992): Methodological requirements for clinical trials in refractory epilepsies – our experience with zonisamide. *Prog. Neuropsychopharmacol. Biol. Psychiatry* **16**, 79–85.

Chapter 39

Therapeutic prospects for novel excitatory amino acid antagonists in idiopathic generalized epilepsy

Astrid G. Chapman

Department of Neurology, Institute of Psychiatry, De Crespigny Park, Denmark Hill, London SE5 8AF, England

Idiopathic generalized epilepsy consists of convulsant and non-convulsant (absence) types of epilepsy, where the two types exhibit very different responses to pharmacological treatment. Clinical absence seizures are traditionally treated with ethosuximide or valproate (Mattson, 1989; Chadwick, 1990), with $GABA_B$-receptor antagonists representing a potential therapeutic approach in experimental absence sizures (Marescaux *et al.*, 1992). GABA agonists and antiepileptic drugs that enhance GABA levels exacerbate absence seizures (Marescaux *et al.*, 1984; Vergnes *et al.*, 1990), and excitatory amino acid antagonists are of relatively limited efficacy in treating experimental absence seizures (Marescaux *et al.*, 1990).

The commonly used antiepileptic drugs for treating convulsant idiopathic generalized epilepsy include valproate, phenytoin and carbamazepine (Mattson, 1989; Chadwick, 1990). In animal models of convulsant idiopathic generalized epilepsy, different classes of excitatory amino acid antagonists have been shown to have potent antiepileptic activity (Chapman, 1991).

Clinical trials of novel anti-epileptic drugs mainly involve patients with refractory epilepsy, where the drug in question is added to existing antiepileptic medication during the trial period. Complex partial seizures predominate among cases of refractory epilepsy and heavily influence the apparent efficacy of the 'add-on' drug; we have therefore relatively little information about the effects of novel antiepileptic drugs in idiopathic generalized epilepsy.

This chapter will review the effects of excitatory amino acid antagonists in animal models of idiopathic generalized epilepsy, as well as discuss the limited amount of information available on drug trials of excitatory amino acid antagonists in human complex partial epilepsy. Furthermore, it has been reported that some novel antiepileptic drugs in clinical use or undergoing clinical trials interact with the excitatory amino acid transmitter system: felbamate has some affinity for the glycine-site at the NMDA receptor (Harmsworth *et al.*, 1993; McCabe *et al.*, 1993; Wasterlain *et al.*, 1993; Rho *et al.*, 1993); the desglycine metabolite of remacemide binds at the channel-site of the NMDA receptor (Palmer *et al.*, 1992); lamotrigine inhibits veratrine-induced release of glutamate (Miller *et al.*, 1986; Leach *et al.*, 1986; Meldrum & Leach, 1994). The efficacy of these novel antiepileptic drugs in clinical and experimental idiopathic generalized epilepsy will be discussed.

Generalized absence epilepsy

Animal seizure models considered to be predictive of efficacy of potential antiepileptic drugs in absence epilepsy include subcutaneous pentylenetetrazol (PTZ) threshold test in rodents (see Macdonald, 1983) or, more recently, rodent strains exhibiting spontaneous spike-and-wave discharge (Vergnes et al., 1990).

Absence seizures in GAERS (genetic absence epilepsy rat from Strasbourg) rats share many characteristics with their human counterpart: a rhythmic spike-and-wave EEG-pattern (8–9 Hz frequency versus 3 Hz frequency in humans) with cortico-thalamic distribution, manifestations of behavioural arrest during seizures, and a very similar pharmacological profile (Vergnes et al., 1990). The functional response of the NMDA receptor (NMDA-evoked calcium influx) is enhanced in GAERS rats, with the laminar profile of optimal calcium influx extending wider to additional layers of the sensory motor cortex in GAERS rats compared to controls (Pumain et al., 1992). A similar functional enhancement has been reported for the hippocampal NMDA receptor in kindled rats (Mody et al., 1988) and in human epileptogenic neocortex (Louvel & Pumain, 1992).

Antagonists acting at the NMDA receptor have been tested for antiepileptic activity in GAERS. Both competitive (2-amino-5-phosphonopentanoic acid (AP5), 200–400 mg/kg; 2-amino-7-phosphonoheptanoic acid (AP7), 100–400 mg/kg; 3-(2-carboxypiperazin-4-yl)propyl-1-phosphonic acid (CPP), 2.5–10 mg/kg) and non-competitive channel-site NMDA antagonists (dizocilpine (MK 801), 0.1–0.5 mg/kg; phencyclidine (PCP) 1–3 mg/kg; N-allylnormetazocine (SKF 10047) 3–20 mg/kg) cause dose-dependent suppression of spike-and-wave discharges (Marescaux et al., 1990). However, the antiabsence efficacy of competitive or non-competitive NMDA antagonists is lower in GAERS rats than in several generalized convulsant seizure models (see Chapman, 1991), and major side effects (EEG-abnormalities, ataxia and stereotyped behaviour) are observed at antiepileptic doses of NMDA antagonists required in this rat strain (Marescaux et al., 1990).

There is no information available on the effect of competitive NMDA antagonists against absence seizures in man. However, felbamate (2-phenyl-1,3-propanediol dicarbamate), which has been shown to interact with the glycine site at the NMDA receptor (Harmsworth et al., 1993; McCabe et al., 1993; Wasterlain et al., 1993; Rho et al., 1993) is reported by Ritter et al. (1993) to be particularly effective in suppressing atypical generalized absence attacks in Lennox–Gastaut syndrome, a syndrome which is normally resistant to antiepileptic drug therapy. An antiabsence effect of felbamate was predicted from preclinical animal studies where felbamate was active in the subcutaneous PTZ seizure threshold test in mice (ED_{50} = 148 mg/kg i.p., ED_{50} = 548 mg/kg p.o.; Swinyard et al. (1986); Leppik & Graves (1989)). High doses of felbamate are required both in patients (1600–3600 mg/day) and animals, however felbamate also appears to have an unusually high therapeutic index (Leppik & Graves, 1989; Theodore et al., 1991; White et al., 1992; Palmer & McTavish, 1993).

Lamotrigine (3,5-diamino-6-(2,3-dichlorophenyl)-1,2,4-triazine), a drug that has a phenytoin-like action at the sodium-channel and also inhibits veratrine-induced release of excitatory amino acids (Miller et al., 1986; Leach et al., 1986; Goa et al., 1993; Meldrum & Leach, 1994), is effective against typical and atypical absence seizures, as well as against tonic/clonic and partial epilepsy (Goa et al., 1993; Schapel et al., 1993). Lamotrigine, in combination with valproate, has likewise been shown to be effective (25–50 mg/day) against absence seizures in a group of patients not controlled by lamotrigine or valproate alone (Panayiotopoulos et al., 1993). A similar combined efficacy of lamotrigine (200–500 mg/day) and valproate (400–800 mg/day) is also observed in patients with refractory partial seizures (Pisani et al., 1993).

Convulsive idiopathic generalized epilepsy

Animal seizure models that represent convulsive idiopathic generalized epilepsy include reflex-induced generalized seizures in rodents and primates, maximal electroshock (MES), as well as various genetic seizure-susceptible syndromes and chemically-induced seizures (Macdonald & Meldrum, 1989). Excitatory amino acid antagonists acting at the AMPA(α-amino-3-hydoxy-5-methylisoxazole-4-proprionic acid)/kainate receptor or at the NMDA receptor (competitively at the agonist binding site, or non-competitively at the channel-site or at the strychnine-insensitive glycine site) have potent anticonvulsant action in many animal models of generalized convulsive epilepsy (Chapman, 1991, Chapman & Meldrum, 1993).

Competitive NMDA antagonists

Selective and potent antagonists (AP7; 3-(2-carboxypiperazin-4-yl)propenyl-1-phosphonic acid, CPPene; *cis*-4-phosphonomethyl-2-piperidine-carboxylic acid, CGS 19755; 2-amino-4-methyl-5-phosphono-3-pentenoic acid, CGP 37849; 2-amino-4-methyl-5-phosphono-3-pentenoate-1-ethyl ester, CGP 39551; 6-phosphono-decahydroisoquinoline-3-carboxylic acid, LY 274614) acting competitively at the NMDA receptor have been available for a number of years, and more information has therefore accumulated about the anticonvulsant properties of this group of antagonists compared to those of other excitatory amino acid antagonists. Despite a relatively poor uptake into the brain, the competitive NMDA antagonists have oral activity and show prolonged and potent anticonvulsant activity against generalized convulsive seizures (reflex-induced, electroshock, chemically-induced seizures) in rodents and primates after intravenous (i.v.), intraperitoneal (i.p.) or oral (p.o.) administration. The competitive NMDA antagonists are comprised of a chemically closely related group of compounds: they are all structural analogues of the excitatory amino acids aspartate and glutamate, where the side-chain carboxylic acid group is replaced with a phosphono- or a tetrazol-group. The anticonvulsant activity of these compounds is stereospecific (the D-isomer being the active enantiomer) and is correlated to their affinities for the NMDA receptor. The most potent members of the group (CPPene, CGS 19755, CGP 37849, LY 274614) have antiepileptic potencies falling within the same range (0.3–3 mg/kg i.p.) in models of generalized convulsant epilepsy (sound-induced seizures in DBA/2 mice, NMDA-induced seizures or electroshock-induced seizures; see Chapman (1991); Rogawski (1992)).

The therapeutic indices (TI) for the competitive NMDA antagonists following acute administration in rodents (TI = 4–20, assessed by rotarod performance; Chapman (1991)) are within the range to those obtained for established antiepileptic drugs (TI = 3–60; Macdonald (1983)). However, Löscher and colleagues have shown that in amygdala-kindled rats (a seizure model considered to be a model of partial epilepsy) the behavioural side-effects of the competitive NMDA antagonists are much more severe than in naive rats (Löscher & Hönack, 1991).

Recently, the competitive NMDA antagonist, D-CPPene (SDZ EAA 494), was shown to be well tolerated in human volunteers following single doses of up to 900 mg orally (Emre, 1992). Chronic (1 week) administration of D-CPPene (500 mg b.d.) was well tolerated in 8/8 control subjects, and 1000 mg b.d. D-CPPene was well tolerated in 6/8 contol subjects (Sveinbjornsdottir *et al.*, 1993). However, when administered as an 'add-on' drug to a group of 8 patients with refractory complex partial seizures patients, D-CPPene caused significant side-effects (poor concentration, sedation, ataxia, depression, amnesia) at lower doses (250 mg–500 mg b.d.), and the study had to be prematurely terminated. No overall improvement was seen in seizure control in this group of patients, and the serum concentration of D-CPPene was much higher than expected based on the pharmacokinetics in the control subjects (Sveinbjornsdottir *et al.*, 1993).

The enhanced susceptibility of the patients with refractory complex partial seizures to the drug-induced side-effects of CPPene resembles the enhanced susceptibility of amygdala-kindled rats to the toxic side-effects of competitive NMDA antagonists compared with control rats (Löscher & Hönack, 1991). A functional up-regulation of the hippocampal NMDA-response has been demonstrated in kindled rats (Mody *et al.*, 1988), which may be related to the enhanced behavioural response to competitive NMDA antagonists. It should be noted that there appears to be no enhanced response to CPPene-induced side-effects in other genetically 'epileptic' rodents (audiogenic DBA/2 mice, audiogenic, genetically epilepsy prone (GEPR) rats) or primates (*Papio papio*, susceptible to photically induced seizures) compared to control animals (see Chapman, 1991). It is not known whether this lack of enhanced sensitivity to CPPene would transfer to humans with photosensitive epilepsy or other forms of generalized seizures. It should also be noted that competitive NMDA antagonists do not consistently substitute for PCP in rodents trained in drug-discrimination tests to identify the psychotomimetic effects of PCP (Willetts *et al.*, 1990). It would be interesting to know how amygdala-kindled rats would perform in such tests.

Finally, the NMDA receptor has recently been shown to consist of a major subunit, NR1, expressed in combination with an additional subunit, NR2, of which there are four different forms, termed A, B, C, or D. These subunit combinations have different regional distribution, developmental profile and different properties (Moriyoshi *et al.*, 1991; Monyer *et al.*, 1992; Nakanishi, 1992). The diversity in NMDA antagonist binding previously detected in autoradiographic binding studies of the NMDA receptor (Beaton *et al.*, 1992; Monaghan *et al.*, 1988) has recently been partly accounted for by different sensitivity of the NR1/NR2 subunit combinations to NMDA antagonist. Competitive NMDA antagonists appear to favor the NR1/NR2A combination (Monaghan *et al.*, 1993; Buller *et al.*, 1993), while MK 801 is more selective for NR1/NR2A or NR1/NR2B compared to NR1/NR2C or NR1/NR2D (Yamakura *et al.*, 1993). The possibility of designing selective antagonists for specific receptor subunit combinations with optimal regional distribution and pharmacological properties is at the present an exciting, but speculative conjecture.

Non-competitive NMDA antagonists acting at the channel site

The non-competitive NMDA antagonists, MK 801 and dextromethorphan, have very potent anticonvulsant activity in a broad range of animal seizure models, but have also very poor therapeutic indices, so that there is little or no separation of therapeutic and toxic doses of drugs (Leander *et al.*, 1988; see Chapman, 1991). Early add-on trials in patients with refractory partial seizures utilized doses of MK 801 (0.6–6 mg/day) or dextromethorphan (120 mg/day) that were 5–10-fold less than those required to suppress seizures in animals, and side-effects prevented the use of higher doses (Troupin *et al.*, 1986; Fisher *et al.*, 1990; Rogawski & Porter, 1990). Recently, some low-affinity, non-competitive NMDA channel site antagonists: 5-aminocarbonyl-10, 11-dihydro-5H-dibenzo[a,d]cycloheptene-5,10-imine (ADCI), an analogue of MK 801; the anti-Parkinsonian drug memantine; remacemide and its desglycine metabolite, have been shown to have anticonvulsant activity and a more favourable therapeutic index than MK 801 (Rogawski *et al.*, 1991; Palmer *et al.*, 1992; Lipton, 1993). Remacemide is active against generalized convusant seizures (MES) in animals, but not against partial seizures (fully amygdala-kindled seizures) and is currently undergoing Phase 2 clinical trials for patients with generalized tonic–clonic and complex partial seizures (Palmer *et al.*, 1992).

Non-competitive NMDA antagonists acting at the glycine site

Ligands acting at the glycine/NMDA site modulates the overall activity of the NMDA receptor. Inhibiting NMDA receptor activity via a modulatory site may provide more flexible and graded inhibition than that achieved using potent, selective antagonists acting competitively directly at the agonist site. The development of selective antagonists acting at the glycine/NMDA site has therefore received considerable attention.

Glycine/NMDA antagonists have anticonvulsant activity in animal models and have been reported to exhibit few toxic side effects following acute administration (Koek & Colpaert, 1990; Saywell *et al.*, 1991; Kemp & Leeson, 1993). Glycine antagonists with appropriate pharmacokinetic properties and blood–brain barrier penetration are only very recently becoming available. A methyl-derivative of HA 966, R-(+)-cis-β-methyl-3-amino-1-hydroxypyrrolid-2-one, L 687,414, has anticonvulsant activity against photically-induced myoclonic seizures in baboon (5–45 mg/kg i.v.; Smith & Meldrum (1992)) and sound-induced clonic and tonic seizures in DBA/2 mice (ED_{50} = 5.1

mg/kg i.p.; Saywell et al. (1991)) following systemic administration. Another systemically active glycine/NMDA site antagonist with potent oral activity is 3-phenyl-4-hydroxy-7-chloro-quinolin-2-(1H)-one, MDL 104,653, which is active both against experimental generalized seizures (sound-induced seizures in DBA/2 mice; ED_{50} = 1.7 mg/kg i.p., 15 min; TI = 4) and partial seizures (fully amygdala-kindled seizures in rats; 20 mg/kg i.p.). The epileptogenic kindling process is also retarded by MDL 104,653 (twice daily, 15 mg/kg, i.p.; Chapman et al. (1993)).

The mechanism of action of the recently introduced antiepileptic compound, felbamate (Leppik & Graves, 1989; Rogawski & Porter, 1990; Ritter et al., 1993), is not fully understood, but the reported interaction with the glycine/NMDA site is being vigorously investigated (Harmsworth et al., 1993; McCabe et al., 1993; Wasterlain et al., 1993; Rho et al., 1993). In addition to being effective in experimental and clinical absence seizures (see above) felbamate is also anticonvulsant in MES and other animal models of generalized convulsant seizures (Swinyard et al., 1986; White et al., 1992), and has antiepileptic activity in refractory partial seizures (Leppik & Graves, 1989; Rogawski & Porter, 1990; Theodore et al., 1991; Palmer & McTavish, 1993; Bourgeois et al., 1993).

Non-NMDA antagonists

AMPA/kainate receptors are responsible for the fast component of glutamatergic excitation. No information is so far available on the action of AMPA/kainate antagonists against clinical convulsant or nonconvulsant generalized epilepsy. In experimental seizure models both competitive (2,3-dihydroxy-6-nitro-7-sulphamoylbenzo(F)-quinoxaline (NBQX); ((3RS,4αRS,6RS,8αRS)-6-[2(1H-tetrazol-5-yl)ethyl]decahydro-isoquinoline-3-carboxylic acid (LY 293558)) and non-competitive (1-(4-aminophenyl)-4-methyl-7,8-methylenediox-5H-2,3-benzodiazepine (GYKI 52466)), AMPA antagonists have anticonvulsant activity against generalized convulsive seizures in rodents and primates (Chapman et al., 1991, 1994; Smith et al., 1991; Rogawski, 1993). In DBA/2 mice the anticonvulsant ED_{50} values (i.p., 30 min, clonic seizures) of the AMPA/kainate antagonists range from 2.7 mg/kg (LY 293558) to 13.6 mg/kg (NBQX); in baboons photically induced myoclonus are inhibited by NBQX (ED_{50} = 3.2 mg/kg i.v., 30 min) and GYKI 52466 (ED_{50} = 2.9 mg/kg i.v., 30 min)(Smith et al., 1991). In addition, these compounds show a promising anticonvulsant action against fully kindled seizures (10 mg/kg i.p.), which is in contrast to the relatively poor anticonvulsant action seen with competitive NMDA antagonists in the same model (Dürmüller et al., 1994), and which might suggest a possible therapeutic application for this group of compounds in temporal lobe epilepsy (see Chapman & Meldrum, 1993).

Like the NMDA receptor, the AMPA/kainate receptor consists of multiple subunits, GluRA, GluRB, GluRC and GluRD, that are assembled in heteromeric combinations with different distribution and different ion conductance (Seeburg, 1993), with preliminary evidence that certain antagonists may be selective for specific subunit combinations (Keller et al., 1993).

Antagonists acting at the metabotropic glutamate receptors

There are multiple metabotropic receptors with a reported wide diversity in function, properties and interaction with other EAA receptors or transmitter systems (see Schoepp & Conn, 1993). A stable up-regulation of metabotropic receptor activity (agonist-induced phosphoinositide hydrolysis) is reported in the amygdala of kindled rats (Akiyama et al., 1992). A number of potent agonists have been identified for this class of receptors, but the currently available antagonists are relatively weak and unselective. Metabotropic agonists exhibit convulsant or pro-convulsant action (Schoepp, 1993; Schoepp & Conn, 1993) and very recent preliminary studies suggest that antagonists acting at different types of metabotropic receptors have anticonvulsant properties, but more potent and selective antagonists need to be synthesized before the role of the metabotropic receptors in epilepsy is clarified.

In conclusion, all known classes of ionotropic excitatory amino acid antagonists (NMDA antagonists acting competitively at the agonist site; glycine/NMDA antagonists; NMDA channel site antagonists; AMPA/kainate antagonists) have anticonvulsant activity in a broad range of experimental seizure models of idiopathic generalized epilepsy, as well as in focal seizure models. The anticonvulsant pharmacological profiles differ between the different classes of antagonists.

The clinical experience with excitatory amino acid antagonists in epilepsy is much more limited. There have been no clinical trials in idiopathic generalized epilepsy. Preliminary small add-on trials in refractory complex partial seizures have been prematurely terminated for the competitive NMDA-antagonist, D-CPPene, due to toxic side-effects, or for the NMDA channel-site antagonist, MK 801, due to lack of antiepileptic effect at tolerated, sub-optimal doses.

Felbamate may be considered a glycine/NMDA antagonist and has been shown to be effective against Lennox–Gastaut syndrome, as well as against refractory partial seizures in man.

References

Akiyama, K., Daigen, A., Yamada, N., Itoh, T., Kohira, I., Ujike, H. & Otsuki, S. (1992): Long-lasting enhancement of metabotropic excitatory amino acid receptor-mediated polyphosphoinositide hydrolysis in the amygdala/pyriform cortex of deep prepiriform cortical kindled rats. *Brain Res.* **569**, 71–77.

Beaton, J.A., Stemsrud, K. & Monaghan, D.T. (1992): Identification of a novel N-methyl-D-aspartate receptor population in the rat medial thalamus. *J. Neurochem.* **59**, 754–757.

Bourgeois, B., Leppik, I.E., Sackellares, J.C., Laxer, K., Lesser, R., Messenheimer, J.A., Kramer, L.D., Kamin, M. & Rosenberg, A. (1993): Felbamate: a double-blind controlled trial in patients undergoing presurgical evaluation of partial seizures. *Neurology* **43**, 693–696.

Buller, A.L., Morrisett, R.A. & Monaghan, D.T. (1993): The NR2 subunit contributes to the pharmacological diversity of native NMDA receptors. *Soc. Neurosci. Abstr.* **19**, 1356.

Chadwick, D.W. (1990): Diagnosis of epilepsy. *Lancet* **336**, 291–295.

Chapman, A.G. (1991): Excitatory amino acid antagonists and therapy of epilepsy. In: *Excitatory amino acid antagonists*, ed. B.S. Meldrum, pp. 265–286. Oxford: Blackwell Scientific.

Chapman, A.G., Smith, S.E. & Meldrum, B.S. (1991): The anticonvulsant effect of the non-NMDA antagonists, NBQX and GYKI 52466, in mice. *Epilepsy Res.* **9**, 92–96.

Chapman, A.G., Dürmüller, N., Parvez, N., Harrison, B.L., Baron, B.M. & Meldrum, B.S. (1993): The anticonvulsant action of a novel NMDA/glycine site antagonist, MDL 104,653, following systemic administration to DBA/2 mice or kindled rats. *Soc. Neurosci. Abstr.* **19**, 197.13.

Chapman, A.G., Smith, S.E., Parvez, N. & Meldrum, B.S. (1994): The effect of aniracetam and cyclothiazide on the anticonvulsant action of 4 AMPA antagonists in rodent seizure models. *Br. J. Pharmacol.* **12**, 14P.

Chapman, A.G. & Meldrum, B.S. (1993): Excitatory amino acid antagonists and epilepsy. *Biochem. Soc. Trans.* **21**, 106–110.

Dürmüller, N., Craggs, M. & Meldrum, B. (1994): The effect of the non-NMDA antagonists GYKI 52466 and NBQX and the competitive NMDA receptor antagonist D-CPPene on the development of amygdala kindling and on amygdala-kindled seizures. *Epilepsy Res.* **17**, 167–174.

Emre, M. (1992): Clinical studies with an NMDA receptor antagonist. *Seizure* **1** (Suppl. A), S6/4.

Fisher, R.S., Cysyk, B.J., Lesser, R.P., Pontecorvo, M.J., Ferkany, J.T., Schwerdt, P.R., Hart, J. & Gordon, B. (1990): Dextromethorphan for treatment of complex partial seizures. *Neurology* **40**, 547–549.

Goa, K.L., Ross, S.R. & Chrisp, P. (1993): Lamotrigine: a review of its pharmacological properties and clinical efficacy in epilepsy. *Drugs* **46**, 152–176.

Harmsworth, W.L., Wolf, H.H., Swinyard, E.A. & White, H.S. (1993): Felbamate modulates glycine receptor function. *Epilepsia* **34** (Suppl. 2), 92–93.

Keller, B.U., Blaschke, M., Rivosecchi, R., Hollmann, M., Heinemann, S.F. & Konnerth, A. (1993): Identification of a subunit-specific antagonist of α-amino-3-hydroxy-5-methyl-4-isoxazolepropionate/kainate receptor channels. *Proc. Natl. Acad. Sci. USA* **90**, 605–609.

Kemp, J.A. & Leeson, P.D. (1993): The glycine site of the NMDA receptor – five years on. *Trends Pharmacol. Sci.* **14**, 20–25.

Koek, W. & Colpaert, F.C. (1990): Selective blockade of N-methyl-D-aspartate (NMDA)-induced convulsions by NMDA antagonists and putative glycine antagonists: relationship with phencyclidine-like behavioral effects. *J. Pharmacol. Exp. Ther.* **252**, 349–357.

Leach, M.J., Marden, C.M. & Miller, A.A. (1986): Pharmacological studies on lamotrigine, a novel potential antiepileptic drug: II. Neurochemical studies on the mechanism of action. *Epilepsia* **27**, 490–497.

Leander, J.D., Rathbun, R.C. & Zimmerman, D.M. (1988): Anticonvulsant effects of phencyclidine-like drugs: relation to N-methyl-D-aspartic acid antagonism. *Brain Res.* **454**, 368–372.

Leppik, I.E. & Graves, N.M. (1989): Potential antiepileptic drugs. Felbamate. In: *Antiepileptic drugs*, 3rd edn. eds. R.H. Levy, F.E. Dreifuss, R.H. Mattson, B.S. Meldrum & J.K. Penry, pp. 983–990. New York: Raven Press.

Lipton, S.A. (1993): Prospects for clinically tolerated NMDA antagonists: open channel blockers and alternative redox states of nitric oxide. *TINS* **16**, 527–532.

Louvel, J. & Pumain, R. (1992): N-methyl-D-aspartate-mediated responses in epileptic cortex in man: an *in vitro* study. In: *Neurotransmitters, seizures and epilepsy IV*, ed. J. Engel, pp. 487–495. Amsterdam: Elsevier.

Löscher, W. & Hönack, D. (1991): Anticonvulsant and behavioral effects of two novel competitive N-methyl-D-aspartate acid receptor antagonists, CGP 37849 and CGP 39551, in the kindling model of epilepsy. Comparison with MK-801 and carbamazepine. *J. Pharmacol. Exp. Ther.* **256**, 432–440.

Macdonald, R.L. (1983): Mechanisms of anticonvulsant drug action. In: *Recent advances in epilepsy*, Vol. 1, eds. T.A. Pedley & B.S. Meldrum, pp. 1–23. Edinburgh: Churchill Livingstone.

Macdonald, R.L. & Meldrum, B.S. (1989): General principles. Principles of antiepileptic drug action. In: *Antiepileptic drugs*, 3rd edn, eds. R.H. Levy, F.E. Dreifuss, R.H. Mattson, B.S. Meldrum & J.K. Penry, pp. 59–83. New York: Raven Press.

Marescaux, C., Micheletti, G., Vergnes, M., Depaulis, A., Rumbach, L. & Warter, J.M. (1984):. A model of chronic spontaneous petit mal-like seizures in the rat: comparison with pentylenetetrazol-induced seizures. *Epilepsia* **25**, 326–331.

Marescaux, C., Vergnes, M., Depaulis, A., Micheletti, G. & Warter, J.M. (1990): Neurotransmission in rats' spontaneous generalized nonconvulsive epilepsy. In: *Neurotransmitters in epilepsy*, ed. G. Avanzini, pp. 453–465. New York: Demos.

Marescaux, C., Vergnes, M. & Bernasconi, R. (1992): $GABA_B$ receptor antagonists: potential new anti-absence drugs. *J. Neural Transm.* **35** (Suppl.), 179–188.

Mattson, R.H. (1989): General principles. Selection of antiepileptic drug therapy. In: *Antiepileptic drugs*, 3rd edn, eds. R.H. Levy, F.E. Dreifuss, R.H. Mattson, B.S. Meldrum & J.K. Penry, pp. 103–115. New York: Raven Press.

McCabe, R.T., Wasterlain, C.G., Kucharczyk, N., Sofia, R.D. & Vogel, J.R. (1993): Evidence for anticonvulsant and neuroprotectant action of felbamate mediated by strychnine-insensitive glycine receptors. *J. Pharmacol. Exp. Ther.* **264**, 1248–1252.

Meldrum, B. & Leach, M. (1994): The mechanisms of action of lamotrigine. *Rev. Contemp. Pharmacother.* **5**, 107–114.

Miller, A.A., Wheatley, P., Sawyer, D.A., Baxter, M.G. & Roth, B. (1986): Pharmacological studies on lamotrigine, a novel potential antiepileptic drug: I. Anticonvulsant profile in mice and rats. *Epilepsia* **27**, 483–489.

Mody, I., Stanton, P.K. & Heinemann, U. (1988): Activation of N-methyl-D-aspartate receptors parallels changes in cellular and synaptic properties of dentate granule cells after kindling. *J. Neurophysiol.* **59**, 1033–1053.

Monaghan, D.T., Olverman, H.J., Nguyen, L., Watkins, J.C. & Cotman, C.W. (1988): Two classes of N-methyl-D-aspartate recognition sites: differential distribution and differential regulation by glycine. *Proc. Natl. Acad. Sci. USA* **85**, 9836–9840.

Monaghan, D.T., Clark, H.C. & Schneider, B.E. (1993): Distribution of NMDA receptor subtypes correspond to specific receptor subunits. *Soc. Neurosci. Abstr.* **19**, 1356.

Monyer, H., Sprengel, R., Schoepfer, R., Herb, A., Higuchi, M., Lomeli, H., Burnashev, N., Sakmann, B. & Seeburg, P.H. (1992): Heteromeric NMDA receptors: molecular and functional distinction of subtypes. *Science* **256**, 1217–1221.

Moriyoshi, K., Masu, M., Ishii, T., Shigemoto, R., Mizuno, N. & Nakanishi, S. (1991): Molecular cloning and characterization of the rat NMDA receptor. *Nature* **354**, 31–37.

Nakanishi, S. (1992): Molecular diversity of glutamate receptors and implications for brain function. *Science* **258**, 597–603.

Palmer, G.C., Murray, R.J., Wilson, T.C.M., Eisman, M.S., Ray, R.K., Griffith, R.C., Napier, J.J., Fedorchuk, M., Stagnitto, M.L. & Garske, G.E. (1992): Biological profile of the metabolites and potential metabolites of the anticonvulsant remacemide. *Epilepsy Res.* **12**, 9–20.

Palmer, K.J. & McTavish, D. (1993): Felbamate: a review of its pharmacodynamic and pharmacokinetic properties, and therapeutic efficacy in epilepsy. *Drugs* **45**, 1041–1065.

Panayiotopoulos, C.P., Ferrie, C.D., Knott, C. & Robinson, R.O. (1993): Interaction of lamotrigine with sodium valproate. *Lancet* **341**, 445.

Pisani, F., Di Perri, R., Perucca, E. & Richens, A. (1993): Interaction of lamotrigine with sodium valproate. *Lancet* **341**, 1224.

Pumain, R., Louvel, J., Gastard, M., Kurcewicz, I. & Vergnes, M. (1992): Responses to *N*-methyl-D-aspartate are enhanced in rats with petit mal-like seizures. *J. Neural Transm.* **35** (Suppl.), 97–108.

Rho, J.M., Donevan, S.D. & Rogawski, M.A. (1993): Mechanism of action of the anticonvulsant felbamate: opposing effects on NMDA and GABAA receptors. *Ann. Neurol.* (in press).

Ritter, F.J. & Felbamate Study Group (1993): Efficacy of felbamate in childhood epileptic encephalopathy (Lennox–Gastaut syndrome). *N. Engl. J. Med.* **328**, 29–33.

Rogawski, M.A., Yamaguchi, S.-I., Jones, S.M., Rice, K.C., Thurkauf, A. & Monn, J.A. (1991): Anticonvulsant activity of the low-affinity uncompetitive *N*-methyl-D-aspartate antagonist ()-5-aminocarbonyl-10,11-dihydro-5H-dibenzo[a,d]cyclohepten-5,10-imine (ADCI): comparison with the structural analogs dizocilpine (MK-801) and carbamazepine. *J. Pharmacol. Exp. Ther.* **259**, 30–37.

Rogawski, M.A. (1992): The NMDA receptor, NMDA antagonists and epilepsy therapy: a status report. *Drugs* **44**, 279–292.

Rogawski, M.A. (1993): Therapeutic potential of excitatory amino acid antagonists: channel blockers and 2,3-benzodiazepines. *Trends Pharmacol. Sci.* **14**,. 325–331.

Rogawski, M.A. & Porter, R.J. (1990): Antiepileptic drugs: pharmacological mechanisms and clinical efficacy with consideration of promising developmental stage compounds. *Pharmacol. Rev.* **42**, 223–270.

Saywell, K., Singh, L., Oles, R.J., Vass, C., Leeson, P.D., Williams, B.J. & Tricklebank, M.D. (1991): The anticonvulsant properties in the mouse of the glycine/NMDA receptor antagonist, L-687,414. *Br. J. Pharmacol.* **102**, 66P.

Schapel, G.J., Beran, R.G., Veijder, F.J., Bertrovic, S.F., Mashford, M.L., Dunnagan, F.M., Yuen, W.C. & Davies, G. (1993): Double-blind placebo controlled, crossover study of lamotrigine in treatment resistant partial seizures. *J. Neurol. Neurosurg. Psychiatry* **56**, 448–453.

Schoepp, D.D. (1993): The biochemical pharmacology of metabotropic glutamate receptors. *Biochem. Soc. Trans.* **21**, 97–102.

Schoepp, D.D. & Conn, P.J. (1993): Metabotropic glutamate receptors in brain function and pathology. *Trends Pharmacol. Sci.* **14**, 13–20.

Seeburg, P.H. (1993): The TINS/TiPS lecture: The molecular biology of mammalian glutamate receptor channels. *Trends Neurosci.* **16**, 359–365.

Smith, S.E., Dürmüller, N. & Meldrum, B.S. (1991): The non-*N*-methyl-D-aspartate antagonists, GYKI 52466 and NBQX are anticonvulsant in two animal models of reflex epilepsy. *Eur. J. Pharmacol.* **201**, 179–183.

Smith, S.E. & Meldrum, B.S. (1992): The glycine-site NMDA receptor antagonist, R-(+)-*cis*-ß-methyl-3-amino-1-hydroxypyrrolid-2-one, L-687,414 is anticonvulsant in baboons. *Eur. J. Pharmacol.* **211**, 109–111.

Sveinbjornsdottir, S., Sander, J.W.A.S., Upton, D., Thompson, P.J., Patsalos, P.N., Hirt, D., Emre, M., Lowe, D. & Duncan, J.S. (1993): The excitatory amino acid antagonist D-CPP-ene (SDZ EAA-494) in patients with epilepsy. *Epilepsy Res.* **16**, 165–174.

Swinyard, E.A., Sofia, R.D. & Kupferberg, H.J. (1986): Comparative anticonvulsant activity and neurotoxicity of felbamate and four prototype antiepileptic drugs in mice and rats. *Epilepsia* **27**, 27–34.

Theodore, W.H., Raubertas, R.F., Porter, R.J., Nice, F., Devinsky, O., Reeves, P., Bromfield, E., Ito, B. & Balish, M. (1991): Felbamate: a clinical trial for complex partial seizures. *Epilepsia* **32**, 392–397.

Troupin, A.S., Mendius, J.R., Cheng, F. & Risinger, M.W. (1986): MK-801. In: *New anticonvulsant drugs. Current problems in epilepsy*, Vol. 4, eds. B.S. Meldrum & R.J. Porter, pp. 191–201. London: John Libbey.

Vergnes, M., Marescaux, C., Depaulis, A., Micheletti, G. & Warter, J.M. (1990): Spontaneous spike-and-wave discharges in Wistar rats: a model of genetic generalized nonconvulsive epilepsy. In *Generalized epilepsy: cellular, molecular, and pharmacological approaches*, eds. M. Avoli, P. Gloor, G. Kostopoulos & R. Naquet, pp. 238–253. Boston: Birkhauser Boston.

Wasterlain, C.G., Wallis, R.A., Adams, L.M. & Panizzon, K.L. (1993): Felbamate is a potent neuroprotective agent. *Epilepsia* **34** (Suppl. 2), 92.

White, H.S., Wolf, H.H., Swinyard, E.A., Skeen, G.A. & Sofia, R.D. (1992): A neuropharmacological evaluation of felbamate as a novel anticonvulsant. *Epilepsia* **33**, 564–572.

Willetts, J., Balster, R.L. & Leander, J.D. (1990): The behavioral pharmacology of NMDA receptor antagonists. *Trends Pharmacol. Sci.* **11**, 423–428.

Yamakura, T., Mori, H., Masaki, H., Shimoji, K. & Mishina, M. (1993): Different sensitivities of NMDA receptor channel subtypes to non-competitive antagonists. *Neuroreport* **4**, 687–690.

Chapter 40

Antiepileptic drugs modulate the seizure threshold for excitatory amino acids in mice

Lechoslaw Turski & David N. Stephens

Research Laboratories of Schering AG, Müllerstr. 178, D-13342 Berlin, Germany

Introduction

Current progress in amino acid research has led to a consensus that L-glutamate-mediated excitation contributes to epileptogenesis (Bradford & Peterson, 1987; Meldrum, 1988). Advances in basic neuroscience have elucidated many of the mechanisms of seizure initiation and spread (Dichter & Ayala, 1987). However, certain aspects of the anticonvulsant action of antiepileptic drugs in current clinical use still remain obscure (Heinemann & Jones, 1990). Current antiepileptic drugs may be classified into three groups according to their ability to (1) inactivate sodium channels (diphenylhydantoin, carbamazepine, sodium valproate), (2) to block calcium currents (ethosuximide, trimethadione), and (3) to enhance γ-aminobutyrate (GABA) mediated inhibition (benzodiazepines, barbiturates) (Macdonald & Meldrum, 1989).

It has long been suspected that many antiepileptic drugs modify L-glutamate mediated excitation (Crawford, 1963; Kleinrok *et al.*, 1980; Stone & Javid, 1980; Meldrum, 1986; Macdonald & Meldrum, 1989). Nevertheless, attempts devoted to establishing a link between *N*-methyl-D-aspartate (NMDA)-dependent processes and the action of antiepileptic drugs have failed (Macdonald & Meldrum, 1989). Although NMDA antagonists have been well characterized as potential antiepileptic compounds (Croucher *et al.*, 1982), antiepileptic drugs currently in use for the treatment of epilepsy do not affect NMDA-mediated excitation (Macdonald & Meldrum, 1989) and only weakly affect NMDA-induced seizures in rodents (Czuczwar *et al.*, 1985; Turski *et al.*, 1991). Much less consensus has been achieved regarding kainate-dependent processes, since specific pharmacological tools are still lacking (Chapman, 1992). Little or no information is available as to whether antiepileptic drugs affect excitation mediated by α-amino-3-hydroxy-5-methyl-4-isoxazolepropionate (AMPA) receptors (Macdonald & Meldrum, 1989).

We report here the development of a method that allows testing the effects of compounds on the threshold for seizures induced by excitatory amino acid agonists activating three subtypes of L-glutamate receptors. Furthermore, we describe the effects of antiepileptic and prototype anticonvulsant drugs – such as diazepam, midazolam, phenobarbital, carbamazepine, diphenylhydantoin, ethosuximide, trimethadione, sodium valproate, 2,3-dihydroxy-6-nitro-7-sulfamoyl-benzo(F)quin-oxaline (NBQX), 1-(4-aminophenyl)-4-methyl-7,8-methylenedioxy-5H-2,3-benzodiazepine (GYKI 52466) and 3-((±)2-carboxypiperazine-4-yl)-propyl-1-phosphonate (CPP) – and convulsants – such as pentylenetetrazol, bicuculline, picrotoxin, 3-mercaptopropionate, strychnine, pilocarpine and methyl–6,7-dimethoxy-4-ethyl-β-carboline-3-carboxylate (DMCM) – on the threshold for seizures induced by excitatory amino acids in mice.

Methods

Animals

Male NMRI mice, 18–22 g in weight, were housed under environmentally controlled conditions (06:00–18:00 h light–dark cycle; 22–24 °C) and permitted free access to food and water. The assignment of mice to experimental groups was random. The observations of seizures took place between 08:00 and 13:00 h. Experimental groups consisted of five to 16 animals.

Drugs and procedure of intracerebral microinfusions

N-Methyl-D-aspartic acid (NMDA; Tocris, Buckhurst Hill, Essex, UK), kainic acid (KA; Sigma, St. Louis, MO, USA) and α-amino-3-hydroxy-5-tertbutyl-4-isoxazolepropionic acid (ATPA; Novo Nordisk, Maaloev, Denmark) were delivered into the lateral brain ventricle of unrestrained mice. The injection setup consisted of a cannula (type 75N) fitted with a stainless-steel circular stop (diameter 4.5 mm) to attain a depth of 3.2 mm. The injection setup was connected with a syringe infusion pump (Harvard Apparatus, South Natick, MA, USA; Model 4400-001) using polyethylene tubing. The injection cannula was placed perpendicular to the surface of the skull according to coordinates derived from the atlas of Montemurro & Dukelow (1972): L 1.0; AP 4.2; V 3.5. The animals were observed for the occurrence of clonic (and tonic) seizures within 180 s. Clonic movements of the limbs lasting more than 5 s scored as a positive response. The beginning of a clonic seizure was used to determine the endpoint indicating that seizure threshold had been reached. Tonic extension of the hindlimbs was used to determine the endpoint indicating that the threshold for tonic seizures had been reached. The dose of the drug required to induce increase/decrease of the seizure threshold by 50 per cent ($THRD_{50}$) was determined in four to six experiments. The $TRHD_{50}$ and the confidence limits were estimated by fitting the data by regression analysis.

Estimation of drug effects on the threshold for seizures induced by excitatory amino acids

For analysis of the action of drugs on the threshold for seizures induced by intracerebral infusions of excitatory amino acids, mice were subjected to clonic convulsions triggered by NMDA, kainic acid and ATPA in the concentration of 1 nmol/5 µl. The infusion rate was kept constant at 5 µl/min. The test drugs were administered i.p. or s.c. before intracerebral administration of amino acids. Diazepam (DIAZ; Hoffmann-La Roche, Basle, Switzerland) was administered in doses of 0.5, 1, 5 and 10 mg/kg (30 min), midazolam (MID; Hoffmann–La Roche) in doses of 5, 10 and 20 mg/kg (30 min), phenobarbital (PHB; Desitin, Hamburg, Germany) in doses of 10, 20, 40 and 80 mg/kg (30 min), valproate (sodium salt; VAL; Desitin) in doses of 100, 200, 300, 400, 500 and 600 mg/kg (30 min), trimethadione (TMD; Abbott, Chicago, IL, USA) in doses of 200, 400 and 800 mg/kg (30 min), ethosuximide (ETX; Goedecke, Berlin, Germany) in doses of 100, 200, 300, 400 and 600 mg/kg (15 min), diphenylhydantoin (DPH; Desitin) in doses of 10, 20, 30 and 40 mg/kg (45 min), carbamazepine (CARB; Ciba–Geigy, Basel, Switzerland) in doses of 10, 20 and 40 mg/kg (45 min), 2,3-dihydroxy-6-nitro-7-sulfamoyl-benzo(F)quinoxaline (NBQX; Novo Nordisk, Maaloev, Denmark) in doses of 0.5, 1, 2, 5, 10 and 50 mg/kg (15 min), 1-(4-aminophenyl)-4-methyl-7,8-methylenedioxy-5H-2,3-benzodiazepine (GYKI 52466; Institute for Drug Research, Budapest, Hungary) in doses of 0.5, 1, 2, 5, 7.5 and 10 mg/kg (15 min), and 3-((±)2-carboxypiperazine-4-yl)-propyl-1-phosphonic acid (CPP; Tocris, Buckhurst Hill, Essex, UK) in doses of 10, 25, 50, 75 and 100 mg/kg (45 min). Pentylenetetrazol (PTZ; Sigma) was administered in doses of 25, 50 and 75 mg/kg (10 min), bicuculline (BIC; Sigma) at a dose of 1 mg/kg (10 min), picrotoxin in doses of 0.5, 1, 2 and

5 mg/kg (10 min), 3-mercaptopropionic acid (3-MP; Sigma) at a dose of 12.5 mg/kg (10 min), strychnine nitrate (STR; Sigma) in the dose of 0.2 mg/kg (10 min), methyl 6,7-dimethoxy-4-ethyl--carboline-3-carboxylate (DMCM, Schering AG, Berlin, Germany) in doses of 0.25, 0.5 and 1 mg/kg (10 min) and pilocarpine hydrochloride (PIL; Sigma) at a dose of 100 mg/kg (15 min).

The dose ranges and time intervals chosen for each antiepileptic drug, excitatory amino acid antagonist, or convulsant were related to maximal efficacy of the respective compound in suppressing/triggering seizures in other experimental models of convulsions (Levy et al., 1989; Dam & Gram, 1991). Furthermore, the anticonvulsant drugs in dose ranges employed in this study produced therapeutic blood levels in NMRI mice (Frey & Schulz, 1970; Frey & Kretschmer, 1971; Frey & Magnussen, 1971; el Sayed et al., 1978; Löscher, 1978; Löscher & Esenwein, 1978; Frey et al., 1979; Frey & Löscher, 1980, 1981; 1982). For intracerebral administration, the drugs were dissolved in saline, while for systemic administration, the drugs were dissolved in saline or 10 per cent (w/v) solution of Cremophor EL (polyethoxylated castor oil; BASF, Ludwigshafen, Germany) in saline.

Statistics

The data from the convulsant tests were statistically analysed by analysis of variance followed by Dunnett's t-test.

Results

Determinations of the threshold for seizures induced by ATPA, kainic acid and NMDA in mice: rationale for concentration, rate and volume of infusions

Figure 1 shows that the excitatory amino acids induced clonic seizures in the course of i.c.v. infusions in mice. The usual convulsive response to excitatory amino acids consisted of staring, twitching of the fore- and/or hindlimbs, hyperventilation and generalized clonic seizures with uncoordination and loss of righting reflex. No qualitative differences in convulsive behaviour were observed in response to ATPA, kainic acid and NMDA. The infusion rate chosen for threshold determinations was set at 5 µl/min and the infusion time was 180 s. These parameters were determined empirically in order to keep the infusion volume into the lateral ventricle of less than 15 µl. The determinations of the threshold for seizures triggered by ATPA showed that it was dependent on the concentration of the amino acid when the infusion rate was kept constant. The latency to seizures using a concentration of 0.25 nmol of ATPA was 133 s, while that for a concentration of 10 nmol 29.8 s (Fig. 1). Comparable results were obtained employing either NMDA or kainic acid (Fig. 1). The delay between the beginning of drug infusion and seizures when using NMDA was 117 s at a concentration of 0.25 nmol, reaching 19 s at a concentration of 10 nmol (Fig. 1). Kainic acid triggered seizures after a delay of 106.2 s at a concentration of 0.25 nmol and after 16.3 s when a concentration of 10 nmol was used (Fig. 1).

These data showed that under pre-determined conditions (rate and volume of infusions), infusion with a concentration of 10 nmol would be useful for detection of anticonvulsant activity of drugs but relatively imprecise for determining possible pro-convulsant effects. Similarly, a concentration of 0.25 nmol could work excellently when determining pro-convulsant actions and would actually fail when working with drugs elevating the seizure threshold. Therefore we tested several other concentrations of all three excitatory amino acids in order to determine which concentration would give an optimal opportunity to assess both seizure threshold elevating and lowering activities. Figure 1 shows that the concentration of 1 nmol for all three amino acids used gave the threshold determinants at about 40–50 s. Such seizure latency offers a convenient opportunity of up and down determinations of the threshold and therefore was chosen for testing the antiepileptic activity of other drugs.

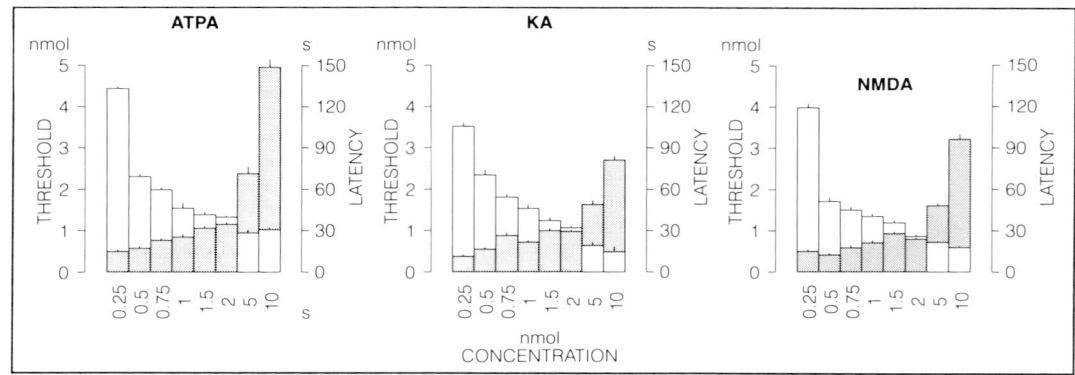

Fig. 1. The threshold (open bars) for and latency (shaded bars) to seizures induced by continuous infusion of different concentrations of excitatory amino acids into the brain lateral ventricle of mice. N-Methyl-D-aspartate (NMDA), kainate (KA) and α-amino-3-hydroxy-5-tertbutyl-4-isoxazolepropionate (ATPA) were infused at a rate of 5 µl/min. The threshold for seizures was determined in nmol ± SEM and latency in s ± SEM. N = 5–8 mice/group.

Effect of drugs on the threshold for seizures triggered by excitatory amino acids

Antiepileptic drugs

The benzodiazepines, diazepam and midazolam, elevated the threshold for kainic acid seizures with an ED_{50} of 4.5 and 11 mg/kg, respectively (Fig. 2; Table 1). No effect of the benzodiazepines on the threshold for ATPA or NMDA seizures was observed up to the dose of 10 mg/kg of diazepam and 20 mg/kg of midazolam. Phenobarbital elevated the threshold for all three amino acids tested, while valproate elevated the threshold for ATPA and kainate seizures. Phenobarbital showed some preference for seizures induced by kainic acid (ED_{50} values of 24 mg/kg)(Fig. 3). Trimethadione elevated the threshold for seizures induced by ATPA and kainic acid (ED_{50} values of 474 and 314.5 mg/kg) and had much less effect against NMDA seizures (ED_{50} 565 mg/kg)(Fig. 4). Ethosuximide consistently elevated threshold for ATPA and kainic acid seizures with ED_{50} values of 334 and 389 mg/kg. The threshold for seizures induced by NMDA was decreased in mice pretreated with

Table 1. Effect of drugs on the threshold for seizures induced by continuous infusion of excitatory amino acids into the lateral brain ventricle of mice ($THRD_{50}$ values)

Treatment	$THRD_{50}$ (mg/kg)					
	ATPA	n	KA	n	NMDA	n
Diazepam	> 10.0	28	4.5 (2.9–7.1)	33	> 10.0	30
Midazolam	> 20.0	18	11.0 (8.5–14.3)	23	> 20.0	23
Phenobarbital	41.4 (34.8–49.4)	31	24.4 (18.2–32.7)	30	34.1 (21.4–54.3)	32
Valproate	345.2 (238–499)	54	250.9 (213–295)	49	> 600	52
Trimethadione	474.4 (410–549)	27	314.5 (242–403)	22	564.9 (390–819)	20
Ethosuximide	333.9 (249–447)	32	388.6 (286–528)	32	> 600	35
Diphenylhydantoin	22.5 (17.3–29.2)	31	> 40.0	30	> 40.0	31
Carbamazepine	13.7 (10.1–18.5)	23	> 40.0	20	> 40.0	24
NBQX	8.0 (5.1–12.5)	42	29.4 (17.7–48.7)	43	> 50.0	34
GYKI 52466	3.5 (1.8–6.9)	36	6.9 (4.0–11.9)	45	8.9 (7.2–10.9)	45
CPP	> 100.0	33	44.4 (30.7–64.2)	30	22.2 (15.0–33.1)	33

NMDA, KA and ATPA were infused in the concentration of 1 nmol/5 µl at a rate of 5 µl/min. The $THRD_{50}$ values and their confidence limits were estimated by fitting the data by non-linear regression analysis and are expressed in mg/kg. n = number of animals.

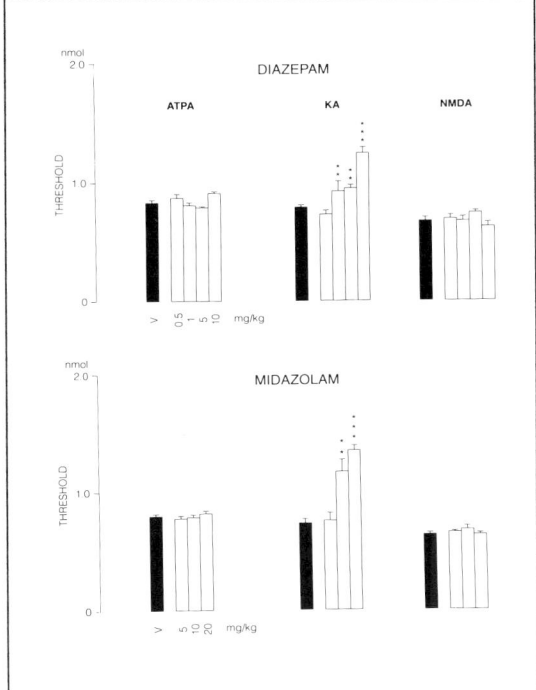

Fig. 2. Effect of diazepam and midazolam on the threshold for seizures induced by continuous infusion of excitatory amino acids into the lateral brain ventricle of mice. N-Methyl-D-aspartate (NMDA), kainate (KA) and α-amino-3-hydroxy-5-tertbutyl-4 isoxazolepropionate (ATPA) were infused with a rate of 5 μl/min. The threshold for seizures was determined in nmol ± SEM. N = number of animals per group = 5–12. **$P < 0.01$; ***$P < 0.001$.

ethosuximide (Fig. 4). Diphenylhydantoin and carbamazepine clearly elevated the threshold for seizures triggered by ATPA (ED_{50} 22.5 mg/kg and 14 mg/kg) but had no effect on kainic acid and NMDA seizures up to the dose of 40 mg/kg (Fig. 5).

The antagonists of excitation mediated by glutamate such as NBQX, GYKI 52466 and CPP were also tested for their effects in the threshold test. NBQX elevated the threshold for ATPA and kainic acid seizures and had no effect on the threshold for NMDA (up to the dose of 50 mg/kg) (Fig. 6; Table 1). GYKI 52466 showed preference for ATPA seizures but also affected seizures induced by kainic acid and NMDA (Fig. 6; Table 1). CPP elevated the threshold for NMDA seizures with an ED_{50} of 22 mg/kg, had little effect on seizures induced by kainate (ED_{50} 44 mg/kg), and no effect on the threshold for seizures triggered by ATPA (up to 100 mg/kg) (Fig. 6).

Convulsant drugs

Pentylenetetrazol lowered the threshold for seizures induced by kainic acid but did not affect the threshold for seizures triggered by ATPA and NMDA (Fig. 7). The GABA antagonist picrotoxin showed a similar effect on seizures triggered by excitatory amino acids as did pentylenetetrazol and lowered the threshold for kainate seizures, while bicuculline, 1 mg/kg, did not affect the threshold for such seizures (Fig. 7). 3-Mercaptopropionic acid, 12.5 mg/kg, and strychnine, 0.2 mg/kg, both had no effect on the threshold for seizures induced by excitatory amino acids (Fig. 8). The β-carboline derivative DMCM lowered the threshold for ATPA seizures and had no effect on the threshold for kainate and NMDA seizures (Fig. 8). Pilocarpine, 100 mg/kg, did not affect the threshold for seizures triggered by excitatory amino acids (Fig. 8).

Discussion

Optimizing the methods for seizure threshold measurements with excitatory amino acids

Analysis of the data obtained with intracerebral infusions of the excitatory amino acids indicates that such a method can be used for determining effects of drugs on the seizure threshold. The seizure susceptibility as determined by the infusion of excitatory amino acids is a variable that depends both on the rate of delivery and the concentration. Higher rates of delivery result in higher threshold determinations when the concentration remains constant. Higher concentration of the amino acids infused with a constant delivery rate also results in elevation of the threshold. Similar observations have been already made when using pentylenetetrazol (i.v.) for determination of the seizure threshold in mice (Nutt et al., 1986). These data indicate that a constant rate of delivery and

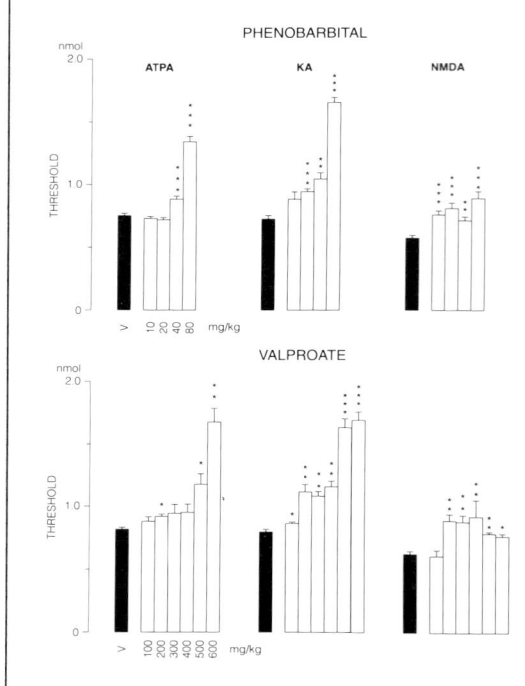

Fig. 3. Effect of phenobarbital and valproate on the threshold for seizures induced by continuous infusion of excitatory amino acids into the lateral brain ventricle of mice. The threshold for seizures was determined in nmol ± SEM. N = number of animals per group = 5–12. *P < 0.05; **P < 0.01; ***P < 0.001.

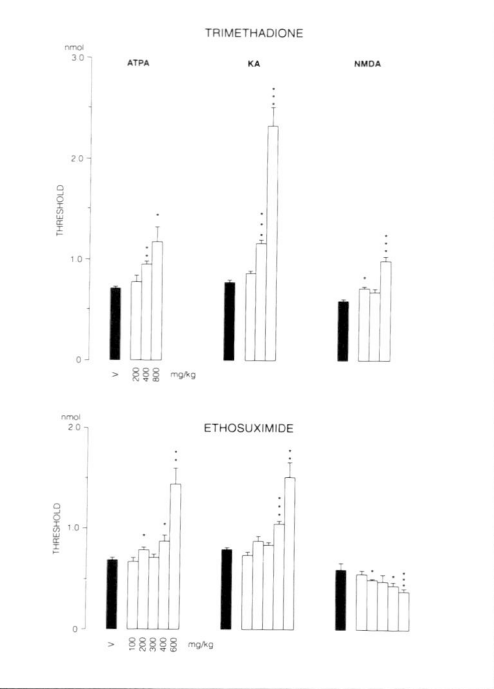

Fig. 4. Effect of trimethadione and ethosuximide on the threshold for seizures induced by continuous infusion of excitatory amino acids into the lateral brain ventricle of mice. The threshold for seizures was determined in nmol ± SEM. N = number of animals per group = 5–11. *P < 0.05; **P < 0.01; ***P < 0.001.

a constant concentration of convulsants is essential for successfully estimating changes in seizure susceptibility. In other words, it is essential for this model system that a reasonable latency to seizures is selected in order to reach a convenient time to threshold to work with. This target may be achieved by means of varying concentrations of drugs in the infusate or by changing infusion rates. Decreasing the concentrations of drug in the infusate or lowering the infusion rate will prolong the latency to seizures. However, increasing the latency in this model will cause an increase in the threshold dose because the infusion time is longer.

In conclusion, the method of threshold determination is convenient for the assessment of anticonvulsant or pro-convulsant activity of drugs. It seems that the intracerebral infusion method may be more advantageous and more valid than systemic infusion technique since when using this method, the limited blood–brain barrier penetrability of the excitatory amino acids does not play any role in estimating drug effects on respective methods. When using a systemic route of administration for both convulsants and experimental drugs, some of the effects observed may be due to competition for or facilitation of the blood–brain barrier penetrability of the excitatory amino acids.

Seizure threshold for excitatory amino acids and activity of drugs

The modulation of the threshold for seizures induced by excitatory amino acids is unknown. Therefore, the principal finding of this research is that antiepileptic drugs differentially modulate

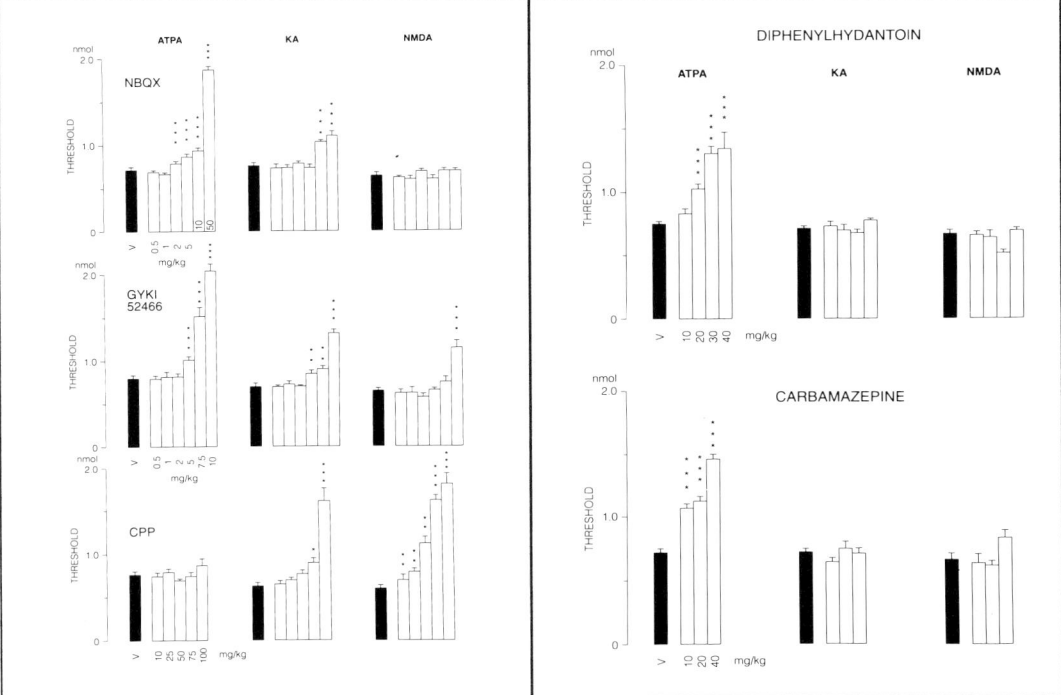

Fig. 5. Effect of diphenylhydantoin and carbamazepine on the threshold for seizures induced by continuous infusion of excitatory amino acids into the lateral brain ventricle of mice. The threshold for seizures was determined in nmol ± SEM. N= number of animals = 7–8. ***$P < 0.001$.

Fig. 6. Effect of excitatory amino acid antagonists on the threshold for seizures induced by continuous infusion of excitatory amino acids into the lateral brain ventricle of mice. The threshold for seizures was determined in nmol ± SEM. N = number of animals per group = 5–11. *$P < 0.05$; **$P < 0.01$; ***$P < 0.001$.

the threshold for such seizures. Diphenylhydantoin and carbamazepine elevated the threshold for seizures induced by the AMPA receptor agonist ATPA and did not affect the seizure threshold for kainate or NMDA. Diphenylhydantoin and carbamazepine were suspected to act on glutamatergic neurotransmission (Skerritt & Johnston, 1984; Meldrum, 1986). However, it is still not known how both drugs may modulate the action of L-glutamate. It is difficult to speculate about the mechanisms of action of diphenylhydantoin and carbamazepine on the threshold for ATPA seizures. What is certainly known is that they do not bind to AMPA receptors (Honore, 1989). It may be that diphenylhydantoin and carbamazepine modulate release of L-glutamate; however, such an action would not explain selectivity against ATPA seizures. It may be speculatively postulated that diphenylhydantoin and carbamazepine modulate activity at AMPA receptors at a novel allosteric site which is different from the AMPA receptor itself and therefore these drugs could be regarded as non-competitive AMPA antagonists. Such an action would also explain, at least in part, clinically relevant effects of diphenylhydantoin and carbamazepine, i.e. their anxiolytic and muscle relaxant actions (Emrich et al., 1983). Alternatively, it may be that both drugs modulate glutamate's action in a different way which is independent of receptors for AMPA or AMPA-gated channels. It is likely that for triggering convulsions NMDA, kainate and ATPA activate different circuitries in the brain, and that diphenylhydantoin and carbamazepine preferentially affect those governed by AMPA receptors, which would also explain the observed selectivity.

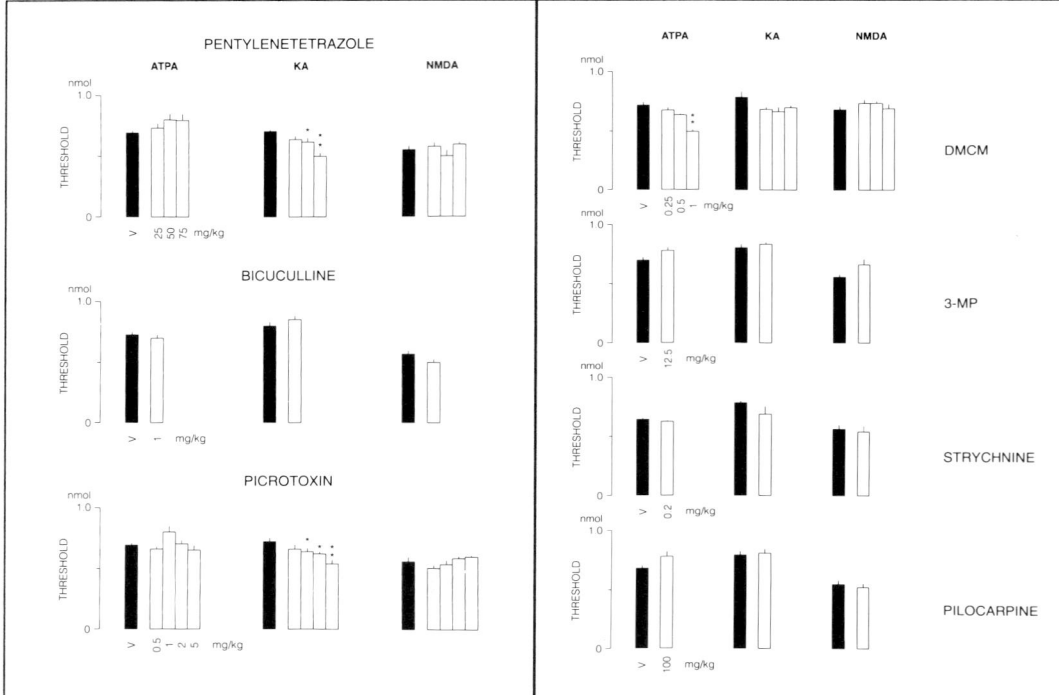

Fig. 7. *Effect of convulsant drugs, pentylenetetrazole, bicuculline and picrotoxin on the threshold for seizures induced by continuous infusion of excitatory amino acids into the lateral brain ventricle of mice. The threshold for seizures was determined in nmol ± SEM. N = number of animals per group = 5–12. *P < 0.05; **P < 0.01.*

Fig. 8. *Effect of convulsant drugs, DMCM, 3-MP, strychnine and pilocarpine on the threshold for seizures induced by continuous infusion of excitatory amino acids into the lateral brain ventricle of mice. The threshold for seizures was determined in nmol ± SEM. N = number of animals per group = 8–10. **P < 0.01.*

The benzodiazepines, diazepam and midazolam, elevated the threshold for kainate seizures but not those for ATPA or NMDA. This selectivity of compounds acting as GABA-receptor modulators is supported by seizure-threshold lowering action of pentylenetetrazol and picrotoxin (GABA antagonists) against kainate. These observations stand in apparent contrast to our previous data on seizures induced by intracerebral administration of excitatory amino acids in mice, since we previously reported that diazepam blocks seizures induced by kainate, quisqualate and NMDA (Turski et al., 1990b). However, in that study diazepam also preferentially affected clonic seizures induced by kainate generating ED_{50} value of 2.2 mg/kg, whereas the ED_{50} value for NMDA was 4.4 mg/kg and that for quisqualate 7.8 mg/kg (Turski et al., 1990b). Furthermore, in that study, midazolam and clonazepam were active only against kainate seizures, and not against seizures triggered by quisqualate or NMDA (Turski et al., 1990a, b). The observations of the threshold modulatory effects of drugs acting on GABA-dependent mechanisms indicate that the benzodiazepines and pentylenetetrazol, and perhaps also picrotoxin, act at a site which modulates kainate receptor/channel complex. This inference is supported by the observation that non-NMDA receptors may be involved in picrotoxin-induced epileptiform activity in the hippocampus (Hablitz & Lee, 1992). At present, little is known about the function and pharmacology of such modulatory sites on glutamate receptors; however, the actions of the benzodiazepines, pentylenetetrazol and picrotoxin on the threshold for kainate seizures reported here imply such a possibility. These observations may gain attention as soon as relevant modulatory sites/proteins at the kainate receptor/channel complex can be identified. Of course, as in the case of the action of diphenylhydantoin or carbamazepine on the thresholds for seizures triggered by ATPA, it is likely that the benzodiazepines preferentially affect circuitries in the brain involved in mediating clonic seizures dependent on kainate receptors, which would also explain their observed selectivity.

Phenobarbital elevated the threshold for seizures induced by all three excitatory amino acids, while valproate was active against seizures induced by ATPA and kainate. Such actions suggest lack of selectivity against either type of excitatory amino acid induced seizures. Phenobarbital and valproate have been reported to affect the release of L-glutamate and L-aspartate (Chapman et al., 1982). It may be that this type of action on glutamate system is mediated by GABA and results in a 'non-selective' elevation of the threshold for ATPA, kainate and NMDA. Although the latter offers an alternative possibility to explain the actions of phenobarbital and valproate on glutamate seizures, the negligible effects of 3-mercaptopropionate on ATPA, kainate and NMDA seizure threshold are not in line with this suggestion. This is because 3-mercaptopropionate, among other actions, is supposed to enhance release of L-aspartate and L-glutamate (Skerritt & Johnston, 1984; Meldrum, 1986).

The actions of trimethadione and ethosuximide on the threshold for seizures induced by different excitatory amino acids were very similar. Both drugs elevated the thresholds for ATPA and kainate seizures, and to a lesser extent, that for seizures induced by NMDA. The important difference was that ethosuximide decreased the threshold for the NMDA seizures. This action was not surprising since ethosuximide has been already reported to enhance susceptibility of mice to clonic seizures induced by NMDA (Turski et al., 1990a). Unfortunately, these observations do not help to explain how both drugs act. It may well be that trimethadione and ethosuximide influence the release of L-glutamate and this could explain the lack of selectivity in their actions, but there is only little evidence to support such a notion (Skerritt & Johnson, 1984; Meldrum, 1986).

Among convulsant drugs, the β-carboline inverse agonist DMCM has been found to be a potent proconvulsant in the ATPA seizure threshold test, while pentylenetetrazol and picrotoxin lowered the threshold for kainic acid seizures. These effects were not seen on the threshold for seizures triggered by NMDA. It seems that DMCM does not act to decrease ATPA seizure threshold at sites which are activated by benzodiazepines, pentylenetetrazol or picrotoxin, since those compounds selectively affected the threshold for seizures induced by kainate and not those triggered by ATPA. The β-carbolines differ from the benzodiazepines in several aspects of their activity in the CNS. It may be that such profiles of action of the β-carbolines and the benzodiazepines depend on different selectivity for GABA-receptor subtypes. Therefore the differences in the selectivity of DMCM and diazepam or midazolam at benzodiazepine receptor subunits may contribute to the observed selectivity of DMCM towards ATPA vs. kainate seizures.

Other convulsants tested, such as bicuculline, 3-mercaptopropionate, strychnine and pilocarpine did not affect the threshold for seizures induced by excitatory amino acids at the doses used.

Conclusions

The method of continuous infusion of excitatory amino acids such as ATPA, kainate and NMDA into the lateral brain ventricle of mice may be used for assessment of drug effects on the threshold for clonic seizures. Such a method offers a novel opportunity for insights into the mechanisms of action of antiepileptic and convulsant drugs. Further work with this seizure model will decide whether it will expand the armamentarium of pharmacologists working in epilepsy research and on drug design.

References

Bradford, H.F. & Peterson, D.W. (1987): Current views of the pathobiochemistry of epilepsy. *Mol. Aspects Med.* **9**, 119–172.

Chapman, A.G. (1992): Effect of NMDA antagonists and non-NMDA antagonists in experimental models of epilepsy. In: *Excitatory amino acids*, ed. R.P. Simon, pp. 265–271. New York: Thieme.

Chapman, A.G., Keane, P.E., Meldrum, B.S., Simiand, J. & Vernieres, J.C. (1982): Mechanism of anticonvulsant action of valproate. *Prog. Neurobiol.* **19**, 315–399.

Crawford, J.M. (1963): The effect upon mice of intraventricular injection of excitant and depressant amino acids. *Biochem. Pharmacol.* **12**, 1443–1444.

Croucher, M.J., Collins, J.F. & Meldrum, B.S. (1982): Anticonvulsant action of excitatory amino acid antagonists. *Science* **216**, 899–901.

Czuczwar, S.J., Frey, H.-H. & Löscher, W. (1985): Antagonism of N-methyl-D-aspartic acid induced by antiepileptic drugs and other agents. *Eur. J. Pharmacol.* **108**, 273–280.

Dam, M. & Gram, L. (1991): *Comprehensive epileptology*. New York: Raven Press.

Dichter, M.A. & Ayala, G.F. (1987): Cellular mechanisms of epilepsy: a status report. *Science* **237**, 157–164.

el Sayed, M.A., Löscher, W. & Frey, H.-H. (1978): Pharmacokinetics of ethosuximide in the dog. *Arch. Int. Pharmacodyn. Ther.* **234**, 180–192.

Emrich, H.M., Altmann, H., Dose, M. & von Zerssen, D. (1983): Therapeutic effects of GABA-ergic drugs in affective disorders. A preliminary report. *Pharmacol. Biochem. Behav.* **19**, 369–372.

Frey, H.-H., Göbel, W. & Löscher, W. (1979): Pharmacokinetics of primidone and its active metabolites in the dog. *Arch. Int. Pharmacodyn. Ther.* **242**, 14–30.

Frey, H.-H. & Kretschmer, B.-H. (1971): Anticonvulsant effect of trimethadione in mice during continued treatment via the drinking water. *Arch. Int. Pharmacodyn. Ther.* **193**, 181–190.

Frey, H.-H. & Löscher, W. (1980): Pharmacokinetics of carbamazepine in the dog. *Arch. Int. Pharmacodyn. Ther.* **243**, 180–191.

Frey, H.-H. & Löscher, W. (1981): Clinical pharmacokinetics of phenytoin in the dog: a reevaluation. *Am. J. Vet. Res.* **41**, 1635–1638.

Frey, H.-H. & Löscher, W. (1982): Anticonvulsant potency of unmetabolized diazepam. *Pharmacology* **25**, 154–159.

Frey, H.-H. & Magnussen, M.P. (1971): A hitherto undescribed feature in the anticonvulsant effect of phenobarbital. *Pharmacology* **5**, 1–8.

Frey, H.-H. & Schulz, R. (1970): Time course of the demethylation of trimethadione. *Acta Pharmacol. Toxicol.* **28**, 477–483.

Hablitz, J.J. & Lee, W.-L. (1992): NMDA receptor involvement in epileptogenesis in the immature neocortex. In: *Neurotransmitters in epilepsy*, eds. G. Avanzini, J. Engel, R. Fariello & U. Heinemann, pp. 139–145. Amsterdam: Elsevier.

Heinemann, U. & Jones, R.S.G. (1989): Neurophysiology. In: *Comprehensive epileptology*, eds. M. Dam & L. Gram, pp. 17–42. New York: Raven Press.

Honore, T. (1989): Excitatory amino acid receptor subtypes and specific antagonists. *Med. Res. Rev.* **9**, 1–23.

Kleinrok, Z., Czuczwar, S.J. & Turski, L. (1980): Prevention of kainic acid-induced seizure-like activity by antiepileptic drugs. *Pol. J. Pharmacol. Pharm.* **32**, 261–264.

Levy, R.H., Dreifuss, F.E., Mattson, R.H., Meldrum, B.S. & Penry, J.K. (1989): *Antiepileptic drugs*. New York: Raven Press.

Löscher, W. (1978): Serum protein binding and pharmacokinetics of valproate in man, dog, rat and mouse. *J. Pharmacol. Exp. Ther.* **204**, 255–261.

Löscher, W. & Esenwein, H. (1978): Pharmacokinetics of sodium valproate in dog and mouse. *Drug Res.* **28**, 782–787.

Macdonald, R.L. & Meldrum, B.S. (1989): Principles of antiepileptic drug action. In: *Antiepileptic drugs*, eds. R. Levy, R. Mattson, B.S. Meldrum, J.K. Penry & F.E. Dreifuss, pp. 59–83. New York: Raven Press.

Meldrum, B.S. (1986): Preclinical test systems for evaluation of novel compounds. In: *New antiepileptic drugs*, eds. B.S. Meldrum & R.J. Porter, pp. 31–48. London: Libbey.

Meldrum, B.S. (1988): What are the future prospects for agents decreasing excitatory neurotransmission as anti-epileptic drugs? In: *Frontiers in excitatory amino acid research*, eds. E.A. Cavalheiro, J. Lehmann & L. Turski, pp. 195–202. New York: Alan Liss.

Montemurro, D.G. & Dukelow, R.H. (1972): *A stereotaxic atlas of the diencephalon and related structures of the mouse.* Mount Kisco, NY: Futura.

Nutt, D.J., Taylor, S.C. & Little, H.J. (1986): Optimizing the pentetrazol infusion test for seizure threshold measurements. *J. Pharm. Pharmacol.* **38,** 697–698.

Skerritt, J.H. & Johnston, G.A.R. (1984): Modulation of excitant amino acid release by convulsant and anticonvulsant drugs. In: *Neurotransmitters, seizures, and epilepsy II*, eds. R.G. Fariello, P.L. Morselli, K.G. Lloyd, L.F. Quesney & J. Engel, pp. 215–226. New York: Raven Press.

Stone, W.E. & Javid, M.J. (1980): Effects of anticonvulsants and glutamate antagonists on the convulsive action of kainic acid. *Arch. Int. Pharmacodyn. Ther.* **23,** 56–65.

Turski, L., Jacobsen, P., Honore T. & Stephens, D.N. (1992): Relief of experimental spasticity and anxiolytic/anticonvulsant actions of the α-amino-3-hydroxy-5-methyl-4-isoxazolepropionate antagonist 2,3-dihydroxy-6-nitro-7-sulfamoyl-benzo(F)quinoxaline.*J. Pharmacol. Exp. Ther.* **260,** 742–747.

Turski, L., Niemann, W. & Stephens, D.N. (1990a): Differential effects of antiepileptic drugs and β-carbolines on seizures induced by excitatory amino acids. *Neuroscience* **39,** 799–807.

Turski, L., Stephens, D.N., Jensen, L.H., Petersen, E.N., Meldrum, B.S., Patel, S., Bondo Hansen, J., Löscher, W., Schneider, H.H. & Schmiechen, R. (1990b): Anticonvulsant action of the β-carboline abecarnil: studies in rodents and baboon, *Papio papio. J. Pharmacol. Exp. Ther.* **253,** 344–352.

Chapter 41

Nitric oxide (NO) and epilepsy

Gérard Rondouin, Marguerite Vergnes* and Mireille Lerner-Natoli

*Laboratoire de Médecine Expérimentale, INSERM U249, CNRS UPR8408, Institut de Biologie, Bd. Henri IV, 34000 Montpellier, France; *Inserm Unité 398, Neurobiologie et Neuropharmacologie des Epilepsies Généralisées, 67084 Strasbourg, France*

Over the past few years, great interest has been shown in nitric oxide (NO), a small diffusible molecule first identified as an air pollutant, but later successively discovered to be involved in several important physiological functions (Lowenstein & Snyder, 1992), and finally assumed to be a novel neuronal messenger. Nitric oxide exerts a potent vasodilative action and was, in fact, demonstrated to play a crucial part in the control of blood pressure (Moncada *et al.*, 1991); it induces relaxation of smooth muscle, governs penile erection, and also controls cerebral blood flow (Iadecola, 1993). It has also been reported that nitric oxide is a cytotoxic molecule produced by macrophages. Moreover, there is some evidence suggesting that in the brain nitric oxide plays a key role in certain basic phenomena of neuronal plasticity, such as long-term potentiation and depression, and it is thus thought to be a major component in the mechanisms of short-term and long-term memory. It seems likely that nitric oxide also contributes to olfactory signalling (Breer *et al.*, 1992), control of pain, and tolerance to morphine (Moore *et al.*, 1991).

Nitric oxide is synthesized peripherally and also in the brain – in neurons and astrocytes – from L-arginine by the enzyme nitric oxide synthase (NOS). In neurons, this enzyme is constitutive, and its activity was shown to be absolutely dependent on Ca^{2+}/calmodulin. Bredt & Snyder (1992) purified the enzyme and mapped the NOS reactivity in the brain. Nitric oxide synthase is present in very specific loci, including the olfactory bulb, cerebellum, colliculi, striatum, hypothalamus, pedunculopontine nucleus, and islands of Calleja. There are also many scattered interneurons with NOS immunoreactivity in the hippocampus and in the cerebral cortex, including the piriform and entorhinal cortices. Since NADPH diaphorase (NADPHd) activity is co-localized with NOS activity (Hope *et al.*, 1991), a majority of neurons producing nitric oxide may also be mapped by the NADPHd histoenzymatic reaction. NADPHd/NOS neurons are remarkable for the wide distribution of their processes (Vincent & Kimura, 1992). In the hippocampus, we (Fig. 1) and others (Vincent & Kimura, 1993; Valtschanoff *et al.*, 1993a) observed multipolar and bipolar cells, sometimes highly stained and displaying large dendritic trees and extensive axonal branching (for a full description of the different types of these neurons see Valtschanoff *et al.* (1993a)). These neurons are essentially present in the dentate gyrus, CA3, and the subiculum, and are also GABA-positive neurons. In the neocortex, scattered neurons are found, a denser innervation being observed in the piriform/entorhinal cortices. Here also, axons, traceable for a long distance from the cell bodies and displaying extensive branching (see Fig. 2), are very characteristic of these neurons. Valtschanoff

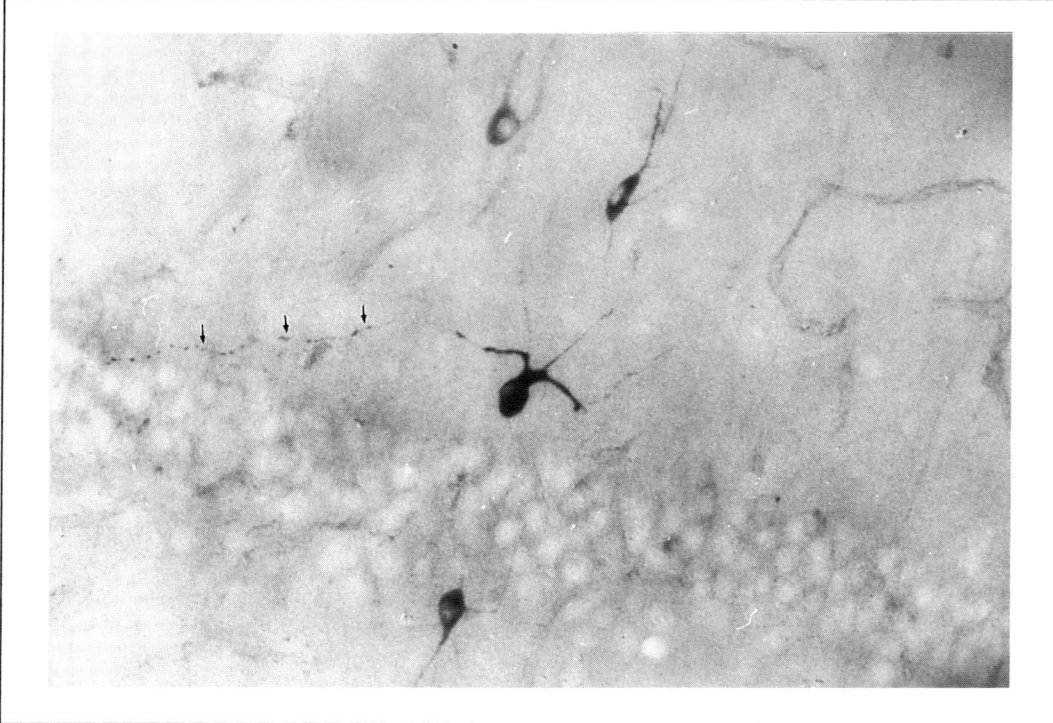

Fig. 1. Stained NADPHd+ neurons in the dentate gyrus. These neurons are close to the cellular bodies of granular cells. Note the remarkable extent of neuronal processes (arrows).

et al. (1993b) also reported co-localization of NADPHd and NOS immunoreactivities with GABA in these neurons, while co-localization with neuropeptide Y and somatostatin has been reported by others (Dawson *et al.*, 1992). Finally, in the present context it must be noted that in rats there is a fairly considerable population of these NOS immunoreactive neurons in the limbic system, particularly in the hippocampus, the medial nucleus of the amygdala, and the piriform/entorhinal cortices. In the thalamus, NADPHd+ neurons are rare and moderately stained; they are found in the paraventricular nucleus. In addition, more or less stained fibre plexus were described in the anteroventral, anteromedial, and submedial nuclei, the reticular nuclei, and the ventroanterior and ventrolateral complex, as well as in the central medial nucleus, the nucleus reuniens, and the laterodorsal nucleus (Vincent & Kimura, 1992). These fibres correspond mainly to terminals of mesopontine cholinergic neurons.

A very important observation was reported by Garthwaite (1991), who demonstrated that activation of glutamate receptors, and especially of NMDA receptors, induced nitric oxide synthesis in the cerebellum. After activation of NMDA receptors (but also of AMPA and metabotropic receptors, and probably indirectly via non-glutamate receptors such as 5-HT$_3$, bradykinin, acetylcholine, and noradrenaline receptors), the resultant influx of Ca^{2+} into the post-synaptic neuron activates the Ca^{2+}/calmodulin-dependent NOS and promotes the synthesis of nitric oxide from L-arginine. Nitric oxide, in turn, can activate soluble guanylate cyclase through binding to a haem moiety in the enzyme. Elevations of cGMP levels result from this activation of the cyclase. Nitric oxide has been reported to stimulate ADP ribosylation of several proteins, including glyceraldehyde-3'-phosphate dehydrogenase (GAPDH) and the GTP-binding proteins through activation of a cytosolic ADP

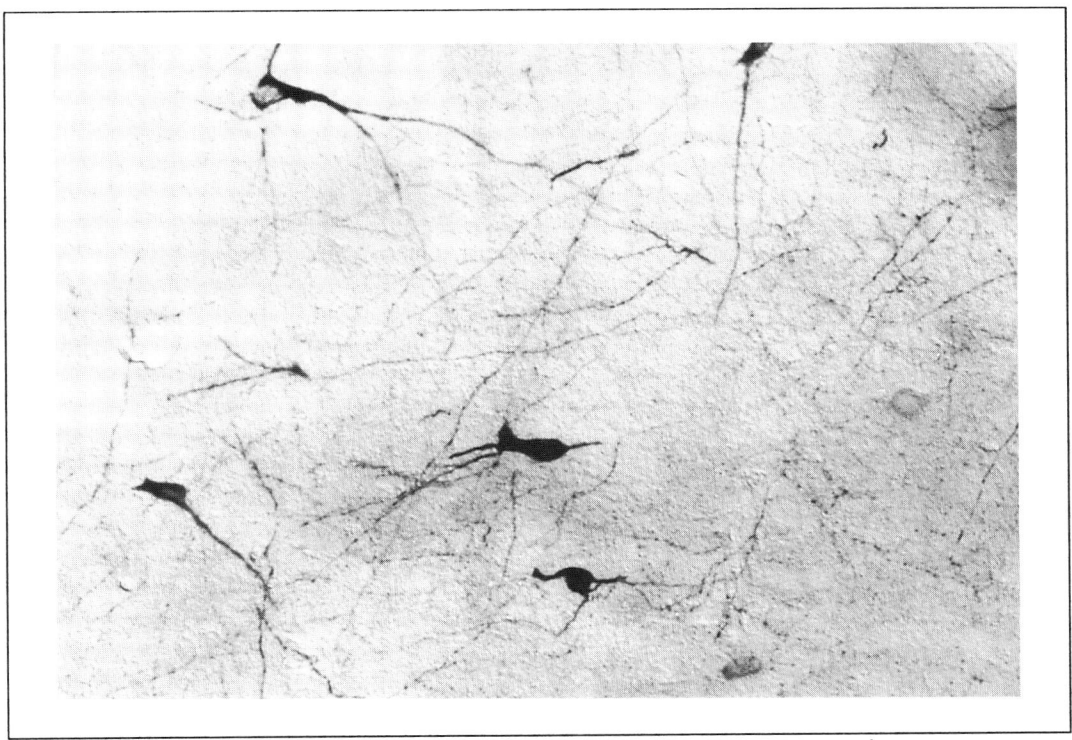
Fig. 2. Stained NADPHd+ neurons in the endopiriform nucleus close to the piriform cortex.

ribosyltransferase (Brune & Lapetina, 1989). In this way nitric oxide could modulate the release of neurotransmitters. Although the areas in which cGMP accumulation was detectable mainly overlapped those expressing NOS, this activation was also observed in neurons other than those producing nitric oxide. Because nitric oxide is a highly diffusible molecule – it has been estimated that nitric oxide diffuses from its native site in a sphere of radius 10 µm (Garthwaite, 1993) – it was proposed that it could cross the membranes and act as an intracellular messenger, exerting at least a paracrine effect on neurons in the neighbourhood (an autocrine effect of nitric oxide, i.e. an effect on the cell in which it is produced, has also been reported). Nitric oxide could serve as an intracellular messenger not only between neurons, but also between neurons and glial cells, and possibly between neurons and blood vessels (Dirnagl et al., 1993).

Additional information about the role of nitric oxide in the brain derived from studies in two models of synaptic plasticity, namely, long-term potentiation (LTP) and long-term depression (LTD). The induction of a long-term potentiation of synaptic transmission observed in hippocampal CA1 after the tetanic stimulation of Schaffer's collateral fibres was blocked by NOS inhibitors (Bon et al., 1992) and also by haemoglobin, a molecule unable to enter the cells, but which is known to trap nitric oxide, whereas SNP, a nitric oxide donor, was reported to induce long-term potentiation by itself (according to recent report by Izumi & Zorumski (1993), but nitric oxide donors, including SNP, induce long-term depression essentially in the hippocampus). Nitric oxide was thus proposed to act as a retrograde messenger (O'Dell et al., 1991) capable of modifying the activity of some enzymes (guanylate cyclase, ADP ribosyl transferase) in the presynaptic terminals, probably resulting in a modification of the release of neurotransmitters (glutamate in this case). Very similar results were obtained in the cerebellum for long-term depression (Shibuki & Okada, 1991).

In patch-clamp and videomicroscopic studies, however, Manzoni et al. (1992) demonstrated that nitric oxide could also block NMDA receptors. Indeed, SIN-1, a nitric oxide donor molecule, was able to block the currents induced by applications of NMDA, but not AMPA. This suggested that there was a negative-feedback loop of nitric oxide on the NMDA receptor. In addition, others reported a down-regulation of NMDA-receptor activity by reaction with thiol groups of the receptor's redox modulatory site, probably based on a reaction with NO^+ (Lei et al., 1992). Some confirmations of this action of nitric oxide were provided by the work of Izumi et al. (1992) showing that the blockade of long-term depression induced by tetanic stimulation by previous application of NMDA was mediated by a nitric oxide mechanism. Moreover, nitric oxide may also inhibit Ca^{2+} currents and reduce cytosolic Ca^{2+} levels (Hoyt et al., 1992).

It has also been reported that in the terminals of the cholinergic neurons in the thalamus nitric oxide may be formed at the presynaptic level (Vincent & Hope, 1992). At all events, the diffusion of nitric oxide outside the neurons in which it originated should be capable of modulating the activity of a more or less large set of neurons, independently of any synaptic transmission.

Insofar as concerns epilepsy, only a few studies have so far addressed this topic and included comparisons with other putative effects of nitric oxide in the brain. It is therefore not surprising that conflicting data have been reported. It is already well known that NMDA receptors are involved in the basic mechanisms of epilepsy (Mody & Heinemann, 1987) and that cGMP levels are increased during a wide variety of seizures (Ferrendelli, 1986). Since nitric oxide is synthesized when NMDA receptors are activated, it is tempting to suppose that the formation of this short-lived molecule and secondarily increased cGMP levels are more or less implicated in epilepsy. Moreover, nitric oxide could also be synthesized by microglia and astrocytes activated during severe epileptic seizures (Wallace & Fredens, 1992)). First of all, some data were reported showing that l-arginine (Mollace et al., 1991; De Sarro et al., 1993) or SNP (De Sarro et al., 1991) could be proconvulsive when injected into specific areas of the brain, whereas a NOS inhibitor (N^G-nitro-l-arginine methyl ester: L-NAME) suppressed this effect. It was proposed that this convulsant effect might be linked to the already demonstrated increase in cyclic GMP during seizures (Ferrendelli, 1986). However, in regard to neurotoxicity, contradictory results were reported: inhibition of the nitric oxide pathway increased the duration of epileptic seizures induced by intracerebroventricular injection of NMDA (Buisson et al., 1993). This effect was also mimicked by methylene blue, which is presumed to be an inhibitor of guanylate cyclase activity, whereas L-arginine or 8-Br-cGMP reversed it. The authors suggested that the increase in cGMP could be linked to the termination of the seizures.

First, we investigated the possible involvement of nitric oxide in partial epilepsy using two models. The first one, the kindling model, is a model of partial secondarily generalized epilepsy (Goddard et al., 1969). Focal seizures secondarily generalized were induced by repeated electrical stimulation (biphasic train of 1 ms pulses, 2 s duration with an intensity ranging from 50 to 200 µA peak to peak) of a limbic structure, the amygdala (see Rondouin et al., 1992, for details). In the second model, seizures were provoked by injection into the amygdala of kainate (2.5 nmoles in 0.5µ l) (Ben Ari et al., 1980), which resulted in sustained epileptic activity in limbic structures (limbic status epilepticus – SE). Our major hypothesis was that if nitric oxide formation is crucial to epilepsy, blockade of nitric oxide synthesis should induce important changes in epileptogenesis.

It is possible, indeed, to block the formation of nitric oxide in the brain by repeatedly injecting twice daily a dose of 25 mg/kg of l-nitro-arginine (L-NOArg). We and others (Dwyer et al., 1991; Rondouin et al., 1992) have shown that this treatment suppresses the formation of cyclic GMP, serving as an index of nitric oxide formation, in response to NMDA activation. However, guanylate cyclase was still activable, as demonstrated by the direct effect of nitric oxide donors.

Under these experimental conditions (see Rondouin et al., 1992 for details), amygdala kindling progressed more rapidly than in untreated animals. The durations of stages 1 and 2 were shortened, whereas the duration of after-discharges was prolonged at these times (Fig. 3). Full kindling was obtained, since no regression was observed when the drug injections were stopped. When adminis-

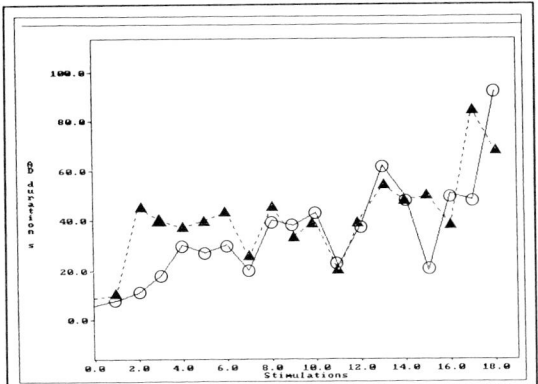

Fig. 3. Effect of L-NOArg on the duration of electrical discharges (AD) in rats during kindling. Note the early increase of AD in the L-NOArg treated rats (black triangles, n = 12) (significant vs control rats, open circles, n = 8, until the 7th stimulation, ANOVA: $P < 0.027$). This early phase of kindling is usually considered to depend on NMDA-receptor-mediated mechanisms.

tered to previously kindled rats, the drug had no effects: neither the duration, nor the severity of the seizures was changed. As the first stages of kindling are generally considered to involve NMDA-receptor stimulation (Stasheff et al., 1989), we proposed that the loss of the negative feed-back of nitric oxide on NMDA receptors was responsible for the facilitation of kindling.

Different results were observed when more severe seizures were induced by injection of kainate into the amygdala. Whereas the initial course of limbic epilepsy provoked by kainate (latency of seizures, EEG patterns) was not modified by L-NOArg, we noted striking differences in the evolution of limbic status epilepticus. A dramatic aggravation of clinical signs, including vocalization and running bouncing fits, was seen 2 h after the beginning of SE, culminating in death after 4 h in the majority of the treated rats. At this time the EEG patterns in treated and untreated animals differed: isolated spikes emerging from low-amplitude EEG were observed in NOArg-treated animals, whereas continuous spiking was present in the EEG of the animals treated with kainate only. An increase in neuropathological lesions was also evident in the animals treated with L-NOArg. Large zones of oedema and the occurrence of eosinophilic neurons (haemalum–eosin staining) were visible in the hippocampal formation of treated animals (4 h after the onset of status), while practically no changes of this nature were seen in the controls (Fig. 4). C-fos immunoreactivity was also increased in the piriform/entorhinal cortices, dentate gyrus and CA1 (see Rondouin et al., 1993, for details). Loss of the negative-feedback loop of nitric oxide on NMDA receptors may also account for these results. Indeed, the observed clinical signs are usually reported after intracerebroventricular injection of NMDA (Matthis & Ungerer, 1992), and c-fos immunoreactivity appeared to be increased in limbic areas with a high density of NMDA receptors.

According to Baron et al. (1989), guanine nucleotides are competitive antagonists of NMDA receptors. It can also be postulated that inhibition of the nitric oxide pathway could prevent this inhibition and thus increase the severity of the seizures. However, the observation that cGMP levels were significantly lower in the treated animals during epilepsy needs to be verified. Moreover, additional effects could be imputed to the loss of nitric oxide control of the regulation of cerebral blood flow (CBF) and brain metabolism in the areas in which neuronal activity was particularly enhanced. Any uncoupling between augmented activity of epileptic neurons and the increase in CBF normally occurring in these conditions (Faraci & Breese, 1993) could presumably lead to an aggravation more closely resembling the conditions seen during ischaemia. Moreover, it is intriguing that the EEG pattern we observed in that condition almost exactly matched the typical pattern in ischaemic, hypoglycaemic conditions. These results are not consistent with the reports (Dawson et al., 1991) of a neuroprotective effect of nitric oxide inhibitors, nor, for that matter, with the findings indicating an epileptogenic effect of nitric oxide donors (De Sarro et al., 1991). These data are also controversial insofar as concerns the involvement of cyclic GMP in epilepsy. A marked increase in cyclic GMP is generally observed before the onset of seizures in various models of epilepsy, and cyclic GMP is generally considered to be proconvulsive (Ferrendelli, 1991). There are only scant data available on the effects of intracerebro-ventricular injections of nitric oxide

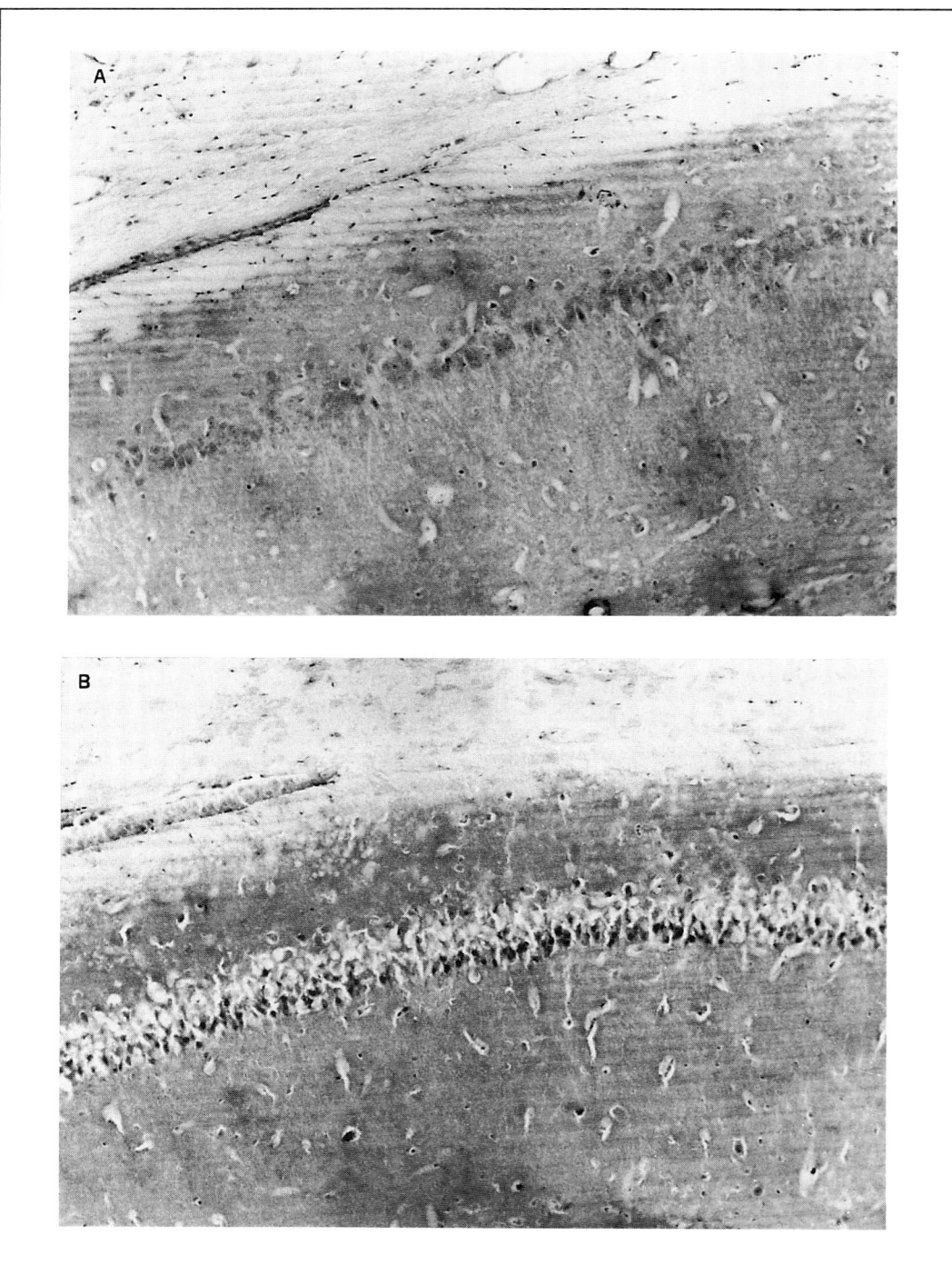

Fig. 4. Hemalun-eosine staining of CA1 pyramidal neurons 4 h after the beginning of limbic status epilepticus in (A) control and (B) in NOArg-treated rats.

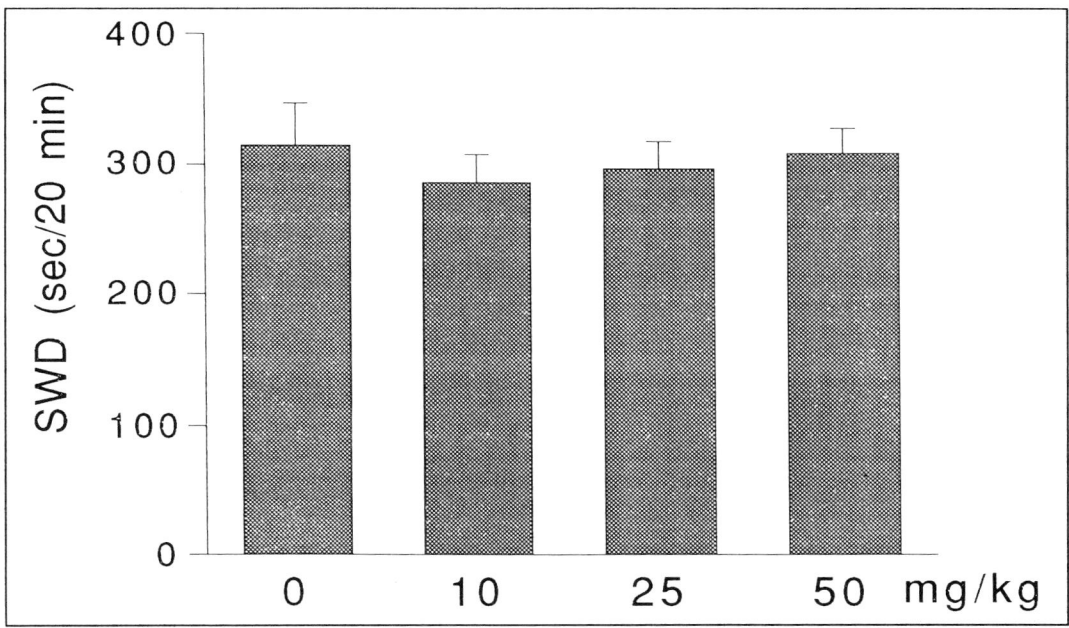

Fig. 5. Mean cumulated duration of spike-and-wave discharges recorded for 1 h after the injection of L-NAME.

donors. Sodium nitroprussiate (SNP) injected into the hippocampus is highly toxic, probably owing to its ability to generate nitric oxide. Severe damage reported by Loiacono et al. (1993) did not appear to be really specific (other nitric oxide donors were without effect), and in these such conditions, it cannot be inferred with any certainty from such observations that nitric oxide is implicated in the aetiology of epilepsy. Moreover, as yet nothing at all is known about the hypothetical epileptogenic effects of the different forms of nitric oxide. As regards neurotoxicity, the various redox states of nitric oxide (Lipton et al., 1993) may have different effects. However, the present results fully agree with those reported by Buisson et al. (1993) and by Haberny et al. (1992), according to which L-NAME aggravates seizures induced by NMDA and quisqualate. They also correlate with the reported increase of (or absence of protection against) glutamate-induced neurotoxicity in neuronal cultures (Pauwels & Leysen, 1992) or in vivo (Lerner-Natoli et al., 1992) and of focal ischaemic infarction by NOS inhibition (Yamamoto et al., 1992), as well as with the persistent elevation of extracellular glutamate concentrations observed in L-NOArg-treated rats after global ischaemia (Zhang et al., 1993). In addition, as postulated by Zhang et al. (1993), inhibitors of NOS may also disturb the balance between superoxide and nitric oxide, thereby increasing the generation of toxic free radicals and thus augmenting the apparent neurotoxicity of EAA.

The possible involvement of nitric oxide in generalized epilepsy was investigated using three different models. In the first model, the seizures induced by a unique injection of a subthreshold dose (20 mg/kg) of pentylenetetrazol (PTZ) are generally considered to closely reflect the pattern of petit mal epilepsy. Cortical electrical activity was recorded through implanted cortical electrodes during 2 h after the injection of PTZ in L-NOArg-treated (n = 10) and control rats (n = 9). Even if a slight tendency to undergo generalized tonic–clonic seizures could be observed in NOArg-treated animals (three out of 10), no statistically significant facilitation of the frequency of occurrence (6–8/min in both groups) or prolongation of the duration (1.5–3 s) of spike-and-wave discharges was demonstrable in this model. Moreover, we failed to demonstrate any facilitation of the effect

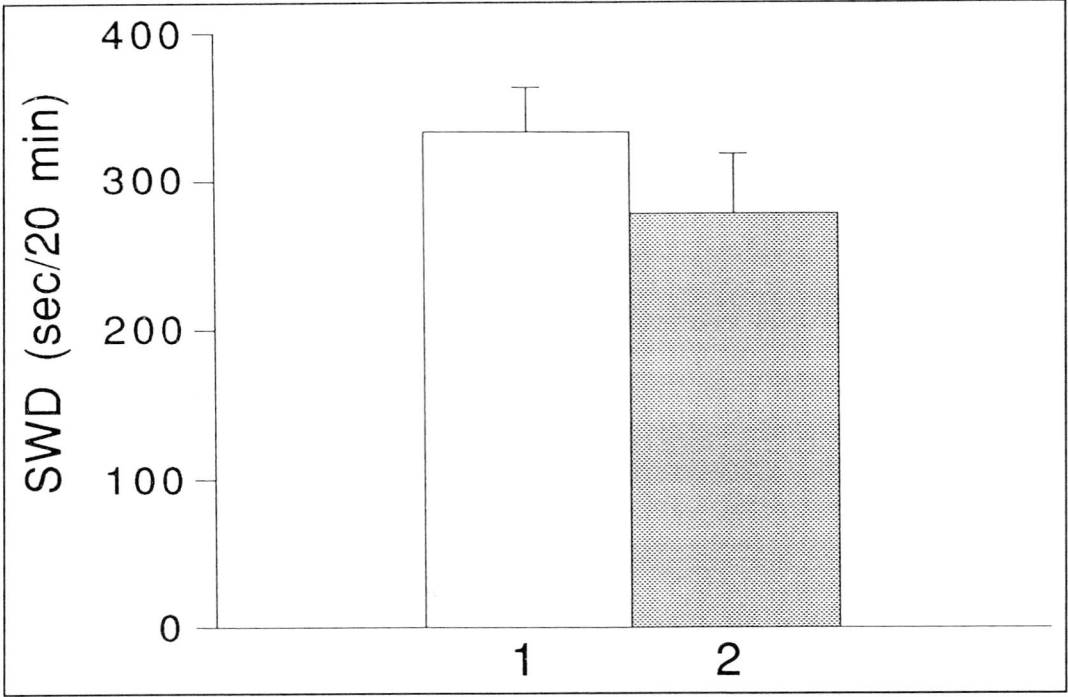

Fig. 6. Mean cumulated duration of spike-and-wave discharges during 1 h (1) after saline injection and (2) after repeated L-NAME injections.

of repeated administration of low doses of PTZ (PTZ kindling) in L-NOArg-treated rats vs controls. These results did not confirm the hypothesis advanced by Pape & Mager (1992) based on the ability of nitric oxide donors to block the physiological oscillations observed in thalamic neurons in cats.

As concerns generalized genetic seizures, additional data were obtained from rats displaying spontaneous absence seizures and from rats susceptible to audiogenic seizures. Adult male Wistar rats from a selected strain with spontaneous absence seizures (genetic absence epilepsy rats from Strasbourg – GAERS) were used. The seizures are characterized by bilateral spike-and-wave discharges (SWD) occurring on the cortical EEG during inactive wakefulness (Vergnes et al., 1982; Marescaux et al., 1992). The EEG was recorded in freely moving animals through four single contact electrodes implanted under pentobarbital (40 mg/kg) anaesthesia over the the fronto-parietal cortex. The rats received intraperitoneal (i.p.) injections of saline or L-NAME, dissolved in 0.9 per cent saline (2 ml/kg). L-NAME was administered either as single injections at the doses of 10, 25 and 50 mg/kg or chronically, twice daily for 4 days at 50 mg/kg. The EEG was recorded for 20 min before and for 1 h after injections. Spike-and-wave discharges were measured and expressed as mean cumulated duration of spike-and-wave discharges for 20 min periods. Single injections of L-NAME in 6 rats at 10, 25 and 50 mg/kg did not change the duration of spike-and-wave discharges for the hour following the injection (Fig. 5). Similarly, repeated injections of 50 mg/kg L-NAME in 11 rats did not significantly reduce the duration of spike-and-wave discharges recorded after the last injection, as compared to the spike-and-wave discharges recorded after a prior saline injection in the same rats (Fig. 6). These results suggest that nitric oxide is not involved in the occurrence of spontaneous spike-and-wave discharges in this genetic model of absence-epilepsy.

Sound-induced seizures in rats are used as a model of generalized convulsive seizures of the brain-stem (Browning, 1985). A strain of Wistar rats susceptible to sound was inbred over 23

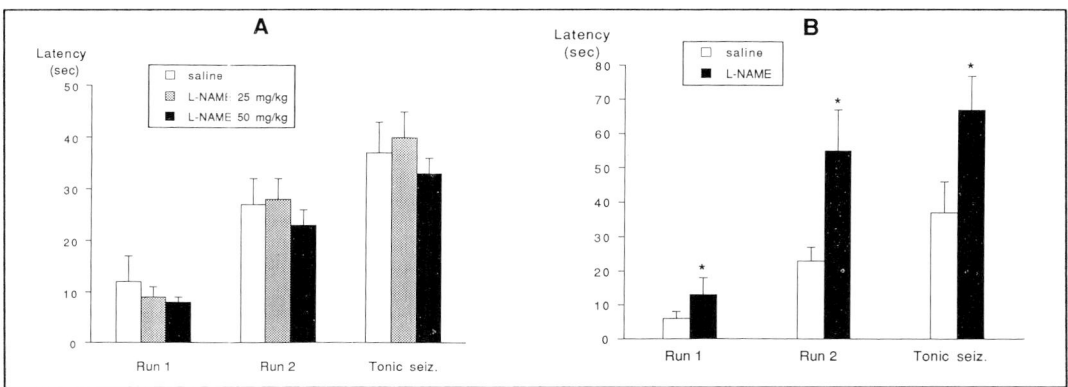

Fig. 7. Sound-induced seizures: mean latency for elicitation of the running phases and the tonic seizure, (A) after acute L-NAME injection, (B) after chronic L-NAME injections. *$P < 0.05$ (Wilcoxon's test).

generations. The animals were exposed to a loud sound (white noise 120 dB, 10–20 kHz) until a seizure was elicited or up to 90 s. The seizures are characterized by one or two episodes of wild running, usually followed by a tonic seizure with dorsal extension of the head (Kiesmann et al., 1988). The latencies of occurrence of the running and tonic phases were noted. No more than two seizures a week were provoked. Rats were exposed to the sound 30 min after the injection of saline or L-NAME at the doses of 25 and 50 mg/kg. Repeated injections of L-NAME 50 mg/kg or saline (twice daily for days) were also performed and animals exposed to sound 30 min after the last injection. Latencies of the running phases and of the tonic seizure were measured. In 16 rats susceptible to audiogenic seizures injected randomly with saline, 25 and 50 mg/kg L-NAME, the mean latencies of the running episodes and of the tonic seizure induced by sound exposure did not differ (Fig. 7a). In a group of 7 rats, repeated L-NAME injections produced increases in the latencies of all phases of the audiogenic seizures elicited at the end of the 4-day treatment, as compared to previous seizures elicited after saline injection (Wilcoxon $P < 0.05$, Fig. 7b). In seven saline-treated paired controls, these latencies were unchanged (results not shown). These results show that nitric oxide may facilitate elicitation of audiogenic seizures, but is not necessary for the different phases of the seizures to occur.

In the Introduction, we pointed out the importance of NADPHd+ neuronal innervation in the limbic system. This could presumably account for the importance of nitric oxide in limbic epilepsy. In addition, our results with nitric oxide inhibition also favour the already proposed hypothesis that primary generalized absence epilepsy involves mechanisms different from those underlying partial epilepsy (indeed they have different pharmacological profiles). Absence epilepsy is thought to be essentially related to GABAergic dysfunction, rather than to EAA-enhanced activation, and PTZ epilepsy preferentially implies GABAergic mechanisms. Unfortunately, it is difficult to devise a good strategic approach to elucidate the role of nitric oxide in epilepsy. As pointed out by Garthwaite (1993), none of the different compounds (i.e. both nitric oxide donors and nitric oxide inhibitors as well as methylene blue) could be considered 'clean' substances completely free of side-effects. Consequently, either systemic or intracerebro-ventricular administration of these compounds could, *per se*, induce neurotoxicity and mask the real mechanisms underlying the involvement of nitric oxide in epilepsy (against this hypothesis is the fact that we observed no lesions in NOArg-treated rats in the kindling experiment).

From all these results, it is at least evident that the formation of nitric oxide is not essential to the induction of seizures and associated neurotoxic effects. Seizures also do not appear to be absolutely dependent on elevations of cyclic GMP levels. Moreover, nitric oxide seems to exert some beneficial effects in the brain during severe, long-lasting seizures, either directly, through NMDA-receptor blockade, or indirectly, through control of cerebrovascular tone and cerebral blood flow. Nitric oxide is a messenger synthesized on demand, and it is not surprising that its principal function in epilepsy could be to modulate a large subset of pathophysiological adaptive mechanisms. That nitric oxide might be an endoconvulsant substance – as provocatively proposed by Buisson et al. (1993) – still remains to be proved.

References

Baron, B.M., Dudley, M.W., McCarthy, D.R., Miller, F.P., Reynolds, I.J. & Schmidt, C.J.J. (1989): Guanine nucleotides are competitive inhibitors of *N*-methyl-D-aspartate at its receptor. *J. Pharmacol. Exp. Ther.* **250**, 162–169.

Ben Ari, Y., Tremblay, E. & Otersen, O.P. (1980): Injections of kainic acid into the amygdaloid complex of the rat: an electrographic, clinical and histological study in relation to the pathology of epilepsy, *Neuroscience* **5**, 515–528.

Bon, C., Böhme, G.A., Doble, A., Stutzman, J.M. & Blanchard, J.C. (1992): A role for nitric oxide in long-term potentiation. *Eur. J. Neurosci.* **4**, 420–424.

Bredt, D.S. & Snyder, S.H. (1992): Nitric oxide, a novel neuronal messenger. *Neuron* **8**, 3–11.

Breer, H., Klemm, T. & Boekhoff, I. (1992): Nitric oxide mediated formation of cyclic GMP in the olfactory system. *Neuroreport* **3**, 1030–1032.

Browning, R. (1985): Role of the brain-stem reticular formation in tonic–clonic seizures: lesion and pharmacological studies. *Fed. Proc.* **44**, 2425–2431.

Brune, B. & Lapetina, E.G. (1989): Activation of a cytosolic ADP-ribosyltransferase by nitric oxide-generating agents. *J. Biol. Chem.* **264**, 8455–8458.

Buisson, A., Lakhmeche, N., Verrechia, C., Plotkine, M. & Boulu, R.G. (1993): Nitric oxide: an endogenous anticonvulsant substance. *Neuroreport* **4**, 444–446.

Dawson, V.L., Dawson, T.M., London, E.D., Bredt, D.S. & Snyder, S.H. (1991): Nitric oxide mediates glutamate neurotoxicity in primary cortical cultures. *Proc. Natl. Acad. Sci. USA* **88**, 6368–6371.

Dawson, T.M., Dawson, V.L. & Snyder, S.H. (1992): A novel neuronal messenger molecule in brain: the free radical nitric oxide. *Ann. Neurol.* **32**, 297–311.

De Sarro, G.B., Di Paola, E.D., De Sarro, A. & Vidal, M.J. (1991): Role of nitric oxide in the genesis of excitatory amino acid-induced seizures from the deep prepiriform cortex. *Fundam. Clin. Pharmacol.* **5**, 503–511.

De Sarro, G., Di Paola, E.D., De Sarro, A. & Vidal, M.J. (1993): l-Arginine potentiates excitatory amino acid-induced seizures elicited in the deep prepiriform cortex. *Eur. J. Pharmacol.* **230**, 151–158.

Dirnagl, U., Lindauer, U. & Villringer, A. (1993): Role of nitric oxide in the coupling of cerebral blood flow to neuronal activation in rats. *Neurosci. Lett.* **149**, 43–46.

Dwyer, M.A., Bredt, D.S. & Snyder, S.H. (1991): Nitric oxide synthase: irreversible inhibition by l-NG-nitroarginine in brain *in vitro* and *in vivo*. *Biochem. Biophys. Res. Commun.* **176**, 1136–1141.

Faraci, F.M. & Breese, K.R. (1993): Nitric oxide mediates vasodilatation in response to activation of *N*-methyl-D-aspartate receptors in brain. *Circ. Res.* **72**, 476–480.

Ferrendelli, J.A. (1986): Roles of biogenic amines and cyclic nucleotides in seizure mechanisms. In: *Advances in neurology*, Vol. 44, eds. A.V. Delgado-Escueta, A.A. Ward, Jr., D.M. Woodbury & R.J. Porter, pp. 393–400. New York: Raven Press.

Garthwaite, J. (1991): Glutamate, nitric oxide and cell–cell signaling in the nervous system. *Trends Neurosci.* **14**, 60–67.

Garthwaite, J. (1993): Nitric oxide signalling in the nervous system. In: *Seminars in the neurosciences*, Vol. 5, ed. J. Garthwaite, pp. 171–180. New York: Academic Press.

Goddard, G.V., McIntyre, D.C. & Leech, C.K. (1969): A permanent change in brain function resulting from daily electrical stimulation. *Exp. Neurol.* **25**, 295–330.

Haberny, K.A., Pou, S. & Eccles, C. (1992): Potentiation of quinolinate-induced hippocampal lesions by inhibition of NO synthesis. *Neurosci. Lett.* **146**, 187–190.

Hope, B.T., Michael, G.J., Knigge, K.M. & Vincent, S.R. (1991): Neuronal NADPH diaphorase is a nitric oxide synthase. *Proc. Natl. Acad. Sci. USA* **88**, 2811–2814.

Hoyt, K.R., Tang, L.H., Aizenman, E. & Reynolds I.J. (1992): Nitric oxide modulates NMDA-induced increases in intracellular Ca^{2+} in cultured rat forebrain neurons. *Brain Res.* **592**, 310–316.

Iadecola, C. (1993): Regulation of the cerebral microcirculation during neural activity: is nitric oxide the missing link? *Trends Neurosci.* **16**, 206–214.

Izumi, Y, Clifford, D.B. & Zorumski, C.F. (1992): Inhibition of long-term potentiation by NMDA-mediated nitric oxide release. *Science* **257**, 1273–1276.

Izumi, Y. & Zorumski, C.F. (1993): Nitric oxide and long-term synaptic depression in the rat hippocampus. *Neuroreport* **4**, 1131–1134.

Kiesmann, M., Marescaux, C., Vergnes, M., Micheletti, G., Depaulis, A. & Warter, J.M. (1988): Audiogenic seizures in Wistar rats before and after repeated auditory stimuli: clinical, pharmacological and electroencephalographic studies. *J. Neural. Transm.* **72**, 235–244.

Lei, S.Z., Pan, Z.H., Aggarwal, S.K., Chen, H.S.V., Hartman, J., Sucher, N.J. & Lipton, S.A. (1992): Effect of nitric oxide production on the redox modulatory site of the NMDA receptor-channel complex. *Neuron* **8**, 1087–1099.

Lerner-Natoli, M., Rondouin, G., De Bock, F. & Bockaert, J. (1992): Chronic NO synthase inhibition fails to protect hippocampal neurones against NMDA toxicity. *Neuroreport* **3**, 1109–1132.

Lipton, A.S., Choi, Y., Pan Z., Lei, S.Z., Chen, H.V., Sucher, N.J., Loscalzo, J., Singel, D.J. & Stamler, J.S. (1993): A redox-based mechanism for the neuroprotective and neurodestructive effects of nitric oxide and related nitroso-compounds. *Nature* **364**, 626–632.

Loiacono, R.E., Jones, N.M. & Beart, P.M. (1993): Nitric oxide (NO) donors result in hippocampal lesions and elevation in transmitter release. *J. Neurochem.* **61**, S274.

Lowenstein, C.J. & Snyder, S.H. (1992): Nitric oxide, a novel biologic messenger. *Cell* **70**, 705–707.

Manzoni, O., Prezeau, L., Marin, P., Deshager, S., Bockaert, J. & Fagni, L. (1992): Nitric oxide-induced blockade of NMDA receptors. *Neuron* **8**, 653–662.

Marescaux, C., Vergnes, M. & Depaulis, A. (1992): Genetic absence-epilepsy in rats from Strasbourg. A review. *J. Neural. Transm. Suppl.* **35**, 37–69.

Matthis, C. & Ungerer, A. (1992): Comparative analysis of seizures induced by intracerebroventricular administration of NMDA, kainate and quisqualate in mice. *Exp. Brain Res.* **88**, 277–282.

Mody, I. & Heinemann, U. (1987): NMDA receptors of dentate gyrus granule cells participate in synaptic transmission following kindling. *Nature* **326**, 701–704.

Mollace, V., Bagetta, G. & Nistico, G. (1991): Evidence that l-arginine possesses proconvulsant effects mediated through nitric oxide. *Neuroreport* **2**, 269–272.

Moncada, S., Palmer, R.M.J. & Higgs, E.A. (1991): Nitric oxide: physiology, pathophysiology, and pharmacology. *Pharmacol. Rev.* **43**, 109–142.

Moore, P.K., Oluyomi, A.O., Babbedge, R.C., Wallace, P. & Hart, S.L. (1991): l-NG-Nitro arginine methyl ester exhibits antinociceptive activity in the mouse. *Br. J. Pharmacol.* **102**, 198–202.

O'Dell, T.J., Hawkins, R.D., Kandel, E.R. & Arancio, O. (1991): Tests of the roles of two diffusible substances in long term potentiation: evidence for nitric oxide as a possible early retrograde messenger. *Proc. Natl. Acad. Sci. USA* **88**, 11285–11289.

Pape, H. & Mager, R. (1992): Nitric oxide controls oscillatory activity in thalamocortical neurons. *Neuron* **9**, 441–448.

Pauwels, P.J. & Leysen, J.E. (1992): Blockade of nitric oxide formation does not prevent glutamate-induced neurotoxicity in neuronal cultures from rat hippocampus. *Neurosci. Lett.* **143**, 27–30.

Rondouin, G., Lerner-Natoli, M., Manzoni, O., Lafon-Cazal, M. & Bockaert, J. (1992): A nitric oxide (NO) synthase inhibitor accelerates amygdala kindling. *Neuroreport* **3**, 805–808.

Rondouin, G., Bockaert, J. & Lerner-Natoli, M. (1993): l-Nitroarginine, an inhibitor of NO synthase, dramatically worsens limbic epilepsy in rats. *Neuroreport* **4**, 1187–1190.

Shibuki, K. & Okada, D. (1991): Endogenous nitric oxide release required for long-term synaptic depression in the cerebellum. *Nature* **349**, 326–328.

Stasheff, S.F., Anderson, W.W., Clark, S. & Wilson, W.A. (1989): NMDA antagonists differentiate epileptogenesis from seizure expression in an *in vitro* model. *Science* **245**, 648–651.

Valtschanoff, J.G., Weinberg, R.J., Kharazia, V.N., Nakane, M. & Schmidt, H.H.W. (1993a): Neurons in rat hippocampus that synthesize nitric oxide. *J. Comp. Neurol.* **333**, 111–121.

Valtschanoff, J.G., Weinberg, R.J., Kharazia, V.N., Schmidt, H.H.H.W., Nakane, M. & Rustioni, A. (1993b): Neurons in rat cerebral cortex that synthetize nitric oxide: NADPH diaphorase histochemistry, NOS immunocytochemistry, and colocalization with GABA. *Neurosci. Lett.* **157**, 157–161.

Vergnes, M., Marescaux, C., Micheletti, G., Reiss, J., Depaulis, A., Rumbach, L. & Warter, J.M. (1982): Spontaneous paroxysmal electroclinical patterns in rat: a model of generalized non-convulsive epilepsy. *Neurosci. Lett.* **33**, 97–101.

Vincent, S.R. & Hope, B.T. (1992): Neurons that say NO. *Trends Neurosci.* **15**, 108–113.

Vincent, S.R. & Kimura, H. (1992): Histochemical mapping of nitric oxide synthase in the rat brain. *Neuroscience* **46**, 775–784.

Wallace, M.N. & Fredens, K. (1992): Activated astrocytes of the mouse hippocampus contain high levels of NADPH-diaphorase. *Neuroreport* **3**, 953–956.

Yamamoto, S., Golanov, E.V., Berger, S.B. & Reis, D.J. (1992): Inhibition of nitric oxide synthesis increases focal ischaemic infarction in rat. *J. Cereb. Blood Flow Metab.* **12**, 717–726.

Zhang, J., Benveniste, H. & Piantadosi, A. (1993): Inhibition of nitric oxide synthase increases extracellular cerebral glutamate concentration after global ischaemia. *Neurosci. Lett.* **157**, 179–182.

Chapter 42

Relevance of the nigral control of seizures in the treatment of generalized epilepsies

Antoine Depaulis

INSERM Unité 398, Neurobiologie et Neuropharmacologie des Epilepsies Généralisées, Centre de Neurochimie du CNRS, 5 rue Blaise Pascal, 67084 Strasbourg Cedex, France

Introduction

Parallel to the studies of the physiopathology of generalized seizures in both animals and humans, several approaches have been taken to elucidate the mechanisms in the central nervous system (CNS) that can intervene to control seizures. Besides the capacity for the neurons underlying the epileptic discharge to correct their abnormal activity by modifying the intracellular and extracellular constituents (e.g. ions and second and third messengers) it is now clear that, as in other physiological processes (e.g. nociception), epileptic seizures can be suppressed by 'remote' endogenous circuits involving several brain structures (for a recent review, see Miller, 1992). In particular, several lines of evidence have converged over the past ten years to demonstrate the existence of a system at least partly involving neurons of the substantia nigra (SN), and which can suppress the generation or propagation of different kinds of seizures in animals (for a recent review see Depaulis *et al.* (1994)). The possibility that neurons of the substantia nigra can be part of an endogenous system controlling different types of seizures was first proposed by Gale in 1985, and the system has often been referred to as the 'nigral control of epilepsy' (NCE). This chapter will review current knowledge of the circuitry and functioning of this system. Because the nigral control of epilepsy appears to intervene in different forms of generalized epilepsy, it affords an interesting approach to the elaboration of new therapeutic strategies for the treatment of idiopathic generalized epilepsies. Data from the literature indicating which neurotransmission systems participates in the nigral control of epilepsy and whether the current antiepileptic compounds act through this system will then be presented in the latter part of the chapter.

Role of the substantia nigra in the control of seizures

The first anatomical evidence for the involvement of the substantia nigra in the control of seizures was reported by Hayashi (1952, 1953): lesions of the rostral midbrain that included the substantia nigra suppressed seizures induced by application of chemical convulsants into the motor cortex. Similar suppression of other types of seizure (e.g. maximal electroshock-induced or bicuculline-in-

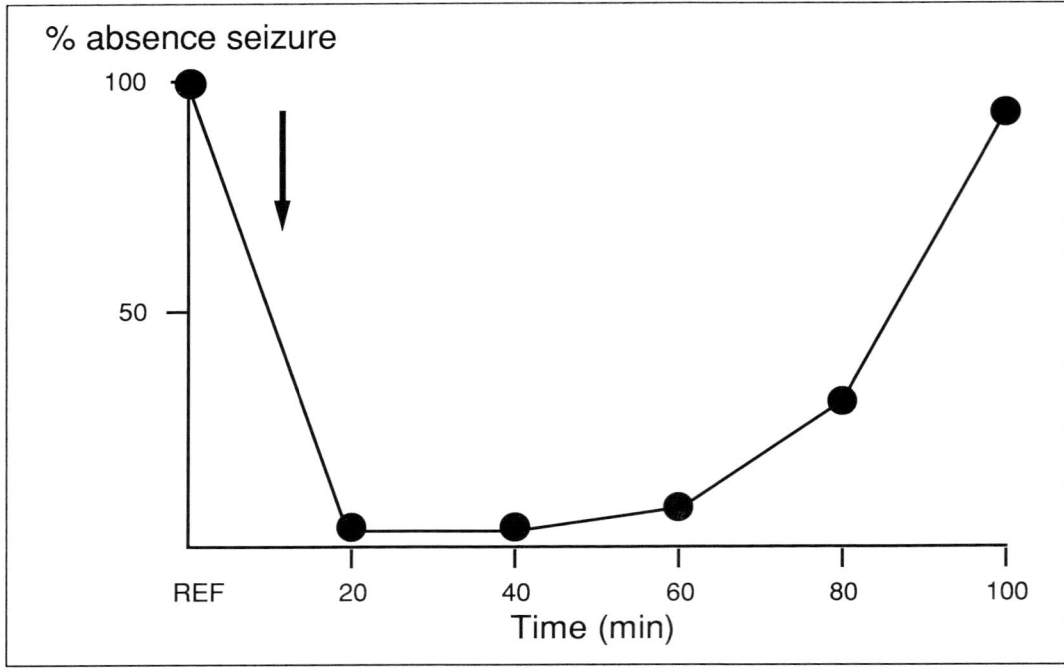

Fig. 1. Time-course of effects of bilateral injections of 2 ng/side of muscimol in the substantia nigra (arrow) on the percentage of absence seizures in a genetic model of generalized non-convulsive epilepsy. The results are expressed in percent of the cumulated duration of seizures as compared to control conditions per 20 min period. Data from Depaulis et al. (1988).

duced seizures, amygdala kindling) was also described after bilateral neurotoxic destruction of the substantia nigra (Garant & Gale, 1983; McNamara et al., 1984). In addition, endogenous γ-aminobutyric acid (GABA) levels were found to be decreased in the SN prior to seizures induced either by methoxypyridoxine (Nitsch & Okada, 1976), or by amygdala kindling (Löscher & Schwark, 1985, 1987). Furthermore (^{3}H)GABA binding was found to be lower in the substantia nigra and the amygdala of kindled rats, whereas it was higher in the striatum (Löscher & Schwark, 1987). In the Mongolian gerbil, which is susceptible to convulsive seizures, the density of GABA-benzodiazepine receptors in the substantia nigra was reported to be lower than in non-susceptible animals (Olsen et al., 1985). This difference was also observed in young animals (i.e. before the occurrence of the first seizure), which suggests that it is not secondary to the recurrence of seizures (Olsen et al., 1985).

Most of the authors who have studied the involvement of the substantia nigra in the control of epileptic seizures have used localized pharmacological manipulations carried out by intracerebral microinjection techniques. Iadarola & Gale (1982) were the first to demonstrate that pharmacological potentiation of GABAergic transmission within the substantia nigra by bilateral microinjections of either muscimol, a GABA agonist, or γ-vinyl GABA (GVG), an inhibitor of GABA transaminase (Lippert et al., 1977), suppressed the seizures in different models of generalized convulsive seizures in the rat. These effects were rapidly confirmed in other models by other research groups (Table 1). As can be seen from Table 1, bilateral activation of GABAergic transmission within the substantia nigra suppresses seizures in very different animal models of epilepsy, e.g. seizures induced by maximal electroshock (Iadarola & Gale, 1982; De Sarro et al., 1985; Mirski et al., 1986; Miller et al., 1987; Platt et al., 1987; Zhang et al., 1991), systemically and intracerebrally applied chemical convulsants (Iadarola & Gale, 1982; Garant & Gale, 1986; Okada et al., 1989; Zhang et al., 1989), flurothyl inhalation (Okada et al., 1986; Toussi et al., 1987; Maggio & Gale, 1989; Sperber et al., 1989; Xu et al., 1991), kindling (Le Gal La Salle et al., 1983; McNamara et al., 1983, 1984; Löscher et al., 1987; Platt et al., 1987; Shin et al., 1987), and systemic injection of pilocarpine (Turski et al., 1986a), as well as genetic or chemically induced absences (Depaulis et al., 1988, 1989). Because of the recurrent nature of the seizures, the genetic model of absence epilepsy provides indications about the time-course of the antiepileptic effects of intranigral injections of a GABA-mimetic. Following bilateral injections of muscimol (2 ng/side), complete suppression of spike-and-wave discharges was observed in epileptic rats, and the inhibitory action remained significant for 60–80 min (Fig. 1: Depaulis et al., 1988). This finding is in agreement with the results of most studies using models of convulsive epilepsy in which suppression of the seizures was observed within the first hour after injection of muscimol.

Table 1. *Effects of bilateral injections of GABA mimetics into the substantia nigra on different models of seizures in adult rats*

Models	Effects
Electroshock	−
Kindling	−
Systemic GABA antagonists	−
Area tempestas	−
Methionine sulfoximine	−
Pilocarpine	−
Fluorothyl	−
Genetic absence	−
Pharmacologically-induced absence	−
Pentylenetetrazol-induced clonic seizures	−
Pentylenetetrazol-induced tonic–clonic seizures	0
Audiogenic seizures	0

− = suppression of seizures; 0 = no suppression of seizures. Data from the literature (see text for references).

The antiepileptic effects reported in Table 1 were always obtained after *bilateral* injections in the substantia nigra; unilateral injections of GABA mimetics had no antiepileptic effects (e.g. Le Gal La Salle et al., 1983; Depaulis et al., 1988; Maggio & Gale, 1989). Furthermore, these effects appear specific to the substantia nigra within the ventral midbrain region. Bilateral injections of GVG into various areas of the brain did not modify maximal electroshock seizures unless they were located in the ventral midbrain (Iadarola & Gale, 1982). Bilateral injections of GABA agonists, which have a more limited diffusion (e.g. Depaulis et al., 1989), within the ventral midbrain, were also shown to be ineffective when performed above, or around the substantia nigra (Iadarola & Gale, 1982; McNamara et al., 1983, 1984; Le Gal La Salle et al., 1983; Toussi et al., 1987; Shin et al., 1987; Depaulis et al., 1988).

Among all the generalized seizures on which the effects of intranigral activation of GABAergic transmission were tested (Table 1), only audiogenic seizures and those induced by high doses of pentylenetetrazol were not consistently suppressed (Frye et al., 1983; Mirski et al., 1986; Miller et al., 1987; Zhang et al., 1989, 1991; Xie et al., 1991; Depaulis et al., 1990b; but see also Gonzalez & Hettinger, 1984). These two forms of seizure are characterized by a predominent tonic component, and it has been suggested that they primarily involve brainstem structures (Browning, 1985). This is in contrast with the other models of generalized epilepsy in which forebrain structures are critical in the generation of the seizures. It has thus been suggested that nigral control of epilepsy is effective on 'forebrain' rather than 'brainstem' seizures (Depaulis et al., 1994).

Furthermore, all the seizures reported in Table 1 are models of *generalized* seizures, or seizures with secondary generalization, as in the case of kindling. Only very few studies have examined the involvement of 'nigral control of epilepsy' in the control of partial seizures. Unilateral intranigral injections of muscimol have been shown to decrease the threshold for seizures induced by low frequency stimulation of the homolateral premotor cortex (Ono & Wada, 1987). This treatment also shortens the latency for generalization of seizures, but does not affect the duration of developed seizures. It is interesting to note the facilitatory effect of intranigral muscimol on this type of model. Further investigations will, however, be necessary to determine whether nigral control of epilepsy is also effective against partial seizures.

Finally, the antiepileptic effects resulting from pharmacological manipulations of the substantia nigra do not appear to be secondary to modifications of sensorimotor processes. These manipulations were clearly shown to be effective not only on the motor aspects of the seizures, but also on the EEG activity (Le Gal La Salle, 1983; Garant & Gale, 1986; Turski et al., 1986a; Depaulis et al., 1988). Moreover, bilateral activation of GABAergic transmission within the substantia nigra also protects against the neuropathological alterations of the limbic circuitry observed in pilocarpine-induced seizures (Turski et al., 1986a).

The foregoing observations thus clearly favour the existence, within the substantia nigra of adult rats, of a population of neurons the inhibition of which leads to antiepileptic effects in different models of generalized epilepsy in which the seizures originate in forebrain structures. This inhibition involves the GABAergic neurotransmission within the substantia nigra, but most probably other neurotransmission systems as well (see below).

The neuroanatomical circuitry of nigral control

The antiepileptic effects observed following pharmacological manipulations within the substantia nigra suggest that either intrinsic neurons or input neurons can, under certain conditions, trigger nigral control of epilepsy. One of the goals in the characterization of nigral control of epilepsy has been to identify the nature of these nigral inputs. Conversely, the fact that inhibition of nigral neurons can protect against very different types of seizure and that the substantia nigra is not a critical structure for the generation of seizures suggests that the antiepileptic effects reported above involve nigral output neurons and cannot be confined to a local phenomenon. Several studies have thus aimed at characterizing the critical nigral outputs involved in nigral control of epilepsy.

Nigral inputs

As indicated by the various data reported above, GABAergic transmission within the substantia nigra appears to play a key role in the triggering of nigral control of epilepsy. GABA, as well as glutamic acid decarboxylase, which is present in a high concentration in the substantia nigra, is derived from nigral afferents rather than from intrinsic interneurons. The major afferent of the substantia nigra is constituted by a massive GABAergic projection from the homolateral striatum (e.g. Oertel et al., 1981; Fisher et al., 1986; Bolam & Smith, 1990). It has been shown that a striatal fibre in the substantia nigra pars reticulata ramifies and frequently terminates on long dendrites of a single nigral neuron (Tokuno et al., 1990). Finally, activation of striatal cells results in GABA release in the substantia nigra, which, in turn, leads to inhibition of the spontaneous firing of pars reticulata cells (e.g. see Chevalier et al., 1985).

Several studies have thus investigated the role of the striatal GABAergic input to the substantia nigra in the control of seizures. Activation of striatal neurons by bilateral injection of low doses of a GABA antagonist or an agonist of one subtype of glutamatergic receptor (e.g. NMDA) into the striatum has been reported to suppress convulsive seizures of different types (e.g. those induced by systemic pilocarpine, bicuculline and kainic acid, amygdala kindling, and local injection of bicuculline into the area tempestas) (Cavalheiro & Turski, 1986; Turski et al., 1985, 1987, 1989). In particular, such injections protect against the EEG and motor components of pilocarpine-induced seizures and the associated brain damage. This treatment appears to be especially effective when the injections are performed in the ventral and posterior part of the caudate putamen (Turski et al., 1987). The involvement of GABAergic striatonigral projections in the antiepileptic effects of NMDA injection into the ventral striatum was confirmed by the fact that these effects were abolished by microinjection of a GABA antagonist into the substantia nigra (Turski et al., 1987).

The substantia nigra receives many other afferent projections from different structures (cortex, subthalamic nucleus, dorsal raphe) with different neurotransmitters (glutamate and aspartate, serotonin, substance P, dynorphin, acetylcholine). However, practically nothing is known about the influence of these different inputs on nigral control of epilepsy. It is very likely that nigral control of epilepsy is not solely modulated by the GABAergic striato-nigral projection, but that its triggering results from an integration of different inputs. In this respect the role of glutamatergic/aspartatergic projections should be further examined, given the effects of intranigral injections of NMDA antagonists (see below).

Nigral outputs

The fact that activation of nigral control of epilepsy protects against very different types of seizures, on the one hand, and that the substantia nigra is not a critical structure in the generation of most seizures, on the other, suggests that nigral control of epilepsy acts rather as a 'remote-control' system than simply as a carrier of 'seizure information' from rostral sites to caudal targets. Neither electrical nor chemical stimulation of the substantia nigra (Gibbs & Gibbs, 1936; Kreindler et al., 1958; Morimoto & Goddard, 1987; Maggio et al., 1990) has provoked seizures. Moreover, there are no strict correlations between seizures and paroxysmal changes in the substantia nigra in kindling or absence seizures (Depaulis, 1990; Vergnes et al., 1990; Bonhaus et al., 1991). It is thus very unlikely that the antiepileptic effects observed after bilateral inhibition of nigral neurons are due to a functional exclusion of this structure. It therefore appeared critically important to determine which nigral outputs were involved in the suppression of seizures reported above.

The nigral outputs can be broadly distinguished as originating from two main populations of neurons: (1) dopaminergic cell bodies, which are located in the pars compacta of the nigral control of epilepsy and project primarily to the neostriatum and foreparts of the brain through the medial forebrain bundle (e.g. Andén et al., 1984; Bentivoglio et al., 1979); (2) GABAergic cell bodies, which are mainly located in the pars reticulata of the substantia nigra and project to (i) the ventromedial thalamic nucleus (e.g. Di Chiara et al., 1979; Deniau & Chevalier, 1992); (ii) the deep and intermediate layers of the superior colliculus (e.g. Bentivoglio et al., 1979; Chevalier et al., 1981; Deniau & Chevalier, 1992), and (iii) the rostral mesencephalic reticular formation and more especially the pedunculopontine nucleus and the ventral peribrachial nuclei (Hopkins & Niessen, 1976; Childs & Gale, 1983; Deniau & Chevalier, 1992). These GABAergic projections appears to exert a tonic inhibition on the target cells (Chevalier et al., 1981, 1985). Furthermore, activation of GABAergic receptors within the substantia nigra results in inhibition of these nigral outputs (Chevalier et al., 1985).

Evidence has accumulated over the last 5 years indicating that the nigrocollicular projection is critical in the circuitry of the nigral control of epilepsy. In a study using maximal electroshock seizures, the anticonvulsant effects of bilateral intranigral injection of muscimol were abolished by a bilateral lesion of the superior colliculus (Garant & Gale, 1987). Similarly, bilateral lesions of this structure, including the superficial, intermediate and deep layers, antagonized the antiepileptic effects on absence seizures resulting from bilateral injections of muscimol into the substantia nigra (Fig. 2; Depaulis et al., 1990c). The critical role of the nigrocollicular pathway is likewise corroborated by the fact that blockade of GABAergic transmission in the superior colliculus suppresses electroshock-induced convulsions (Dean & Gale, 1989; Redgrave et al., 1992; Weng & Rosenberg, 1992), absence seizures (Depaulis et al., 1990a,c) and focally evoked limbic motor seizures (Gale

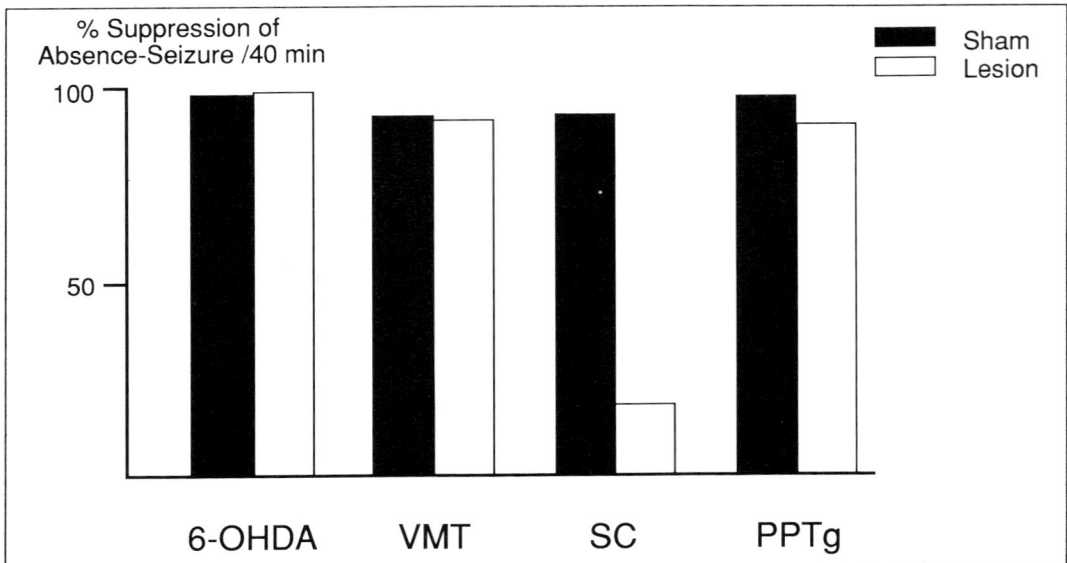

Fig. 2. Suppressive effects of a bilateral injection of 2 ng/side of muscimol in the SN on absence seizures in a genetic model of generalized nonconvulsive epilepsy after lesions of the different nigral outputs. The percentage of suppression is calculated by comparing the cumulated duration of spike-and-wave discharges over 40 min after injection of muscimol versus saline. 6-OHDA = bilateral lesions of dopaminergic output by 6-hydroxydopamine injection into the hypothalamus; VMT = bilateral lesion of the ventromedial nucleus of the thalamus; SC = bilateral lesion of the superior colliculus; PPTg = bilateral lesion of the pedunculopontine nucleus of the tegmentum. Data from Depaulis et al. (1990).

et al., 1993). Moreover, direct activation of cell bodies induced by microinjections of excitatory amino acids into the superior colliculus suppresses both spontaneous (Depaulis et al., 1990c) and PTZ-induced absence seizures (Redgrave et al., 1988).

The critical involvement of the nigro-collicular projection is confirmed by the findings that interruption of the other pathways, or lesions of their target structures, always failed to block the antiepileptic effects observed after bilateral injections of GABA-mimetics in the substantia nigra. For instance, after neurotoxic destruction of nigral dopaminergic cells by 6-hydroxydopamine, resulting in a depletion of dopamine levels in the forebrain or unilateral section of the medial forebrain bundle, bilateral injections of muscimol into the substantia nigra still significantly suppressed absence seizures (Fig. 2; Depaulis et al., 1990c). Moreover, it was still possible to suppress absence seizures in spontaneously epileptic rats by intranigral injection of muscimol after extensive bilateral electrolytic lesioning of the ventromedial nucleus of the thalamus or the pedunculopontine nucleus of the tegmentum (Fig. 2; Depaulis et al., 1990c; Depaulis et al., in preparation).

Although the complete circuitry of the nigral control of epilepsy is far from being understood, there is now little doubt about the critical roles of the GABAergic striato-nigral input and the GABAergic nigro-tectal connections. According to our knowledge of the functioning of the striato-nigro-tectal pathway (see Chevalier et al., 1985), we submit that this 'two-GABAergic-neuron' system constitutes one of the key components of the nigral control of epilepsy. Activation of GABAergic striato-nigral neurons increases the release of GABA in the pars reticulata of the substantia nigra. This results in inhibition of the nigro-collicular GABAergic neurons, which leads to activation of collicular neurons by a disinhibitory process (Fig. 3). These collicular neurons may in turn, by an as yet unknown mechanism, exert an inhibitory influence on generalized seizures.

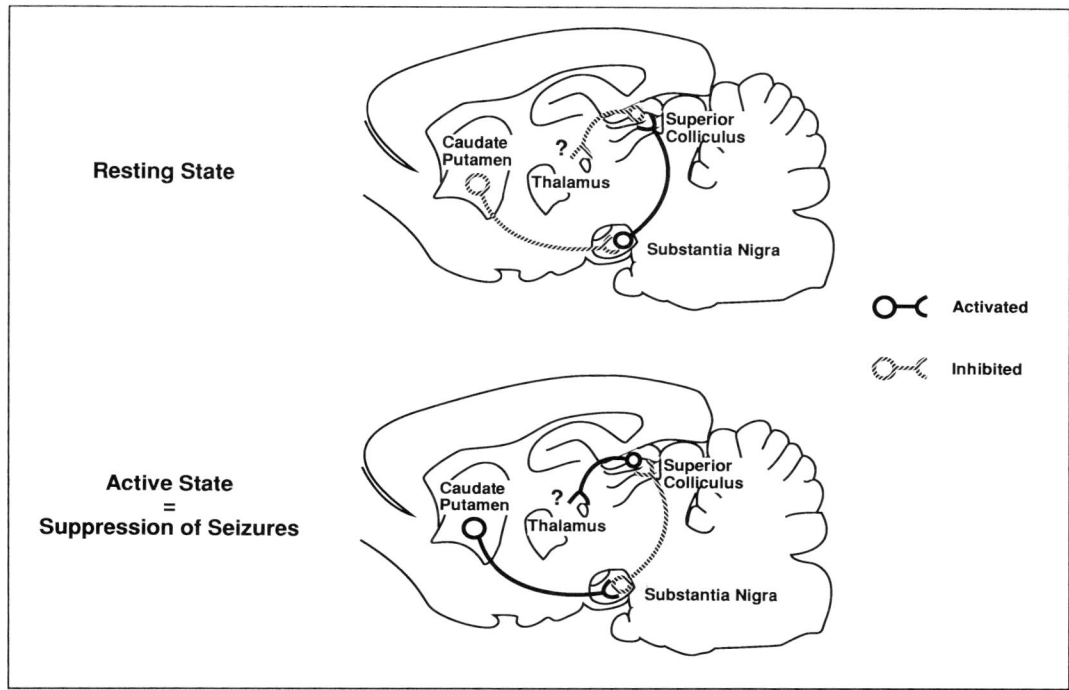

Fig. 3. Schematic diagram illustrating on a saggital view of a rat brain the hypothetical functioning of the nigral control of epilepsy during the resting state (i.e. no suppression of seizures) and active state (suppression of seizures).

Relevance of nigral control in the treatment of generalized epilepsies

Nigral control as a wide-spectrum antiepileptic mechanism

Several authors have reported antiepileptic effects following intracerebral microinjections of different pharmacological agents and, in particular, GABA agonist compounds, in various structures of the brain besides the substantia nigra. For example, microinjections of GABA agonists in the inferior colliculus suppress audiogenic seizures (Frye et al., 1983); in the entopeduncular nucleus, they suppress pilocarpine-induced seizures (Patel et al., 1986); and in different parts of the thalamus they can block diverse types of convulsive or non-convulsive seizure, according to the region of injection (Mirski et al., 1986; Miller et al., 1987; Lee et al., 1989; Liu et al., 1991). However, each of these antiepileptic effects is specific to a given type of seizure and appears to result from an interaction with the underlying neural substrate.

Although nigral control of epilepsy is not a 'universal' control system for epilepsies, it is interesting to note, from the therapeutic point of view, that antiepileptic effects have been obtained in a wide variety of seizure models after inhibition of nigral neurons. In particular, suppressant effects occurred after bilateral injections of muscimol in both convulsive and non-convulsive seizures (see Table 1). Opposite results have always been observed following global manipulations of GABA neurotransmission: models of convulsive seizures are generally suppressed by systemic injections of GABA mimetics (for review see Meldrum, 1989), whereas *non-convulsive* seizures are aggravated (Vergnes et al., 1984). Similarly, only valproate and the benzodiazepines are effective on both types of seizure, whereas opposite effects are obtained with most other anti-epileptic compounds (e.g. ethosuximide, carbamazepine).

Neurotransmissions involved

The initial results reported by Iadarola & Gale (1982) indicated that bilateral activation of GABAergic receptors within the SN led to suppression of seizures. The GABAergic nature of this treatment was confirmed in several reports and especially in a study performed in the genetic model of absence epilepsy (Depaulis *et al.*, 1988). The various data collected suggest the preferential involvement, in adult rats, of the $GABA_A$ receptor. For instance, flurothyl-induced seizures, which have been shown to be blocked in adult rats by bilateral intranigral injection of muscimol, are not suppressed even by high doses (up to 400 ng/side) of the $GABA_B$-receptor agonist, baclofen, injected at the same sites (Sperber *et al.*, 1989). The anticonvulsant effects of intranigral injection of benzodiazepines also confirm the preferential involvement of the $GABA_A$-receptor complex (King *et al.*, 1987; Zhang *et al.*, 1991). It must be noted, however, that very few studies have compared the involvement of the two types of GABA receptor, and further experiments using new ligands of the $GABA_B$ receptor are, however, necessary to further examine a possible specificity of $GABA_A$ receptors.

Other neurotransmission mechanisms within the substantia nigra are certainly also involved in the triggering of nigral control of epilepsy. In particular, several data suggest the involvement of excitatory amino acid transmission. Bilateral injections into the SN of 2-amino-7-phosphonoheptanoate, an NMDA-receptor antagonist, suppress electroshock-induced seizures (De Sarro *et al.*, 1985), seizures evoked by injection of bicuculline into the area tempestas (Maggio & Gale, 1989), audiogenic seizures (Meldrum *et al.*, 1988), flurothyl-induced seizures (Wurpel *et al.*, 1992), and pentylenetetrazol-induced clonic seizures (Xie *et al.*, 1991) and also afford protection against the behavioural, electrographic and morphological features of seizures induced by pilocarpine (Turski *et al.*, 1986b) (Table 2). More recently, it was shown that intranigral bilateral injection of CGP 40116 or MK801, two NMDA-receptor antagonists, suppressed spontaneous absence seizures. By contrast, microinjections at similar sites of 6-cyano-7-nitroquinoxaline-2,3-dione, an antagonist of non-NMDA receptors, or of 2,3-dihydroxy-6-nitro-7-sulphamoylbenzo(F)-quinoxaline, an antagonist of receptors sensitive to α-amino-3-hydroxy-5-methyl-4-isoxazolepropionate, were without effects on the seizures, even at doses up to 2 nmol/side (Deransart *et al.*, 1994). These data suggest a preferential involvement of NMDA receptors in these suppressive effects. Moreover, the fact that bilateral injection of NMDA antagonists into the substantia nigra triggers nigral control of epilepsy suggests the existence of a tonic influence of excitatory amino acid inputs on nigral neurons. In this respect, the glutamatergic projection from the subthalamic nucleus to pars reticulata cell bodies deserves further investigations. Finally, bilateral intranigral injection of opiates also protects against maximal electroshock seizures and absence seizures (Garant & Gale, 1985; Depaulis, 1990), and injection of dynorphin-1-3 suppresses kindled seizures with a potency comparable to that of intranigral muscimol (Bonhaus *et al.*, 1987) (Table 2).

Table 2. *Effects of bilateral injections of antagonists of the NMDA receptor or agonist of the opioid receptor into the SN on different models of seizures in adult rats*

Models	NMDA antagonists	Opiate agonists
Electroshock	−	−
Kindling		−
Area tempestas	−	
Pilocarpine	−	
Fluorothyl	−	
Genetic absence	−	−
Pentylenetetrazol-induced clonic seizure	−	
Audiogenic seizure	−	

− = suppression of seizures. Data from the literature (see text for references).

Activation by antiepileptic drugs

The existence within the central nervous system of an endogenous system that controls a great variety of seizures is of great interest for the design of new antiepileptic drug treatments. Several studies have explored the possibility that antiepileptic compounds can activate nigral control of epilepsy either directly or indirectly, for example, by increasing the release of GABA within the substantia nigra.

After bilateral microinjection of different antiepileptics directly into the substantia nigra, no consistent picture emerges (Table 3). Bilateral injections of high doses of benzodiazepines, ethosuximide, or valproate did not modify the spike-and-wave discharges in the genetic model of absence epilepsy (Depaulis, 1990). Similarly, bilateral injections of carbamazepine or phenytoin into the substantia nigra had no effects on electroshock seizures (Chen et al., 1989), and injection of ethosuximide was without effects on amygdala-kindled seizures (Leite et al., 1990). By contrast, intranigral injection of antiepileptic drugs like phenobarbitone, benzodiazepines and GVG suppresses the seizures in different animal models (Iadarola & Gale, 1982; McNamara et al., 1984; Turski et al., 1986a, 1990; King et al., 1987; Löscher et al., 1987; Chen et al., 1989; Zhang et al., 1989, 1991). These latter drugs, however, are known to activate GABAergic transmission either by potentiation of the $GABA_A$ receptor complex or by inhibition of GABA degradation. It is interesting to note that intranigral bilateral injection of trimethadione, which apparently has no effect on GABAergic transmission, suppresses pilocarpine-induced seizures (Turski et al., 1990).

Table 3. Effects of bilateral injections of different antiepileptic drugs into the SN on different models of seizures in adult rats

	Models			
Antiepileptics	Electroshock	Kindling	Pilocarpine	Genetic absence
Benzodiazepines	–	–	–	0
Valproate				0
Barbiturates	–		–	
Ethosuximide		0	+	0
Trimethadione			–	
Carbamazepine	0			
Phenytoin	0		0	

– = suppression of seizures; 0 = no suppression of seizures; + = aggravation of seizures. Data from the literature (see text for references).

Some antiepileptic drugs could act by triggering nigral control of epilepsy through indirect inhibition of nigral neurons. Systemic administration of valproate, diazepam, trimethadione, and phenobarbitone has been shown to partially decrease the spontaneous firing of pars reticulata neurons (Waszczak et al., 1986; Farrant & Webster, 1989) and potentiate the striatal-evoked inhibition of these cells, an effect which is correlated with the time-course of the drug in epilepsy models (Farrant & Webster, 1989). Systemic administration of carbamazepine, phenytoin, or ethosuximide, by contrast, did not modify, and sometimes even increased, the activity of nigral cells (Waszczak et al., 1986). It was also shown that systemic administration of valproate increases endogenous GABA levels specifically at the substantia nigra nerve terminals (Iadarola & Gale, 1981; Löscher & Vetter, 1984, 1985; Farrant & Webster, 1989), an effect most likely to be due to an increase in the rate of GABA synthesis (Löscher, 1989). However, the concentration of GABA in the substantia nigra was not increased until 60 min after injection, whereas antiepileptic effects of valproate start 10–15 min post injection (Farrant & Webster, 1989). Similarly, the anticonvulsant activity of GVG on kindling seizures was not concomitant with the increase in GABA levels induced in the substantia nigra nerve terminal by this compound (Löscher *et al.*, 1989). Finally, it was demonstrated by a push-pull technique that systemic administration of valproate does not modify the release of GABA in the substantia nigra (Farrant & Webster, 1989). The possibility remains, however, that some drugs (e.g. valproate) increase the release of GABA or reduce its re-uptake in the substantia nigra significantly enough to modify the activity of the pars reticulata cells, but not to allow detection by current techniques (Farrant & Webster, 1989). It is also possible that antiepileptic drugs trigger nigral control of epilepsy through the modification of another nigral input (e.g. excitatory amino acid, ankephalins) and/or at another level of nigral control of epilepsy (e.g. the superior colliculus).

From the data collected so far, it appears very unlikely that antiepileptics exert a direct effect on nigral cells. However, the possibility that some of these compounds act through the nigral control of epilepsy by modulating the activity of some nigral inputs remains to be demonstrated. Because of the similarity between its activity spectrum and nigral control of epilepsy, valproate appears to be the best candidate.

Conclusions and perspectives

Evidence has accumulated over the past 10 years that demonstrates the existence, within the central nervous system, of a control mechanism exerting an inhibitory influence on various forms of generalized seizure. More precisely, the findings suggest that this inhibitory control system involves GABAergic neurons with cell bodies localized in the pars reticulata of the substantia nigra and with nerve terminals in the superior colliculus. Disinhibition of collicular neurons results in an increase in their firing, which, in turn, suppresses seizures by a mechanism that remains to be characterized.

The key of a further understanding of nigral control of epilepsy now lies in characterizing the exact population of neurons constituting the circuitry of this control system and whether this circuitry is the same for all types of seizures that are controlled. Although the existence of nigral control of epilepsy in human is yet not possible to confirm, studies in higher species than the rat are required. Because it controls a wide variety of generalized seizures, nigral control of epilepsy may participate in the mode of action of some wide spectrum antiepileptics. It also constitutes a very promising approach in the design of new drugs and/or new therapeutic strategies that could selectively activate parts of the circuitry of nigral control of epilepsy.

Acknowledgement

I wish to thank Marguerite Vergnes and Christian Marescaux for their comments on the manuscript.

References

Andén, N.E., Carlsson, A., Dahlström, A., Fuxe, K., Hillarp, N.A. & Larsson, K. (1984): Demonstration and mapping out of nigro-neostriatal dopamine neurons. *Life Sci.* **3**, 523–530.

Bentivoglio, M., Van der Kooy, D. & Kuypers, H.G.J.M. (1979): The organization of the efferent projections of the substantia nigra in the rat. A retrograde fluorescent double labeling study. *Brain Res.* **174**, 1–17.

Bolam, J.P. & Smith, Y. (1990): The GABA and substance P input to dopaminergic neurones in the substantia nigra of the rat. *Brain Res.* **529**, 57–78.

Bonhaus, D.W., Rigsbee, L.C. & McNamara, J.O. (1987): Intranigral dynorphin 113 supresses kindled seizures by a naloxone- insensitive mechanism. *Brain Res.* **405**, 358–363.

Bonhaus, D.W., Russell, R.D. & McNamara, J.O. (1991): Activation of substantia nigra pars reticulata neurons: role in the initiation and behavioral expression of kindled seizures. *Brain Res.* **545**, 41–48.

Browning, R.A. (1985): Role of the brain stem reticular formation in tonic–clonic seizures: lesions and pharmacological studies. *Fed. Proc.* **44,** 2425–2431.

Cavalheiro, E.A. & Turski, L. (1986): Intrastriatal N-methyl-D-aspartate prevents amygdala kindled seizures in rats. *Brain Res.* **377,** 173–176.

Chen, L.S., Millington, D.S., Maltby, D.A. & McNamara, J.O. (1989): Effects of intranigral applications of clinically-effective anticonvulsants on electroshock-induced seizures. *Neuropharmacology* **28,** 781–786.

Chevalier, G., Thierry, A.M., Shibazaki, T. & Feger, J. (1981): Evidence for a GABAergic inhibitory nigro-collicular pathway in the rat. *Neurosci. Lett.* **21,** 67–70.

Chevalier, G., Vacher, S., Deniau, J.M. & Desban, M. (1985): Disinhibition as a basic process in the expression of striatal functions. I. The striato-nigral influence on tecto-spinal/tecto-diencephalic neurons. *Brain Res.* **334,** 215–226.

Childs, J.A. & Gale, K. (1983): Neurochemical evidence for a nigrotegmental GABAergic projection. *Brain Res.* **258,** 109–114.

Dean, P. & Gale, K. (1989): Anticonvulsant action of GABA receptor blockade in the nigro-collicular target region. *Brain Res.* **477,** 391–395.

Deniau, J.M. & Chevalier, G. (1992): The lamellar organization of the rat substantia nigra pars reticulata: distribution of projection neurons. *Neuroscience* **46,** 361–377.

Depaulis, A. (1990): Etude neuropharmacologique du controle inhibiteur par la substance noire des crises d'épilepsie généralisée non-convulsive chez le rat. PhD dissertation, Louis Pasteur University, Strasbourg.

Depaulis, A., Vergnes, M., Marescaux, C., Lannes, B. & Warter, J.M. (1988): Evidence that activation of GABA receptors in the substantia nigra suppresses spontaneous spike-and-wave discharges in the rat. *Brain Res.* **448,** 20–29.

Depaulis, A., Snead, O.C., III, Marescaux, C. & Vergnes, M. (1989): Suppressive effects of intranigral injection of muscimol in three models of generalized non-convulsive epilepsy induced by chemical agents. *Brain Res.* **498,** 64–72.

Depaulis, A., Liu, Z., Vergnes, M., Marescaux, C., Micheletti, G. & Warter, J.M. (1990a): Suppression of spontaneous generalized non-convulsive seizures in the rat by microinjection of GABA antagonists into the superior colliculus. *Epilepsy Res.* **5,** 192–198.

Depaulis, A., Marescaux, C., Liu, Z. & Vergnes, M. (1990b): The GABAergic nigrocollicular pathway is not involved in the inhibitory control of audiogenic seizures in the rat. *Neurosci. Lett.* **111,** 269–274.

Depaulis, A., Vergnes, M., Liu, Z., Kempf, E. & Marescaux, C. (1990c): Involvement of the nigral output pathways in the inhibitory control of the substantia nigra over generalized non-convulsive seizures in the rat. *Neuroscience* **39,** 339–349.

Depaulis, A., Vergnes, M. & Marescaux, C. (1994): Endogenous control of epilepsy: the nigral inhibitory system. *Prog. Neurobiol.* **44,** 33–52.

Depaulis, A., Danober, L., Deransart, C., Vergnes, M. & Marescaux, C. The nigral control of absence seizures in the rat does not involve the mesopontine projection, in preparation.

Deransart, C., Depaulis, A., Vergnes, M. & Marescaux, C. (1994): Blockade of N-methyl-D-aspartate receptors in the substantia nigra suppresses absence seizures in a genetic model in the rat. XIXth Collegium Internationale Neuro-Psychopharmacologicum Congress, Washington.

De Sarro, G., Meldrum, B.S. & Reavill, C. (1985): Anticonvulsant action of 2-amino-7-phosphonoheptanoic acid in the substantia nigra. *Eur. J. Pharmacol.* **106,** 175–179.

Di Chiara, G., Porceddu, M.L., Morelli, M., Mulas, M.L. & Gessa, G.L. (1979): Evidence for a GABAergic projection from the substantia nigra to the ventromedial thalamus and to the superior colliculus of the rat. *Brain Res.* **176,** 273–284.

Farrant, M. & Webster, R.A. (1989): Neuronal activity, amino acid concentration and amino acid release in the substantia nigra of the rat after sodium valproate. *Brain Res.* **504,** 49–56.

Fisher, R.S., Buchwald, N.A., Hull, C.D. & Levine, M.S. (1986): The GABAergic striatonigral neurons of the cat: demonstration by double peroxidase labeling. *Brain Res.* **398,** 148–156.

Frye, G.D., McCown, T.J. & Breese, G.R. (1983): Characterization of susceptibility to audiogenic seizures in ethanol-dependent rats after microinjection of gamma-aminobutyric acid (GABA): agonists into the inferior colliculus, substantia nigra and medial septum. *J. Pharmacol. Exp. Ther.* **227,** 663–670.

Gale, K. (1985): Mechanisms of seizure control mediated by gamma aminobutyric acid: role of the substantia nigra. *Fed. Proc.* **44**, 2414–2424.

Gale, K., Pazos, A., Maggio, R., Japikse, K. & Pritchard, P. (1993): Blockade of GABA receptors in superior colliculus protects against focally evoked limbic motor seizures. *Brain Res.* **603**, 279–283.

Garant, D.S. & Gale, K. (1983): Lesions of the substantia nigra protect against experimentally induced seizure. *Brain Res.* **273**, 156–161.

Garant, D.S. & Gale, K. (1985): Infusion of opiates into substantia nigra protects against maximal electroshock seizures in rats. *J. Pharmacol. Exp. Ther.* **234**, 45–48.

Garant, D.S. & Gale, K. (1986): Intranigral muscimol attenuates electrographic signs of seizure activity induced by intravenous bicuculline in rats. *Eur. J. Pharmacol.* **124**, 365–369.

Garant, D.S. & Gale, K. (1987): Substantia nigra-mediated anticonvulsant actions: role of nigral output pathways. *Exp. Neurol.* **97**, 143–159.

Gibbs, F.A. & Gibbs, E.L. (1936): The convulsive threshold of various parts of the cat's brain. *Arch. Neurol. Psychiatry* **35**, 109.

Gonzalez, L.P. & Hettinger, M.K. (1984): Intranigral muscimol suppresses ethanol withdrawal seizures. *Brain Res.* **298**, 163–166.

Hayashi, T. (1952): A physiological study of epileptic seizures following cortical stimulation in animals and its application to human clinics. *Jpn. J. Pharmacol.* **3**, 46–64.

Hayashi, T. (1953): The efferent pathway of epileptic seizures following cortical stimulation differs from that for limbs. *Jpn. J. Pharmacol.* **4**, 306–321.

Hopkins, D.A. & Niessen, L.W. (1976): Substantia nigra projections to the reticular formation, superior colliculus and central gray in the rat, cat and monkey. *Neurosci. Lett.* **2**, 253–259.

Iadarola, M.J. & Gale, K. (1981): Cellular compartments of GABA in brain and their relationship to anticonvulsant activity. *Mol. Cell. Biochem.* **39**, 305–330.

Iadarola, M.J. & Gale, K. (1982): Substantia nigra: site of anti-convulsant activity mediated by gamma-aminobutyric acid. *Science* **218**, 1237–1240.

King, P.H., Shin, C., Mansbach, H.H., Chen, L.S. & McNamara, J.O. (1987): Microinjection of a benzodiazepine into substantia nigra elevates kindled seizure threshold. *Brain Res.* **423**, 261–268.

Kreindler, A., Zuckermann, E., Steriade, M. & Chimion, D. (1958): Electroclinical features of convulsions induced by stimulation of brain stem. *J. Neurophysiol.* **21**, 430–436.

Le Gal La Salle, G., Kaijima, M. & Feldblum, S. (1983): Abortive amygdaloid kindled seizures following microinjection of gamma-vinyl-GABA in the vicinity of substantia nigra in rats. *Neurosci. Lett.* **36**, 69–74.

Lee, R.J., Depaulis, A., Lomax, P. & Olsen, R.W. (1989): Anticonvulsant effect of muscimol injected into the thalamus of spontaneously epileptic mongolian gerbils. *Brain Res.* **487**, 363–367.

Leite, J.P., Bortolotto, Z.A. & Cavalheiro, E.A. (1990): Bilatral microinjection of ethosuximide into the substantia nigra does not prevent amygdala-kindled seizures. *Braz. J. Med. Biol. Res.* **23**, 1139–1141.

Lippert, B., Metcalf, B.W., Jung, M.J. & Casara, P. (1977): 4-amino-hex-5-enoic acid, a selective catalytic inhibitor of gamma-aminobutyric acid aminotransferase in mammalian brain. *Eur. J. Biochem.* **74**, 441–445.

Liu, Z., Vergnes, M., Depaulis, A. & Marescaux, C. (1991): Evidence for a critical role of GABAergic transmission within the thalamus in the genesis and control of absence seizure in the rat. *Brain Res.* **545**, 1–7.

Löscher, W., Czuczwar, S.J., Jakel, R. & Schwarz, M. (1987): Effect of microinjections of gamma-vinyl GABA or isoniazid into substantia nigra on the development of amydala kindling in rats. *Exp. Neurol.* **95**, 622–638.

Löscher, W. & Schwark, W.S. (1985): Evidence for impaired GABAergic activity in the substantia nigra of amyloidal kindled rats. *Brain Res.* **339**, 146–150.

Löscher, W. & Vetter, M. (1984): Drug-induced changes in GABA content of nerve endings in 11 rat brain regions. Correlation to pharmacological effects. *Neurosci. Lett.* **47**, 325–331.

Löscher, W. & Vetter, M. (1985): *In vivo* effects of aminooxyacetic acid and valproic acid on nerve terminal (synaptosomal): GABA levels in discrete brain areas of the rat. *Biochem. Pharmacol.* **34**, 1747–1756.

Löscher, W. (1989): Valproate enhances GABA turnover in the substantia nigra. *Brain Res.* **501**, 198–203.

Löscher, W. & Schwark, W.S. (1987): Further evidence for abnormal GABAergic circuits in amygdala-kindled rats. *Brain Res.* **420**, 385–390.

Löscher, W., Jackel, R. & Müller, F. (1989): Anticonvulsant and proconvulsant effects of inhibitors of GABA degradation in the amygdala-kindling model. *Eur. J. Pharmacol.* **163**, 1–14.

Maggio, R. & Gale, K. (1989): Seizures evoked from area tempestas are subject to control by GABA and glutamate receptors in substantia nigra. *Exp. Neurol.* **105**, 184–188.

Maggio, R., Liminga, U. & Gale, K. (1990): Selective stimulation of kainate but not quisqualate or NMDA receptors in substantia nigra evokes limbic motor seizures. *Brain Res.* **528**, 223–230.

McNamara, J.O., Galloway, M.T., Rigsbee, L.C. & Shin, C. (1984): Evidence implicating substantia nigra in regulation of kindled seizure threshold. *J. Neurosci.* **4**, 2410–2417.

McNamara, J.O., Rigsbee, L.C. & Galloway, M.T. (1983): Evidence that substantia nigra is crucial to neural network of kindled seizures. *Eur. J. Pharmacol.* **86**, 485–486.

Meldrum, B.S. (1989): GABAergic mechanisms in the pathogenesis and treatment of epilepsy. *Br. J. Clin. Pharmacol.* **27**, 3S–11S.

Meldrum, B.S., Millan, M., Patel, S. & De Sarro, G. (1988): Anti-epileptic effects of focal micro-injection of excitatory amino acid antagonist. *J. Neural Transm.* **72**, 191–200.

Miller, J.W. (1992): The role of mesencephalic and thalamic arousal systems in experimental seizures. *Prog. Neurobiol.* **39**, 155–178.

Miller, J.W., McKeon, A.C. & Ferrendelli, J.A. (1987): Functional anatomy of pentylenetetrazol and electroshock seizures in the rat brainstem. *Ann. Neurol.* **22**, 615–621.

Mirski, M.A., McKeon, A.C. & Ferendelli, J.A. (1986): Anterior thalamus and substantia nigra: two distinct structures mediating experimental generalized seizures. *Brain Res.* **397**, 377–380.

Morimoto, K. & Goddard, G.V. (1987): The substantia nigra is an important site for the containment of seizure generalization in the kindling model of epilepsy. *Epilepsia* **28**, 1–10.

Nitsch, C. & Okada, Y. (1976): Differential decrease of GABA in the substantia nigra and other discrete regions of the rabbit brain during the preictal period of methoxypyridoxine-induced seizures. *Brain Res.* **105**, 173–178.

Oertel, W.H., Schmechel, D.E., Brownstein, M.J., Tappaz, M.L., Ransom, D.H., & Kopin, I.J. (1981): Decrease of glutamate decarboxylase (GAD)immunoreactive nerve terminals in the substantia nigra after kainic acid lesion of striatum. *J. Histochem. Cytochem.* **29**, 977–980.

Okada, R., Moshé, S.L., Wong, B.Y., Sperber, E.F. & Zhao, D. (1986): Age-related substantia nigra-mediated seizure facilitation. *Exp. Neurol.* **93**, 180–187.

Okada, R., Negishi, N. & Nagaya, H. (1989): The role of the nigrotegmental GABAergic pathway in the propagation of pentylenetetrazol-induced seizures. *Brain Res.* **480**, 383–387.

Olsen, R.W., Wamsley, J.K., McCabe, R.T., Lee, R.J. & Lomax, P. (1985): Benzodiazepine/gamma-aminobutyric acid receptor deficit in the midbrain of the seizure-susceptible gerbil. *Proc. Natl. Acad. Sci. USA* **82**, 6701–6705.

Ono, K. & Wada, J.A. (1987): Facilitation of premotor cortical seizure development by intranigral muscimol. *Brain Res.* **405**, 183–186.

Patel, S., Millan, M.H., Mello, L.M. & Meldrum, B.S. (1986): 2-Amino-7-phosphonoheptanoic acid (2-APH) infusion into entopeduncular nucleus protects against limbic seizures in rats. *Neurosci. Lett.* **64**, 226–230.

Platt, K., Butler, L.S., Bonhaus, D.W. & McNamara, J.O. (1987): Evidence implicating Alpha-2 adrenergic receptors in the anticonvulsant action of intranigral muscimol. *J. Pharmacol. Exp. Ther.* **241**, 751–754.

Redgrave, P., Dean, P. & Simkins, M. (1988): Intratectal glutamate suppresses pentylenetetrazole-induced spike-and-wave discharges. *Eur. J. Pharmacol.* **158**, 283–287.

Redgrave, P., Simkins, M., Overton, P. & Dean, P. (1992): Anticonvulsant role of nigrotectal projection in the maximal electroshock model of epilepsy – I. Mapping of dorsal midbrain with bicuculline. *Neuroscience* **46**, 379–390.

Shin, C., Silver, J.M., Bonhaus, D.W. & McNamara, J.O. (1987): The role of substantia nigra in the development of kindling: pharmacologic and lesion studies. *Brain Res.* **412**, 311–317.

Sperber, E.F., Wurpel, J.N.D., Zhao, D.Y. & Moshé, S.L. (1989): Evidence for the involvement of nigral GABA$_A$ receptors in seizures of adult rats. *Brain Res.* **480**, 378–382.

Tokuno, H., Nakamura, Y., Kudo, M. & Kitao, Y. (1990): Laminar organization of the substantia nigra pars reticulata in the cat. *Neuroscience* **38**, 255–270.

Toussi, H.R., Schatz, R.A. & Waszczak, B.L. (1987): Suppression of methionine sulfoximine seizures by intranigral gamma-vinyl GABA injection. *Eur. J. Pharmacol.* **137**, 261–264.

Turski, L., Cavalheiro, E.A., Turski, W.A. & Meldrum, B.S. (1985): Anticonvulsant action of excitatory amino acid in the rat striatum. *Epilepsia* **26**, 507–514.

Turski, L., Cavalheiro, E.A., Schwarz, M., Turski, W.A., De Moraes Mello, L.E.A., Bortolotto, Z.A., Klockgether, T. & Sontag, K.H. (1986a): Susceptibility to seizures produced by pilocarpine in rats after microinjection of isoniazid or gamma-vinyl-GABA into the substantia nigra. *Brain Res.* **370**, 294–309.

Turski, L., Cavalheiro, E.A., Turski, W. & Meldrum, B.S. (1986b): Excitatory neurotransmission within substantia nigra pars reticulata regulates threshold for seizures produced by pilocarpine in rats: effect of intranigral 2-amino-7-phosphonoheptanoate and *N*-methyl-D-aspartate. *Neuroscience* **18**, 61–77.

Turski, L., Meldrum, B.S., Cavalheiro, E.A., Calderazzo-Eilho, L.S., Bortolotto, Z.A., Ikonomidou-Turski, C. & Turski, W.A. (1987): Paradoxical anticonvulsant activity of the excitatory amino acid *N*-methyl-D-aspartate in the rat caudate-putamen. *Proc. Natl. Acad. Sci. USA* **84**, 1689–1693.

Turski, L., Cavalheiro, E.A., Calderazzo-Filho, L.S., Bortolotto, Z.A., Klockgether, T., Ikonomidou, C. & Turski, W.A. (1989): The basal ganglia, the deep prepyriform cortex, and seizure spread: bicuculline is anticonvulsant in the rat striatum. *Proc. Natl. Acad. Sci. USA* **86**, 1694–1697.

Turski, L., Andrews, J.S., Loschmann, P.A., Bressler, K., Bortolotto, Z.A., Calderazzo-Fihlo, L.S. & Cavalheiro, E.A. (1990): Substantia nigra regulates action of antiepileptic drugs. *Brain Res.* **520**, 232–239.

Vergnes, M., Marescaux, C., Micheletti, G., Depaulis, A., Rumbach, L. & Warter, J.M. (1984): Enhancement of spike and wave discharges by GABA mimetic drugs in rats with spontaneous petit-mal-like epilepsy. *Neurosci. Lett.* **44**, 91–94.

Vergnes, M., Marescaux, C. & Depaulis, A. (1990): Mapping of spontaneous spike and wave discharges in Wistar rats with genetic generalized non convulsive epilepsy. *Brain Res.* **523**, 87–91.

Waszczak, B.L., Lee, E.K. & Walters, J.R. (1986): Effects of anticonvulsant drugs on substantia nigra pars reticulata neurons. *J. Pharmacol. Exp. Ther.* **239**, 606–611.

Weng, X. & Rosenberg, H.C. (1992): Infusion of bicuculline methiodide into the tectum: model specificity of pro- and anticonvulsant actions. *Epilepsy Res.* **12**, 1–8.

Wurpel, J.N.D., Sperber, E.F. & Moshé, S.L. (1992): Age-dependent differences in the anticonvulsant effects of 2-amino-7-phosphono-heptanoic acid or ketamine infusions into the substantia nigra of rats. *Epilepsia* **33**, 439–443.

Xie, X.H., Tietz, E.I. & Rosenberg, H.C. (1991): Anti-pentylenetetrazol effect of intranigral 2-amino-7-phosphonoheptanoate attenuated by muscimol. *Brain Res.* **544**, 331–334.

Xu, S.G., Garant, D.S., Sperber, E.F. & Moshé, S.L. (1991): Effects of substantia nigra gamma-vinyl-GABA infusions on fluorothyl seizures in adult rats. *Brain Res.* **566**, 108–114.

Zhang, H., Rosenberg, H.C. & Tietz, E.I. (1989): Injection of benzodiazepines but not GABA or muscimol into pars reticulata of substantia nigra suppresses pentylenetetrazol seizures. *Brain Res.* **488**, 73–79.

Zhang, H., Rosenberg, H.C. & Tietz, E.I. (1991): Anticonvulsant actions and interaction of GABA agonists and a benzodiazepine in pars reticulata of substantia nigra. *Epilepsy Res.* **8**, 11–20.

Chapter 43

Gene therapy: perspectives in epilepsy

Gildas Le Gal La Salle[*] and Jacques Mallet[†]

[*]*Institut Alfred Fessard, Centre National de la Recherche Scientifique (CNRS), 91198 Gif sur Yvette, France;*
[†]*Laboratoire de Génétique Moléculaire de la Neurotransmission et des Processus Dégénératifs, CNRS, 91198 Gif-sur-Yvette, France*

Introduction

Gene therapy involves either correcting a deficient gene or producing a protein of therapeutic value by delivering the genetic information into the affected cells or organs. Thus, in its full meaning, gene therapy is not limited to diseases with a genetic origin and may be applicable to any disorder. DNA, which is the agent used for gene therapy, can be introduced into appropriate cells *in vitro* before subsequent grafting, or directly into the tissue of interest *in vivo*.

Although some progress has been made in the development of gene therapy in some areas of clinical medicine (Friedmann, 1989, 1993; Roemer & Friedmann, 1992; Mulligan, 1993), the exploitation of this approach is only just starting for neurological diseases (Friedmann & Hyder, 1993). The delay in this field was mainly due to two related reasons: the specificity of the CNS itself, as compared to other organs, and the lack of appropriate tools for targeting therapeutic genes into the brain. The recent discovery of efficacious virus vectors for the delivery of foreign genes to neuronal or glial cells *in vivo* (Breakefield, 1993; Neve, 1993) has opened new avenues for the development of gene therapy for neurological disorders. The feasibility of applying gene transfer methods to basic research and therapy for brain dysfunctions can now be assessed. Although disorders like Parkinson's disease and tumours have been more extensively investigated, there is now the hope that epilepsy could be susceptible to gene therapy.

In this chapter, we will discuss how gene therapy could become an alternative to currently available therapeutic tools for epilepsy treatment. We will concentrate on the use of virus-mediated gene transfer methods which, for several reasons, constitute a promising approach for future therapy.

Is the central nervous system (CNS) amenable to gene therapy?

Strategies developed for gene therapy of a wide range of clinical diseases are not directly transposable to the treatment of central nervous system disorders. Gene therapy for the central nervous system poses a number of unique problems and is subject to various constraints not encountered in other organs. Indeed, there are additional specific conceptual and technical issues to be addressed when dealing with brain disorders that could be amenable to correction at the genetic level. In particular, the bony encasement of the brain and the presence of a functional blood–brain barrier physically prevent vectors bearing therapeutic genes from having good access to the neuronal cells. Furthermore, in contrast with most other organs, the central nervous system is a rather heterogeneous tissue composed of a variety of distinct cell types which are intermingled in complex neuronal networks. Both normal and abnormal functions of these cells and networks are still poorly characterized, in spite of rapid progress. In addition, a great number of the disorders affecting the central nervous system are probably multigenic or multifactorial, thus preventing a single gene replacement or correction. Finally and most importantly, neurons are fully differentiated post-mitotic cells which cannot be transfected using retroviral vectors, the most commonly used gene transfer method. In recent years, this has led to the development of transplantation experiments using genetically-modified neuronal or surrogate cells previously transfected with retroviral vectors. A well-documented example is grafting engineered cells for producing tyrosine hydroxylase to Parkinson-like disease in animal models (Horellou et al., 1990; Gage et al., 1991; Jiao et al., 1993).

In parallel to this cellular gene therapy, new approaches based on the direct introduction of a transgene into the central nervous system in vivo is being developed using gene transfer techniques and viruses as neurotropic vectors. It has been shown that post-mitotic differentiated neuronal, glial or ependymal cells in rodents are able to express a foreign gene introduced using herpes or adenovirus vectors. This technique has been mainly described using reporter and not therapeutic genes and there is no evidence yet for any specific correction in animal models. Nevertheless, the apparent technical feasibility of the approach has opened new avenues for further developments in gene therapy of the brain.

Which vectors for gene transfer?

During the past decade, the development of powerful methods for delivering foreign genes into mammalian cells has opened new perspectives for manipulating genomic expression and for treating a number of human diseases by gene therapy (see Mulligan, 1993). The choice of the vector system to deliver the genetic material to the central nervous system is of critical importance. A number of characteristics such as tropism, size of insert, expression of the transgene, efficiency, safety, etc. are currently being investigated.

Until now, retroviruses have been the most widely used vector system in gene therapy (Varmus, 1988). However, they have several limitations which render them inappropriate for in vivo gene transfer into the central nervous system. Indeed, interfering with gene expression in fully differentiated cells that do not further divide involves problems which require new developments and strategies.

One approach that can circumvent the limitations of retroviruses is the use of neurotropic viruses. Herpes vectors were the first viruses used to directly transfer genes into nerve cells (Geller & Breakefield, 1988). Nevertheless, the herpes simplex virus (HSV) has not proved to be fully adequate, for reasons of both efficacy and pathogenicity (for review see Breakefield & DeLuca, 1991). Although new recombinant herpes simplex virus mutants with reduced neurocytotoxicity has been developed, this remains a problem and represents a major disadvantage of the herpes virus. Another drawback of herpes simplex virus viral vectors is their low titre which results in low infectivity. In spite of substantial improvement in the characteristics of new herpes simplex virus constructs, they retain these limitations which compromise their use for gene therapy in humans.

The adenoviral vector: a promising tool for basic research and gene therapy

The possibility of using adenoviral vectors for transfecting foreign genes into the nervous system was recently demonstrated in vitro in various cell lines and in primary neural cell cultures and in situ, following direct stereotactic injection into the brain parenchyma (Le Gal La Salle et al., 1993;

Chapter 43 Gene therapy: perspectives in epilepsy

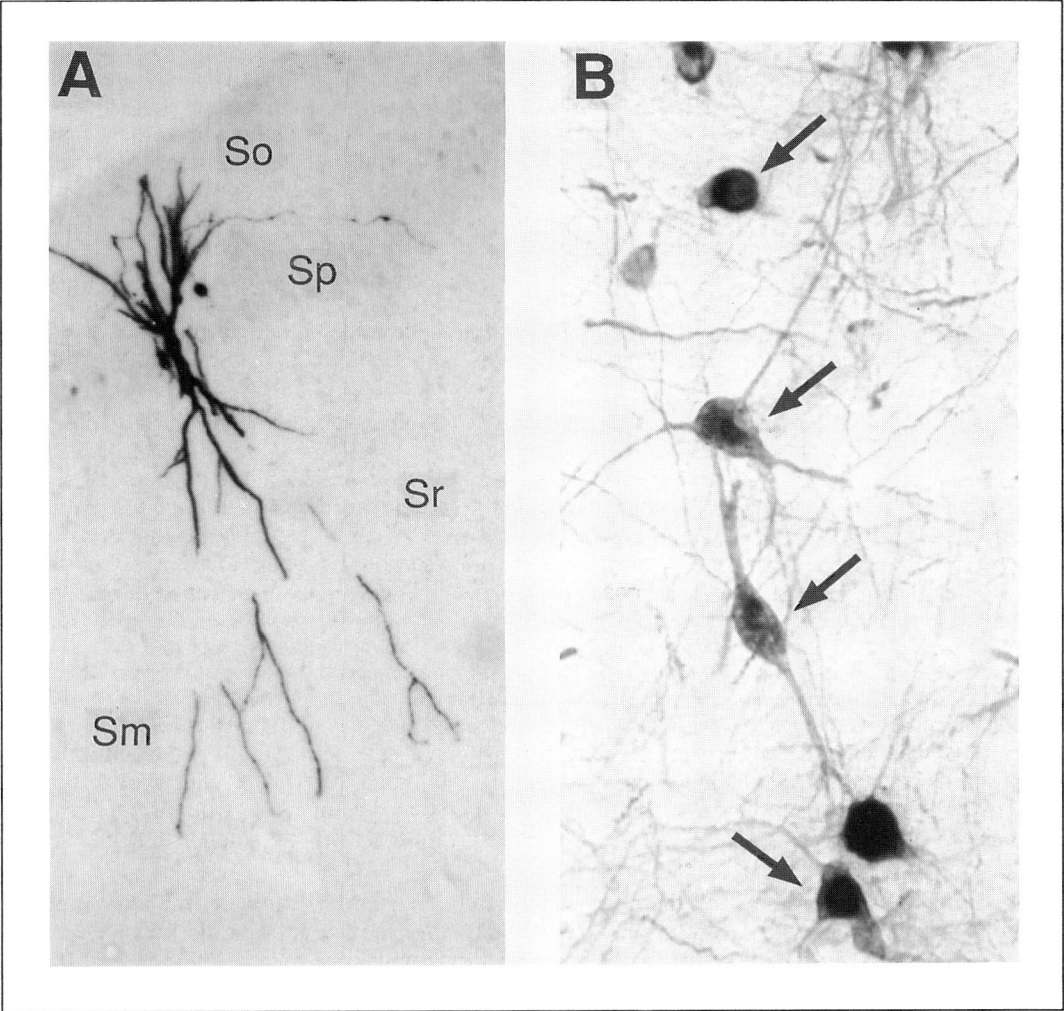

Fig. 1. Example of neurons infected by direct in vivo inoculation with an adenovirus carrying a reporter gene encoding β-galactosidase. Dense blue staining was detectable in a pyramidal cell of the CA1 stratum pyramidale of the dorsal hippocampus (a) and in nigral cells, most of which were also labelled with tyrosine hydroxylase monoclonal antibodies. sm = stratum moleculare; so = stratum oriens; sp = stratum pyramidale; sr = stratum radiatum (see also colour plate).

Akli et al., 1993; Bajocchi et al., 1993; Davidson et al., 1993). Some of the native properties of this vector, including efficacy, safety, low pathogenicity and long-term expression of the transfected genes make it a particularly promising subject for future gene studies.

Adenoviruses share a number of similarities with herpes simplex viruses. It can be made replication-defective by deleting the immediate early viral genome E1 which plays a role in viral genomic transcription and the E3 gene region which codes for products preventing cytolysis by cytotoxic T-cells and the tumour necrosis factor (Stratford-Perricaudet et al., 1990). Adenovirus has a large genome such that foreign genes up to 7.5 kb long can be introduced. Titres as high as 10^{10} or 10^{11}

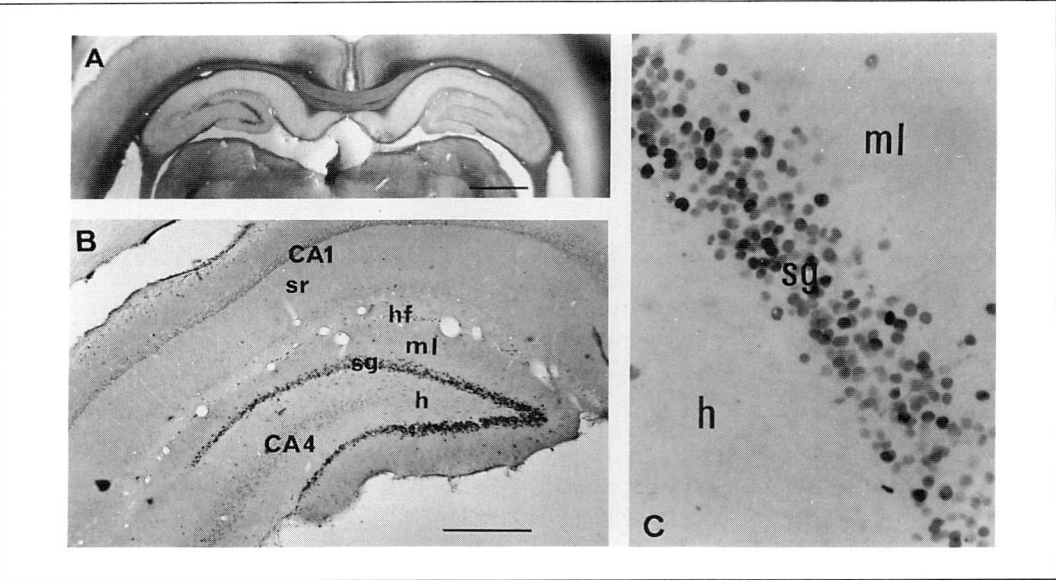

Fig. 2. Distribution of β-galactosidase-positive cells in the dorsal hippocampus 1 month after stereotaxic inoculation with recombinant adenovirus. (A) Photomicrograph stained for β-galactosidase expression with X-gal histochemistry. The cells that are stained blue were observed in the dentate gyrus of the injected left hippocampus. Scale bar, 1 mm. (B) Dentate localization of the infected cells was confirmed immunohistochemically using an antibody against β-galactosidase. Scale bar, 300 μm. (C) High magnification view showing the large number of densely packed immunoreactive (anti-β-gal antibodies) cells in the granular cell layer of the dentate gyrus. h = hilus; hf = hippocampal fissure; ml = molecular layer; sg = stratum granulosum; sr = stratum radiatum. (From Le Gal La Salle et al., 1993) (see also colour plate)

pfu/ml can be obtained. The viral genes are introduced in an episomal form, without DNA integration into the host genome. Finally the pathogenicity of adenoviruses in human is low.

The vector currently used was derived from the human adenovirus serotype 5, whose natural target is not the nervous system but the respiratory epithelium (see Jaffe et al., 1992; Quantin et al., 1992; Rosenfeld et al., 1991, 1992). We have used a replication-defective adenovirus, Ad-RSV-β-gal, which expressed a nuclearly targeted β-galactosidase cDNA under the control of the Rous sarcoma virus long terminal repeat (RSV LTR) promoter (Stratford-Perricaudet et al., 1992). This vector was able to infect various cells in culture, including cell lines and nerve cells (neurons and astrocytes) taken from different embryonic tissues in the rat. In all these *in vitro* experiments (Caillaud et al., 1993; Le Gal La Salle et al., 1993), inoculation of the Ad-RSV-β-gal virus resulted in β-galactosidase activity in between two-thirds and all the cultured cells. The transgene was more efficiently and rapidly expressed in glial cells than in neurons.

The feasibility of directly transferring genes *in vivo* to the nervous system using replication-deficient recombinant adenoviruses was also demonstrated (Akli et al., 1993; Bajocchi et al., 1993; Davidson et al., 1993; Le Gal La Salle et al., 1993). The virus was introduced by stereotactic intracerebral inoculation into a variety of brain structures, including the hippocampus and the substantia nigra of adult rats, both structures known to play a role in the pathology of several neurological diseases. As early as 24 h after Ad-RSV-β-gal inoculation, a large number of neural cells around the injected site were infected and expressed high levels of β-galactosidase activity.

Anatomical, morphological and immunohistochemical investigations showed that the cells infected were microglial cells, astrocytes and neurons. In a few cases, probably depending on the β-galactosidase concentration, some cells were stained with a Golgi-like profile. An example of this is shown in Fig. 1a for a CA1 pyramidal cell in the dorsal hippocampus. When the adenovirus was inoculated in the substantia nigra, a proportion of cells expressing the transgene was also immunoreactive for tyrosine hydroxylase (Fig. 1b). This demonstrates that it is possible to infect neurons in the intact animal. Interestingly, the transgene has been also shown to be expressed in remote dopaminergic nigral neurons after retrograde transport from axon terminals located in the striatum, at the site of injection (Ridoux et al., 1994b).

The number and the extent of labelled cells was correlated to both the volume and the titre of the viral solution administered, as well as to the structure into which it was injected. Indeed, local anatomical features, such as the presence of fibres, affect the diffusion of the viral particles which tend to spread through tissues of lesser resistance.

Several studies have shown that transgenes introduced in adenovirus vectors are expressed for prolonged periods. For example, expression of β-galactosidase was detected for up to 6 months following intrahippocampal inoculation. One month after inoculation, the β-galactosidase activity remained restricted to the granule cells of the dentate gyrus (Fig. 2). Dentate location of infected cells was further confirmed by immunohistochemical β-galactosidase detection. This prolonged expression is a further advantage in gene therapy. One to 6 months after inoculation of the virus, there was no apparent sign of cell loss among the infected cells. Even for high titre suspensions, no cytopathogenicity was apparent, except immediately adjacent to the injection site.

These early results are sufficiently encouraging to allow the expectation that it will be possible to transfer therapeutic genes into cerebral areas known to be implicated in specific neurological dysfunction or diseases. The treatment of epilepsy, or at least certain forms with a well-known anatomical focus may eventually be able to use this new therapeutic approach.

Cellular gene therapy

Although the present report is mostly focused on direct *in vivo* gene transfer using viral vectors, it is interesting to consider the *ex vivo* strategy involving the use of genetically-modified cells as vehicles for foreign gene expression after transplantation into the central nervous system in animal models of epilepsy. Attempts to graft engineered cells (or embryonic tissue) to prevent epileptic seizures have been rare and the results rather disappointing (see Lindvall & Björklund, 1992). Except from a very few studies (Fine et al., 1990; Miyamoto et al., 1993), there is no clear direct evidence of any seizure protection following transplantation. GABA-producing cells grafted into the substantia nigra of kindled or kainate-treated animals and genetically seizure-prone rats did not prevent seizures (unpublished personal results). Our interpretation of these results is that GABA production was too low to exert the expected anticonvulsant effect, or subject to down-regulation after grafting *in vivo*.

In recent work (Ridoux et al., 1994a), we used the adenovirus to transfer genetic material into cultured cells before their subsequent grafting into a host brain. Thus, primary astrocytes taken from new-born rat brains were transfected with the reporter gene encoding β-galactosidase. After transplantation of these cells into various brain structures, they exhibited a good survival rate and expressed the transgene for several months. These results demonstrate that adenovirus-mediated gene expression is particularly efficient for inducing long-lasting expression of a transgene in intracerebrally grafted nerve cells and thus represents an attractive method for genetic graft therapy. However, it has been reported that grafting cells into some brain structures may induce paroxysmal activity (Buszaki et al., 1991). Thus this technique may increase the epileptogenic risk in an already epileptic brain, and therefore has serious disadvantages.

Before trying to develop gene-therapy strategies for epilepsy, we need to examine whether or not epilepsy can indeed be treated by *in vivo* gene-transfer methods.

Is epilepsy amenable to gene therapy?

Even if the techniques are now available for intervening and manipulating genes in the brain, are the procedures generally used in gene therapy feasible and acceptable for the treatment of some forms of epilepsy? We will first consider genetic forms of epilepsy with particular reference to idiopathic generalized epilepsy. We will then discuss how some presumed acquired epilepsies may be also amenable to gene therapy.

Genetic epilepsy

Techniques in molecular genetics have developed rapidly and this has led to evidence that genetic factors play an important role in the aetiology of some seizure disorders (see Gardiner, 1990). A number of apparently hereditary aspects of familial epilepsies have been genetically demonstrated. However, the highest estimations indicate that inherited forms may account for no more than 20 per cent of all epilepsies. Idiopathic (mostly generalized) epilepsies are characterized by a strong genetic background. As reported in several chapters of this book, characterization of the genes responsible for various idiopathic generalized epilepsies (including juvenile absence epilepsy, juvenile myoclonic epilepsy, benign myoclonic epilepsy, benign familial neonatal convulsions) is likely in the near future and thus will obviously help the choice of therapeutically relevant genes.

Nevertheless, cases for which a single responsible gene has been demonstrated are rare and genetic heterogeneity has been reported for a number of epileptic phenotypes (benign familial neonatal convulsions, juvenile myoclonic epilepsy). It is suspected that most of the genetic epilepsies might be due to a combination of genetic predisposition and environmental factors and are thus multifactorial. In fact there might be very few single-gene inherited epileptic syndromes. It is now accepted that genetic predisposition plays a predominant role in the appearance of idiopathic generalized epilepsy. This factor might also contribute significantly to other forms, including temporal lobe epilepsy. Finally, there are about one hundred diseases (e.g. tuberous sclerosis of Bourneville) with a genetic origin where epilepsy is just one symptom. In these cases, epilepsy is a manifestation of a complex neurological genetic disorder.

It is not yet clear whether the identification of a defective gene responsible for a given form of epilepsy can be translated into an effective therapy for prevention or cure. Nevertheless, it is possible that in some cases a single therapeutic gene could notably improve the symptomatology of a multigenic disease, without directly interfering on the genetic causes.

Non-genetic epilepsy

Theoretically, every disease susceptible to cure or improvement by the presence of a protein should be amenable to gene therapy. Therefore, gene therapy may be just as applicable to acquired diseases as to inherited diseases.

About 20 per cent of the total population of all epileptic syndromes are forms of presumed acquired epilepsy, which are refractory to anticonvulsant medication. Most of them cause partial seizures (for review see Pedley, 1993). For cases where high-dose polytherapy does not control the seizures, surgical treatment is more and more frequently proposed. However, a number of epilepsies with complex partial seizures cannot be operated, either because they have a too diffusely located or bilateral focus, or because they involve areas exerting critical functions. Thus, new therapeutic strategies would be of great value, particularly for intractable temporal lobe epilepsy. In addition to the therapeutic potential of these techniques they also promise rapid advances in the understanding of the pathophysiology of these epilepsies.

For gene therapy of medically intractable epilepsy it is of the utmost importance to identify accurately the epileptogenic focus. Usually, it is delineated by various complementary methods assessing the electrical, functional and morphological aspects of the epilepsy. Sometimes, presurgical evaluation includes invasive methods, such as intracerebral stereotaxic depth-electrode recorordings. Thus, gene therapy may well be no more invasive than preoperative procedures in cases of intractable seizures which are candidates for ablative surgery. In addition, the use of gene therapy techniques (for example antisense strategy) can be envisaged to explore further the function of the epileptic focus before surgical intervention.

What indications for gene therapy?

Epilepsy is a particularly heterogeneous group of disorder with at least 48 identified clinical types (Commission, 1989). Indications for potential gene therapy are therefore numerous and various. Therapeutic indications for gene therapy in epilepsy would be first, complete failure of the anticonvulsant drugs that are currently available, second, severe and frequent seizures, and third, serious impairment of the quality of life of the patient.

Complete abolition of seizures with appropriate anticonvulsant drugs can be expected in up to 80–90 per cent of epileptic patients. Furthermore, it is also expected that the number of medically intractable epilepsies will diminish in the future, owing to a better utilization of the drugs already available, the discovery of new ones and improvements in surgical techniques. Thus, the proportion of cures requiring adjunctive strategies will be small. Assuming that central nervous system gene therapy will be perfected, it may eventually be used for up to 5–10 per cent of the epileptic population.

Most idiopathic generalized epilepsies are sensitive to standard antiepileptic medication and patients with intractable idiopathic generalized epilepsy are very much less numerous than those with partial epilepsy. Thus, patients with intractable partial epilepsy are the best candidates for gene therapy.

Another indication could be when the drug therapy, even if effectively stopping seizures, is not well tolerated and induces undesirable effects. Prediction of severe postoperative memory impairment in preoperative neuropsychological evaluations might be also a good indication for alternative therapy.

Interestingly, in frequent, particularly severe and disabling epilepsies, gene therapy may be used to exert palliative rather than curative effects. In such case, different strategies and therapeutic genes could be required. When patients with severe medically-refractory seizures cannot be cured by surgery of the primary focus, a possible alternative solution is to try to reduce the frequency and the intensity of the seizures. This technique is best suited to generalized epilepsies with no recognized epileptogenic focus, which may thus be among the candidates for gene therapy.

Finally, it may also be possible to treat directly the cause of the dysfunction rather than the epilepsy itself, in cases of epilepsy induced by certain external factors. A possible example is that of intraparenchymal neoplasms which are a major aetiological factor in partial seizure disorders refractory to medical treatment: curing the tumour should stop the seizures.

Which therapeutic genes?

Theoretically, there are two situations to consider for gene therapy of medically refractory epilepsy.

(1) The neurological disease results from an abnormality of one or several genes. The 'good' gene(s) can thus be transfected into the target cells to correct the genetic defect. Recent findings suggest that this approach will mainly involve idiopathic epilepsies. A number of genes specific for particular forms of inherited epilepsies are likely to be identified in the near future. However, as most of this group of epilepsies can be satisfactorily treated with anticonvulsant drugs, few are likely to be candidates for gene therapy.

(2) The disease is acquired and does not involve any particular genetic defect. The strategy to adopt will depend on the characteristics of the type of epilepsy to be treated. The anatomo-functional data available today (in particular on the structures involved in genesis, propagation or arrest of seizures, as well as the neurotransmitters which are implicated: see Meldrum

(1990)) will guide both the choice of the relevant genes and the cerebral structures in which these genes may be able to act.

Irrespective of whether the epilepsy is genetic or acquired, the genes suspected to exert a therapeutical effect could interfere with the regulation of gene expression. Such gene activity could replace functions that are missing, or correct those that are aberrant. In addition, understanding how seizures correlate with the expression of specific genes may suggest novel therapeutic approaches.

In the light of current knowledge, two classes of molecules normally present in the brain deserve a special interest. First, the neurotransmitters exerting a general inhibitory effect on the cerebral activity (for example GABA or glycine) or those inhibiting excitatory synaptic transmission, and second, the growth factors involved in the development and maintenance of the nervous system, during both development and also processes following different cerebral insults, such as trauma, ischaemia or epilepsy (Goedert et al., 1986; Kromer, 1987; Gall et al., 1991). The growth factor family includes nerve growth factor (NGF), brain-derived neurotrophic factor (BDNF), ciliary neurotrophic factor (CNTF), neurotrophin-3 (NT3), etc.

The gene coding for glutamic acid decarboxylase (GAD), the enzyme synthesizing the inhibitory neurotransmitter γ-aminobutyric acid (GABA), may have a general interest for gene therapy in epilepsy (see reviews of Snodgrass, 1992; Gale, 1993; Martin & Rimvall, 1993). GABA exerts a local control over neuronal excitability and there is increasing evidence that elevation of GABA levels in particular brain areas can decrease or even prevent the triggering of a seizure. Thus, increasing the level of GABA in an epileptic focus is expected to prevent the generation of the seizures. This has already been demonstrated in some experimental models (Le Gal La Salle & Feldblum, 1983; Faingold et al., 1994). GABA may also act in critical neuronal networks outside an epileptic focus, by being involved in different functions, such as propagation of paroxysmal discharges or mechanisms of arrest of the seizures. In this context, an important seizure network site is the substantia nigra which can inhibit generalized epilepsies (Le Gal La Salle et al., 1983; Gale, 1985; Depaulis et al., 1990).

Finally, classes of genes that may play critical roles in seizure generation and propagation are those coding for receptors (glutamate or GABA receptors for example) and channels (potassium channel for example), and those which regulate receptor and channel function (such as second and tertiary messengers).

How to treat?

It is clear that the blood–brain barrier is a major obstacle to the delivery of recombinant viruses to the brain via systemic administration. Therefore, the brain has to be accessed by direct injection into the brain parenchyma.

The spread of adenoviral particles in the brain tissue appears to be limited. This feature could be very useful for targeting a foreign gene into a specific, well-circumscribed brain area and this is of particular relevance for epilepsies with an anatomically well-identified focus. In contrast, the poor diffusion of the virus will impede applications when the therapeutic activity is aimed at a widespread population of neuronal cells as, for example, in the case of large epileptic scars. Repeated administration of the virus at several sites may be necessary for increasing the volume of tissue in contact with the virus. In addition, refinements of the technique by favouring diffusion and cell penetration of the virus can be expected in the near future. Nevertheless, regional administration of the adenovirus will remain inadequate when larger brain areas need to be infected. Interestingly, the ability of the adenovirus to infect ependymal cells lining the ventricles following intracerebroventricular injection may offer a suitable route for delivering the transgene into the cerebroventricular fluid, provided that the gene product can cross the brain-ventricular barrier. Compared with the direct infusion of a given therapeutic gene product into the cerebrospinal fluid (CSF) which is rapidly turned over, adenovirus-mediated gene transfer into ependymal cells may provide a sustained, long-lasting production. Thus, this approach has potential for global correction of some neurological disorders. Osmotic disruption of the blood–brain barrier is another possible route for global delivery of genetic material. (Neuwlet *et al.*, 1991).

Finally another potentially interesting way of delivering foreign genes is through retrograde transport towards a selected cell population. The feasibility of this method has been demonstrated for dopaminergic nigral cells following striatal microinjection of a viral solution (Ridoux *et al.*, 1994b).

Some critical issues that remain to be solved

Gene transfer to the brain using direct injection of recombinant viruses has to fulfil several criteria to be therapeutically valuable: the two key areas are efficacy and safety.

First, the therapeutic gene has to be expressed at a level which can produce the desired effect. A prerequisite for successful gene therapy is long-term expression and stability of the transgene. This problem is of particular significance for a number of neurotransmitters, like GABA for example. The experimental reference data are deduced from pharmacological results where the therapeutic doses are much higher than those expected to result from *in vivo* gene transfer. However, the effect of low expression might be compensated for by reliable targeting of the foreign gene into the appropriate tissue, or even into the relevant cells, for example neurons *vs* glia. Cell specific expression can be achieved using promoters with the cell-specific activity. The method using adenovirus has mainly been assessed using strong ubiquitously active viral promoters (often a viral long terminal repeat or cytomegalovirus promoters). The next step will be the use of more specific promoters, for example housekeeping or tissue-specific promoters. Factors governing the regulation of promoters are also important for optimizing expression. More room in the viral genome may therefore be required for inserting regulatory sequences. At present a limitation of the adenovirus vector system is the size of exogenous DNA which can be accommodated, making difficult the insertion of promoter and regulatory sequences with the therapeutic gene. However, it should be possible to develop vectors with a theoretical insert capacity of about 35 kb by deleting more of the viral genome. Obviously, the appearance of cytotoxic effects associated with the development of an immunological reaction against viral proteins would be a major drawback. Generation of new constructs by deletion of immunogenic zones of the viral genome could prevent this type of immunological problem.

Finally, safety is of paramount importance. Adenoviral vectors would have to be as safe as possible for the successful development and application of gene therapy. In the near future the safety of these vectors will have to be clearly established and further improved. Although replication-deficient, the recombinant adenovirus might be transcomplemented if there were coinfection with wild non-defective viruses. To eliminate or to significantly reduce this potential risk it is proposed to use viruses of other species than human (canine for example), or to modify the packaging sequences. Nevertheless, adenoviruses are already considered sufficiently safe to have been approved by the Food and Drug Administration in the USA for small-scale gene therapy trials.

In conclusion, it should be pointed out that gene therapy for epilepsy will not become available before the viral vector system is completely mastered, in particular in terms of efficacy and safety. Other critical issues will be the choice of the appropriate therapeutic gene and the appropriate delivery of the viral vector into selected brain areas. Direct intracerebral microinjection of the viral solution is a method which provokes little damage at the injection site but the risks associated with this must be evaluated. However, whatever the future refinements of the technique, the neurophysiological background of the epilepsy to be treated should be perfectly understood to ensure a fully adapted approach to its treatment. Thus, before any clinical trial can be envisaged for any type of epilepsy, the proof of the efficacy of gene therapy must be demonstrated in animal models and its possible application in human medicine must be carefully investigated. The way is now open.

Acknowledgements

We would like to thank Dr R. Naquet for critical and helpful discussions. This study was supported by grants from Human Frontier Science Organization, The Association Française contre la Myopathie and the Fondation Française pour la Recherche sur l'Epilepsie.

References

Akli, S., Caillaud, C., Vigne, E., Stratford-Perricaudet, L.D., Poenaru, L., Perricaudet, M., Kahn, A. & Peschanski, M.R. (1993): Transfer of a foreign gene into the brain using adenovirus vectors. *Nature Genet.* **3**, 224–228.

Bajocchi, G., Feldman, S.H., Crystal, R.G. & Mastrangeli, A. (1993): Direct *in vivo* gene transfer to ependymal cells in the central nervous system using recombinant adenovirus vectors. *Nature Genet.* **3**, 229–234.

Breakefield, X.O. (1993): Gene delivery into the brain using virus vectors. *Nature Genet.* **3**, 187–189.

Breakefield, X.O. & DeLuca, N.A. (1991): Herpes simplex virus for gene delivery to neurons. *New Biologist* **3**, 203–218.

Buzsaki, G., Masliah, E., Chen, L.S., Horvath, Z., Terry, R. & Gage, F.H. (1991): Hippocampal grafts into intact brain induce epileptic patterns. *Brain Res.* **554**, 30–37.

Caillaud, C., Akli, S., Vigne, E., Koulakoff, A., Perricaudet, M., Poenaru, L., Kahn, A. & Berwald-Netter, Y. (1993): Adenoviral vector as a gene delivery system into cultured rat neuronal and glial cells. *Eur. J. Neurosci.* **5**, 1287–1291.

Commission on Classification and Terminology of the International League against Epilepsy (1989): Proposal for revised classification of epilepsies and epileptic syndromes. *Epilepsia* **30**, 389–399.

Davidson, B.L., Allen, E.D., Kozarsky, K.F., Wilson, J.M. & Roessler, B.J. (1993): A model system for *in vivo* gene transfer into the central nervous system using an adenoviral vector. *Nature Genet.* **3**, 219–223.

Depaulis, A., Vergnes, M., Liu, Z., Kempf, E. & Marescaux, C. (1990): Involvement of nigral output pathways in the inhibitory control of the substantia nigra over generalized non-convulsive seizures in the rat. *Neuroscience* **39**, 339–349.

Faingold, C.L., Marcinczyk, M.J., Casebeer, D.J., Randall, M.E., Arneric, S.P. & Browning, R.A. (1994): GABA in the inferior colliculus plays a critical role in control of audiogenic seizures. *Brain Res.* **640**, 40–47.

Fine, A., Meldrum, B.S. & Patel, S. (1990): Modulation of experimentally induced epilepsy by intracerebral grafts of fetal GABAergic neurons. *Neuropsychologia* **28**, 627–634.

Friedmann, T. (1989): Progress toward human gene therapy. *Science* **244**, 1275–1281.

Friedmann, T. (1993): Gene therapy a new kind of medicine. *Tibtech.* **11**, 156–159.

Friedmann, T. & Hyder, A.J. (1993): Gene therapy for disorders of the nervous system. *Tibtech.* **11**, 192–197.

Gage, F.H., Kawaja, M.D. & Fisher, L.J. (1991): Genetically-modified cells – applications for intracerebral grafting. *Trends Neurosci.* **14**, 328–333.

Gale, K. (1985): Mechanisms of seizure control mediated by GABA: role of the substantia nigra. *Fed. Proc.* **44**, 2414–2424.

Gale, K. (1993): GABA and epilepsy: basic concepts from preclinical research. *Epilepsia* **33**, (Suppl. 5), 3–12.

Gall, C., Murray, K. & Isackson, P.J. (1991): Kaïnic acid induced seizures increased expression of nerve growth factor mRNA in rat hippocampus. *Mol. Brain Res.* **9**, 113–123.

Gardiner, R.M. (1990): Genes and epilepsy. *J. Med. Genet.* **27**, 537–544.

Geller, A.I. & Breakefield, X.O. (1988): A defective HSV-1 vector expresses *Escherichia coli* β-galactosidase in cultured peripheral neurons. *Science* **241**, 1667–1669.

Goedert, M., Fine, A., Hunt, S.P. & Ullrich, A. (1986): Nerve growth factor mRNA in peripheral and central rat tissues and in human nervous system: lesion effects in the rat brain and levels in Alzheimer disease. *Mol. Brain Res.* **1**, 85–92.

Horellou, P., Brundin, P., Kalen, P. & Mallet, J. (1990): *In vivo* release of DOPA and dopamine from genetically engineered cells grafted to the denervated rat striatum. *Neuron* **5**, 393–402.

Jaffe, H.A., Danel, C., Longenecker, G., Metzger, M., Setoguchi, Y., Rosenfeld, M.A., Gant, T.W., Thorgeirsonn, S.S., Stratford-Perricaudet, L.D., Perricaudet, M., Pavirani, A., Lecocq, J.P. & Crystal, R.G. (1992): Adenovirus-mediated in vivo gene transfer and expression in normal rat liver. *Nature Genet.* **1**, 372–378.

Jiao, S., Gurevich, V. & Wolff, J.A. (1993): Long-term correction of rat model of Parkinson's disease by gene therapy. *Nature* 362, 450–453.

Kromer, L.F. (1987): Nerve growth factor treatment after brain injury prevents neuronal death. *Science* 235, 214–216.

Le Gal La Salle, G. & Feldblum, S. (1983): Role of the amygdala in development of hippocampal kindling in the rat. *Exp. Neurol.* 82, 447–455.

Le Gal La Salle, G., Kaijima, M. & Feldblum, S. (1983): Abortive amygdaloid kindled seizures following microinjection of γ-vinyl-GABA in the vicinity of substantia nigra in rats. *Neurosci. Lett.* 36, 69–74.

Le Gal La Salle, G., Robert, J.J., Berrard, S., Ridoux, V., Stratford-Perricaudet, L.D., Perricaudet, M. & Mallet, J. (1993): Adenovirus as a potent vector for gene transfer in neurons and glia in the brain. *Science* 235, 986–988.

Lindvall, O. & Björklund, A. (1992): Intracerebral grafting of inhibitory neurons: a new strategy for seizure suppression in the central nervous system. In: *Advances in neurology*, Vol. 57, eds. P. Chauvel, A.V. Delgado-Escueta *et al.*, pp. 561–569. New York: Raven Press.

Martin, D.L. & Rimvall, K. (1993): Regulation of γ-aminobutyric acid synthesis in the brain. *J. Neurochem.* 60, 395–407.

Meldrum, B.S. (1990): Anatomy, physiology and pathology of epilepsy. *Lancet* 336, 231–234.

Miyamoto, O., Itano, T., Yamamoto, Y., Tokuda, M., Matsui, H., Janjua, N.A., Suwaki, H., Okada, Y., Murakami, T.H., Negi, T. Nakahara, S. & Hatase, O. (1993): Effect of embryonic hippocampal transplantation in amygdaloid kindled rat. *Brain Res.* 603, 143–147.

Mulligan, R.C. (1993): The basic science of gene therapy. *Science* 260, 926–932.

Neuwelt, E.A., Pagel, M.A. & Dix, R.D. (1991): Delivery of ultraviolet-inactivated 35S-herpesvirus across an osmotically modified blood-brain barrier. *J. Neurosurg.* 74, 475–479.

Neve, R.L. (1993): Adenovirus vectors enter the brain. *TINS* 16, 251–253.

Pedley, T.A. (1993): The challenge of intractable epilepsy. In: *New trends in epilepsy management*, ed. D. Chadwick, pp. 3–12. Royal Society of Medicine Services Limited.

Quantin, B., Perricaudet, L.D., Tajbakhsh, S. & Mandel, J.L. (1992): Adenovirus as an expression vector in muscle cells *in vivo*. *Proc. Natl. Acad. Sci. USA* 89, 2581–2584.

Ridoux, V., Robert, J.J., Zhang, X., Perricaudet, M., Mallet, J. & Le Gal La Salle, G. (1994a): The use of adenovirus vectors for intracerebral grafting of transfected nervous cells. *Neuroreport* 5, 801–804.

Ridoux, V., Robert, J.J., Zhang, X., Perricaudet, M., Mallet, J. & Le Gal La Salle, G. (1994b): Adenoviral vectors as functional retrograde neuronal tracers. *Brain Res.* (in press).

Roemer, K. & Friedmann, T. (1992): Concepts and strategies for human gene therapy. *Eur. J. Biochem.* 208, 211–225.

Rosenfeld, M.A., Siegfried, W., Yoshimura, K., Yoneyama, K., Fukayama, M., Stier, L.E., Pääkkö, P.K., Gilardi, P., Stratford-Perricaudet, L.D., Perricaudet, M., Jallat, S., Pavirani, A., Lecocq, J.-P. & Crystal, R.G. (1991): Adenovirus-mediated transfer of a recombinant α1-antitrypsin gene to the lung epithelium *in vivo*. *Science* 252, 431–434.

Rosenfeld, M.A., Yoshimura, K., Trapnell, B.C., Yoneyama, K., Rosenthal, E.R., Dalemans, W., Fukayama, M., Bargon, J., Stier, L.E., Stratford-Perricaudet, L.D., Perricaudet, M., Guggino, W.B., Pavirani, A., Lecocq, J-P. & Crystal, R.G. (1992): *In vivo* transfer of the human cystic fibrosis transmembrane conductance regulator gene to the airway epithelium. *Cell* 68, 142–155.

Snodgrass, S.R. (1992): GABA and epilepsy: their complex relationship and the evolution of our understanding. *J. Child Neurol.* 7, 77–86.

Stratford-Perricaudet, L.D., Levreto, M., Chase, J.F., Perricaudet, M. & Briand, P. (1990): Evaluation of the transfer and expression in mice of an enzyme-encoding gene using a human adenovirus vector. *Hum. Gene Ther.* 1, 241–256.

Stratford-Perricaudet, L.D., Makeh, I., Perricaudet, M. & Briand, P. (1992): Widespread long-term gene transfer to mouse skeletal muscles and heart. *J. Clin. Invest.* 90, 626–630.

Varmus, H. (1988): Retroviruses. *Science* 240, 1427–1435.

List of Contributors

Leah E. ADAMS-CURTIS
Department of Basic Sciences
University of Illinois
College of Medicine at Peoria
PEORIA IL 61656 - USA

Eric AKAWIE
Epilepsy Research Lab
Department of Medicine
Duke University and Durham Veterans Administration
Medical Centers
508 Fulton Street
DURHAM NC 27707 - USA.

Frederick ANDERMANN
Montreal Neurological Hospital & Institute
3801 University Street
MONTREAL, Quebec - Canada H3A 2B4

V. Elving ANDERSON
Epilepsy Clinical Research Program
University of Minnesota
MINNEAPOLIS, MN 55455 - USA

Massimo AVOLI
Montreal Neurological Hospital & Institute
3801 University Street
MONTREAL, Quebec - Canada H3A 2B4

Jean de BARRY
Laboratoire de Neurobiologie Cellulaire
Centre de Neurochimie du CNRS
5 rue Blaise Pascal
67000 STRASBOURG - France

Cesira BATINI
Laboratoire de Physiologie de la Motricité, CNRS et
Université P. et M. Curie
9 Quai Saint Bernard
75005 PARIS - France

Gertrud BECK-MANAGETTA
Universitatsklinikum Rudolf Virchow der Freien
Universität Berlin
Standort Charlottenburg
Neurologie
Spandauer Damm 130
1000 BERLIN 19 - Germany

Yehezkel BEN-ARI
INSERM U29
123 Boulevard de Port-Royal
75014 PARIS - France

Raymond BERNASCONI
INSERM U398
Faculté de Médecine
Rue Humann
67000 STRASBOURG - France

Colin BINNIE
The Maudsley Hospital
Department of Clinical Neurophysiology
Denmark Hill SE5 8AZ
LONDON - England

Helmut BITTIGER
Research and Development Department
Pharmaceutical Division
Ciba-Geigy
BASEL - Switzerland.

Anne BLANC-PLATIER
INSERM U398
Faculté de Médecine
Rue Humann
67000 STRASBOURG - France

Dominique BROGLIN
Clinique Paul Castaigne,
Groupe Hospitalier Pitié-Salpêtrière,
47–83 Blvd de l'Hôpital,
75651 PARIS Cedex 13 - France
and
Sanofi Winthrop
9 rue du Président Allende
94258 GENTILLY Cedex - France

Chapter 43 List of Contributors

Ronald A. BROWNING
Department of Physiology and Pharmacology
Southern Illinois University School of Medicine
CARBONDALE, IL 62901 - USA

Michelle BUREAU
Centre Saint Paul
300, Boulevard de Sainte Marguerite
13009 MARSEILLE - France

Zhen CAO
Epilepsy Research Lab
Department of Medicine
Duke University and Durham Veterans Administration
Medical Centers
508 Fulton Street
DURHAM NC 27707 - USA

Astrid G. CHAPMAN
Department of Neurology
Institute of Psychiatry
De Crespigny Park, Denmark Hill
LONDON SE5 8AF - England

Catherine CHIRON
Service de Neuropédiatrie
Hôpital Saint Vincent de Paul
74, Avenue Denfert Rochereau
75674 PARIS Cédex 14 - France

Douglas A. COULTER
Department of Neurology
PO Box 980 599
Medical College of Virginia
Virginia Commonwealth University
RICHMOND, VA 23298 - 0599 USA

Vincenzo CRUNELLI
Department of Physiology
University of Wales, PO Box 902
Museum Avenue
CARDIFF CF1 1SS, Wales - UK

John W. DAILEY
Department of Basic Sciences
University of Illinois
College of Medicine at Peoria
PEORIA IL 61656 - USA

Mogens DAM
University Clinic of Neurology
Hvidovre Hospital
DK-2650 HVIDOVRE - Denmark

Jean-François DARTIGUES
72, rue Gambetta
33200 BORDEAUX - France

Antonio V. DELGADO-ESCUETA
California Comprehensive Epilepsy Program
and Neurological and Research Service
Suite 3405
West Los Angeles VA Medical Center (W127B)
Wilshire and Sawtelle Boulevards
WEST LOS ANGELES, CA 90073 - USA

Antoine DEPAULIS
Laboratoire de Neurophysiologie et Biologie des
Comportements
Centre de Neurochimie du CNRS
5 rue Blaise Pascal
67084 STRASBOURG Cedex - France

Isabelle DESGUERRE
Service de Neuropédiatrie
Hôpital Saint Vincent de Paul
74, Avenue Denfert Rochereau
75674 PARIS Cédex 14 - France

Charlotte DRAVET
Centre Saint Paul
300, Boulevard de Sainte Marguerite
13009 MARSEILLE- France

Olivier DULAC
Service de Neuropédiatrie
Hôpital Saint Vincent de Paul
74, Avenue Denfert Rochereau
75674 PARIS Cédex 14 - France

Noureddine FADLALLAH
Laboratoire de Physiologie de la Motricité, CNRS et
Université P. et M. Curie
9 Quai Saint Bernard
75005 PARIS - France

Wolfgang FROESTL
Research and Development Department
Pharmaceutical Division
Ciba-Geigy
BASEL - Switzerland

Mark GEE
California Comprehensive Epilepsy Program
and Neurological and Research Service
Suite 3405
West Los Angeles VA Medical Center (W127B)
Wilshire and Sawtelle Boulevards
WEST LOS ANGELES, CA 90073 - USA

Pierre GENTON
Centre Saint Paul
300, Boulevard de Sainte Marguerite
13009 MARSEILLE- France

Pierre GLOOR
Montreal Neurological Hospital & Institute
3801 University Street
MONTREAL, Quebec - Canada H3A 2B4

Giuseppe GOBBI
Servizio di Neuropsichiatria Infantile
Divisione di Pediatria
Arcispedale S. Maria Nuova
Viale Risorgimento 80
42100 REGGIO EMILIA - Italy

Maria del Socorro GONZALES SANCHEZ
Andador Vista Alegre 2744
Col. Seattle, GUADALAJARA
Jalisco, Mexico

David GREENBERG
Department of Psychiatry
Mount Sinai School of Medicine
One Gustave L. Levy Place
NEW YORK, NY 10029 - USA

Renzo GUERRINI
Istituto Neuropsichiatria Infantile
Via dei Giacinti, 2
56018 CALAMBRONE DI PISA - Italy

Nicolas GUY
Laboratoire de Physiologie de la Motricité, CNRS et
Université P. et M. Curie
9 Quai Saint Bernard
75005 PARIS - France

Alice GUYON
Département de Neurobiologie Cellulaire
Institut des Neurosciences
Université P. et M. Curie
9 Quai Saint Bernard
75005 PARIS - France

Thomas HILDMANN
Heinrich Neitzel Institut für Humangenetik
Heubnerweg 6
1000 BERLIN 19 - Germany

Edouard HIRSCH
INSERM U398
Faculté de Médecine
Rue Humann
67000 STRASBOURG - France

Gregory HOLMES
Department of Neurology
Children's Hospital and Harvard Medical School
300 Longwood Ave
BOSTON MA02115 - USA

David A. HOSFORD
Epilepsy Research Lab
Department of Medicine
Duke University and Durham Veterans Administration
Medical Centers
508 Fulton Street
DURHAM NC 27707 - USA

Alex HUIN
Epilepsy Research Lab
Department of Medicine
Duke University and Durham Veterans Administration
Medical Centers
508 Fulton Street
DURHAM NC 27707 - USA

Dieter JANZ
Universitatsklinikum Rudolf Virchow der Freien
Universität Berlin
Standort Charlottenburg
Neurologie
Spandauer Damm 130
1000 BERLIN 19 - Germany

Phillip C. JOBE
Department of Basic Sciences
University of Illinois
College of Medicine at Peoria
PEORIA IL 61656 - USA

Dorothee KASTELEIJN-NOLST-TRENITÉ
Instituut voor Epilepsiebestrijding
Postbus 21
2100 AA HEEMSTEDE - The Netherlands

Peter E. KEANE
Sanofi Recherche
195 route d'Espagne
31036 TOULOUSE Cedex - France

Kwang Ho. KO
Department of Pharmacy
College of Pharmacy
Seoul National University
SEOUL 151-742 - South Korea

Diana L. KRAEMER
Epilepsy Research Lab
Department of Medicine
Duke University and Durham Veterans Administration
Medical Centers
508 Fulton Street
DURHAM NC 27707 - USA

Michel KHRESTCHATISKY
INSERM U29
123 Boulevard de Port-Royal
75014 PARIS - France

Carlos LAHOZ
Servicio de Neurologia

Hospital General de Asturias
33006 OVIEDO - Spain

Nicole-M. LE DOUARIN
Institut d'Embryologie Cellulaire et Moléculaire
CNRS et Collège de France
NOGENT SUR MARNE - France

Gildas LE GAL LA SALLE
Institut Alfred Fessard, CNRS
Avenue de la Terrasse
91198 GIF-SUR-YVETTE Cedex - France

Mark F. LEPPERT
Eccles Institute of Human Genetics
Building 533
University of Salt Lake City
SALT LAKE CITY, UT 84112 - USA

Nathalie LERESCHE
Département de Neurobiologie Cellulaire
Institut des Neurosciences
Université P. et M. Curie
9 Quai Saint Bernard
75005 PARIS - France

Mireille LERNER-NATOLI
Laboratoire de Médecine Expérimentale
INSERM U429, CNRS UPR 8408
Institut de Biologie
Boulevard Henri IV
34060 MONTPELLIER - France

Fu-hsiung LIN
Epilepsy Research Lab
Department of Medicine
Duke University and Durham Veterans Administration Medical Centers
508 Fulton Street
DURHAM NC 27707 - USA

Dick LINDHOUT
Department of Clinical Genetics
Faculty of Medicine
P.O. Box 1738
3000 DR ROTTERDAM - The Netherlands

Amy LIU
California Comprehensive Epilepsy Program
and Neurological and Research Service
Suite 3405
West Los Angeles VA Medical Center (W127B)
Wilshire and Sawtelle Boulevards
WEST LOS ANGELES, CA 90073 - USA

Jérôme LOISEAU
Department of Neurology

Bordeaux University Hospital
Hôpital Pellegrin-Tripode
33076 BORDEAUX Cédex - France

Pierre LOISEAU
Department of Neurology
Bordeaux University Hospital
Hôpital Pellegrin-Tripode
33076 BORDEAUX Cédex - France

Alain MALAFOSSE
Laboratoire de Médecine Expérimentale
Institut de Biologie
34060 MONTPELLIER - France

Jacques MALLET
UMR 9923
CNRS
Avenue de la Terrasse
91198 GIF-SUR-YVETTE Cedex - France

Jean-Louis MANDEL
Laboratoire de Génétique
Faculté de Médecine
67000 STRASBOURG - France

Christian MARESCAUX
INSERM U398
Faculté de Médecine
Rue Humann
67000 STRASBOURG - France

Pascal MATHIVET
INSERM U398
Faculté de Médecine
Rue Humann
67000 STRASBOURG - France

Bruno MATON
Clinique Neurologique
Unité d'EEG et d'Epileptologie
Hôpital Cantonnal Universitaire de Genève
1211 GENÈVE - Switzerland

Marco T. MEDINA
California Comprehensive Epilepsy Program
and Neurological and Research Service
Suite 3405
West Los Angeles VA Medical Center (W127B)
Wilshire and Sawtelle Boulevards
WEST LOS ANGELES, CA 90073 - USA

Christian MENINI
Institut Alfred Fessard
Avenue de la Terrasse
91198 GIF SUR YVETTE Cedex - France

Stewart MICKEL
Research and Development Department
Pharmaceutical Division
Ciba-Geigy
BASEL - Switzerland

Pravin K. MISHRA
Department of Basic Sciences
University of Illinois
College of Medicine at Peoria
PEORIA IL 61656 - USA

Joëlle MOREAU
INSERM U29
123 Boulevard de Port-Royal
75014 PARIS - France

Solomon MOSHE
Albert Einstein College of Medicine
Rose F. Kennedy Center
1410 Pelham Parkway
South Bronx, NEW YORK 10461 - USA

Robert NAQUET
Institut Alfred Fessard, CNRS
Avenue de la Terrasse
91198 GIF SUR YVETTE Cedex - France

Astrid NEHLIG
INSERM U398
Faculté de Médecine
Rue Humann
67000 STRASBOURG - France

Jérôme NIQUET
INSERM U29
123 Boulevard de Port-Royal
75014 PARIS - France

Jeffrey L. NOEBELS
Department of Neurology
Baylor College of Medicine
One Baylor Plaza
HOUSTON, TX 77030 - USA

Luis OLLER-DAURELLA
Escuelas Pias 89
8017 BARCELONA - Espagne

Luis OLLER FERRER VIDAL
Neurologia Y Neurofisiologia Clinica
Escuelas Pias, 89
08017 BARCELONA - Spain

Chrysotomos P. PANAYIOTOPOULOS
Department of Clinical Neurophysiology and Epilepsy
St Thomas'Hospital
LONDON SE1 7EH - England

Perrine PLOUIN
Service d'Explorations Fonctionnelles du Système Nerveux
Hôpital Saint Vincent de Paul
74, Avenue Denfert Rochereau
75674 PARIS Cédex 14 - France

Hélène POLLARD
INSERM U29
123 Boulevard de Port-Royal
75014 PARIS - France

Alfonso REPRESA
INSERM U29
123 Boulevard de Port-Royal
75014 PARIS - France

Stefano RICCI
Ospedale Pediatrico "Bambino Gesù"
Piazza San Onofrio, 4
00165 ROMA - Italy

Joseph ROGER
116, rue Edmond Rostand
13006 MARSEILLE - France

Gérard RONDOUIN
Laboratoire de Médecine Expérimentale
INSERM U429, CNRS UPR 8408
Institut de Biologie
Boulevard Henri IV
34060 MONTPELLIER - France

Stephen G. RYAN
Department of Pediatrics
University of Texas, Health Science Center
7703 Floyd Curl Drive
SAN ANTONIO, TX 78284 - USA

Xavier SALAS-PUIG
Servicio de Neurologia
Hospital General de Asturias,
33006 OVIEDO - Spain

Amalia SALTARELLI
Centro Regionale per l'Epilessia
Ospedale San Paolo
Via Di Rudini 8
20142 MILANO - Italy

Thomas SANDER
Universitatsklinikum Rudolf Virchow der Freien
Universität Berlin
Standort Charlottenburg

Neurologie
Spandauer Damm 130
1000 BERLIN 19 - Germany

Jose SERRATOSA
California Comprehensive Epilepsy Program
and Neurological and Research Service
Suite 3405
West Los Angeles VA Medical Center (W127B)
Wilshire and Sawtelle Boulevards
WEST LOS ANGELES, CA 90073 - USA

Carmen SILVA-BARRAT
Institut Alfred Fessard
Avenue de la Terrasse
91198 GIF SUR YVETTE Cedex - France

Simone SIMLER
INSERM U398
Faculté de Médecine
Rue Humann
67000 STRASBOURG - France

O. Carter SNEAD
Department of Neurology
University of Southern California
Children's Hospital, Box 82
4650 Sunset Boulevard
LOS ANGELES, CA 90027- USA

Ortrud STEINLEIN
Institut für Humangenetik und Anthropologie
im Neuenheimer Feld 328
69120 HEIDELBERG - Germany

David N. STEPHENS
Research Laboratories of Schering AG
Müllerstr. 178
D-13342 BERLIN - Germany

Takeo TAKAHASHI
Yaotome Clinic
Yaotome 2-12-2, Izumiku
SENDAI 981 -31 - Japan

Marie-Aimée TEILLET
Institut d'Embryologie Cellulaire et Moléculaire
CNRS et Collège de France
NOGENT SUR MARNE - France

Pierre THOMAS
Service de Neurologie
du Pr Chatel
Hôpital Pasteur
Avenue de la Voie Romaine
B.P. 69
06002 NICE Cédex - France

Lucy J. TREIMAN
California Comprehensive Epilepsy Program
and Neurological and Research Service
Suite 3405
West Los Angeles VA Medical Center (W127B)
Wilshire and Sawtelle Boulevards
WEST LOS ANGELES, CA 90073 - USA

Alberto TUÑON
Servicio de Neurologia
Hospital General de Asturias,
33006 OVIEDO - Spain

Jonathan P. TURNER
Department of Physiology
University of Wales, PO Box 902
Museum Avenue
CARDIFF CF1 1SS, Wales - UK

Lechoslaw TURSKI
Research Laboratories of Schering AG
Müllerstr. 178
D-13342 BERLIN - Germany

Walter Van EMDE BOAS
Instituut voor Epilepsiebestrijding
Postbus 21
2100 AA HEEMSTEDE - The Netherlands

Marguerite VERGNES
INSERM U398
Faculté de Médecine
Rue Humann
67000 STRASBOURG - France

Libor VELISEK
Albert Einstein College of Medicine
Rose F. Kennedy Center
1410 Pelham Parkway
South Bronx, NEW YORK 10461 - USA

Federico VIGEVANO
Ospedale Pediatrico "Bambino Gesù"
Piazza San Onofrio, 4
00165 ROMA - Italy

Juhn A. WADA
Divisions of Neurosciences and Neurology
University of British Columbia
VANCOUVER BC V6T 2A1- Canada

Stephan WALTZ
Klinikum der Christian-Albrechts-Univers ität zu Kiel
Kinderklinik
Schwanenweg 20
2300 KIEL 1 - GERMANY

Karen WEISSBECKER
California Comprehensive Epilepsy Program
and Neurological and Research Service
Suite 3405
West Los Angeles VA Medical Center (W127B)
Wilshire and Sawtelle Boulevards
WEST LOS ANGELES, CA 90073 - USA

Stephen R. WILLIAMS
Department of Physiology
University of Wales, PO Box 902
Museum Avenue
CARDIFF CF1 1SS, Wales - UK

John T. WILSON
Epilepsy Research Lab
Department of Medicine
Duke University and Durham Veterans Administration
Medical Centers
508 Fulton Street
DURHAM NC 27707 - USA

Peter WOLF
Epilepsie-Zentrum Bethel
Klinik für Anfallskranke - Mara 1
Maraweg 21
4800 BIELEFELD 13 (Bethel) - Germany

Yin YIN
Epilepsy Research Lab
Department of Medicine
Duke University and Durham Veterans Administration
Medical Centers
508 Fulton Street
DURHAM NC 27707 - USA

Yun-fu ZHANG
Department of Neurology
PO Box 980 599
Medical College of Virginia
Virginia Commonwealth University
RICHMOND, VA 23298 - 0599 USA

Index

A

Absence seizures 73–227
  action of AEDs on excitatory amino acid
    antagonists 449–451
  age of onset 90
  with cerebral blood flow 172–173
  cholinergic mechanisms 140
  classification 75–85
    relevant criteria in French study 87–93
  clinical spectrum 75–85
  compared in humans and rats 154
  definition 75
    EEG SWD 75
    typical/atypical 75
  excitatory amino acid-mediated in
  GABA-mediated mechanisms 138–139
  experimental
    lethargic mouse model 187–200
    pharmacology 142
  GABA-mediated mechanisms 137–138
  $GABA_B$ receptor antagonists, therapy in
  experimental epilepsy 463
  gamma-hydroxybutyrate (GHB)-mediated 140–142
  generalized tonic–clonic seizures 90
  hyperventilation 12
  monoaminergic mechanisms 139–140
  phantom 84
  photosensitivity 84
  prognosis 91
  reflex 84
  with single, non-rhythmic myoclonia 83
  see also Absences, typical; Animal models;
Genetic absence epilepsy rat of Strasbourg
Absence status
  de novo form 95–106
  late-onset 84,95–109
    case histories 98–99
    precipitating factors, 97–8, 102–6
    prognosis 98
    pseudonyms in literature 102
    triggering by benzodiazepines 98, 102–106
Absences
  atypical, defined 75
  typical
    defined 75
    symptomatic and secondary 84
  see also Absence seizures; Childhood absence
epilepsy; Eyelid myoclonia; Juvenile absence epilepsy;
Juvenile myoclonic epilepsy; Myoclonic absence
epilepsy; Perioral myoclonia; Stimulus–sensitive
absence epilepsy
Acetylcholine, SWD in GAERS 160
Adenoviral vector, gene therapy in epilepsy 512–515
Adult onset absence status 95–109
AEDs *see* Antiepileptic drugs
N-Allylnormetazocine, selective antagonist,
  NMDA receptors 464
2-Amino-5-phosphonopentanoic acid (AP5) 464
2-Amino-7-phosphoheptanoic acid (AP7),
  selective antagonist, NMDA receptors 353,464
AMPA type glutamate receptor antagonists 434
AMPA/kainate receptors, glutamatergic
  excitation 467
Amygdalar kindling experiments 351
  callosal bisection 351–352
  ultimate pattern 352
  Wistar AS rats 416
Anatomy of convulsive seizures 399–413
Animal models
  absence seizures, pharmacology 142
  absence seizures in rats 133–150
    criteria 136
  avian FEpi reflex epilepsy 375–383
  baboon models 331–348
  brain metabolism, cerebral blood flow 169–176
  brain structure, seizure-induced changes 433–445
  cat dorsal lateral geniculate nucleus
  intrinsic pacemaker 202
  chicken model of genetic epilepsy 375–383
  drug-induced epilepsy 51–64
  excitatory amino acid antagonists,
  therapeutic prospects 463–471
  feline generalized penicillin epilepsy 111–121
  genetic absence epilepsy rat of Strasbourg 136–139
  GEPR model of epilepsy 385–398
  ILS(intermittent light stimulation)
    feline studies 360–362
    primate studies 362–366
  lethargic mouse model, absence seizures 187–200
  minimal electroshock threshold (MES) 60
  partial onset secondarily generalized
  convulsion (kindling model) 350
  primate models 331–348, 349–373
    see also Baboon
  state dependency 133
  SWD, genetic transmission 162–165

thalamocortical circuitry	133–135	ILS-induced seizures, summary	360
thalamocortical rhythms	123–132	kindling time	352
Wistar AS rats, audiogenic seizures	415–422	nonepileptic myoclonus	331–332,334–338
Anti-epileptic drugs		photosensitivity	331–348
action, mechanisms	447–454	Baclofen, $GABA_B$ receptor agonist	177,181,189
in animal models		Barbiturates	
development aspects	51–64	efficacy, impulsive petit mal	243
modulation of seizure threshold		resistance by GAs	133
for EAAs	473–483	see also Phenobarbitone	
effects on substantia nigra, rat models	504	Batrachotoxin, induction of sodium influx	
excitatory amino acid antagonists, novel	463–471	into synaptosomes	448
FEpi reflex epilepsy	375–383	Benign familial infantile convulsions	
future prospects	429	age of onset	47,49
GEPR, model for studies	391–292	case analysis	45–46
long-term outcome	428–429	coincidence with BFNC	48
mechanisms of action	423–424	EEGs	47
summary	451	epilepsy in relatives	47
modulation of seizure threshold for EAAs		multicentre study	46–47
in mice	473–483	sex ratio	46
novel drugs, mechanisms of action	455–461	see also Benign familial neonatal convulsions	
seizure threshold in mice, results	476	Benign familial myoclonic convulsions	
short-term outcome	425–428	chromosome 20q	65–66,67
absence seizures	427	gene mapping	65–71
GTCSs	426	Benign familial neonatal convulsions	39–44
myoclonic seizures	427	age of cessation	65
photosensitive epilepsies	428	age of onset	39,65
2-APH, selective antagonist to NMDA		APGAR score	39,65
receptors	353,464	cases and families	40
Area tempestas, effects on NMDA receptors,		defined	9
substantia nigra	504	DNA analysis, parental counselling	70
ATPA, seizure threshold in mice, AEDs	474–478	EEGs	41–43,67
Atropine, induction of myoclonus	336	gene mapping	65–71
Audiogenic seizures		genetics	28
cerebral blood flow	173–176	inheritance	42–43,65
effects on NMDA receptors, substantia nigra	504	linkage analysis	66–67
Wistar AS rats	415–422	locus heterogeneity	67
effects on c-fos expression	417–420	lod score	66
effects on cerebral blood flow	420–421	questions for future	67–8
positive transfer to hippocampal and		RFLP markers	42,66
amygdalar kindling	417	seizure type	40–43,67
Avian FEpi reflex epilepsy	375–383	sex ratio	39
brain anatomy	375	see also Benign familial infantile convulsions	
EEG and EMG of ILS-induced seizures	378–381	Benign myoclonic epilepsy in infancy	268–269
prosencephalon and mesencephalon	381	as an IGE	20
		defined	9
B		EEG criteria	11
Baboon model of epilepsy		reflex form	269–270
kindling time	352	similarity to childhood-onset myoclonic	
sensitivity to amygdaloid-kindled seizures	352	epilepsy	270–271
Baboon models of epilepsy		syndromic classification	16
forebrain convulsive mechanisms:		Benign neonatal convulsions	
claustrum	349–373	age of onset	10
GABAergic neurotransmission	335	as an IGE	20
genetic transmission of ILS myoclonus	341–342	defined	9
idiopathic generalized epilepsy	331–348	Benzodiazepines	
ILS-induced myoclonus	332–334,335,339–340	absence seizures	427

in absence seizures	138
abuse	98
acute withdrawal	98,102–103
baboon myoclonus	331,335
blockade by physostigmine	336
and cholinergic system	338
EEG normalization	98
effects on substantia nigra, rat models	504
ILS-induced myoclonus blockade and nonepileptic myoclonus induction	335–336
mechanisms of action, myoclonic seizures	448–489
seizure threshold in mice	474–478
specific antagonists of	335,337–338
BF-HLA loci, chromosome 6p	283–285
BFIC *see* Benign familial infantile convulsions	
BFNC *see* Benign familial neonatal convulsions	
Bicuculline	
EEG seizures	56
motor seizures	54–56
pathology	56
pharmacology	57
seizure threshold in mice,data	480
Bilateral spike-wave complexes	19
BMEI *see* Benign myoclonic epilepsy in infancy	
BNC *see* Benign neonatal convulsions	
Brain chimaeras, avian FEpi reflex epilepsy	376–378
Brain metabolism, animal models	169–176
Brain structure, seizure-induced changes	433–445
induction phase	433–437
maintenance phase	437–442
Brainstem seizures, triggering forebrain seizures	409
Brainstem structures	
brainstem and forebrain separation of seizure substrates	399–401
pathways of propagation	408
remote systems, regulatory control	408
running/bounding (R/B) clonic and tonic convulsions	400–403,406–408

C

c-fos expression, Wistar AS rats, effects of audiogenic seizures	417–420
Calcium channels, and anticonvulsants	335
Calcium conductance, SWD	119
Carbamazepine	
effects on substantia nigra, rat models	504
generalized tonic–clonic seizures	426
mechanisms of action, tonic–clonic seizures	448
resistance by GAs	133
seizure threshold in mice	476
data	479
spontaneous rhythms	129
3-(2-Carboxypiperazin-4-yl)propyl-1-phosphonic acid (CPP)	
seizure threshold in mice	476
selective antagonist, NMDA receptors	464
Cerebellum, R/B clonic and tonic convulsions	406–407
Cerebral blood flow	
with absence seizures	172–173
animal models	169–176
autoradiography	169–170
audiogenic seizures	173–176
Laser–Doppler flowmetry	170,173–175
Wistar AS rats, effects of audiogenic seizures	420–421
CGP-35348, SWD seizures, blockade	221
CGP-54626 and CGP-27492, GABA$_B$-antagonist radioligands	178–184
Chicken models of epilepsy, convulsive seizures	375–383
Childhood absence epilepsy	
defined	9
EEG criteria	11–12,13–14
exclusion criteria	78–79
France	22
frequency	15
inclusion criteria	77–78
syndromic classification	16
Childhood-onset myoclonic epilepsy	10,270–271
Cholinergic mechanisms, absence seizures	140
Chromosome 6	
BF-HLA loci	283–285
JME and photosensitivity	302
linkage with marker, JME	290
Chromosome 20q, benign familial myoclonic convulsions	65–66,67
CMM6 (D20S19) marker	68
markers	286
RMR6 (D20S20) marker	69
Chromosome 21	
markers	286
PME	326
Classification	
absences	75–85
relevant criteria in French study	87–93
International (1989) ILAE	8,9–10
Claustrum	
discussion	368
lesioning in primate studies	362–366
transformation of ILS-induced visual afferents	360–368
Clonazepam	
EEG normalization	100
in lethargic mice	191
mechanisms of action, myoclonic seizures	427,448
Clorazepate, EEG normalization	98
CMM6 (D20S19) marker, chromosome 20q	68
Convulsant drugs, seizure threshold in mice	477
data	480
Convulsive seizures	
anatomy of	399–413
chicken model	375–383

GEPR model	385–398	Epilepsy with generalized tonic–clonic seizures on awakening, defined	9
myoclonus in baboon	331–348	Ethosuximide	
novel excitatory amino acid antagonist, action in animal models	464–468	absence seizures	89,172,425
pathophysiology of	329–421	animal models	128,476,478,504
primate model of forebrain mechanisms	349–373	in lethargic mice	191
propagation of	415–421	effects on substantia nigra, rat models	504
Corneal electroshock, GEPRs compared with non-epileptic animals (table)	388–389	mechanisms of action	
		absence seizures	449
Corneal kindling		release of γ-hydroxybutyrate (GHB)	450
GEPRs compared with non-epileptic animals (table)	388–389	seizure threshold in mice	476
		data	478
transcorneal and transauricular stimulation compared	401	site and mechanism of action	208
		Excitatory amino acid antagonists	
Corpus callosum		novel, therapeutic prospects	463–71
role in convulsive seizure bilateralization and generalization	354–355	seizure threshold in mice, data	479
		see also Felbamate; Lamotrigine; Remacemide;	
discussion	369–370	Excitatory amino acid neurotransmitters	424,434
CPP see 3-(2-Carboxypiperazin-4-yl)propyl-1-phosphonic acid		EAA-mediated mechanisms in absence seizures	138–139
Cryptogenic epilepsy, myoclonic absence epilepsy	76	glutamate	161
		bursting activity	434
D		seizure thresholds modulated by AEDs in mice	473–483
2DG autoradiographic mapping	404		
Dimethadione, spontaneous rhythms	128–129	see also ATPA; Kainate; NMDA;	
Diphenylhydantoin see Hydantoins		Eyelid myoclonia with absences	76,77–79
Dizocilpine (MK 801), selective antagonist, NMDA receptors	464	criteria, French study	89
		definition	82–83
DNA polymorphisms		prognosis	91
positional cloning	33–34	see also Childhood absence epilepsy	
tandem repeat polymorphisms	34	**F**	
VNTRs	34	Facial and forelimb clonus, forebrain structures	404–406
Dopamine, SWD in GAERS	160		
Drug-induced epilepsy, animal models	51–64	Familial neonatal and infantile convulsions	37–71
Drugs, novel, role of GEPR	393	see also Benign familial	
E		Faroes, epilepsy	21
EAA see Excitatory amino acid		Felbamate	
Earclip electroshock, GEPRs compared with non-epileptic animals (table)	388–389	characteristics and mechanisms of action	458
		clinical studies	464
EEG characteristics		glycine-site, NMDA receptor	463
idiopathic generalized epilepsy	7–18	Feline generalized penicilin epilepsy	111–121
low-voltage, genetic study	68–69	comparisons with other models	117–119
EEG criteria		roles of thalamus and cortex	113–117
benign myoclonic epilepsy in infancy	11	spindles and SWD	112–113
childhood absence epilepsy	11–12,13–14	Feline studies, ILS	360–362
idiopathic generalized epilepsy	11	FEpi reflex epilepsy	
IGEs, shortcomings	19–20	AED	375–383
juvenile myoclonic epilepsy	12–13	as model of primary GCE	375–383
Elderly patients		FGPE see Feline generalized penicilin epilepsy	
idiopathic generalized epilepsy	95–109	Flumenazil	300
IGEs, myoclonic forms	10	Fluorothyl	
Electroshock, effects on NMDA receptors, substantia nigra	504	EEG seizures	58–59
		effects on NMDA receptors, substantia nigra	504
Embryological techniques, avian FEpi reflex epilepsy	381	motor seizures	57–58
		pathology	59–60
Epidemiology, idiopathic generalized epilepsy	19–25	pharmacology	60–61

Forebrain and brain-stem separation of seizure substrates	399–401
Forebrain structures	
facial and forelimb clonus	404–406
remote systems, regulatory control	408
France	
absence epilepsy, criteria	87–93
N epidemiological survey	22–24
SW, epidemiological survey	22–24
Frontal cortex, epilepsy and non-epileptic myoclonus	339–40

G

G proteins	
binding by Gpp(NH)p	178
coupling to $GABA_B$ binding sites	192
GABA	
potentiation by valproate	449
SWD in GAERS	161–162
GABA autoradiograms	
baclofen-displaceable	190–191,194
seizures in lh/lh mice	193–195
GABA-mediated mechanisms, absence seizures	137–138
Gabaculine, intra-SI injection	353–354
GABAergic neurotransmission	
anti-absence compounds	450
baboon	335
Gabapentin, characteristics and mechanisms of action	458
$GABA_A$ IPSP-mediated oscillations, thalamic	201–213
$GABA_A$ receptors	161
effect of benzodiazepines	448–449
$GABA_B$ receptor antagonists, absence seizures	463
$GABA_B$ receptors	161,177–185
absence seizures, pharmacology manipulation	207–208
activation, lethargic mouse model, absence seizures	187–200
antagonist radioligands, CGP	178–185
binding by Gpp(NH)p	178
compounds acting, seizures in lh/lh mice	192
GAERS, and non-epileptic controls	177–185
role in SWD	424
GAERS see Genetic absence epilepsy rat of Strasbourg	
Gamma-hydroxybutyrate (GHB)	
mechanisms of action, absence seizures	449–450
mediation, in absence seizures	140–142
Gamma-vinyl GABA (GVG), in GAERS	137
Gaucher's disease	326
Gene mapping	27–36
benign familial myoclonic convulsions	65–71
Gene therapy in epilepsy	511–521
cellular gene therapy	511–512,515
genetic epilepsy	516
non-genetic epilepsy	516–517
critical issues	519
indications	517
mode of delivery	518–519
relevant genes	517–518
retroviral vectors	512–515
Generalized absence (GA) see Absence seizures	
Generalized convulsive seizures	399–413
Generalized tonic–clonic seizures	
action of AEDs	447–448
age on onset	10
age-dependency	20–21
France	22
syndromic classification	16–17
Genetic absence epilepsy rat of Strasbourg	136–139
absence seizures, novel excitatory amino acid antagonists	463
cortical spreading depression	155
EEG and behavioural characteristics	152–154
inbred status	151
as isomorphic model	154
pathophysiological mechanisms	151–168
as predictive model	155
SWD	
bilateralization and synchronization	158–160
genetic transmission	162–165
networks involved	155–158
neurotransmitters involved	160–162
pharmacology	154–155
TC cells	208–210
thalamic electrolytic lesions	157
Genetic linkage, APM and ASP methods, linkage analysis	32
Genetic transmission, SWD, animal models	162–5
Genetically epilepsy-prone rat (GEPR)	385–398
comparison with non-epileptic animals (table)	388–389
convulsive seizures	385–398
facial and forelimb (F&F) clonus, forebrain structures	399–400,404–406
GEPR-3 and GEPR-9 compared	402–404
innate seizure predisposition model	387–390
innately determined, age-dependent epileptogenesis	390
moderate seizure GEPR-3 and severe seizure GEPR-9, seizure predisposition	386–387
moderate seizure GEPR-3 and severe seizure GEPR-9	385
running/bounding (R/B) clonic and tonic convulsions brainstem structures	400–403,406–408
stimulus-exacerbated genetically determined seizure predisposition	391
three predominant motor patterns	399–401
transcorneal and transauricular stimulation	401
Genetics	
basic principles	28–30
positional cloning	30–34
Germany, absence seizures, prevalence	21

GHB *see* Gamma-hydroxybutyrate	
Glial reaction, and loss of neurones	437–438
Glucose	
2DG method (radiolabelled 2-deoxyglucose)	169
local cerebral metabolic rates (LCMR glc)	169–170
with absence seizures	170–172
Glutamate	
in bursting activity	434
SWD in GAERS	161
Glutamatergic receptors	
antagonists, AMPA type	434
changes after seizures	440–442
metabotropic, antagonists acting	467–468
Glutamic acid decarboxylase blockade, pyridoxine	335
Gpp(NH)p binding	178,181–183
Graft techniques, avian FEpi reflex epilepsy	381
GTC *see* Generalized tonic–clonic seizures	
GVG *see* Gamma-vinyl GABA	
GYKI 52466	
non-NMDA antagonist	467
seizure threshold in mice	476

H

Haloperidol, cerebral effects	172
Herpin–Janz syndrome *see* Juvenile myoclonic epilepsy	
Hexafluorodiethyl ether *see* Flurothyl	
Hippocampal kindling, Wistar AS rats	416
Hippocampal mossy fibres, reactive sprouting	438–440
Historical aspects	
idiopathic generalized epilepsy	3–6
juvenile myoclonic epilepsy	229–231
HLA antigens	32–33
Human Gene Mapping, 11th Workshop	33–34
Hydantoins	
efficacy, impulsive petit mal	243
seizure threshold in mice	476
data	478
6-Hydroxydopamine	
lesions	139
stargazer mutant	221
Hyperventilation, absence epilepsy	12

I

Idiopathic generalized epilepsy	3–36
age of onset	10
age-dependency	20–21
baboon model	331–348
classification	
in clinical practice	13–17
seizure types	16
special groups	15–16
syndromic classification	16
clinical aspects	7–18
clinical criteria	9–10
definition, methodological problems	20–31
definitions of syndromes	9
EEG characteristics	7–18
EEG criteria	11
elderly patients, late-onset	95–109
epidemiology	19–25
literature data	21
European studies	21–24
incidence, age-related	23
influence of drugs on outcome	425–433
nigral control	497–510
novel excitatory amino acid antagonist action in animal models	464–468
phenotypic variability	287–291
three types of seizure	9
IGEs *see* Idiopathic generalized epilepsy	
ILAE *see* Classification	
ILS	
anatomical substrate involved	357–360
feline studies	360–362
ILS-induced seizures, avian FEpi reflex epilepsy	378–381
primate studies	362–366
Impulsive grand mal	236
Impulsive petit mal	229–251
Infantile convulsions,familial,benign	45–50
Inferior colliculus, R/B clonic and tonic convulsions	407
Innate seizure predisposition model	387–390
Innately determined age-dependent epileptogenes, GEPR model	390
Intermittent light stimulation *see* ILS	
Iodoantipyrine, radiolabelled,IAP technique	170
IPS (intermittent photic stimulation)	297
Isoniazid, GABA synthesis impairment	335
Italy, epilepsy, prevalence	21

J

Jerks, hypnagogic	235–236,242
Juvenile absence epilepsy	
defined	9,79,81
exclusion criteria	81
inclusion criteria	80–81
syndromic classification	16
Juvenile myoclonic epilepsy	227–293
absences in	81–82
clinical aspects	253–265
clinical and EEG affectedness	281–282
defined	9
EEG criteria	12–13
frequency	15
genetics	30
heterogeneity?	287–288
historical aspects	229–231
HLA DQ A1 locus	291–293
idiopathic generalized epilepsy with myoclonus	267–280
impulsive petit mal	229–251
linkage mapping: chr 6p	283–285

phenotypic variability	289–290
and photosensitivity	325–326
plus symptoms	287–288
refinement of map position of EJM1	291–293
relatives, prevalence of clinical forms	288
segregation analysis	282–283
seizures	81–82
subgroups I-VIII	282
subphenotypes I, IIA and IIB	285–286
Juvenile syndromes, differentiation	17

K

Kainate, seizure threshold in mice, AEDs	474–478
Kindling, effects on NMDA receptors, substantia nigra	504
Kindling model	
defined	351
experiments, summary	356–357
as model with partial onset secondarily generalized convulsion	350

L

Lamotrigine	300,427
characteristics and mechanisms of action	456–457
interaction with excitatory amino acid transmitter system	463
Laser-Doppler flowmetry, cerebral blood flow	170,173–175
Late-onset, absence status	84,95–109
Lennox–Gastaut syndrome	275
Lethargic mouse model, absence seizures	187–200
Light stimulation *see* ILS	
Limbic kindling, GEPRs compared with non-epileptic animals (table)	388–389
Linkage analysis	31–32
affected pedigree (APM) method	32
affected sib pain (ASP) method	32
benign familial neonatal convulsions	66–67
Linkage mapping: chr 6p, juvenile myoclonic epilepsy	283–285
Lod-scores and significance tests	31–32
Loreclezole	300
Low-voltage, EEG	68–69
LY 293558, non-NMDA antagonist	467

M

MAE *see* Myoclonic absence epilepsy	
Magnesium perfusion, thalamocortical slices	125–127
Massa intermedia	
discussion	368
role in convulsive seizure bilateralization and generalization	356
Mesencephalon, avian FEpi reflex epilepsy	381
Minimal electroshock threshold (MES), animal models	60
Minor seizures	
characteristics	232
rhythmicity	232–234

see also Petit mal	
MK 801 (dizocilpine)	464
Molecular mapping, epilepsy genes	27–36
Monoaminergic mechanisms, absence seizures	139–140
Mouse	
lethargic mutant	187–200,220
stargazer mutant	215–225
SWD autosomal recessive gene loci	216
SWD epilepsies	215–225
tottering mutant, allelic heterogeneity	217–218
see also Animal models	
Myoclonic absence epilepsy	76
definition	82
Myoclonic seizures	
action of AEDs	448–449
historical aspects	229–231
Myoclonic–astatic epilepsy	267,272–275
Myoclonus	
baboon, convulsive seizures	331–348
EEG characteristics	242
generalized	271–272
in IGEs	267
as sole defining symptom	267

N

NBQX	
non-NMDA antagonist	467
seizure threshold in mice	476
Neonatal convulsions	
familial, benign	39–44
gene mapping	65–71
see also Benign familial neonatal convulsions	
Netherlands, BFNC study	69–70
Neurones, loss, and glial reaction	437–438
Neurotransmitters	
SWD in GAERS	160
see also EAA	
Nigral control	
idiopathic generalized epilepsy	497–510
see also Substantia nigra	
Nitric oxide, second messenger	424,485–496
blockade	488
inhibition of pathway	489–490
involvement in epilepsy	491–494
location of synthesis	485–487
role in brain	487–488
NMDA	
blockade	335
seizure threshold in mice, AEDs	474–478
NMDA receptors	
action of novel excitatory amino acid antagonists	464–468
competitive antagonists, anticonvulsive properties	465–466
complex, ligand binding	139
non-competitive antagonists acting at channel site	466

535

non-competitive antagonists acting at glycine site	466–467
selective antagonists	
2-amino-5-phosphonopentanoic acid (AP5)	464
2-amino-7-phosphoheptanoic acid (AP7)	353,464
3-(2-carboxypiperazin-4-yl)-propyl-1-phosphonic acid (CPP)	464
dizocilpine (MK 801)	464
effects on substantia nigra	504
N-allylnormetazocine	464
phencyclidine (PCP)	464
Noradrenaline, SWD in GAERS	160
Noradrenergic neurotransmission	139–140
Novel drugs, mechanisms of action	455–461
Nucleus reticularis thalami (NRT)	123
IPSPs	128

O

Occipital cortex and projection	
corpus callosum, role	359–360
corticectomy	358
discussion	367
disruption of occipito-frontal projection	359
putative role	358–360
6-OHDA *see* 6-Hydroxydopamine	
Opiate receptors, effects of agonists on substantia nigra	504
Oxcarbazepine, characteristics and mechanisms of action	455

P

Papio anubis	334
Papio cynocephalus	351
insensitivity to amygdaloid-kindled seizures	352
Papio hamadryas	334
Papio papio see Baboon model of epilepsy	
Paroxysmal depolarizing shifts (PDSs), thalamocortical slices	126–127
Partial epilepsy, discussion	366–370
Pathophysiology of convulsive seizures	329–421
Penicillin-induced epilepsy in cat (FGPE)	111–121
Pentylenetetrazol	
EEG seizures	53–54
motor seizures	51–53
pharmacology and pathology	54
PTZ-induced seizures	129
Pentylenetetrazole	
GEPRs compared with non-epileptic animals (table)	388–389
seizure threshold in mice, data	480
threshold test	464
Pentylenetetrazole-induced clonic seizure, effects on NMDA receptors, substantia nigra	504
Perioral myoclonia with absences	76,77–79
criteria, French study	89
definition	83
prognosis	91
see also Childhood absence epilepsy	
Petit mal, *see also* Juvenile myoclonic epilepsy; Minor seizures	
Petit mal, impulsive	229–251
aetiology	234
age of onset	234
constitution of patients	237–239
course	235–236
differential diagnosis	244–245
distribution and aetiology	231
EEG findings	239–242
impulsive grand mal	236
inheritance	234–235
pathophysiology and nosology	245–249
prevalence	234
prognosis	244
treatment	242–244
triggering factors	237
Petit mal status *see* Absence status	
Phantom absence	84
Phencyclidine, selective antagonist, NMDA receptors	464
Phenobarbital	
for absence seizures	133
for absence status	98
for BFIC	46
Phenobarbitone	
effects on substantia nigra, rat models	504
generalized tonic–clonic seizures	426
mechanisms of action, myoclonic seizures	448–449
myoclonic seizures	425
seizure threshold in mice	476
data	478
Phenytoin	
effects on substantia nigra, rat models	504
efficacy, impulsive petit mal	243
generalized tonic–clonic seizures	426
long-term	100
mechanisms of action, tonic–clonic seizures	447–448
resistance by GAs	133
spontaneous rhythms	129
Photosensitivity	295–328
absences	84
baboon models of epilepsy	331–348
definition	317–319
establishing	298
female preponderance	302
genetic approach	317–328
genetics	
family studies	324
genetic marker	302
mode of inheritance	324–325
molecular approach	325–326
twin studies	324
human model of epilepsy	297–303
incidence	319–321

and juvenile myoclonic epilepsy	325–326
model for AED studies	299–302
in pathogenesis of epilepsy	321–322
pathophysiological mechanisms	305–315
photoparoxysmal response, (types 1-4)	318–319,320
and progressive myoclonus epilepsy	326
ranges	298–299
in relatives, seizure risk	323–324
visual stimulation experiments	305–312
see also ILS	
Picrotoxin, seizure threshold in mice, data	480
Pilocarpine, effects on NMDA receptors, substantia nigra	504
PME see Progressive myoclonus epilepsy	
Positional cloning	30–34
DNA polymorphisms	33–34
linkage analysis, lod-scores and significance tests	31–32
nonparametric method	32–33
Pregnancy, inhibition of seizures	237–238
Premotor area (PMA) kindling	350
Primary generalized epilepsy see Idiopathic generalized epilepsy	
Primate studies	
claustral lesioning, ILS-induced seizures	362–366
ILS	362–366
model of forebrain mechanisms, convulsive seizures	349–373
see also Baboon	
Primidone	
generalized tonic–clonic seizures	426
myoclonic seizures	425
Progabide	299
Propagation of convulsive seizures	415–421
Prosencephalon and mesencephalon, avian FEpi reflex epilepsy	381
Psychoactive drugs, proconvulsant and anticonvulsant potential	392–393
Psychotropic drugs, and absence status	97–98
Pyknolepsy see Childhood absence epilepsy	
Pyridoxine	
dependency/deficiency, familial convulsions	47
glutamic acid decarboxylase blockade	335

Q

Quinuclidinyl benzylate, induction of myoclonus	336–337

R

Ranitidine, toxic encephalopathy	98–99
Rat brain	
SWD mapping	156
thalamic and CC lesions	156
see also Animal models; Genetic absence epilepsy rat of Strasbourg; GEPR	
Reflex absence	84
Remacemide, interaction with excitatory amino acid transmitter system	463
Retroviral vectors, gene therapy in epilepsy	512–515
RMR6 (D20S20) marker, chromosome 20q	69
Running/bounding (R/B) clonic and tonic convulsions, brainstem structures	400–403,406–408

S

School performance, children with IGEs	24
Second messengers, nitric oxide, role	424,485–496
Seizure predisposition, aetiology, model	391
Serotonin, SWD in GAERS	160
SI see Substantia innominata	
Single, non-rhythmic myoclonia, seizures with	83
Situation-induced absence status	95–106
Skull, abnormalities, impulsive petit mal	237–238
Sleep	
onset, normal physiological jerks	235
typology, petit mal	238
Sodium currents, voltage-gated, sodium valproate	119
Sodium influx, into synaptosomes, batrachotoxin action	448
Sodium valproate, absence seizures	427
for absence seizures	89,133
for benign myoclonic epilepsy	269
for BFIC	46
effects on substantia nigra, rat models	504
for generalized tonic–clonic seizures	426
mechanisms of action	
absence seizures	449
myoclonic seizures	448–449
release of -hydroxybutyrate (GHB)	450
tonic–clonic seizures	448
myoclonic seizures	427
in photosensitivity	297,306
reduction of GABA release	450–451
seizure threshold in mice	474–478
data	478
sodium currents, voltage-gated	119
Stargazer mutant, mouse	215–225
Strasbourg rat see GAERS	
Stroboscopy	305
Subcortical structures, epilepsy and non-epileptic myoclonus	340–341
Substantia innominata	
discussion	367
role in convulsive seizures	353–354
Substantia nigra	
activation, by AEDs	505–506
animal models, R/B clonic and tonic convulsions	407
GABAergic neurons	424
neuroanatomical circuitry	500
neurotransmitters involved	504–505
nigral control of idiopathic generalized epilepsy	497–510
nigral inputs and outputs	500–502
relevance of nigral control, treatment of	

537

epilepsies	503
role in control of seizures	497–500
Superior colliculus	
animal models, R/B clonic and tonic convulsions	407–408
role	358
SWD epilepsies	221
pharmacology, variation	221–222
seizure-induced gene expression	222
in feline generalized penicillin epilepsy	112–119
in GAERS	151,154
genetic transmission, animal models	162–165
inherited	215–225
age of onset variability	219
allelic heterogeneity	217–218
gene dose	218–219
genetic and phenotypic diversity	216
in vitro network excitability defects	221
locus heterogeneity	216–217
neurotransmitter imbalances	220–221
pharmacology, variation	221–222
morphology of SWD	219–220
regional cerebral synchronization	220
transformation to GTC discharge	349
transition to GTC, intracortical inhibition	118–119
Sweden, epilepsy	21
Symptomatic and secondary typical absences	84
Synaptosomes, batrachotoxin, induction of sodium influx	448

T

Terminology, historical aspects	3–6
Thalamocortical mechanisms	
absence seizures	157–158
and AED	119
FGPE cat	113–117
$GABA_A$ IPSP-mediated oscillations	201–213
intracortical inhibition	118–119
SWD and information processing	118
Thalamocortical neurons	
$GABA_B$ receptor-mediated oscillations	205–206
genetic absence epilepsy rat of Strasbourg	208–210
intrinsic oscillations	203–205
thalamic oscillations	201–203
Thalamocortical rhythms	
functional aspects	134–150
generation *in vitro*	123–132
intracellular recordings	125
Thalamocortical slices, magnesium perfusion	125–127
paroxysmal depolarizing shifts (PDSs)	126–127
Thalamus, role in convulsive seizure bilateralization and generalization	356
Thiosemicarbazide, GABA synthesis impairment	335
Tiagabine, characteristics and mechanisms of action	458–459
Tizanidine, action	335
Tonic–clonic seizures *see* Generalized tonic–clonic seizures	
Tottering mutant, mouse	217–218
Toxic encephalopathy, ranitidine	98–99
Transcription factors, activation	435–437
Triggering modalities, GEPRs compared with non-epileptic animals (table)	388–389
Trimethadione	
absence seizures	133,427
effects on substantia nigra, rat models	504
in lethargic mice	191
seizure threshold in mice	476
data	478
spontaneous rhythms	128–129
Trophic factors, activation	435–437
Tuberous sclerosis	10

U

ucbL059	300
UK, epilepsy, incidence	21
Unverricht–Lundborg disease	28–30,229–231,244
see also Progressive myoclonus epilepsy	
US, epilepsy, incidence	21

V

Valproate *see* Sodium valproate	
VAPSEs	33
Variants affecting protein structure or expression	33
Vigabatrin, characteristics and mechanisms of action	458–459
Visual stimulation	
discussion	312–315
full-field	308
hemifield	308–311
precipitating factors	311–312
Visual stimulation experiments	305–312
VNTRs, DNA polymorphisms	34
VPA *see* Sodium valproate	

Z

Zonisamide, characteristics and mechanisms of action	457–458